NEURORADIOLOGY

Second Edition

RUTH G. RAMSEY, M.D.

Professor of Radiology, Rush Medical College;
Senior Attending Physician, Section of Neuroradiology,
Rush-Presbyterian-St. Luke's Medical Center,
Chicago, Illinois

1987

W. B. SAUNDERS COMPANY

Philadelphia, London, Toronto, Mexico City, Rio de Janeiro, Sydney, Tokyo, Hong Kong

W. B. Saunders Company: West Washington Square
Philadelphia, PA   19105

Library of Congress Cataloging-in-Publication Data

Ramsey, Ruth G.

Neuroradiology.

Rev. ed. of: Neuroradiology with computed tomography. 1981.

Bibliography: p.

Includes index.

1. Nervous system—Radiography.   I. Ramsey, Ruth G.
Neuroradiology with computed tomography.   II. Title.
[DNLM: 1. Nervous System—radiography. WL 141 R183n]

RC349.R3R35 1987   616.8′047572   86–6639

ISBN 0–7216–1827–8

Acquisition Editor: John Dyson

Developmental Editor: David Kilmer

Copy Editor: Donna Walker

Production Manager: Frank Polizzano

Indexer: Bonnie Boehme

Neuroradiology   ISBN   0-7216-1827-8

Last digit is the print number: 9   8   7   6   5   4   3   2   1

To
Michael M. Ramsey

PREFACE

There have been considerable advances in neuroradiology since the first edition of this book. Most recently the introduction of magnetic resonance (MR) imaging has greatly influenced and altered the approach to the diagnosis and evaluation of diseases affecting the central nervous system. Even now, advancements continue in both the hardware and software of magnetic resonance equipment. However, the technique of MR is sufficiently mature to justify publication at this time. This text is intended to review the various radiologic tests available for evaluation of neurologic disease, from plain skull and spine radiographs through the more sophisticated invasive and noninvasive types of studies that are available.

Although angiography is still performed, it has become less critical as a diagnostic test. The development of computed tomography (CT) and MR have obviated the need for angiography in a large number of cases. Many patients have either definitive surgical resection or stereotactic biopsy based on these noninvasive tests. For this reason, a small number of older cases, with angiographic and CT correlation, have been preserved because of their teaching value. Likewise, occasional older CT scans are preserved when they demonstrate particular value as a teaching case or there is pathologic correlation.

There is sufficient discussion of the physics of magnetic resonance to make the technique understandable. The emphasis of this book is on the practical and clinical usefulness of the technique of magnetic resonance as well as other neuroradiologic techniques in the evaluation and diagnosis of neurologic disease. The esoteric, unusual, and rare cases have been de-emphasized in favor of common neuroradiologic processes and uncommon presentations of common diseases.

Magnetic resonance has been incorporated chapter by chapter rather than as a single, separate chapter. Correlation is made with other neuroradiologic diagnostic techniques whenever available. The technique for the performance of the MR examination is included with a large percentage of magnetic resonance scans so that the student, resident, or practitioner can have a basis for interpretation and/or performance of the various studies. The spine chapter has been expanded and includes a large number of magnetic resonance scans. There is a chapter devoted to neuroradiologic evaluation of degenerative and metabolic diseases.

This text allows the medical student and the resident in radiology, neurology, neurosurgery, or other specialty, as well as the practicing radiologist or clinician, to become familiar with the older as well as newer techniques of diagnosis and to correlate the various types of studies. The text is extensively illustrated and can also be used as an atlas and convenient guide to diagnosis of cases seen on a daily basis.

The "students" of the neurosciences at all levels—professor, resident, medical student, clinician, and technologist—truly provide the inspiration for this text. Thanks also to my sons Thomas and Timothy for their encouragement and understanding. To my colleagues and friends, to the professional and technical staff of the Department of Radiology, and to the staff of the medical photography department, I owe my thanks. Thanks also to my editor, John Dyson, and the staff at W. B. Saunders for their help and patience, and to my secretary Ameedah Munir, who works so hard and never complains. And, truly to my own residents and fellows in neuroradiology, whose constant questions remind me that there is not only a lot to learn, but also a lot to teach.

RUTH G. RAMSEY

This book is supported in part by the Robert R. McCormick Foundation.

CONTENTS

1

THE ORDER OF NEURORADIOLOGIC PROCEDURES

Selecting the most effective sequence of neuroradiologic procedures from the variety available today is not always an easy matter. A thoughtful approach to the problems unique to each individual patient is required. In some cases only one examination may be necessary before instituting therapy; others may require all of the several examinations if a correct diagnosis is to be determined.

In general, the work-up of a patient should begin with noninvasive studies. The patient's symptoms may serve as a guide, dictating the order of testing to a certain extent. Unfortunately, even patients with sizeable tumor masses may have minimal symptoms. Therefore, diagnostic acumen and judgment also contribute ·significantly to choosing the order of testing. Of course, all thorough diagnostic work must begin with a history of the present illness and significant past history and with a thorough physical and neurologic examination. Whether the patient's illness is acute or chronic is very important—particularly if alteration of mentation has occurred following head trauma.

SKULL RADIOLOGY

A routine skull examination will demonstrate the presence or absence of bony metastatic deposits, areas of reactive bone formation, intracranial calcification, skull fractures, sinusitis,

changes in size of the sella turcica, and such metabolic changes as those of Paget's disease, fibrous dysplasia, or the hemoglobinopathies.

ELECTROENCEPHALOGRAPHY

A discussion of the electroencephalogram is beyond the scope of this book. This study can be helpful in certain patients, particularly those with a seizure disorder.

RADIONUCLIDE SCAN

The radionuclide brain scan has been a very helpful diagnostic tool, although since the introduction of the CT scan the indications for its use are less clear. The radionuclide angiogram may show decreased flow through the carotid arteries in a patient with suspected occlusive vascular disease. Following a stroke it may provide evidence of decreased perfusion in the area of infarction, which after several days will demonstrate an area of increased uptake secondary to breakdown of the blood-brain barrier. In the presence of an acute subdural hematoma the radionuclide angiogram may show an area of poor perfusion over the cerebral convexity, while the static scan is normal. With a chronic subdural hematoma the scan reveals a crescentic area of increased activity. Brain tumors

1

demonstrate areas of increased activity on the scan, as do areas of abscess formation. Computed tomography and magnetic resonance scanning have essentially eliminated the need for radionuclide brain scans.

POSITRON EMISSION TOMOGRAPHY

Positron emission tomography (PET) requires the use of a positron emitting radionuclides that are tagged to various brain metabolites such as glucose. After these substances are administered, their presence in the brain is detected by a scanning device similar to those used for other radionuclide studies. These PET studies evaluate the function of the brain. Clinical research studies reveal that, for example, when an individual listens to music certain areas of the brain become more metabolically active than other areas and demonstrate increased activity with PET scanning.

In clinical application, PET has been shown to be helpful in the evaluation of Alzheimer's disease, in which there is decreased metabolism of certain glucose metabolites as compared to normal individuals.

The expense of the cyclotron for manufacture of the radioactive materials and the limited clinical applications indicate that PET may remain a research tool.

COMPUTED TOMOGRAPHY

Brain Tumors

It is not unreasonable to say that the introduction of computed tomography of the brain has revolutionized our approach to the diagnosis of neurologic disorders. The CT scan demonstrates the size of the lesion, its location, its configuration, and its relationship to any surrounding edema. From its appearance on the scan we can tell whether the mass is solid or cystic, space-occupying or not, of CSF density or of a density equal to normal brain tissue (isodense) or of higher or lower density than normal brain. The CT scan also demonstrates any evidence of ventricular enlargement and/or cortical sulcus enlargement. Additionally, the scan also demonstrates shift of the ventricles that may be secondary to cerebral edema or a mass lesion.

All patients with suspected brain metastases should have a CT examination both with and without infusion. The contrast material is the same as that used for intravenous pyelography.

It is necessary to administer 40 grams of iodine. The brand of contrast material is of no consequence. It can be administered as an infusion of 300 cc of 30 per cent contrast (one half infused rapidly prior to scanning, the remainder during the scan) or as an injection of 150 cc of 60 per cent contrast material.

Subarachnoid Hemorrhage

Following subarachnoid hemorrhage, blood can be seen in the basilar cisterns, the interhemispheric fissure, over the cerebral cortex, and occasionally within the ventricular system. The CT scan accurately reflects the presence of blood in the subarachnoid space in approximately 80 to 90 per cent of cases. Patients with severe headaches, photophobia, a stiff neck, and an alteration in mental status without or with focal neurologic findings require a lumbar tap if the CT scan does not show evidence of a subarachnoid hemorrhage. The CT scan does not accurately demonstrate the presence of an aneurysm unless it is very sizeable (probably over 2 cm); therefore, angiography is necessary to establish or rule out aneurysm.

Angiography is necessary for the evaluation of patients with subarachnoid hemorrhage. None of the other ancillary tests will reveal the size and position of the aneurysm, nor whether there is or is not evidence of vascular spasm. In approximately 15 per cent of cases the cause of subarachnoid hemorrhage will not be found.

Intracerebral Hematoma

Intracerebral hematoma is readily demonstrated using the CT scan, and even small areas of hemorrhage can easily be identified. The areas of hemorrhage may be in any portion of the cerebral hemispheres, particularly in patients suffering from coagulopathies. Hypertensive hemorrhages occur most commonly in the region of the basal ganglia and cerebellum but also may involve the brain stem. Often the CT scan will be the only examination to demonstrate these abnormalities.

Intracerebral hemorrhage may be associated with an element of intraventricular hemorrhage; thus, the clinical appearance of headache, photophobia, altered mental status, and stiff neck may mimic that of a subarachnoid hemorrhage. The CT scan reveals the true nature of the problem, although at times an aneurysm may cause an intracerebral hematoma.

If an acute intracerebral hematoma is suspected, a CT scan is the examination of choice.

Atrophy

When a possible diagnosis of atrophy is entertained, the CT or MR is the examination of choice. The size of the lateral ventricles and cortical sulci is readily demonstrated. It appears that there is some increase in the size of both the ventricles and the cortical sulci with increasing age, but precise guidelines are not yet available. The CT scan also rules out the presence of an unsuspected brain tumor or chronic subdural hematoma.

Trauma

In the patient who has sustained head trauma the CT scan is also the procedure of choice. With acute head trauma and a change in mentation and/or focal physical findings an immediate scan should be performed. This can be performed with the patient sedated or, in the uncooperative patient, under general anesthesia. It cannot be overemphasized that all efforts should be made to obtain a diagnostic examination so that prompt treatment can be instituted as needed. In acute subdural or epidural hematoma the neurosurgeon commonly undertakes an operative procedure without an angiogram or any other work-up. Indeed, in rare instances, a single scan through the mid-portion of the brain to confirm the existence of a hematoma, followed by rapid evacuation, may be a life-saving procedure. If computed tomography is not available, angiography may be necessary for evaluation.

MAGNETIC RESONANCE

Magnetic resonance imaging is the newest diagnostic tool to become available. MR has proved to be most useful in the diagnosis of abnormalities of the central nervous system. The method does not require the use of ionizing radiation and is a noninvasive diagnostic technique. MR is more sensitive than CT for the diagnosis of intracranial pathology, although the specificity is yet to be determined. At the present stage of our technology, MR is based upon hydrogen proton imaging, although additional substances may be used in the future. Hydrogen is abundant in biologic systems and therefore is an ideal nuclear proton to study. In the central nervous system, most pathologic

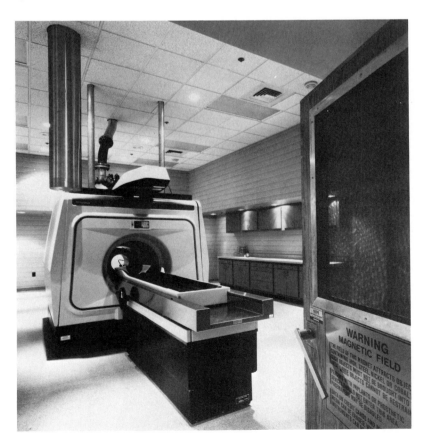

FIGURE 1–1. The magnetic resonance installation at the Rush-Presbyterian-St. Luke's Hospital in Chicago, Illinois. This unit is a 5-kilogauss (0.5 Tesla) superconductive scanner. (Courtesy of Technicare Corporation, Cleveland, Ohio.)

states result in an increase in the amount of water—edema—in the abnormal area. Therefore, the MR scan is readily able to detect these abnormalities.

In addition to increased sensitivity, MR has certain advantages over CT. One of the major advantages is the absence of artifact from the bony structures. The hydrogen protons present in the bone are not "mobile" protons because they are firmly locked into the crystal lattice of the bone. Because of the absence of mobile protons, the bone appears as an area of low signal intensity. While this poor visibility is at times a disadvantage, the absence of bony artifact far outweighs this disadvantage. There is excellent visualization of the middle cranial fossa and posterior fossa. The artifact-free visibility of these areas is a great advantage over other diagnostic methods. There is no "Hounsfield" artifact between the petrous bones which often degrades the CT scans so much that they are nondiagnostic. The MR scans of the posterior fossa are excellent and are the diagnostic examination of choice.

MR also has the capability of multiplanar imaging without the need to manipulate the position of the patient. This capability is particularly helpful in the examination of the posterior fossa where the sagittal images provide an anatomic evaluation of the structures. This is also helpful in the examination of the sella and parasellar regions. This multiplanar imaging of the region around the pituitary fossa allows one to directly visualize the intrasellar and parasellar structures and reveals any variations from

normal. Again, the lack of need for the injection of contrast material—either intravenous or water soluble—in the subarachnoid space is a great advantage. Also, there is no artifact from the surrounding bone. It appears that MR will replace other diagnostic tests for evaluation of the sella turcica.

Evaluation of the spinal column and its contents is also possible with MR. There is a distinct advantage to the use of MR for evaluation of the spinal vertebral column and spinal cord. MR allows direct visualization of the spinal cord and surrounding CSF. Again, this is possible in any plane desired and does not require the use of contrast material. Changes similar to those seen on myelography are easily identified, with the CSF providing the outline of the spinal cord in a way similar to the contrast instilled into the subarachnoid space. MR of the spine is useful for evaluation of metastatic disease of the vertebral bodies, fractures (both post-traumatic and pathologic), paraspinal masses, postradiation change, spinal cord tumors, and various congenital anomalies. Because of the excellent visualization of the posterior fossa structures and region around the foramen magnum, MR often provides the definitive study for the various Chiari malformations. Although MR is noninvasive, it provides better visualization of these abnormalities than does any other method and is usually the only examination that is necessary prior to surgery.

There are no known biologic effects with magnetic resonance. MR has proved to be the diagnostic procedure of choice, particularly with the demyelinating diseases, and is complemen-

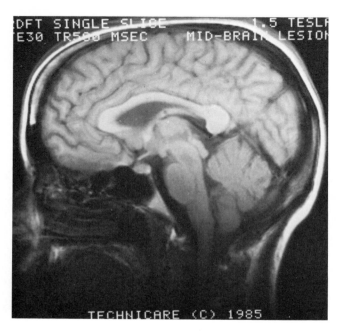

FIGURE 1—2. A midsagittal image of the brain using a 15-kilogauss (1.5 Tesla) superconductive magnetic resonance scanner. (Courtesy of the Technicare Corporation, Cleveland, Ohio.)

tary to CT and other diagnostic methods for the evaluation of various disease processes. The future of MR is assured, and future advances will only improve its diagnostic capabilities.

ANGIOGRAPHY

In general, angiography is performed following the noninvasive examinations. Definitive morbidity and even mortality can follow angiography, and this examination should be performed only after adequate consideration.

Angiography is needed whenever the operating surgeon feels that it is necessary to outline the vascular supply to the tumor—and, just as important, to demonstrate the position and relationship of the major intracerebral vessels to the tumor mass. This is especially true of the cortical veins, which serve as markers for the surgeon as the surgical approach is planned.

If the tumor is a meningioma, the blood supply usually is from the external carotid artery, although the tentorial artery arises from the internal carotid artery and may supply a posterior fossa or tentorial meningioma.

At times posterior fossa tumors can be operated upon without the benefit of angiography. This is especially true of acoustic neurinomas.

General Indications for Angiography

1. For evaluation of intracranial mass lesions identified by other diagnostic methods.
2. In patients with vascular abnormalities, e.g., arteriovenous malformations, subarachnoid hemorrhage, transient ischemic attacks, certain intracerebral hematomas, and cerebral venous thrombosis.
3. With cerebral trauma when computed tomography is not available.

General (Relative) Contraindications to Angiography

1. Patients with "stroke in evolution" or a progressing stroke.
2. Inadequate equipment or technical personnel.
3. Untrained or inexperienced operators to perform the procedures without adequate supervision.
4. Allergy to contrast material.
5. Professional help should be available to deal with any abnormalities found in a way that will benefit the patient. Without such assistance, angiography should not be performed.

PNEUMOENCEPHALOGRAPHY

Pneumoencephalography as it was previously performed is no longer necessary. Metrizamide cisternography is now used to evaluate the basilar cisterns and the region of the sella turcica, although MR has essentially eliminated the need for cisternography. Air cisternography, using approximately 5 cc of room air, is an excellent technique for evaluating a cerebellopontine angle mass. This technique requires the instillation of approximately 5 cc of air via lumbar puncture, followed by CT scanning to determine the presence or absence of a mass (see Chapter 13, The Posterior Fossa).

2

THE PLAIN SKULL FILM

For many years the plain film examination of the skull served as one of the main diagnostic tools in the work-up of the patient with suspected intracranial pathology. Careful examination of the plain skull film may reveal important information that will be helpful in diagnosis. Skull fractures, intracranial air, intracranial calcification, and alterations in the bony calvaria are only a few of the pathologic changes that can be seen on plain films. Even today, after the introduction of such diagnostic tools as pneumoencephalography, arteriography, radionuclide scanning, and, most recently, CT and MR of the brain, plain skull films continue to be an important diagnostic tool, although the newer techniques are more informative and more accurate in their evaluation of intracranial pathology.

These developments led to a decreased emphasis on the skull film, and some clinicians have even suggested that there is no longer a need for the plain skull examination. While it is true that other diagnostic tools have added greatly to our ability to diagnose intracranial disorders, the plain skull examination continues to provide excellent data about the structure of the bony calvaria. It should not be discarded, and routine radiography should be correlated with other diagnostic tools.

DEFINITION

Routine radiographs of the skull are known as the "plain skull" examination, as opposed to roentgen examinations of the skull which are not "plain" but either involve the administration of contrast material or are altered in some other manner. The routine set of films varies from institution to institution, but most employ approximately the same set of standard films. The routine examination is set up in such a fashion that all the parts of the skull that are of interest in the case at hand are visualized on one or more films. In our department the routine set includes a right and left lateral, a Towne's view, a posteroanterior view with the internal auditory canal projected through the mid-portion of the orbit, and a submentovertex view of the skull. Each of these views provides a unique look at some area of the skull that is of particular interest and that is not as well visualized on the other views. Some departments routinely include a stereo lateral view of the skull for evaluation of intracranial calcifications or skull fractures. The Caldwell view also may be included as part of the routine series.

Although some authors have questioned the need for routine skull films since the advent of computed tomography of the brain, a more conservative approach would indicate that skull films can be of great value and generally should be obtained whenever intracranial pathology is suspected. They are particularly helpful in cases of head trauma. In addition, close examination of the series occasionally will reward the physician by providing diagnostic clues. If nothing else, they may be of importance in planning which examinations should be performed next in order to arrive at the diagnosis expeditiously.

6

When reviewing routine skull films it is helpful to have a brief but pertinent clinical history as a guide. In general, when reviewing the skull for evidence of trauma one is looking for a fracture. Particular attention should be paid to the area showing external signs of trauma when a clinical history or positive physical findings are not available. Lacking a history, "bright lighting" the film may give a clue to the area of interest by revealing a localized area of soft tissue swelling.

If a skull fracture is found, one should be aware of the possibility of an associated traumatic pneumocephalus (see Chapter 13). The sphenoid sinus should be checked for an air-fluid level indicating either blood or cerebrospinal fluid leakage into the sinus. When air-fluid levels are found secondary to trauma or sinusitis, skull radiography in the upright position is strongly suggested. If the patient is prone or supine, these abnormalities may not be visualized. If the patient is too ill to sit upright for routine radiographs, lateral skull films with the patient supine may be obtained for initial evaluation (see Chapter 13).

POSTEROANTERIOR VIEW OF THE SKULL (FIG. 2–1, p. 13)

This view is obtained with the patient lying prone with the forehead closest to the film. The patient is positioned in such a way that the internal auditory canals are projected into the mid- or lower portion of the orbit. The central ray is angled 10 degrees rostrally in relation to the anthropologic base line. This view is used to evaluate the internal auditory canals and for inspection of the orbits and the frontal bone. The lambdoid suture will be projected lower than the coronal suture in this view. The posterior parietal and upper portion of the occipital bone are also readily visualized with this position.

OCCIPITAL OR TOWNE-CHAMBERLAIN VIEW (FIG. 2–2, p. 14)

The patient is placed in the supine position and the central ray is directed at an angle of 25 to 35 degrees caudad with respect to the orbitomental line. This Towne's view of the skull provides the best view of the occipital bone. It also allows for evaluation and comparison of the size of the internal auditory canals, which are readily seen in this view. Evaluation of the petrous bones and mastoid air cells can also be made on the Towne's view. Lesions of the frontal lobes of the brain will be seen to project lower in the Towne's view than in the posteroanterior view; this may help to better localize a lesion that is visible only on anteroposterior or posteroanterior views. In addition, the orbits will also be projected more inferiorly on this view, allowing for visualization of the inferior orbital fissure. The zygomatic arches are frequently seen in silhouette on this view. If a base-of-skull fracture is suspected, careful inspection of the occipital bone on the Towne's view may reveal a linear fracture that extends forward to involve the temporal bone. The foramen magnum is well visualized on this view, and the dorsum sellae and the posterior clinoids should project into the foramen magnum in a well-positioned Towne's view.

LATERAL VIEW (FIGS. 2–3 and 2–4, pp. 15 and 16)

The right and left lateral views of the skull are obtained first with the patient's right side and then with the patient's left side closest to the film. It should be noted that the patient may be "off lateral" in one or two planes in the lateral projection. The patient may tilt the head to one side or the other, resulting in one orbital roof being higher than the other, or the patient may turn the head slightly to the right or the left, resulting in failure of superimposition of the greater wings on the sphenoid bone on the radiograph (see illustration). These "off lateral" positions can easily be evaluated by inspecting the radiograph. This is most important when the tilting of the head may give the false appearance of a double floor of the sella. The right and left lateral views are especially helpful in evaluating a possible skull fracture; i.e., if a linear skull fracture is present on the right side it will appear sharpest on the right lateral view of the skull. Conversely, inspection of the left lateral view will reveal that the fracture line is less distinct and appears wider because of the magnification that occurs through the width of the skull. Obviously the reverse will be true when a fracture is present on the left side.

Stereoscopic lateral views also may be helpful in this instance and in other cases in which localization of an area of calcification is needed. Since CT became available we no longer obtain stereo views of the skull in our department.

SUBMENTOVERTEX OR BASE VIEW OF THE SKULL (FIG. 2–5, p. 17)

This view is obtained by placing a film at the top of the skull, hyperextending the patient's neck, and angling the tube slightly toward the front of the head with the tube in front of the patient's chest. It should be noted that this view may be difficult to obtain in elderly patients, particularly in those with degenerative arthritis of the cervical spine, which limits mobility. This view may also be difficult or impossible to obtain in combative or unconscious patients.

The base view gives particularly excellent images of the clivus and of the multiple foramina at the base of the skull, which are not visible on any other projection. The pterygoid plates are also well seen (see illustration).

The three lines of the middle cranial fossa are also visualized on the base view. With this view one looks tangentially down the greater wing of the sphenoid bone, which forms a curvilinear line on either side of the skull outlining the anterior margin of the middle cranial fossa (13). The curvilinear line anterior to this, which will be seen to form an "S" configuration and to be continuous with the zygomatic bone laterally, is the bony margin of the back wall of the maxillary sinus (22). A mnemonic useful for remembering this is that the "S" line outlines the back wall of the sinus. This "S"-shaped line is to be differentiated from the straight line that forms the back wall of the orbit (23). This straight line will be seen to course from medial-posterior to lateral-anterior (see illustration).

The base view of the skull also provides an opportunity for an additional look at the maxillary sinuses when they are not well seen on the routine views and when it cannot be decided whether they are indeed normal or abnormal.

The submentovertex view is also particularly helpful when trying to evaluate varying degrees of asymmetry of the cranial vault. CT scans simulate the base position and can be correlated with the plain film base view. In addition, evaluation can be made of the internal auditory canals, the jugular foramen, and the mastoid air cells. Since metastatic carcinoma and primary nasopharyngeal carcinomas often involve the base of the skull, the base view will be helpful to the oncologist or radiotherapist for evaluation of bony erosions. Indeed, radiographic tomographic studies of the base of the skull may be performed for the purpose of evaluating a metastatic lesion or local invasion of the base of the skull.

This view also lends itself well to oral and written certification examinations because of the multiple anatomic landmarks that are visible.

NORMAL SELLA CONFIGURATION (FIGS. 2–6 and 2–7, p. 18)

Figure 2–6 illustrates three separate lines of the posterior portion of the sella which frequently can be demonstrated in an individual case. These lines are the clivus, the anterior margin of the dorsum sellae, and the anterior margin of the posterior clinoids, which wrap forward around the sella and project anterior to the dorsum sellae.

The depth of the sella (Fig. 2–7) is measured by drawing a line between the tuberculum sellae (T) and the dorsum sellae (D) and then dropping a perpendicular to this line at the deepest part of the sella. The depth of the sella should not exceed 14 mm.

The anteroposterior dimension of the sella is measured by drawing a line from the anterior margin of the sella turcica to the dorsum sellae at the longest part of the sella (A-P). This measurement should not be oblique and should not be taken from the tuberculum to the lowest portion of the dorsum sellae. The anteroposterior measurement should not exceed 17 mm.

Note that the posterior clinoid processes extend superior and anterior to the dorsum sellae.

The standard chest radiograph measures 14 × 17 inches—thus providing a good way to remember the upper limits of the size of the sella.

In actual fact, sellae even larger than these measurements are sometimes seen, and no detectable abnormality can be found in the patient. In these cases one can hypothesize an arrested pituitary adenoma, which was probably functioning at one time but is no longer active.

Osteochondromas arise from the base of the skull, which develops from endochondral bone. They are rare and resemble osteochondromas found elsewhere (no example shown).

The presence of basilar impression can be judged by measurements taken from the plain skull film using the lateral view (see Fig. 2–58, p. 62). These measurements are known as Chamberlain's line and McGregor's line. In some cases, notably the normal, Chamberlain's line and McGregor's line are superimposed; in others they are widely separated.

McGregor's Line. When a line is drawn from the posterior margin of the hard palate to the most inferior margin of the occipital squama, the odontoid should not extend more than 4 to

Table 2–1. Important Cranial Structures and Foramina

1. *Cavernous Sinus*
   a. Internal carotid artery
   b. Third cranial nerve (III)
   c. Fourth cranial nerve (IV)
   d. Ophthalmic branch of the fifth cranial nerve (V^1)
   e. Maxillary branch of the fifth cranial nerve (V^2)
   f. Sixth cranial nerve (VI)

2. *Superior Orbital Fissure*
   a. Superior ophthalmic vein
   b. Third cranial nerve (III)
   c. Fourth cranial nerve (IV)
   d. Sixth cranial nerve (VI)
   e. Ophthalmic branch of the fifth cranial nerve (V^1)

3. *Inferior Orbital Fissure*
   a. Maxillary branch of the fifth cranial nerve (V^2)
   b. Infraorbital artery and vein
   c. Sympathetic nerves

4. *Foramen Ovale*
   a. Mandibular branch of the fifth cranial nerve (V^3)

5. *Foramen Spinosum*
   a. Middle meningeal artery

6. *Foramen Rotundum*
   a. Maxillary branch of the fifth cranial nerve (V^2)

7. *Foramen Lacerum*
   a. Sympathetic nerves

8. *Carotid Canal*
   a. Carotid artery

9. *Jugular Foramen*
   a. Internal jugular vein
   b. Ninth cranial nerve
   c. Tenth cranial nerve
   d. Eleventh cranial nerve

10. *Internal Auditory Canal*
    a. Seventh cranial nerve
    b. Eighth cranial nerve

11. *Stylomastoid Foramen*
    a. Facial nerve

12. *Supraorbital Foramen*
    a. Ophthalmic division of the fifth cranial nerve (V^1)
    b. Supraorbital artery and vein

13. *Infraorbital Foramen*
    a. Infraorbital nerve (V^2)

5 mm above this line. If the odontoid protrudes farther than 4 to 5 mm, basilar impression is present (see Fig. 2–58, p. 62).

Platybasia. Platybasia (not illustrated) is an entity entirely different from basilar impression. Platybasia refers to the basal angle of the skull. The basal angle is measured by connecting the nasion to the tuberculum sellae and then to the anterior margin of the foramen magnum. The angle formed is normally 125 to 143 degrees. If the angle is greater than 143 degrees there is flattening of the base of the skull, or platybasia. If the angle formed is less than 125 degrees there is basilar kyphosis.

Platybasia may be congenital, may occur in association with the Chiari malformation and may be acquired following suboccipital craniectomy in childhood.

Platybasia and basilar impression may be seen in association with one another.

THE ABNORMAL SELLA

General Appearance. In the absence of trauma, plain skull evaluation is generally done to demonstrate the presence of primary or metastatic disease to the bony calvaria or cranial contents, metabolic disease, pituitary tumor, or evidence of sellar erosion.

Erosion of the sella secondary to increased intracranial pressure can be demonstrated quite early by plain film examination. The earliest signs of erosion secondary to increased intracranial pressure are erosion of the anterior-inferior aspect of the dorsum sellae and demineralization of the dorsum sellae. Over a period of time these changes of demineralization will come to involve the entire sella and may even affect the planum sphenoidale. With time, there will be not only demineralization of the floor sella but also thinning and truncation of the uppermost portion of the dorsum sellae and the posterior clinoids. These changes are secondary to nonspecific changes of increased intracranial pressure; they do not necessarily indicate a tumor adjacent to the sella itself. Indeed, the tumor may be quite remote from the region of the sella.

Even more remote changes may be seen, but are found less frequently in today's practice, because patients seek medical care earlier in the course of their illness and do not suffer from increased intracranial pressure long enough to exhibit these marked changes. In addition, better diagnostic techniques make early diagnosis of intracranial lesions possible.

On the other hand, the changes seen in the sella may be secondary to continued erosion by the anterior recesses of a dilated third ventricle as the transmitted pulsations of both respiration and heart beat produce erosion of the very top of the dorsum sellae, resulting in truncation of the dorsum as well as demineralization.

This type of change is seen in the presence of a space-occupying lesion that leads to the production of hydrocephalus secondary to obstruction at or below the level of the posterior portion of the third ventricle. Most commonly, this is secondary to a posterior fossa mass lesion, to a pineal tumor, or, occasionally, to adult onset of symptoms of aqueduct stenosis.

In the pediatric age group the changes of increased intracranial pressure are reflected in splitting of the sutures, usually without changes in the sella turcica. After 10 to 12 years of age, the sutures become functionally closed, and the changes of increased pressure are reflected in alterations of the sella turcica. Between the ages of 1 year and 10 to 12 years the sutures should not be more than 2 mm wide.

In the presence of changes of increased intracranial pressure, other findings will be helpful and may suggest a diagnosis; e.g., if the pineal gland is shifted, the lateralization of a supratentorial tumor mass may be possible (see Fig. 2–11, p. 22).

Care must be taken in measuring the shift of the midline structures, and the use of a measured ruler rather than trusting the eye is strongly suggested. Because of possible asymmetric calcification of the pineal, a shift of the pineal of up to 2 mm is considered within normal limits.

Other diagnostic clues are the presence of tumor calcification secondary to pinealoma, oligodendroglioma, astrocytoma, dermoid, cholesteatoma, aneurysm, calcified granuloma, and a variety of other disorders. There may likewise be localized areas of hyperostosis secondary to the presence of a meningioma. Again, a pertinent clinical history may be helpful.

Evaluation of the absolute size of the sella should be made during the course of the skull examination. This is not only because the sella may be enlarged secondary to increased intracranial pressure, but also because the presence of intrasellar tumors will lead to an enlarged sellae. Depending on the age group, the pituitary tumor is probably the most common cause of sellar enlargement. There are, however, multiple other causes of enlargement of the sella.

These include:

1. Pituitary adenoma
2. Carotid artery aneurysms
3. Meningiomas adjacent to the sella
4. Teratoma
5. Craniopharyngioma
6. Optic glioma
7. Increased intracranial pressure
8. Empty sella syndrome
9. Chordoma
10. Metastases

This list of relatively common and some less common causes of sellar enlargement should be committed to memory. In addition, there are other more obscure and more rare lesions that also lead to similar changes in the sella.

Empty Sella Syndrome

The empty sella syndrome is a clinical entity that has been associated with enlargement of the sella and subsequent demonstration of the entrance of air or contrast material into the enlarged sella. There appears to be absence or incompetence of the diaphragma sellae. These patients may be symptomatic, complaining of visual difficulties—apparently because the optic nerves are able to "fall" into the empty sella. Commonly, headache is their main complaint. This syndrome has been seen more often in women than in men, and it has been postulated that the sella may enlarge following swelling of the pituitary gland in response to pregnancy. This initial swelling later shrinks, leaving the "empty sella."

Amipaque Cisternography

The recent introduction of Amipaque has led to a new method for the diagnosis of a suprasellar mass lesion or even for the evaluation of the empty sella syndrome. Additional clinical experience and expertise has eliminated the need for pneumoencephalography for lesions around the sella.

Amipaque can be introduced into the lumbar subarachnoid space using 6 cc of a 180 mg/ml concentration. The patient is placed immediately in the 45-degree head-down position and the contrast medium is allowed to flow cephalad and to accumulate in the basilar cisterns. With the patient in the standard position, the scan is then performed. If a sellar tumor with suprasellar extension is present, there will be a lucent defect—the tumor—surrounded by the higher density Amipaque in the suprasellar cistern. With an "empty sella," the Amipaque will be identified within the confines of the sella.

With thin section tomography a fairly accurate estimate of the size of the lesions can be made. In addition, the patient can be scanned using coronal sections for direct visualization of the size of the tumor. This may be unsatisfactory because metallic fillings in the teeth will interfere with the scanning device and degrade the image.

Pituitary Adenomas

Chromophobe Adenoma. Of the pituitary adenomas the chromophobe adenoma causes the greatest amount of sellar enlargement and may even progress to cause total destruction of the sella. Massive destructive changes of the sella may be present, with complete erosion of the dorsum sellae and posterior clinoids. These tumors may extend downward through the floor of the sella, eroding the sphenoid sinus and causing a nasopharyngeal mass. Calcification of these tumors is very rare. The clinical syndrome is usually that of panhypopituitarism secondary to pressure obliteration of the remainder of the gland, and the classic physical finding is the presence of a bitemporal hemianopia secondary to pressure on the optic chiasm.

CT scanning of these tumors may be helpful for diagnosis, and scans obtained in coronal projection and/or reconstruction tomography is also helpful for better evaluation of the suprasellar extent of the mass. Such studies have eliminated the need for pneumoencephalography for sellar lesions. High resolution CT scanning with 3- to 5-mm slices should be obtained in the coronal projection for accurate evaluation. Depending upon the clinical presentation, CT may be performed postinfusion only or both pre- and postinfusion. If a microadenoma of the pituitary (less than 1 cm in size) is suspected, a postinfusion only scan should be performed following rapid bolus injection. The microadenoma usually appears as low density in a gland with an upwardly convex superior margin.

If the tumor is a macroadenoma (greater than 1 cm in size), the postinfusion only scan in the coronal projection usually demonstrates dense homogeneous enhancement of the tumor, although cystic areas may also occur in these tumors. If a craniopharyngioma is suspected, the scan should be performed both pre- and postinfusion because the enhancement may obscure small areas of calcification. (See Chapter 13.) MR may eliminate the need for additional work-up. Even microadenomas of the pituitary are well demonstrated by MR.

Basophilic Adenoma. Basophilic adenomas of the pituitary gland rarely cause sellar enlargement. The clinical picture is that of Cushing's disease. The one exception to this would be following bilateral adrenalectomy, when the sella may enlarge secondary to an ACTH-producing tumor. Changes in the sella with this rare disease may be only those seen with Cushing's disease—i.e., diffuse demineralization.

In actual fact, any cell type of pituitary adenoma may demonstrate any of the clinical syndromes, and there is a great deal of crossover between the various types of tumors.

BRAIN TUMORS

Meningioma. The incidence of radiographically visible calcification has been reported to be as high as 18 per cent, but 10 per cent or less is the most commonly reported figure. As with other types of calcified brain tumors, it seems that the incidence of visible calcifications on plain skull films is lower than previously reported. This is because brain tumors in general are being diagnosed earlier and are therefore smaller in size. On the other hand, CT scans are able to detect areas of calcification not visible on the plain film examination.

The meningiomas contain psammomatous calcification, and these calcifications frequently are small stippled areas distributed homogeneously throughout the tumor. They may be distributed only peripherally or may calcify only in a portion of the tumor (see Chapter 9).

These tumors also may exhibit reactive bone formation.

Tumors. A variety of brain tumors and inflammatory processes may lead to intracranial calcification. Table 2–2 lists most of the causes of intracranial calcification. Examples of these calcifications are given in the illustrations at the end of this chapter.

Oligodendroglioma. These tumors exhibit calcification in most cases, but are uncommon. Over one half of these tumors calcify. The calcification may be amorphous and/or speckled; however, the author has frequently seen "boomerang-shaped" areas of calcification in these oligodendrogliomas; this is exhibited in the present example (Fig. 2–86, p. 88).

The calcification is readily demonstrated on the CT scan, even when it is only faintly visible on the plain skull examination. In this case the abnormal area is much more readily identified on the CT scan than on the plain skull examination.

Gliomas. As a group, the gliomas represent approximately 50 per cent of all the primary brain tumors. They demonstrated microscopic

Table 2—2. Intracranial Calcifications

1. Meningioma	16. Dermoid
2. Astrocytoma	17. Epidermoid
3. Oligodendroglioma	18. Tuberous sclerosis
4. Glioblastoma	19. Cytomegalic inclusion disease
5. Abscess	20. Toxoplasmosis
6. Infarct	21. Rubella
7. Arteriovenous malformation	22. Herpes simplex
8. Aneurysm	23. Parasite infestations:
9. Basal ganglia calcification	(a) cysticercosis
10. Hematoma	(b) paragonimiasis
11. Granuloma	(c) *Trichinella spiralis*
12. Gumma	24. Sturge-Weber syndrome
13. Ependymoma	25. Craniopharyngioma
14. Pinealoma	26. Pituitary adenoma (rare)
15. Teratoma	27. Aneurysm of the vein of Galen

calcification in one third of the cases when reported in 1914. However, at the present time it appears that the incidence of calcification is far less than that previously reported. This is presumably because computed tomography and other diagnostic techniques have made diagnosis possible much earlier in the course of the disease. The calcification is due to the focal areas of necrosis that result as the tumor outgrows its normal blood supply. The calcification is amorphous and may proceed asymmetrically within the tumor mass. There may be solitary areas of calcification or large clusters.

These areas of calcification are readily detected by CT scanning, even if not visible on plain skull radiographs.

Astrocytoma—Grades I and II. Calcifications are detectable in approximately one fifth of cases. These tumors frequently have a cystic component, and calcifications also may occur in the walls of the cyst.

METASTASES

Although osteoblastic metastatic deposits may be seen with prostatic carcinoma, with treated osteolytic lesions (in the healing phase), or in healing hyperparathyroidism, most metastatic deposits in the cranial vault are osteolytic. The lesions frequently are of varying size, with poorly defined irregular margins. Differentiation from multiple venous lakes may be difficult.

Any tumor known to metastasize may spread to the bony calvaria; however, metastatic breast carcinoma is seen most commonly in daily practice. These lesions may be demonstrated on the CT scan of the calvaria; however, the routine skull series is a more efficient and reliable examination for the diagnosis of metastatic disease.

DEFINITIONS

Burr hole: A small (approximately 1.5 cm) opening made with a metal "burr" for trephination of the skull. It is used to drain chronic subdural hematomas, for ventriculogram studies, and for placement of shunt tubes.

Craniotomy: The opening of the bony calvaria—usually by connecting strategically placed burr holes. Following the operative procedure, the bony flap is replaced in its original position.

Craniectomy: Following a craniotomy the bony calvaria is not replaced—a craniectomy. This is frequently seen following operative procedures on the posterior fossa.

Post-op changes: The appearance of the skull following a surgical procedure will depend upon the type of surgery performed.

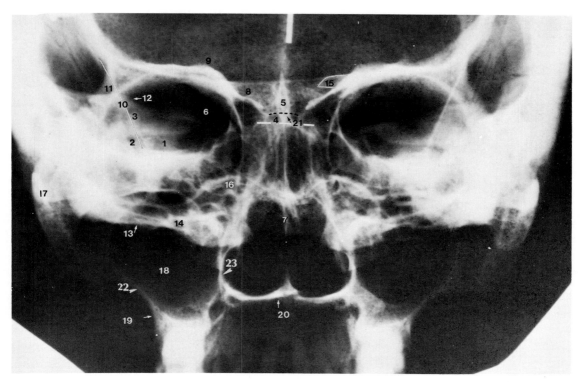

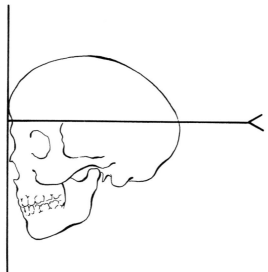

FIGURE 2–1. Posteroanterior view with internal auditory canals viewed through the orbit.

1 Internal auditory canal.	13 Floor of posterior cranial fossa.
2 Vestibule.	14 Infraorbital canal.
3 Superior semicircular canal.	15 Anterior clinoid process.
4 Floor of sella turcica.	16 Foramen rotundum.
5 Crista galli.	17 Zygomatic arch.
6 Superior orbital fissure.	18 Maxillary sinus.
7 Nasal septum.	19 Alveolar ridge of maxilla.
8 Roof of ethmoid sinus.	20 Hard palate.
9 Roof of orbit.	21 Cribriform plate.
10 Linea innominata.	22 Lateral wall of maxillary sinus.
11 Zygomatic process of frontal bone.	23 Medial wall of maxillary sinus.
12 Arcuate eminence.	

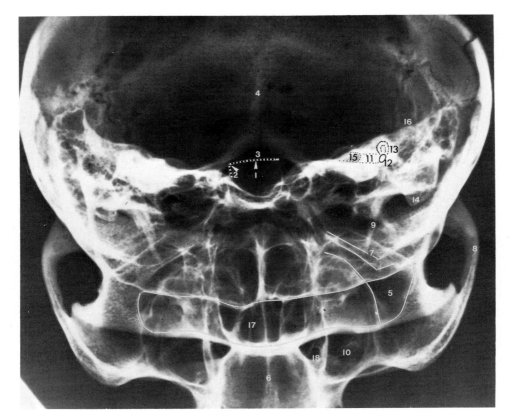

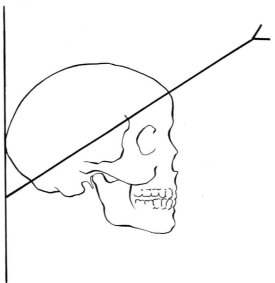

FIGURE 2–2. Towne's view.

1 Dorsum sellae.
2 Posterior clinoid process.
3 Posterior margin of foramen magnum.
4 Internal occipital crest.
5 Inferior orbital fissure.
6 Nasal septum.
7 Floor of middle cranial fossa.
8 Zygomatic arch.
9 Styloid process.
10 Maxillary sinus.
11 Internal auditory canal.
12 Vestibule.
13 Superior semicircular canal.
14 Tip of mastoid process.
15 Posterior wall of porus acusticus internus.
16 Posterior surface of petrous pyramid.
17 Frontal sinus.
18 Nasal lacrimal duct canal.

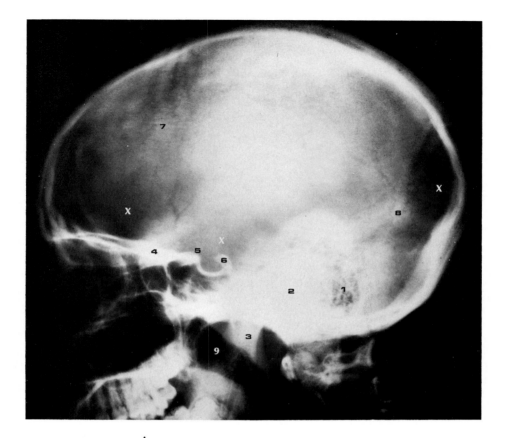

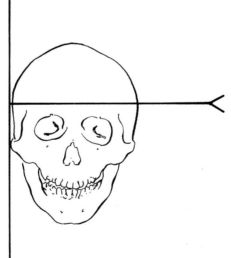

FIGURE 2–3. Lateral view.

1 Mastoid air cells.
2 External auditory canal.
3 Nasopharyngeal soft tissues.
4 Roof of orbits.
5 Tuberculum sellae.

6 Posterior clinoids and dorsum sellae.
7 Coronal suture.
8 Lambdoid suture.
9 Nasopharyngeal air shadow.
X Areas of physiologic thinning of the calvarium.

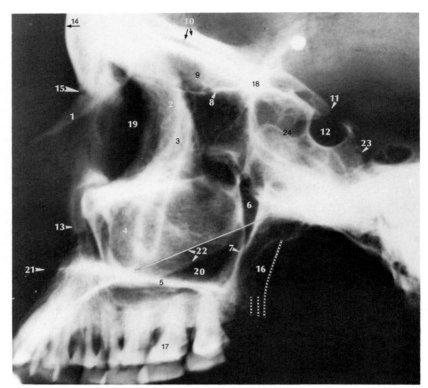

FIGURE 2–4. Lateral view of facial bones.

1 Nasal bone.
2 Zygomatic process of frontal bone.
3 Frontal process of zygomatic bone.
4 Zygomatic recess of maxillary antrum.
5 Hard palate.
6 Pterygomaxillary space.
7 Posterior wall of maxillary antrum.
8 Cribriform plate.
9 Roof of ethmoid sinuses.
10 Roof of orbits.
11 Anterior clinoid processes.
12 Sella turcica.
13 Anterior wall of maxillary antrum.
14 Anterior wall of frontal sinus region.
15 Nasofrontal suture.
16 Pterygoid plates.
17 Floor of maxillary antrum.
18 Greater wing of sphenoid bone (anterior margin of middle cranial fossa).
19 Orbit.
20 Maxillary sinus.
21 Anterior maxillary spine.
22 Inferior margin of zygomatic bones.
23 Upper margin of clivus.
24 Sphenoid sinus.

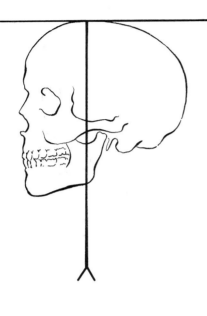

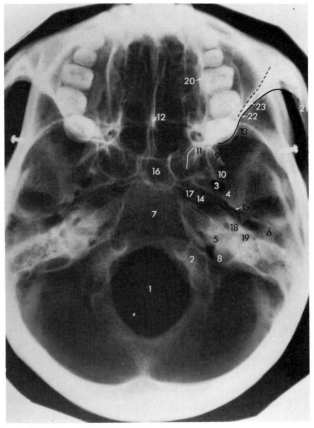

FIGURE 2–5. The submentovertex view.

1 Foramen magnum.
2 Hypoglossal canal.
3 Foramen ovale.
4 Foramen spinosum.
5 Internal auditory canal.
6 External auditory canal.
7 Clivus.
8 Jugular foramen.
9 Lateral pterygoid.
10 Inferior portion of lateral pterygoid.
11 Medial pterygoid.
12 Nasal septum.
13 Greater wing of sphenoid bone (anterior margin of middle cranial fossa).
14 Carotid canal.
15 Bony portion of eustachian tube.
16 Air cells of sphenoid sinus around sella turcica.
17 Foramen lacerum.
18 Cochlea.
19 Vestibule.
20 Medial wall of maxillary sinus.
21 Zygomatic arch.
22 Posterolateral wall of maxillary sinus.
23 Posterior wall of orbit.

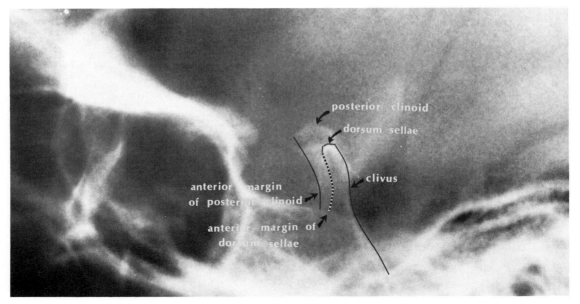

FIGURE 2–6. Normal lateral view of the sella turcica.

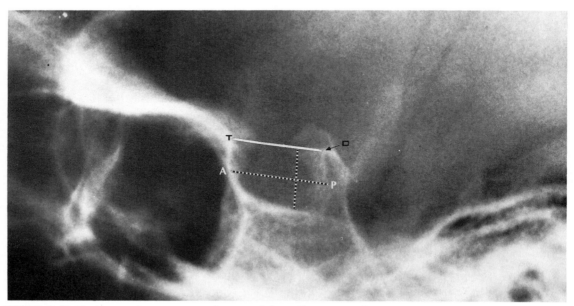

FIGURE 2–7. Technique for measuring the size of the sella turcica. The anteroposterior measurement should not exceed 17 mm, and the depth should not exceed 14 mm.

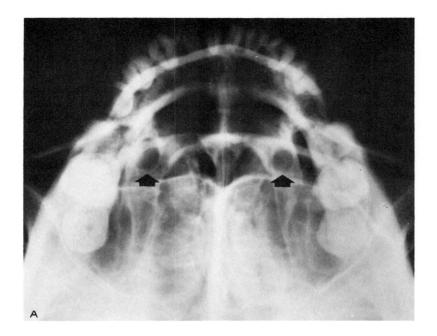

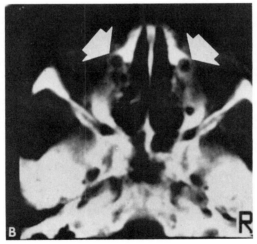

FIGURE 2–8. *Nasolacrimal Duct Canal:* This submentovertex view of the skull (A) demonstrates the nasolacrimal duct canal (*arrows*). They lie along the medial inferior margin of the orbit. The patient is positioned so that the nasolacrimal duct canal projects in a direct line with the aerated frontal sinus and just behind the mandible. The nasolacrimal canal also can be seen on the CT scan (B), where it appears as rounded foramina (*white arrows*).

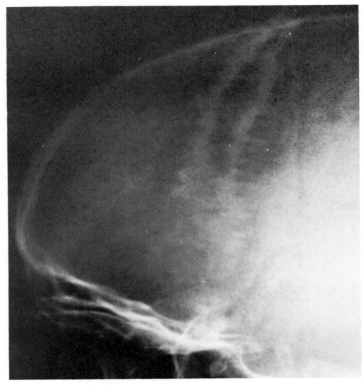

FIGURE 2–9. *Perisutural Sclerosis:* The suture lines as they fuse together frequently exhibit perisutural sclerosis, which gives the suture lines a very dense appearance. This patient is turned slightly so that each coronal suture is seen independently. The suture of the outer table of the skull exhibits large interdigitations, whereas the suture of the inner table is relatively straight. The inner table suture line should not be mistaken for a linear skull fracture.

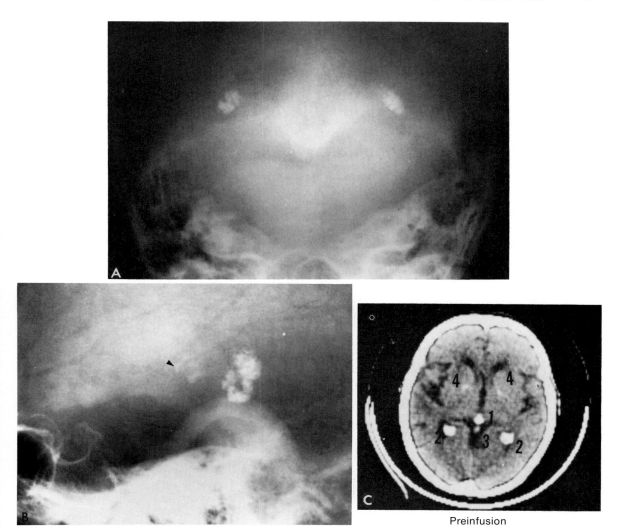

Preinfusion

FIGURE 2–10. *Habenular Commissure:* The habenular commissure calcifies in its anterior margin and forms a curvilinear line convex posteriorly just anterior to the pineal gland (*black arrow* in B). The habenula may be mistaken for pineal calcification and may itself calcify without calcification of the pineal.

Pineal: The pineal gland is calcified in 55 per cent of white adults over the age of 20 years. The normal pineal may measure up to 15 mm in size. The gland may be evaluated for changes in its anteroposterior and superoinferior position by comparing its position radiographically with the anticipated normal position originally described by Vastine and Kinney. Various modifications of the Vastine-Kinney charts have been made since the original charts were described; however, recent advances in neuroradiologic techniques, especially CT scanning, have made these measurements less important than previously. The measurements are reliable only in the normally shaped skull; and, of course, not all masses create a displacement of the pineal gland.

On the other hand, the side-to-side displacement of the pineal is very useful in daily practice for rapid and convenient evaluation of the shift of midline structures. This is especially true of Emergency Room patients and others with head trauma, where rapid evaluation of the shift of the midline structures is necessary (see Fig. 2–11).

The anteroposterior view (A) demonstrates the calcifications in the glomus of the choroid plexus bilaterally. They are located in the atrium of the lateral ventricles. On the lateral view (B) the calcifications in the glomus of the choroid plexus project posterior to the pineal gland. The patient is tilted slightly for this examination so that the calcifications project one slightly higher than the other.

C, The CT scan reveals the calcified pineal gland (1) and the well-calcified glomus in the atrium of the lateral ventricles bilaterally (2). The vein of Galen is also visualized because of the injection of contrast material; it projects just posterior to the pineal gland (3). Tiny areas of calcification are also present bilaterally in the basal ganglia. This small amount of basal ganglia calcification is not visible on plain skull films (4).

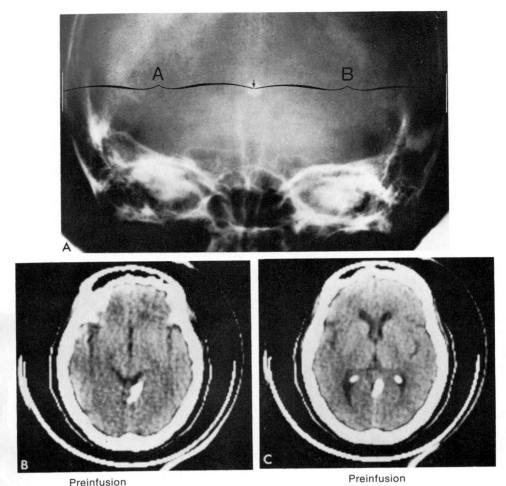

Preinfusion   Preinfusion

FIGURE 2–11. *Pineal Gland Measurements:* Shift of the pineal gland from side to side is determined on the frontal views of the skull (A). A small dot is placed in the center of the pineal gland and the distance from this point to the outer table on one side is compared to the distance from this point to the outer table on the contralateral side. One half the difference between these two measurements represents the actual shift of the pineal gland; i.e., ½ (A − B) = amount of shift. The pineal gland may be shifted up to 2 mm and still be considered to be within normal limits because the gland may calcify asymmetrically. Obviously, a noncalcified pineal is of no value for measurement, and bilateral symmetric lesions will not cause a shift of the pineal gland.

If there is a question of possible intracranial pathology, a CT scan should be obtained for evaluation. Indeed, the availability of CT scanning has greatly decreased the importance of all these measurements.

B and C, The CT scans demonstrate a large area of calcification which projects to the right of the midline. The calcification is actually in the tentorium, but could be mistaken for a shifted pineal gland on plain film examination. A tentorial calcification usually is flattened to follow the dura, whereas the pineal gland usually has a rounded configuration.

FIGURE 2–12. *Pinealoma:* The lateral view of the skull (A) reveals that the pineal gland is obviously displaced posteriorly and inferiorly (*arrow*). The sella turcica reveals truncation of the dorsum sellae and demineralization of the floor of the sella, particularly along the anterior inferior margin of the dorsum sellae.

The CT scans (B) reveal a mass in the region of the pineal gland that is of higher density than normal brain tissue; it also shows that the pineal gland (*arrow*) has calcified and has been displaced posteriorly and surrounded by the mass. The mass is slightly larger on the right side than on the left, and it flattens the posterior portion of the third ventricle. There is moderately severe obstructive hydrocephalus because the tumor blocks the outlet of the third ventricle and the aqueduct of Sylvius. The postinfusion scans reveal marked homogeneous enhancement of the tumor, which was found surgically to be a germinoma.

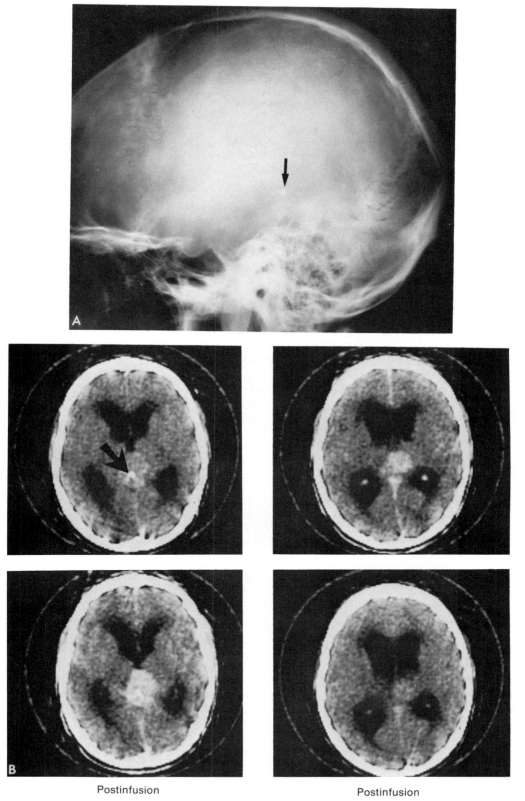

Postinfusion

Postinfusion

FIGURE 2–12. *See legend on the opposite page.*

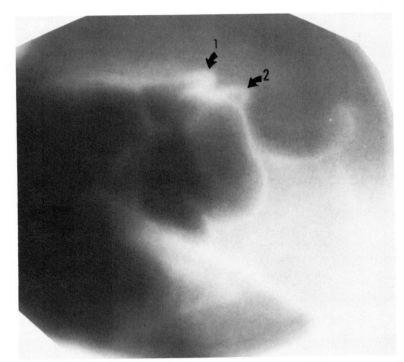

FIGURE 2–13. *Limbus and Tuberculum Sellae:* (1) The *limbus sphenoidalis* represents the most posterior extent of the planum sphenoidale. It is most commonly fused with and inseparable from the tuberculum sellae. However, as in this case, total fusion does not always occur. (2) The tuberculum sellae represents the actual anterior boundary of the pituitary fossa in the midline. The chiasmatic groove is of variable size and lies between the limbus and tuberculum; fusion of the two may result in flattening of the tuberculum sellae.

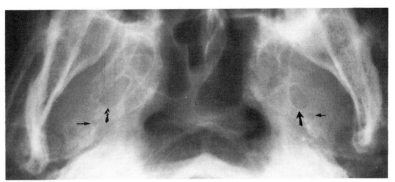

FIGURE 2–14. *Asymmetric Foramen Ovale:* The mandibular branch of the fifth cranial nerve passes through the *foramen ovale*. The size of the foramen normally may vary from side to side, and may be divided by a calcified ligament (*large arrows*). In this case we see that the right foramen ovale is larger than the left and has a somewhat more oval configuration. This is a normal variation.

Foramen Spinosum: The middle meningeal artery passes through this foramen, which may also vary in size from side to side. In the presence of a meningioma the foramen spinosum may enlarge unilaterally to accommodate an enlarged middle meningeal artery, but this is not a reliable sign, particularly if other supporting evidence is lacking. In this case, the foramen spinosum is larger on the left side (*small arrows*), a normal variation.

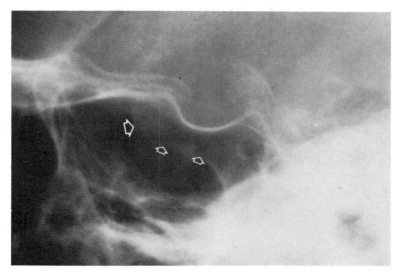

FIGURE 2–15. *Carotid Groove:* The arrowheads mark the bony fossa, which contains the carotid artery as it courses on either side of the sella turcica. If this groove is positioned higher it may be mistaken for a double floor of the sella. This is called the "pseudo–double floor" of the sella.

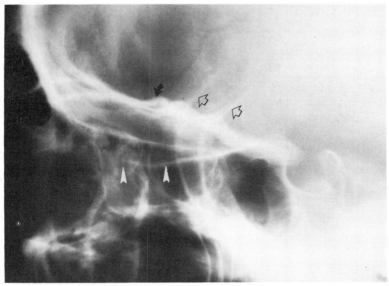

FIGURE 2–16. *Anterior Cranial Fossa:* The black arrow points to the irregular roofs of the orbits, which are superimposed in this view. The white arrowheads show the planum sphenoidale posteriorly and its anterior continuation, the cribriform plate. The cribriform plate is a very thin bone with multiple perforations; therefore, it is rarely seen on routine skull films and only infrequently demonstrated on tomograms. The tiny bony line between the orbital roofs and the planum sphenoidale/cribriform plate is the roof of the ethmoid sinuses. The open arrowheads indicate the upper portions of the greater wings of the sphenoid bone bilaterally. In a true lateral projection these curvilinear lines will be superimposed.

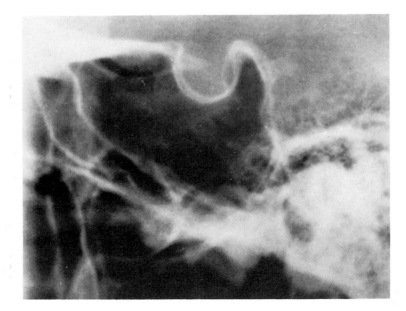

FIGURE 2–17. *Aerated Sphenoid Bone:* The entire sphenoid bone is aerated and surrounds the sella turcica.

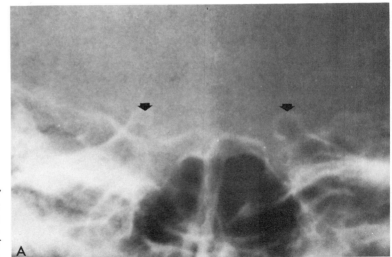

FIGURE 2–18. *Aerated Anterior Clinoids:* The posteroanterior view of the skull (A) reveals the aerated anterior clinoids (*arrowheads*) bilaterally. The low cut of the CT scan (B) reveals both the aerated anterior clinoids (*arrows*) and the aerated dorsum sellae. Note that the mastoid air cells are particularly well developed and well aerated in this case.

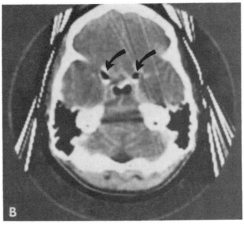

Postinfusion

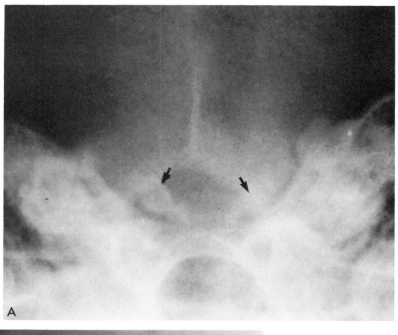

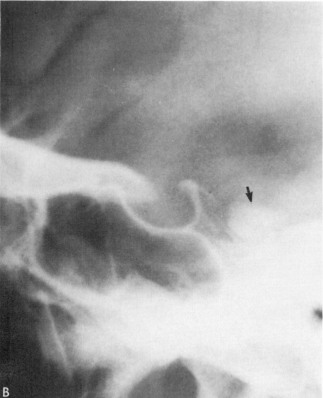

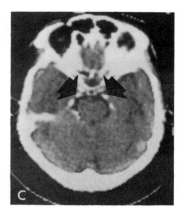

FIGURE 2–19. *Petroclinoid Ligament:* This dural reflection extends from the posterior clinoid process on each side posterolaterally to the petrous bone. It is frequently calcified and more commonly appears as a linear area of calcification. If the calcification takes on a globular appearance, it is known as "horsetail" calcification of the petroclinoid ligament. In the case shown, the horsetail calcification (*arrows*) is seen clearly on both the Towne's (*A*) and the lateral (*B*) views. A small area of linear calcification is seen on the lateral view just anterior to the larger globular area of calcification. The CT scan (*C*) also demonstrates the petroclinoid ligament calcification (*arrowheads*).

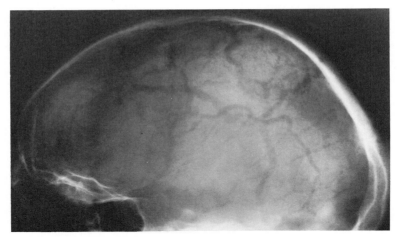

FIGURE 2–20. *Normal Prominent Vascular Pattern:* The veins in the diploic space can appear very prominent in some cases. Extensive venous markings and multiple venous lakes, known as phlebectasia, are of no significance. At times it is difficult or impossible to differentiate these from multiple metastases.

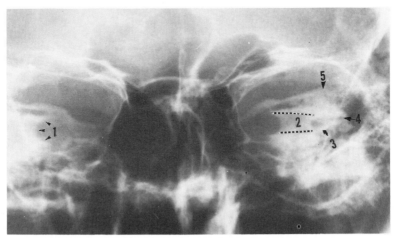

FIGURE 2–21. *Ear Structures on Plain Film Examination:* The normal ear structures are readily visualized on the standard posteroanterior skull films, particularly when the internal auditory canals (2) are projected through the center of the orbit. The posterior margin of the internal auditory canal is readily demonstrated (1). The internal auditory canal abuts on the vestibule (3), and the horizontal semicircular canal extends laterally from the vestibule (4). The superior (5) semicircular canal extends superiorly from the vestibule; it is frequently, but not always, located just below the arcuate eminence of the petrous bone.

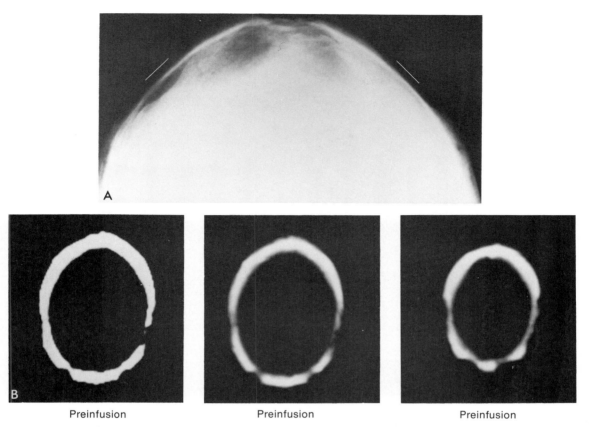

Preinfusion   Preinfusion   Preinfusion

FIGURE 2–22. *Biparietal Thinning:* Biparietal thinning affects the outer table of the skull; it is of no pathologic significance and its occurrence may be familial. (A) The plain skull film reveals bilateral thinning of the outer table of the skull. The white lines represent the anticipated position of the outer table of the skull. (B) CT scans of the bony calvaria demonstrate the thinning of the skull bilaterally. Note that this affects only the outer table and leaves the inner table intact.

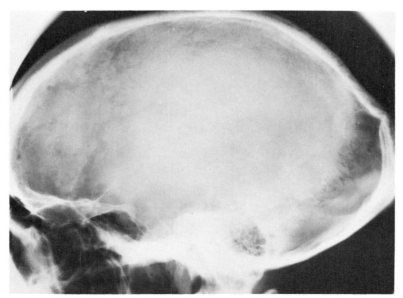

FIGURE 2–23. *Bathrocephaly:* The occipital bone is seen on the lateral view to protrude more posteriorly than the parietal bone at the level of the lambdoid suture. This is a normal anatomic variation.

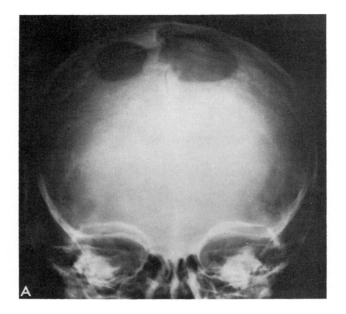

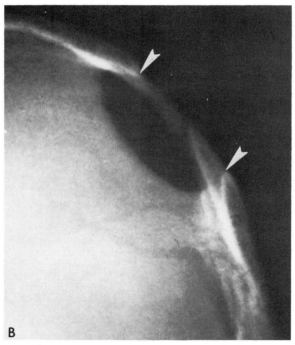

FIGURE 2–24. *Biparietal Foramina:* These openings in the parietal region involve both the inner and outer tables of the skull. They vary in size from very small to large and are of no pathologic significance. The lateral view (*B*) demonstrates the foramina and also shows the point of meeting of the inner and outer tables of the skull (*arrows*). These foramina are also visible on CT scans.

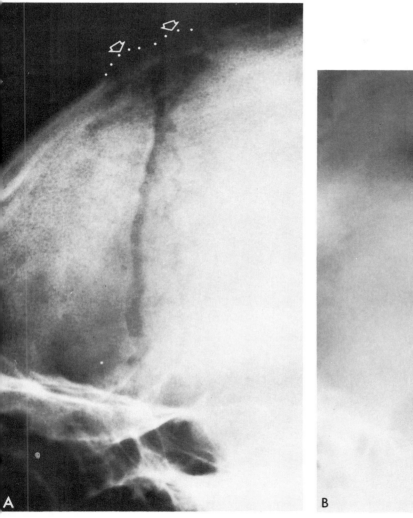

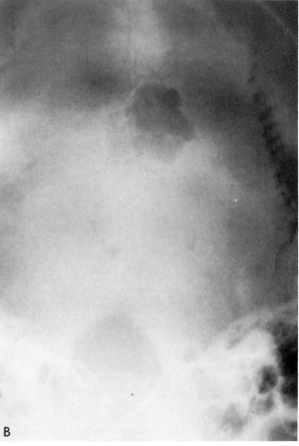

FIGURE 2–25. *Pacchionian Granulations:* *A,* The arachnoid villi protrude through the dura and function to resorb the cerebrospinal fluid. These villi erode the inner table of the skull in a localized fashion (*arrows*). These areas of thinning usually are situated within 3 cm of the midsagittal plane in the frontal and parietal regions; they may at times be very prominent.

In the case shown, a large venous structure in the diploic space—the phenoparietal sinus—is seen draining the pacchionian granulations in the posterior frontal region (*arrows*).

B, Pacchionian granulations also may be seen in the region of the torcular, where they may be quite prominent.

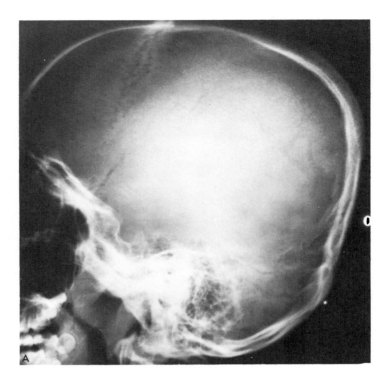

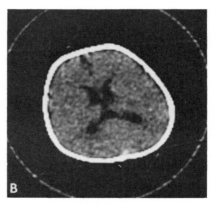

Preinfusion

FIGURE 2–26. *Brachiocephaly:* This malformation may be developmental or may be secondary to premature closure of the coronal or lambdoidal suture, which results in decreased anteroposterior length and increases in the width and height of the skull.

In this example (*A*), the head is short and wide, giving a brachiocephalic appearance; however, the back of the vault is flattened. The brachiocephalic appearance in this case, a mentally retarded patient, is secondary to prolonged periods spent lying supine.

The CT scan (*B*) is of a different patient whose brachiocephaly was developmental. Note that the cranial contents and the lateral ventricles are normal.

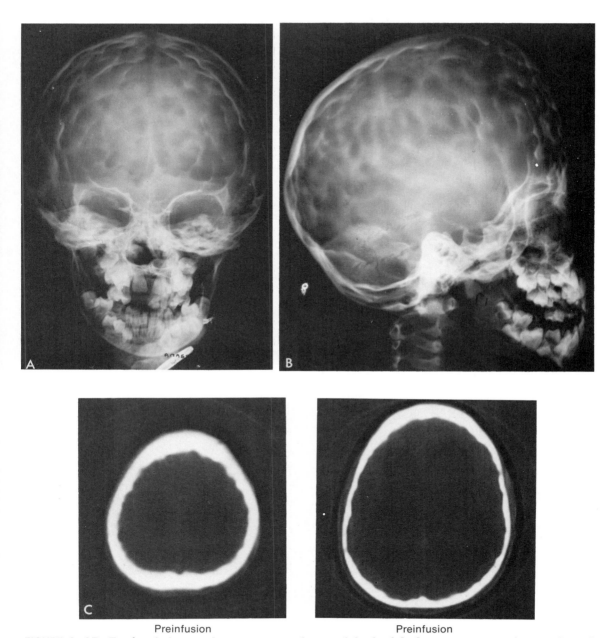

Preinfusion   Preinfusion

FIGURE 2–27. *Turricephaly:* *A* and *B*, Premature closure of the lambdoid suture causes a short, wide and high cranial vault. Note also the marked prominence of the digital markings of the skull. The CT scans (*C*) also demonstrate these pronounced digital markings.

Trigonocephaly results in a pointed appearance of the forehead. It is secondary to premature closure of the metopic suture. (No example shown.)

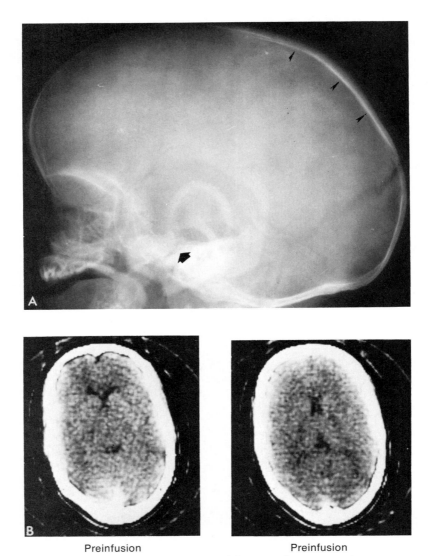

Preinfusion   Preinfusion

FIGURE 2–28. *A, **Dolichocephaly:*** Premature closure of the sagittal suture results in compensatory excessive growth of the sutures perpendicular to it (i.e., coronal and lambdoid). This results in an elongated but narrow skull, i.e., dolichocephalic craniostenosis. In some individuals a mild degree of dolichocephaly appears to be developmental, as there is no premature suture closure.

B, CT scans reflect the radiographic appearance of the bony calvaria, but the cranial contents otherwise appear to be normal.

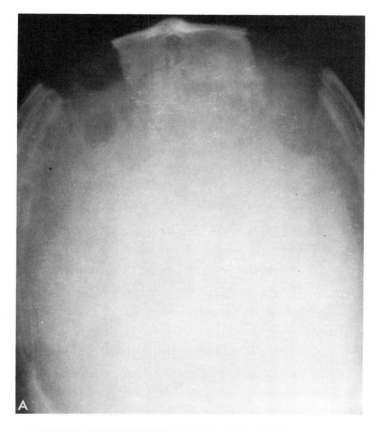

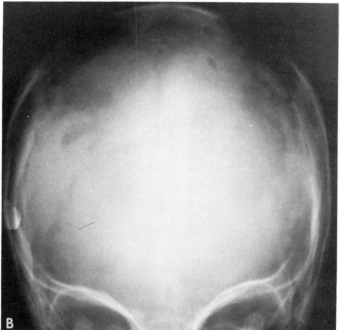

FIGURE 2–29. *Morcellation Procedure:* *A,* The surgical treatment for dolichocephalic craniostenosis involves placement of long cuts in the skull in the parasagittal areas bilaterally. This allows the skull to grow in the transverse direction. A later film (*B*) demonstrates partial bony overgrowth of the surgical incisions. (Case courtesy of Drs. Oscar Sugar and Glen Dobben.)

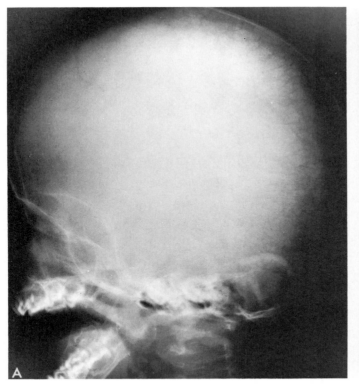
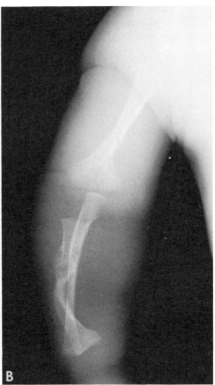
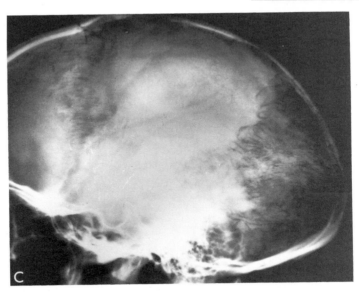

FIGURE 2–30. *Wormian Bones:* These intrasutural bones are small, irregular islands of bones that occur most commonly in the lambdoid suture. The number of bones is highly variable, and bones may be found in normal individuals. They are also found in other conditions such as cleidocranial dysostosis, cretinism, osteogenesis imperfecta, and chronic hydrocephalus, as well as less common disease processes.

A, In this example, the patient, in addition to multiple wormian bones, also has marked thinning of the bony calvaria secondary to osteogenesis imperfecta.

B, The same patient demonstrates multiple long bone fractures following minimal trauma.

C, Innumerable wormian bones are present in the coronal, sagittal, and lambdoid sutures. The etiology is unknown in this normal individual. (Case courtesy of Dr. Kenneth D. Schmidt.)

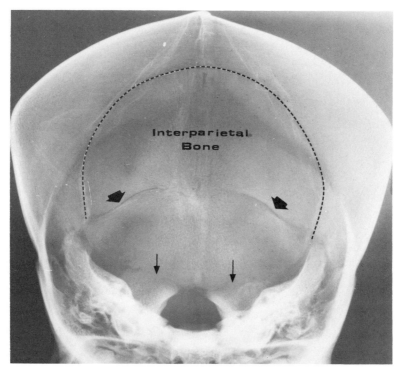

FIGURE 2–31. *Occipital Bone:* The dotted line follows the lambdoid suture. The large black arrowheads demonstrate the mendosal suture. The interparietal portion of the occipital bone develops in membranous bone; if the mendosal suture fails to fuse, this portion of the occipital bone becomes known as the interparietal bone. Beneath the mendosal suture the supraoccipital portion of the occipital bone is seen; it is separated from the exoccipital portion of the occipital bone by the synchondrosis between the two (*small arrows*). Both the synchondrosis and the mendosal suture may be mistaken for fractures. The mendosal suture may be present unilaterally, in which case differentiation from fracture may be quite difficult.

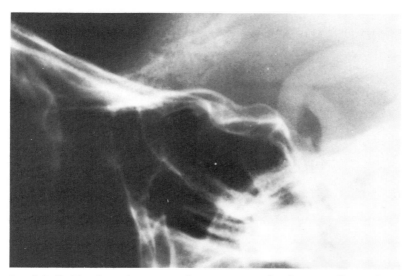

FIGURE 2–32. *Small Sella Turcica:* This patient demonstrates a developmentally small sella of no pathologic significance. In this case there is also calcification of the interclinoid ligament.

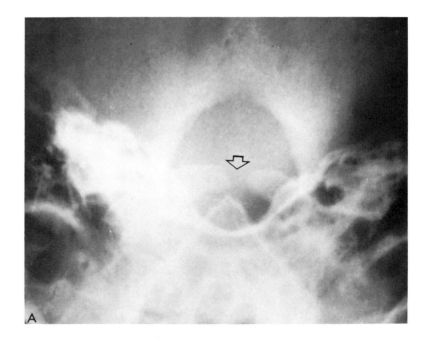

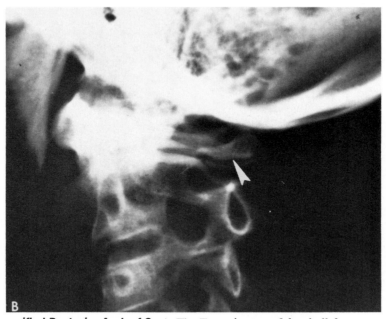

FIGURE 2–33. *Unossified Posterior Arch of C₁:* A, The Towne's view of the skull demonstrates the unossified mid-portion of the posterior arch of C_1. The posterior arch of C_2 can be seen just inferior to the arch of C_1.

B, The lateral view in another patient demonstrates that the white line marking the point of fusion between the laminae of either arch is not present, owing to a failure of fusion of the posterior margin of the arch similar to that demonstrated in A. This is of no pathologic significance, and the visualized bony structures are held in place by fibrous bands.

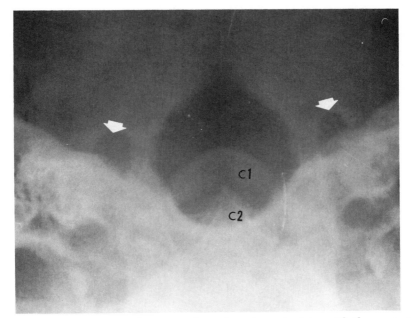

FIGURE 2–34. *Condyloid Foramen:* At the point where the atlas articulates with the occiput there is a fossa for the lateral masses of the atlas. In some cases (*arrows*) a foramen actually develops. The foramen is bridged by fibrous tissue and should not be mistaken for lytic lesions of the skull. The posterior arch of both C_1 and C_2 can be seen through the foramen magnum.

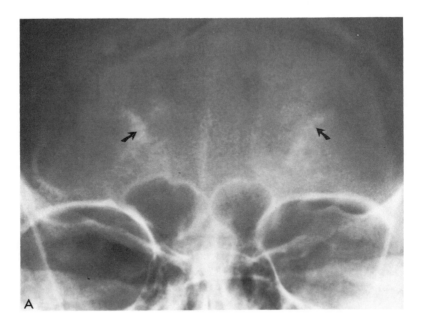

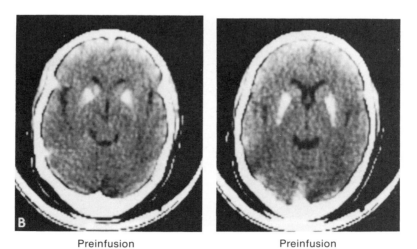

Preinfusion   Preinfusion

FIGURE 2–35. *Basal Ganglia Calcification:* A, These calcifications may be readily visible (*arrows*) or, more commonly, only faintly visible or invisible on skull radiographs. These areas of calcification may also present in the dentate nucleus of the cerebellum.

B, The calcifications are readily visible on the CT scans—even when they are seen only faintly or not at all on plain film radiography. Basal ganglia calcifications may be seen with a variety of conditions, including hypoparathyroidism, pseudohypoparathyroidism, Fahr's disease, Cockayne's syndrome, and other less common diseases. It also may be idiopathic.

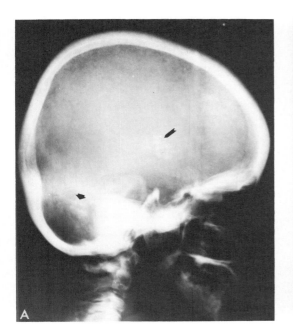
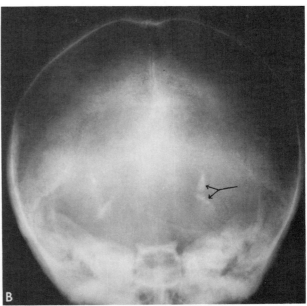
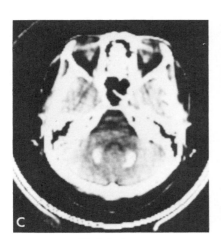
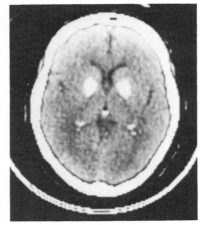

Preinfusion   Preinfusion

FIGURE 2–36. *Basal Ganglia and Dentate Nucleus Calcification:* A, The lateral view of the skull demonstrates readily visible basal ganglia and dentate nucleus calcification (*arrows*).

B, The Towne's view of the skull reveals that the two areas of calcification are now superimposed (*double-headed arrows*).

C, Small areas of calcification not apparent on the skull film may be demonstrated on the CT scan. At times, even relatively extensive areas of calcification may be present which are not readily apparent on skull films except, perhaps, in retrospect. The patient shown here had a clinical diagnosis of progeria.

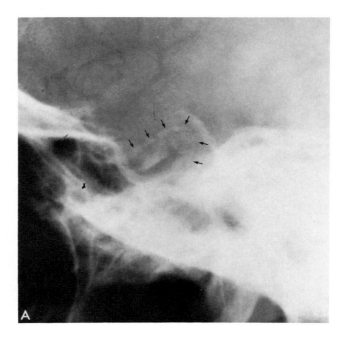

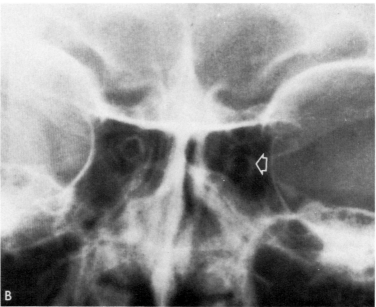

FIGURE 2–37. *Calcified Cavernous Carotid Artery:* *A,* The curvilinear areas of calcification of the cavernous carotid artery are readily visualized in this example.

B, On the posteroanterior views they are viewed end-on and appear as rounded circles of calcification—in this case seen bilaterally through the sphenoid sinus in the parasellar area (arrow is on the left-sided calcification).

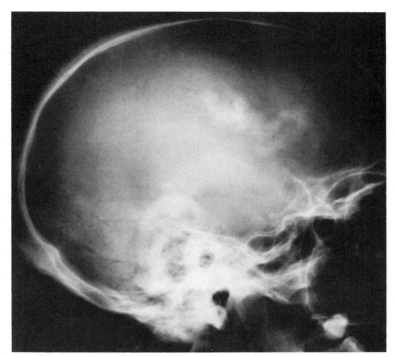

FIGURE 2–38. _Braids of Hair:_ Braided locks of hair may project over the skull and give the appearance of osteoblastic metastatic lesions. However, their appearance is changeable and not reproducible on multiple views, and close examination of the films reveals their true nature. These hair braids may be multiple, and better evaluation of the bony calvaria can be obtained if the hair is unbraided before radiography.

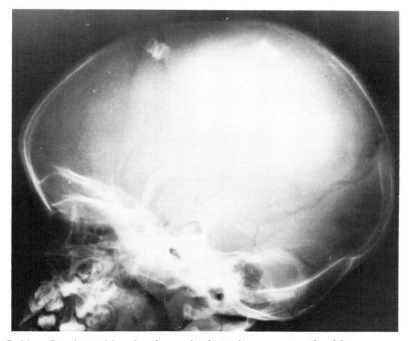

FIGURE 2–39. _Rubber Bands:_ Rubber bands on the hair also may give the false appearance of metastatic lesions involving the bony calvaria.

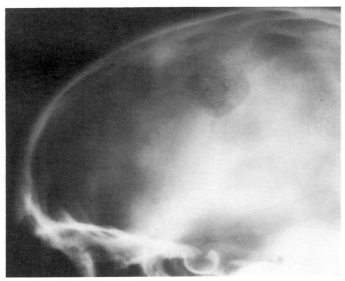

FIGURE 2–40. *Cavernous Hemangioma:* The lesion is lucent with a border that is smooth and well-defined but not sclerotic. The area of lucency frequently has a granular or salt-and-pepper appearance. Hemangiomas may demonstrate a "spoke-wheel" appearance. These are benign lesions and vary greatly in size. There may be a vascular groove that drains away from the hemangioma. Hemangiomas are diplopic lesions and expand the inner and outer tables of the skull.

FIGURE 2–41. *Cavernous Hemangioma and Osteoma:* There is a lucent defect in the midfrontal region with a well-defined border and a granular appearance. In addition, there is an osteoma that involves the outer table of the skull just posterior to the hemangioma. The osteoma is typical in that the density is quite high and the border is well-defined; however, it is not typical because the border is irregular—not rounded, as is usually the case.

Osteomas usually involve the outer table of the skull; they may involve the inner table and, rarely, the diploë. A tangential view may reveal a radiolucent line at the base of the osteoma. Osteomas are very dense, have a well-defined margin, and arise abruptly from the bony calvaria. An osteoma of the inner table may be difficult to differentiate from a meningioma without the aid of a CT scan.

The CT scan reveals a well-defined high-density bony lesion arising from the outer or inner table of the skull. Osteomas may also be identified in the diploë of the skull on the CT scan.

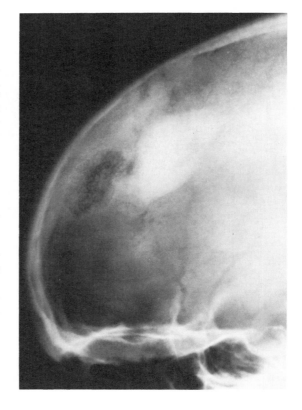

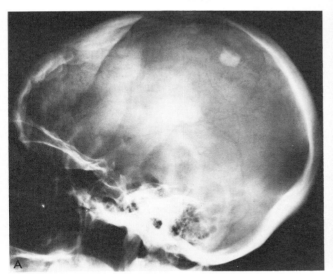

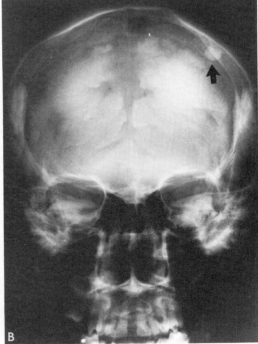

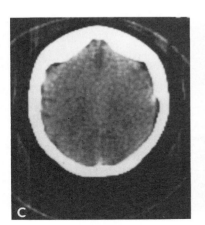

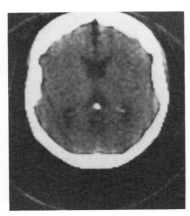

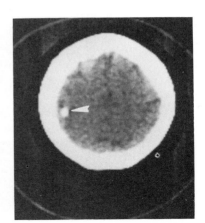

Preinfusion   Preinfusion   Preinfusion

FIGURE 2–42. *Osteoma of the Inner Table of the Skull and Diffuse Hyperostosis:* *A*, The plain skull film demonstrates a small osteoma in the midparietal region on the lateral view.

B, The osteoma also can be seen arising from the inner table of the skull on the posteroanterior view.

C, CT scans also reveal the osteoma high in the left parietal region (*arrow*). The osteoma is of high density, is not associated with edema, and does not change following the infusion of contrast material.

In addition to the osteoma, there is marked thickening of the inner table of the skull in the frontal region bilaterally. Note that in the posteroanterior view the hyperostosis does not cross the midline. This is a typical appearance of "hyperostosis frontalis interna," a process that affects the inner table of the skull, has curvilinear margins, and does not cross the midline because of the dural reflection of the falx. This process of hyperostosis is more common in older women and is most common in the frontal region. This process of hyperostosis may affect other areas of the skull—as seen in this case, in which the parietal and temporal areas are involved along with the frontal region. If other areas are affected it should not be considered a separate process, but rather a process similar to that seen in the frontal region.

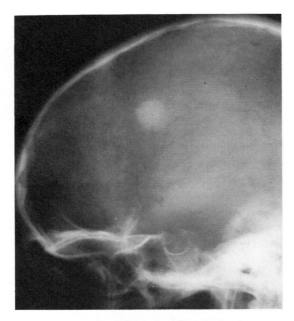

FIGURE 2–43. *Sebaceous Cyst:* The plain skull series reveals a high-density lesion; but the density is not that of bone, and the margins are rather indistinct. This is a sebaceous adenoma of the scalp. It could be readily palpated and moved with the skin of the scalp. It may be difficult to differentiate the two radiographically.

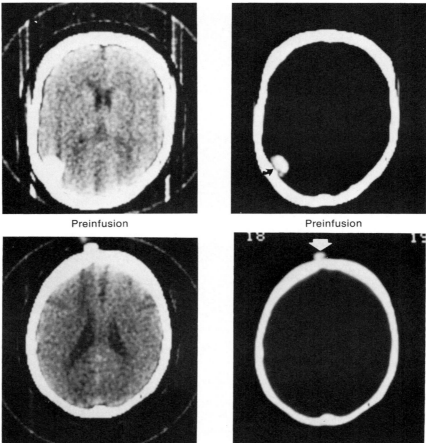

Preinfusion   Preinfusion

Preinfusion   Preinfusion

FIGURE 2–44. *CT of an Osteoma:* The osteoma (*arrowhead*) is of bone density, and the thin radiolucent line can be identified at the base of the lesion on the high window level views. The appearance is typical of an osteoma.

In these examples from different individuals, one osteoma arises from the inner table of the skull; another arises from the outer table.

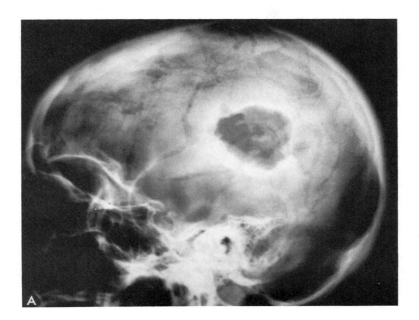

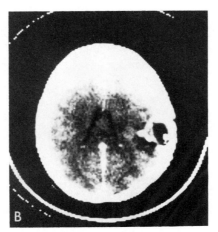

FIGURE 2–45. *Epidermoids of Bony Calvaria:* These present as lucent lesions (A) with well-defined, scalloped margins that have a characteristic sclerotic appearance. They expand the diploë, contain desquamated dermal tissues, and may be called cholesteatomas of the skull. They are most common in the vault but may occur in the orbital region.

The CT scan (B) demonstrates the lucent, low-density expansile nature of the lesion, which tends to protrude more intracranially than extracranially. The sclerotic high-density margin is also well-demonstrated. (Case courtesy of Dr. Kenneth D. Schmidt.)

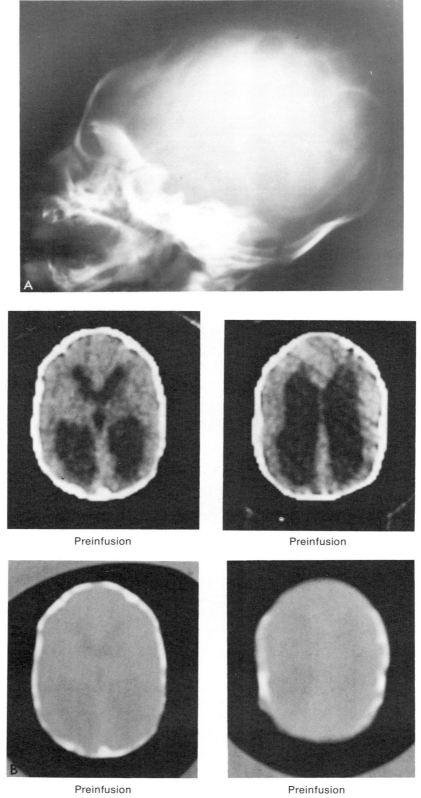

Preinfusion   Preinfusion

Preinfusion   Preinfusion

FIGURE 2–46. *See legend on the opposite page.*

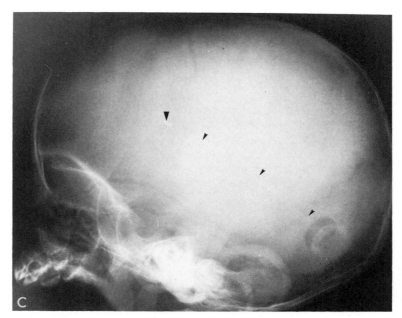

FIGURE 2–46. *Craniolacunia (Lückenschädel):* A, This abnormal honeycomb appearance of the calvaria is caused by areas of dense bone separated by radiolucent areas of very thin or absent bone. This congenital abnormality is present at birth and is usually seen in patients who have a meningocele or meningoencephalocele. The etiology is unknown, but it may be related to increased intracranial pressure in utero.

B, CT scans reveal the honeycomb appearance of the bony calvaria with multiple areas of bony thinning. In addition, there is hydrocephalus secondary to the obstruction of the aqueduct in this patient with a Chiari II malformation. The patient demonstrates typical craniolacunia and had a meningomyelocele. The abnormal appearance disappears soon after birth and is followed by changes of increased intracranial pressure. The craniolacunia disappear, the head enlarges, and the sutures widen because of continued enlargement of the lateral ventricles.

C, The skull film at six months of age reveals the enlarged skull with the widened suture and the absence of the craniolacunia. A shunt tubing device is in place (*arrows*).

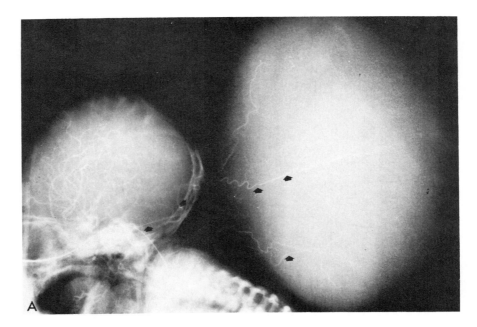

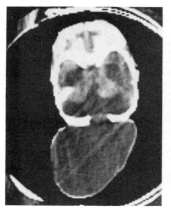

Postinfusion

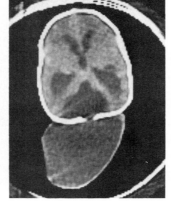

Postinfusion

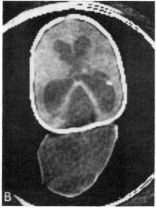

Postinfusion

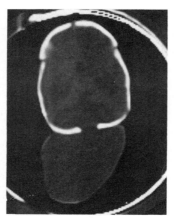

Postinfusion

FIGURE 2–47. *Meningoencephalocele:* A varying amount of meningeal and/or brain tissue may protrude through an abnormal opening in the bony calvaria—usually in the midline. If the protruding tissue is made up only of the meninges, it is called a meningocele; with both brain tissue and meninges, it is a meningoencephalocele. *A*, The lateral arteriographic view reveals a large meningoencephalocele in the occipital region. The vertebral arteries (*arrows*) can be seen to supply the brain tissue that is outside the cranial vault.

B, CT scans in a different patient reveal a large occipital meningocele. The material in the meningocele is of CSF density, and no brain tissue is present. In addition there is hypoplasia of the cerebellum with posterior fossa structures that appear to be abnormal. There is moderate hydrocephalus—probably secondary to aqueduct stenosis. The bony defect is readily identified at the midline in the posterior fossa.

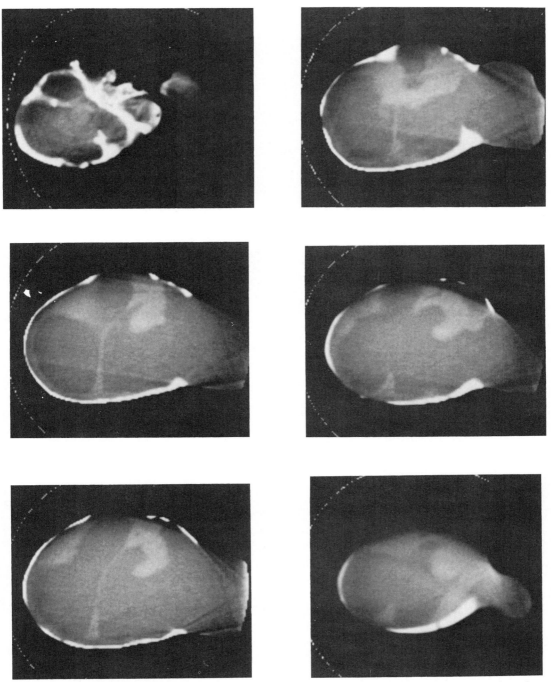

FIGURE 2–48. *Meningoencephalocele:* Clinically, this patient had a grossly misshapen cranial vault, and only one eye was identifiable. The CT scans reveal a large right frontal meningoencephalocele that communicates with the right lateral ventricle. In addition, there is severe hydrocephalus with deformity of the intracranial structures. A large bony defect is seen in the right lateral wall of the bony calvaria. Except for pathologic examination, the CT scan provides a much more accurate impression of the intracranial structures than is possible with any other neuroradiologic examination. In most cases of hydrocephalus, the only examination necessary before undertaking appropriate treatment is the CT scan of the cranial contents.

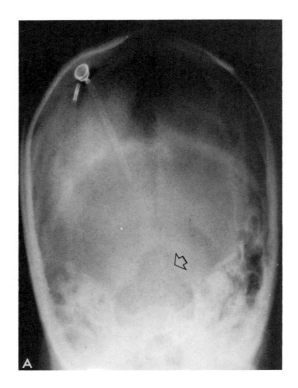

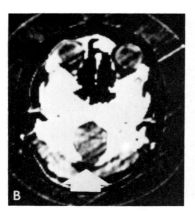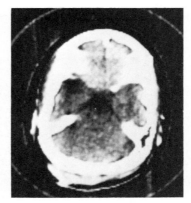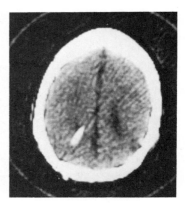

Preinfusion   Preinfusion   Preinfusion

FIGURE 2–49. *Chiari Type II: A*, There is downward displacement of the posterior fossa structures into the upper cervical region; because of this, there is enlargement of the foramen magnum (*arrow*) to accommodate the additional structures. Because there is also an associated aqueduct stenosis, the patient developed hydrocephalus, and a shunt tubing device can be seen in place on the right side.

B, CT scans on the same patient demonstrate the large foramen magnum. The posterior margin is actually intact, but because of the projection of the cut appears to be open posteriorly. The fourth ventricle is never seen because it is positioned down in the cervical region. The upper cuts reveal the shunt tubing device in place and adequate decompression of the lateral ventricles.

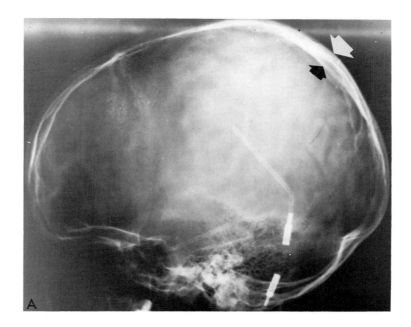

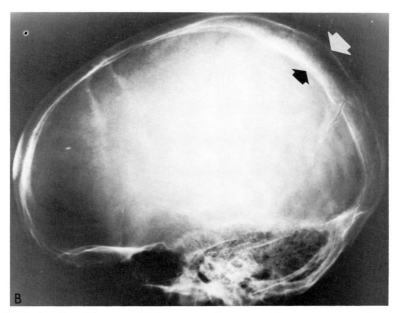

FIGURE 2–50. *Post-shunting Changes:* With increased intracranial pressure secondary to hydrocephalus, widening of the sutures occurs that is most marked in the coronal and sagittal sutures. The lambdoid suture is frequently spared. There may also be an increase in the digital markings.

Post-shunting, the sutures will no longer be widened; in response to a decrease in the intracranial pressure on the cranial vault there may be an increase in the thickness of the bony calvaria. *A,* The early skull film reveals a shunt in place and a mild increase in the thickness of the cranial vault secondary to the initial shunting procedure. *B,* After additional shunt revisions, a skull film obtained at a later date shows a marked increase in the thickness of the bone in the parietal and occipital regions (*arrows*). (Case courtesy of Drs. O. Sugar and G. Dobben.)

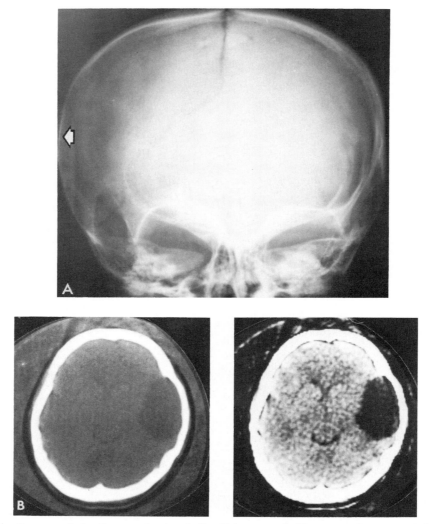

FIGURE 2–51. *Porencephaly:* Frequently the skull will be normal. There may be areas of thinning of the bone over the porencephalic cysts because they appear to exert some pressure on the bony calvarium. The CT scan demonstrates these areas to excellent advantage, and, in fact, the areas of bone thinning seen on the CT scan may not be appreciated on the skull series.

By definition, a porencephalic cyst is lined by ependyma and is an outpouching from the lateral ventricles. Through the years this definition has been broadened to include cystic lesions that communicate with the lateral ventricle, the subarachnoid space, or a "closed" porencephalic cyst that lies deep within the cerebral substance and does not communicate with either.

Porencephaly in a general sense implies any lesion of cerebrospinal fluid density that is nonmalignant. These lesions may be caused by germ plasm abnormalities, birth trauma, anoxia, hemorrhage, vascular thrombosis, or embolism, both postinflammatory and postsurgical.

A, The skull film demonstrates an area of bony expansion and thinning over a porencephalic cyst. This PA view demonstrates bulging of the skull in the right temporal and parietal regions with thinning of the bone. These changes are long-standing and secondary to an underlying cyst. The cyst may be a porencephalic cyst or a temporal arachnoid cyst. (Case courtesy of Drs. O. Sugar and G. Dobben.)

B, The CT scan demonstrates a well-defined, cerebrospinal fluid–containing lesion that has caused a thinning of the overlying bony calvaria. This example is of a temporal arachnoid cyst, not a porencephalic cyst. At times, as in this case, it is difficult to differentiate between the two. These arachnoid cysts are lined by an arachnoid-like membrane.

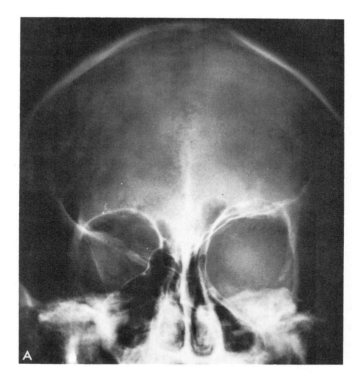

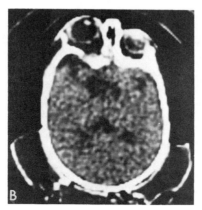

Preinfusion

FIGURE 2–52. *Neurofibromatosis:* This disease is characterized by developmental abnormalities of mesenchymal tissues, even in the absence of soft tissue neurofibromas. Skull films frequently demonstrate changes secondary to orbital and middle cranial fossa dysplasias. The sella turcica may be enlarged. The developmental abnormality that affects the sphenoid wings results in elevation of the orbital roof and absent or marked thinning of the greater wing of the sphenoid. This is a mesenchymal abnormality and is not related to the presence of a neurofibroma. The orbit appears "empty" on the skull films (*A*)—the "harlequin eye." Exophthalmos may be present on the affected side. The entire orbit may be enlarged, as it is in this case.

The CT scan (*B*) reflects these changes, but does not demonstrate a mass lesion.

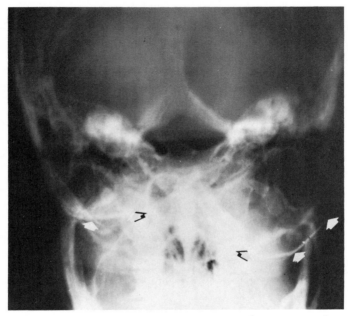

FIGURE 2–53. *Middle Cranial Fossa Dysplasia of Neurofibromatosis:* The Towne's view of the skull reveals a normal middle cranial fossa on the right side and an enlarged and ballooned middle cranial fossa on the left side (*arrowheads*).

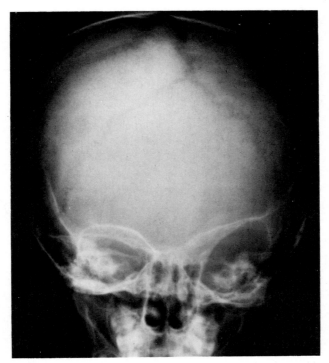

FIGURE 2–54. *Plagiocephaly:* This irregularly shaped deformity of the cranial vault is often due to unilateral premature closure of the coronal or lambdoidal suture. It may also be seen with generalized premature craniostenosis.

Premature closure of one coronal suture elevates the roof of the orbit on the ipsilateral side, creating an appearance similar to that seen in hemiatropy or in dysplasias secondary to neurofibromatosis. Note that the hemicranium on the left side demonstrates a sloping cranial vault because the entire left hemicranium is smaller than the right, secondary to premature suture closure.

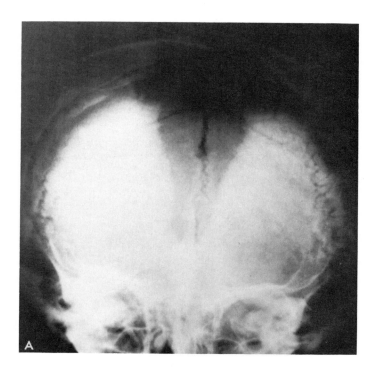

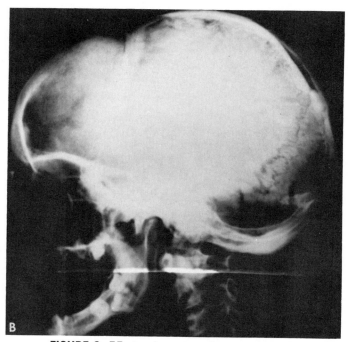

FIGURE 2–55. *See legend on the opposite page.*

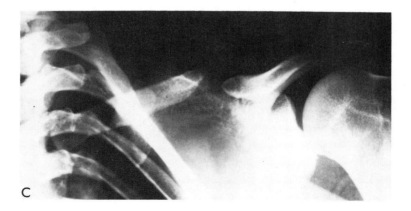

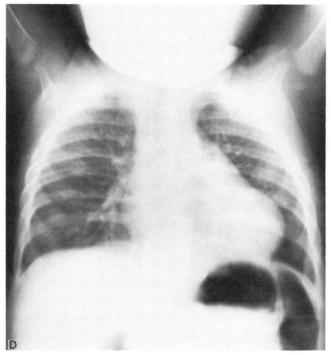

FIGURE 2–55. *Cleidocranial Dysostosis:* *A* and *B*, The skull abnormalities include midline defects with wide sutures and numerous wormian bones. There is delayed closure of the fontanelles. All these findings are present in this case. In addition, dental abnormalities are a major part of this syndrome. There are multiple defects of the teeth, with retention of deciduous teeth, delayed eruption, and enamel defects. Note the retained teeth in the mandible and maxilla.

As the name suggests, there are congenital ossification defects in the clavicles that may be partly (*C*) or completely absent (*D*). These patients may be intellectually intact. (Case courtesy of Drs. Glen Dobben and Oscar Sugar.)

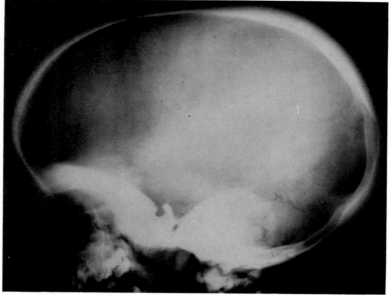

FIGURE 2–56. *Osteopetrosis:* There is an increased density of all the bones of the body, including the bones of the base of the skull. This may result in encroachment upon the foramina of the base of the skull and may result in visual problems, including blindness when it involves the optic foramina.

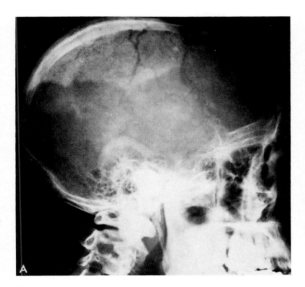

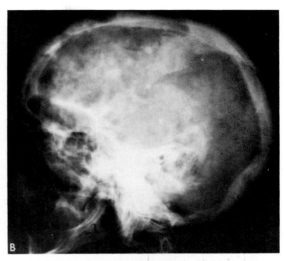

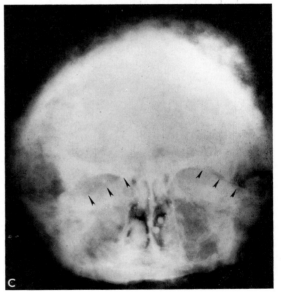

FIGURE 2–57. *Paget's Disease (Osteitis Deformans, Osteoporosis Circumscripta):* The initial phases of Paget's disease of the skull may reveal a diffuse osteolysis of a large, well-defined area of the calvarium (A). This process usually begins in the frontal-parietal and occipital areas, while the vertex appears of normal density. The area of demineralization is often large, with a well-defined but irregular border that crosses the sutures.

B, With time, osteoporosis circumscripta or the lytic phase of Paget's disease may be combined with the productive or blastic phase of the disease, resulting in biphasic Paget's disease (*B*).

With the biphasic form of Paget's disease there is thickening of the skull with widening of the diploic space. This process preferentially involves the outer table and diploë, but, less frequently, the inner table also may be involved. The calvarium becomes involved with rounded areas of increased and decreased density in a patchy distribution described as the "cotton-wool" appearance.

The incidence of bony metastases to the calvaria is decreased in the presence of Paget's disease. For a long time this was felt to be caused by rapid blood flow with arteriovenous shunting. However, it has been shown recently that A-V shunting does *not* take place in Paget's disease, and the reason for the decreased incidence of metastases is unknown.

An increased incidence of osteogenic sarcoma is associated with Paget's disease of the bone.

C, As a result of softening of the base of the skull, basilar invagination (basilar impression) may develop. Note the upward tilting (*arrowheads*) of the medial ends of the petrous bones.

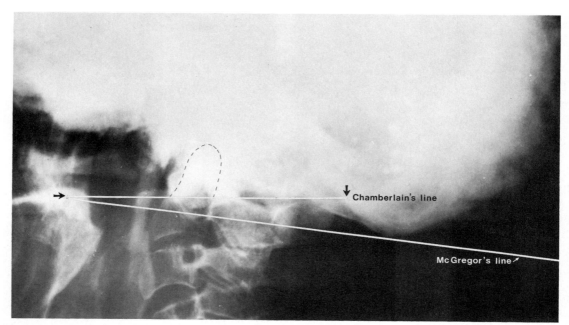

FIGURE 2–58. *Chamberlain's Line:* When a line connecting the posterior margin of the hard palate to the posterior margin of the foramen magnum is drawn, basilar impression is present if one half or more of the odontoid projects above this line. This upward displacement of the odontoid reflects elevation of the posterior portion of the base of the skull. Basilar impression can be seen with atlanto-occipital fusion, which is a congenital deformity, or with acquired conditions such as Paget's disease (as in this case), osteogenesis imperfecta, hyperparathyroidism, and osteomalacia. It reflects a softening and pliability of the bones of the base of the skull. Basilar impression may be present congenitally in patients with the Chiari malformation.

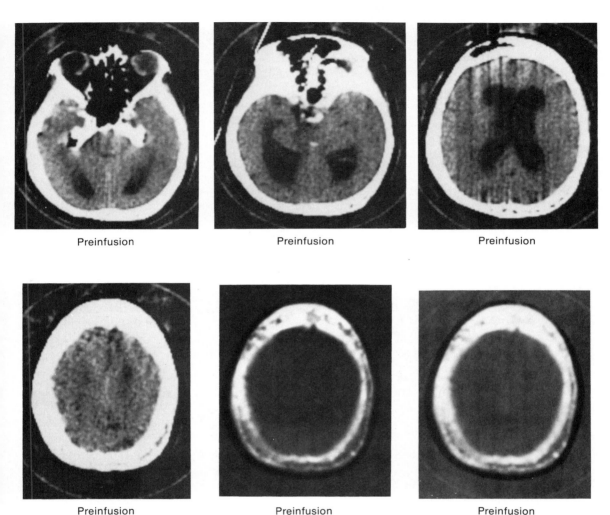

Preinfusion   Preinfusion   Preinfusion

Preinfusion   Preinfusion   Preinfusion

FIGURE 2–59. *Paget's Disease with Basilar Impression and Obstructive Hydrocephalus:* CT scans reveal that the petrous apices are displaced superiorly and are visualized on the same cut with the sella. Because they are pushed so high, the occipital horns of lateral ventricles are also seen on the same cut. There is thickening of the bony calvaria which involves mainly the outer table and the diploë but also compromises the inner table. The typical cotton-wool appearance is also apparent on CT scans at high window widths and window levels.

There is dilatation of the lateral ventricles because of the obstruction of the ventricular system which results when the basiocciput is elevated and the cerebral tonsils become impacted in the foramen magnum, thus preventing free flow of cerebrospinal fluid out of the foramina of Magendie and Luschka.

FIGURE 2–60. *Atlanto-occipital Fusion:* The atlas may fuse with the base of the skull. This results in upward displacement of the odontoid into the foramen magnum, causing basilar impression and compromise of the size of the foramen magnum.

There may be partial or complete fusion of the atlas. The anterior arch of C_1 becomes incorporated into the clivus. The lateral mass is fused to the base of the skull on either side of the foramen magnum, and the posterior arch of the atlas fuses to the squama of the occiput. Because the vertebral artery normally lies in a groove along the upper margin of C_1 before entering the foramen magnum, a separate foramen must be formed to allow the artery to enter the cranial vault.

Because of the narrowing of the spinal canal at the level of the foramen magnum, pressure may be exerted on the spinal cord and medulla. The patient may develop symptoms simulating multiple sclerosis, amyotrophic lateral sclerosis, syringomyelia, and other neurologic disorders.

A, The lateral view of the cervical spine reveals that C_1 is fused (*white arrow*) to the base of the skull, and the second cervical vertebra and the odontoid process are displaced superiorly. In addition, there is narrowing of the disk space at C_3–C_4, and degenerative changes are present. This is probably secondary in part to the abnormal relationship of C_1 to the base of the skull.

B, The midline lateral tomogram reveals that the odontoid process rests *above* the level of the foramen magnum, with its tip resting at the inferior margin of the medulla and markedly narrowing the foramen magnum (*arrow*).

C, The AP tomogram reveals that the lateral mass of C_1 is fused to the base of the skull and is actually incorporated into the base of the skull (*large arrowhead*). In addition, the foramen for the vertebral artery is also visible in this projection (*small arrow*).

D, A tomogram through the lateral masses of C_1 and C_2 reveals that C_1 is incorporated into the base of the skull, and the foramen (*open arrowhead*) for the vertebral artery is readily demonstrated. The degenerative changes are also seen at the C_3–C_4 level.

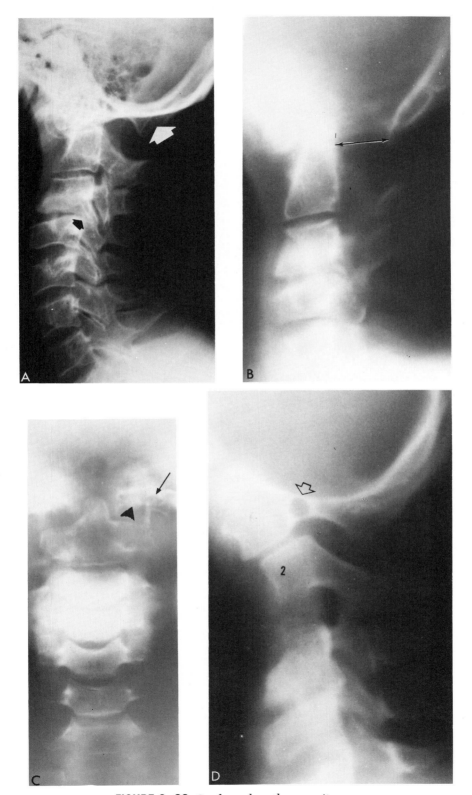

FIGURE 2–60. *See legend on the opposite page.*

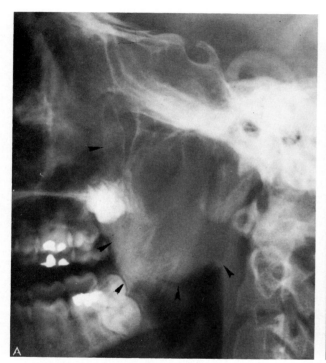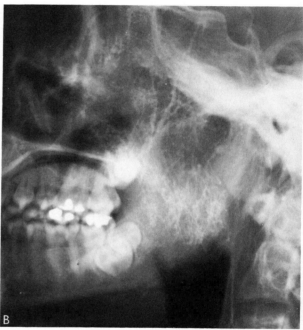

FIGURE 2–61. *Juvenile Angiofibroma:* These patients are almost always in the second decade of life; they present clinically with recurrent epistaxis; marked male predominance.

A, Radiographs demonstrate a soft tissue mass in the nasopharynx with marked forward bowing of the posterior wall of the maxillary sinus (*arrows*). The pterygomaxillary space is present only on the contralateral side; it has been destroyed on the side of the mass.

The blood supply is via the internal maxillary artery and its branches. The highly vascular mass frequently feeds from both external carotid arteries.

B, The lateral arterial film of a selective external carotid arteriogram reveals a markedly vascular tumor that fed primarily from the internal maxillary artery. This appearance is very typical.

A choanal polyp may have a similar soft tissue appearance on the plain radiographs but demonstrates only minimal vascularity with arteriography.

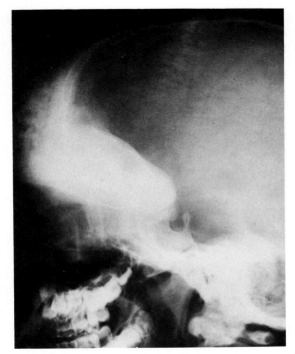

FIGURE 2–62. *Fibrous Dysplasia:* This entity may present in many forms. A purely sclerotic form frequently involves the orbits and the base of the skull (see illustration). The clinical picture is that of "lion-like facies" because of the involvement and thickening of the bony structures of the face. The extensive homogeneous increase in density is typical of fibrous dysplasia, although lesser degrees of involvement may be impossible to differentiate from the reactive sclerosis secondary to a meningioma. If other bones are involved, as in polyostotic fibrous dysplasia, differentiation from meningioma is easier.

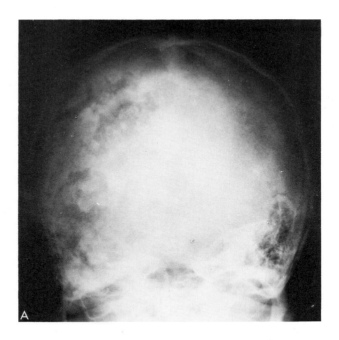

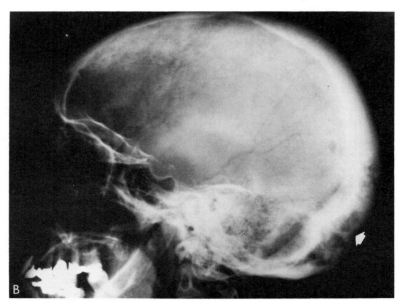

FIGURE 2–63. *Fibrous Dysplasia:* The mixed sclerotic and radiolucent type of fibrous dysplasia is more common in the cranial vault than in the long bones. This gives the "soap bubble" appearance typical of fibrous dysplasia. This type of fibrous dysplasia may be mistaken for Paget's disease.

Fibrous dysplasia can present a variety of appearances and perhaps should be mentioned in the differential diagnosis of any obscure skull lesion.

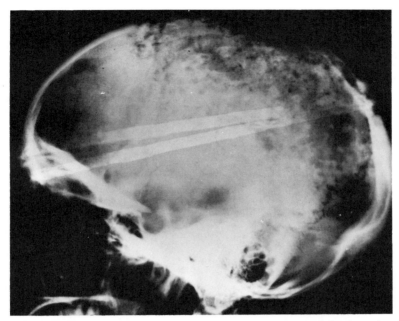

FIGURE 2–64. *Osteomyelitis:* The entire parietal bone as well as portions of the frontal and occipital bones is involved with a diffuse osteolytic process that presents as multiple lucent areas with poorly defined margins. A history of an infected scalp wound is frequently obtained in these patients. In addition, osteomyelitis can be seen following a severe frontal sinusitis.

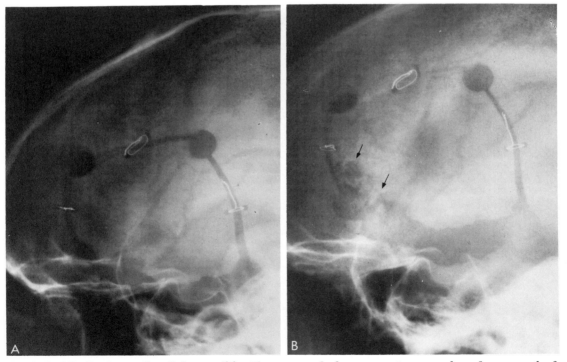

FIGURE 2–65. *Postoperative Osteomyelitis:* This patient had an operative procedure for removal of a sphenoid wing meningioma. *A,* Immediately postoperatively, the skull films reveal a craniotomy flap with well-defined margins. The patient developed a wound infection and the follow-up skull films six weeks later (*B*) reveal that the anterior inferior margin of the flap is now poorly defined. The bone on either side of the craniotomy line is also poorly defined and has a mottled appearance (*arrows*)—findings consistent with osteomyelitis. The skull films may not reveal the true extent of the bony involvement, and wide surgical excision is necessary to remove the affected bone.

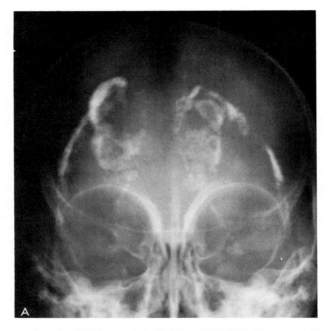

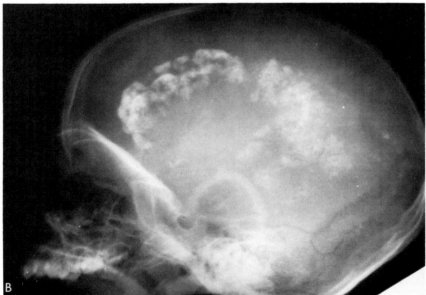

FIGURE 2–66. *See legend on the opposite page.*

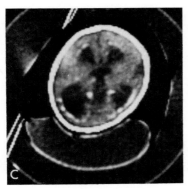
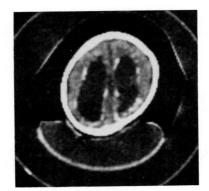

Preinfusion   Preinfusion

FIGURE 2–66. *Cytomegalic Inclusion Disease:* This disease is caused by a cytomegalovirus from the herpes family. The disease is often subclinical and may be acquired in utero. The skull films (*A* and *B*) reveal multiple intracranial periventricular calcifications. The infection results in destruction of the cerebral tissues and microcephaly secondary to loss of cerebral substance. It is associated with enlargement of the lateral ventricles.

The calcifications may be periventricular or may occur in any portion of the brain substance. Differentiation from toxoplasmosis by radiography is impossible. The CT scans (*C*) reveal multiple periventricular calcifications associated with microcephaly and ventricular dilatation. Both the microcephaly and the ventricular dilatation are secondary to loss of brain substance. (The skull films are courtesy of Drs. O. Sugar and G. Dobben.)

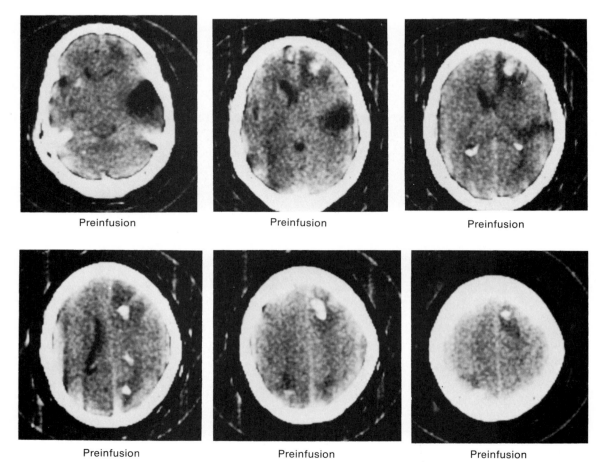

Preinfusion   Preinfusion   Preinfusion

Preinfusion   Preinfusion   Preinfusion

FIGURE 2–67. *Cysticercosis:* This disease results from the ingestion of eggs of the pork tapeworm, *Taenia solium.* The larvae become encysted in muscles and brain and cause multiple areas of calcification. The pig is the usual host, with man the intermediate host following ingestion of poorly cooked pork. However, when sanitation is poor, man becomes the primary host.

Skull films (not illustrated) show multiple small scattered intracranial calcifications. The CT scans reveal similar findings. In this case the areas of calcification are surrounded by edema. There is also a cystic lesion in the right temporal region.

Diagnosis rests on a strong clinical history or tissue diagnosis. The disease is prevalent in Latin America, Mexico, and the West Indies.

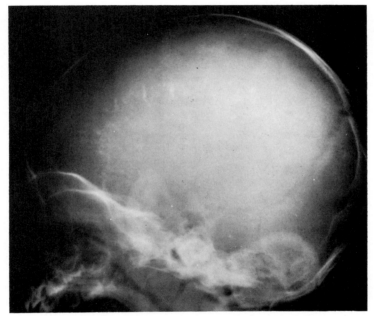

FIGURE 2–68. *Toxoplasmosis:* This encephalitis is secondary to a protozoan infestation seen in utero or in early life. Radiographs reveal calcifications scattered throughout the parenchyma; these form within areas of necrosis and granuloma formation. The radiologic appearance cannot be differentiated from that of cytomegalic inclusion disease. The calcifications may be periventricular in distribution, as demonstrated in this case. Because of brain destruction there is associated microcephaly and enlargement of the lateral ventricles.

The CT scan (not shown) readily demonstrates these areas of calcification.

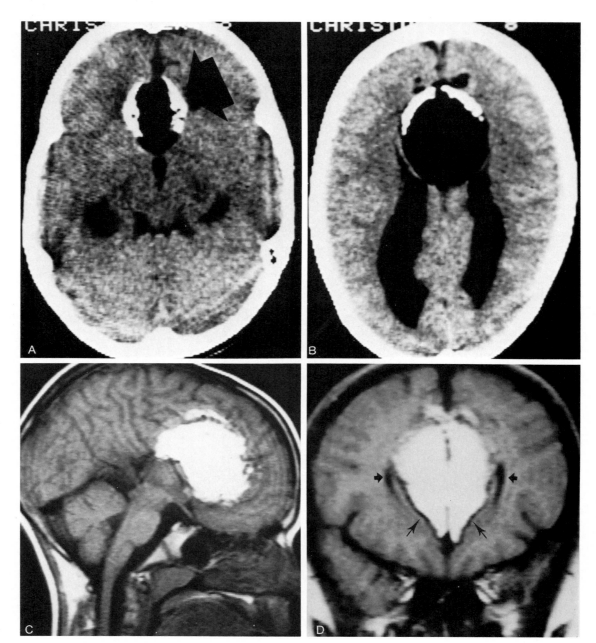

FIGURE 2–69. *CT and MR of Lipoma of the Corpus Callosum:* *A* and *B*, CT scans demonstrate a low-density mass in the midline in the region of the corpus calllosum. The mass measures approximately −50 Hounsfield units. There is peripheral calcification of the lipoma, not an uncommon finding (*arrow*). The frontal horns of the lateral ventricles are splayed apart, and there is often an associated partial agenesis of the corpus callosum. There are several smaller lipomas projecting anterior to the calcification on *B* that appear as low-density areas.

C, Midsagittal TR530/TE30 SE image demonstrates the very large lipoma of the corpus callosum with the typical high signal intensity of fat on the T-1 weighted image. The lipoma is irregularly marginated and is surrounded by multiple small lipomas.

D, Coronal TR530/TE30 SE image demonstrates the lipoma, the multiple smaller lipomas that project superior to it, and the laterally splayed frontal horns of the lateral ventricles (*arrowheads*). The peripherally calcified areas are only faintly demonstrated by MR (*long arrows*). Note that the fat in the subcutaneous tissue and in the marrow of the clivus is similar in signal intensity.

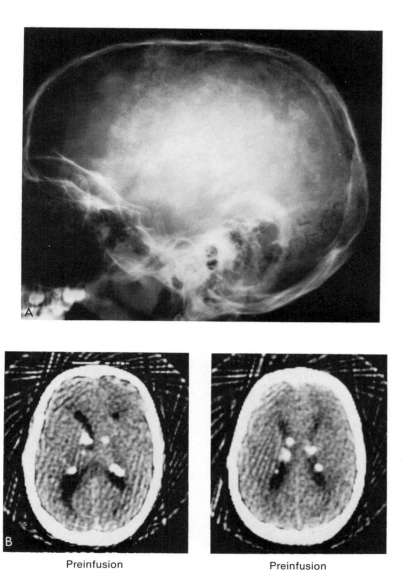

Preinfusion   Preinfusion

FIGURE 2—70. *Tuberous Sclerosis* (Bourneville's disease): Skull films demonstrate multiple scattered calcifications in a periventricular distribution. Scattered random intracranial calcifications also may occur. The subependymal periventricular calcifications are associated with giant glial cells and subependymal astrocytomas, which frequently degenerate into glioblastomas. The calcifications usually appear after two years of age.

Localized areas of increased or decreased density also occur in the bony calvaria in a large percentage of cases, and differentiation from intracranial calcification may be difficult (A). Computed tomography (B) readily demonstrates the periventricular areas of calcification, and many degenerate into gliomas.

Cystic changes may occur in the hand; hamartomas (angiomyolipomas) may be present in the kidneys. Hamartomas also may occur in the liver.

The clinical syndrome is that of mental retardation, seizures, and sebaceous adenomas of the face with a "butterfly" distribution.

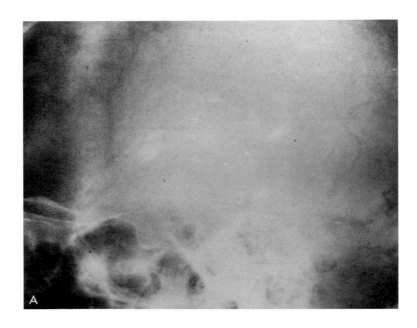

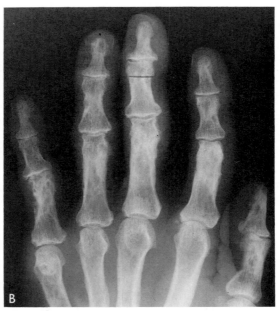

FIGURE 2–71. *A*, The lateral view of a patient with tuberous sclerosis reveals multiple intracranial calcifications in a periventricular distribution.

B, Multiple small cystic lesions are scattered throughout the phalanges.

Illustration continued on the opposite page

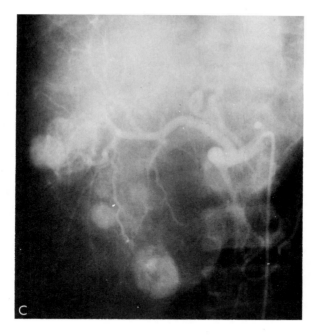

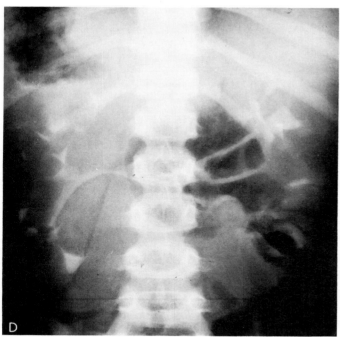

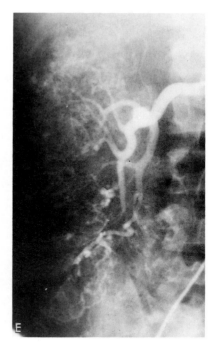

FIGURE 2–71 *Continued.*

C, The selective hepatic arteriogram demonstrates hepatomegaly with multiple hypervascular, nodular hamartomas of the liver.

D, The intravenous pyelogram reveals marked enlargement of the kidney bilaterally. The calices are distorted and splayed apart. The infundibula are elongated.

E, The renal arteriogram demonstrates intrinsically abnormal blood vessels supplying multiple vascular hamartomas throughout the greatly enlarged kidney.

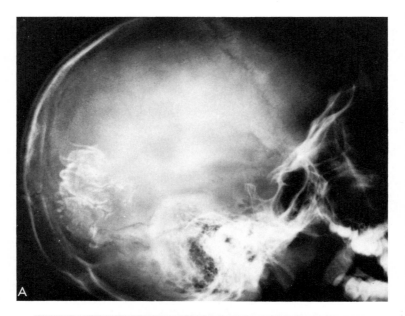

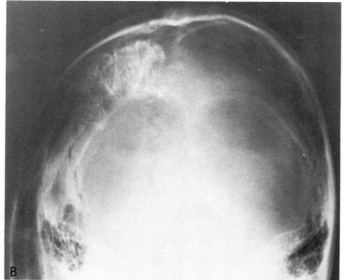

FIGURE 2–72. *Sturge-Weber Syndrome:* This entity is one of the neurocutaneous syndromes, which include von Recklinghausen's disease (neurofibromatosis), tuberous sclerosis, von Hippel-Lindau's disease, Sturge-Weber syndrome, and ataxia-telangiectasia.

Sturge-Weber is associated with a hemangioma in the ophthalmic distribution of the fifth cranial nerve, mental retardation, hemiatrophy of the skull on the same side as the facial hemangioma, and intracranial calcification—usually in the occipital region and also on the same side. The calcifications are in a venous angioma of the brain and usually are described as railroad-track calcifications because the curvilinear lines are paired and run parallel to one another.

The hemiatrophy (*A* and *B*) is characterized by a sloping hemicranium and elevation of the petrous bone and greater wing of the sphenoid bone, enlargement of the frontal sinus on the side of the atrophy, and tilting of the crista galli toward the atrophic side. The hemiatrophy picture was originally described by Davidoff and Dyke in patients with chronic relapsing subtemporal hematomas.

The CT scans (*C*) in the same patient demonstrate the asymmetry of the cranial vault, with fattening of the posterior portion of the hemicranium. Curvilinear areas of calcification deep in the substance of the brain correspond to the plain skull findings.

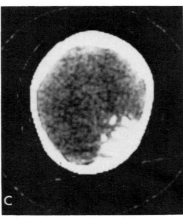

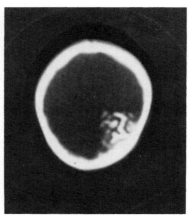

Preinfusion   Preinfusion

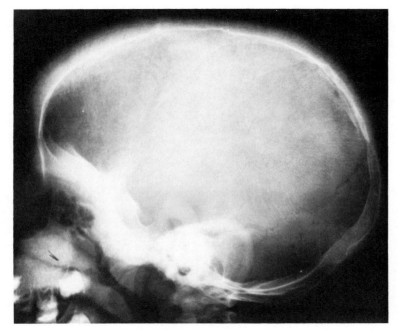

FIGURE 2–73. *Thalassemia:* The appearance is similar to that of sickle cell disease, with expansion of the diploic space and a "hair-on-end" appearance of the bony spicules. With thalassemia, however, there may be involvement of the maxillary sinuses and mastoid regions with hematopoiesis—not seen in sickle cell anemia.

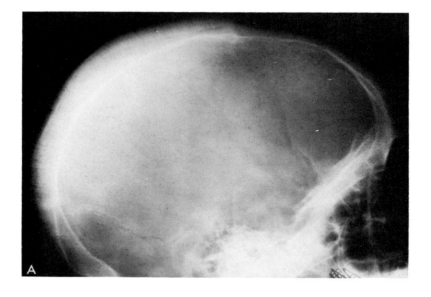

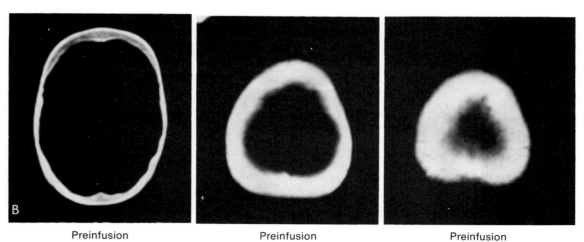

Preinfusion Preinfusion Preinfusion

FIGURE 2–74. *Sickle Cell Anemia:* *A,* Because of hyperplasia of the bone marrow, there is expansion of the diploic space. The spicules of bone are arranged in a radial pattern perpendicular to the inner table—apparently in an attempt to support the diploic space and outer table, which are weakened and thinned.

B, These changes are also apparent on CT scans of the bony calvaria.

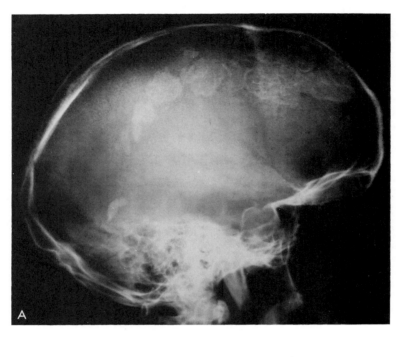

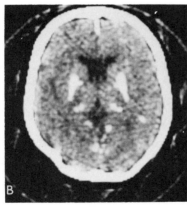
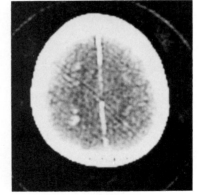

Preinfusion   Preinfusion

FIGURE 2–75. *Secondary Hyperparathyroidism:* The plain skull lateral view (A) demonstrates diffuse deossification of the bony calvaria. In addition, there is extensive calcification of the falx cerebri and tentorium cerebelli.

The CT scan (B) also demonstrates the falx and tentorial calcification. In addition, extensive calcification of the basal ganglia and thalamus is seen which is not visible on the plain films. The calcium deposition is typical of *secondary* hyperparathyroidism.

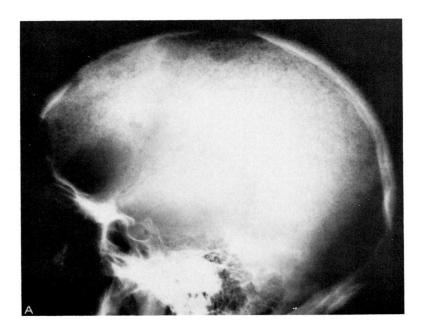

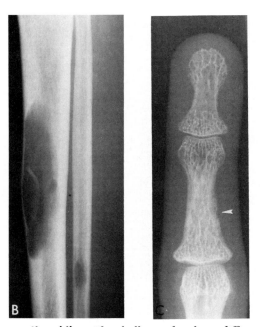

FIGURE 2–76. *Primary Hyperparathyroidism:* The skull may develop a diffuse granular (*A*) "salt and pepper" appearance becase of a combination of bone production and destruction. In addition, cystic brown tumors may also involve the bony calvaria. Demonstration of brown tumors in the long bones (*B*) and subperiosteal bony resorption along the radial side of the phalanges (*C*) also substantiate the diagnosis of hyperparathyroidism. The changes in this patient are secondary to a functioning parathyroid adenoma. Laboratory data are necessary for complete evaluation.

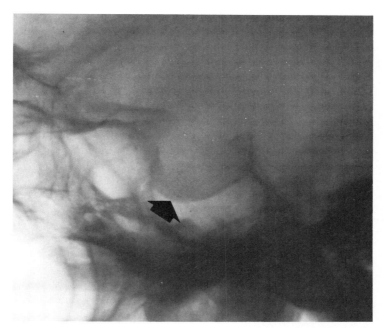

FIGURE 2–77. *Demineralization of the Dorsum Sellae Secondary to Increased Intracranial Pressure:* There is marked demineralization of the floor of the sella, especially in its anterior, inferior margin (*arrow*). The sella is also minimally expanded.

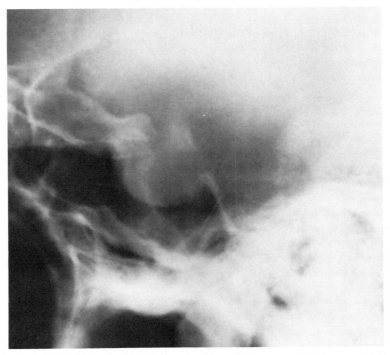

FIGURE 2–78. *Marked Sella Changes Secondary to Chronic Increased Intracranial Pressure:* There is almost complete dissolution of the floor of the sella; the dorsum sellae is truncated, and the posterior clinoids are markedly demineralized and almost completely destroyed. These changes are secondary to an enlarged, dilated third ventricle protruding into the sella. (Case courtesy of Dr. Gregory I. Shenk; see also Chapter 10.)

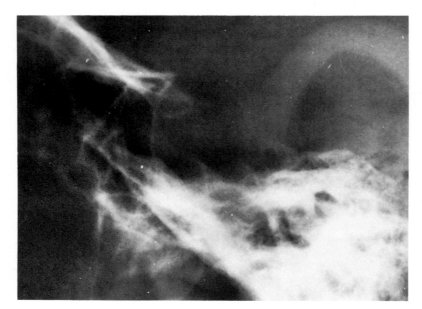

FIGURE 2–79. *Pituitary Adenoma:* The sella is greatly enlarged, and there is destruction of the dorsum sellae and posterior clinoids. There is "undercutting" of the anterior clinoids, which also demonstrate a pointed appearance secondary to the expansion of an intrasellar adenoma—in this case a chromophobe adenoma.

FIGURE 2–80. *Acromegaly* (Eosinophilic adenoma): In acromegaly there may or may not be enlargement of the sella turcica secondary to an eosinophilic tumor of the pituitary. There may be a diffuse increase in calvarial thickness, or the process may be confined to the frontal region—as opposed to hyperostosis frontalis interna, which spares the midline. This hyperostosis crosses the midline. One may also detect enlargement of the frontal sinuses and of the external occipital protuberance, and an increase in the angle of the jaw, with prognathism and enlarged spaces between the teeth. This case demonstrates all these findings; in addition, there is an increase in the degenerative changes in the spine—a finding also seen with acromegaly. Other changes that may be detected include enlargement of the ungual tufts of the fingers and accentuation of the dorsal kyphosis of the spine.

In the younger age groups, excess secretion of growth hormone results in pituitary gigantism.

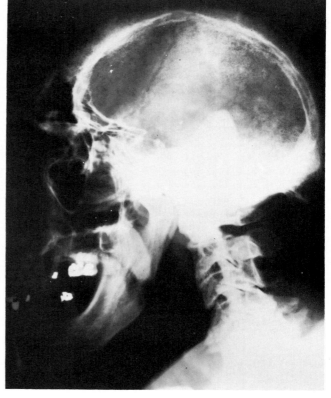

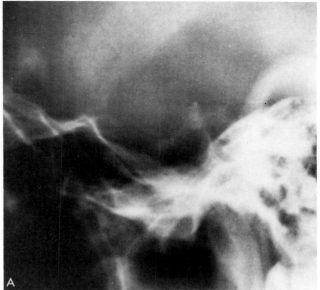

FIGURE 2–81. *Enlarged Sella Secondary to Dilated Third Ventricle: A,* The sella is greatly enlarged, especially in its posterior inferior portion, and is markedly demineralized throughout. The dorsum sellae is thinned and displaced posteriorly.

B, The contrast ventriculogram demonstrates dilatation of the lateral and third ventricles and obstruction of the dilated aqueduct (*arrowhead*). The dilated third ventricle exactly conforms to the abnormal shape of the sella.

This patient was an adult with adult aqueduct obstruction.

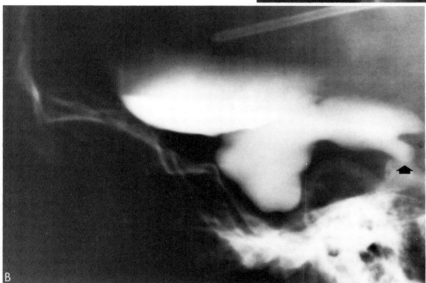

FIGURE 2–81 *Continued.*

C, Midsagittal MR TR530/TE30 SE image demonstrates the occluded aqueduct with the dilated proximal portion (*arrow*). The third ventricle is greatly dilated, and the optic chiasm and optic tracts are stretched and displaced anteriorly. The sella turcica is enlarged. The appearance is remarkably similar to that of a different patient illustrated in *B.* The advantage of MR in cases such as this is obvious. The diagnosis is readily made without the use of ventricular needles or catheters and without the use of contrast material. (Case courtesy of Drs. L. Berlin and G. Novetsky. Reprinted from the Journal of Computerized Axial Tomography, Vol. 18, No. 6, 1984.)

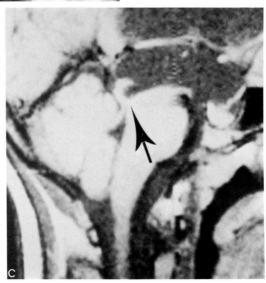

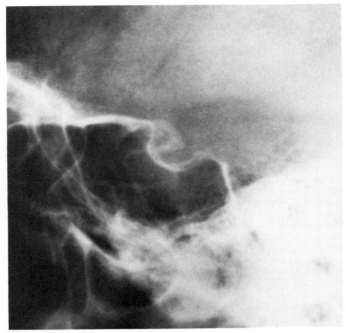

FIGURE 2–82. *Amputation of Dorsum Sellae:* Because of the nonspecific changes of chronic increased intracranial pressure, there is total amputation of the dorsum sellae and the posterior clinoid processes. Note that the size of the sella is otherwise unchanged in this example.

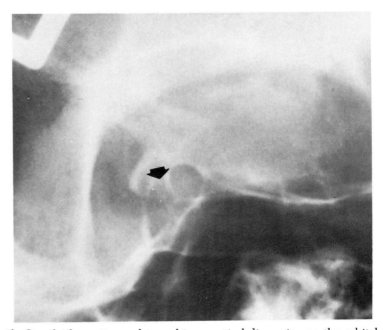

FIGURE 2–83. *Optic Canal:* The optic canal is oval in a vertical dimension on the orbital side, round in the midportion, and oval in a horizontal dimension on the brain side. The optic canals should never exceed 7 mm in diameter. The maximum difference between the two sides should not exceed 2 mm. The "sphenoid strut" (*arrowhead*) separates the optic canal from the superior orbital fissure.

The optic canal may be enlarged by such processes as an optic glioma or chronic increased intracranial pressure or decreased in size secondary to optic atrophy or encroachment by osteopetrosis.

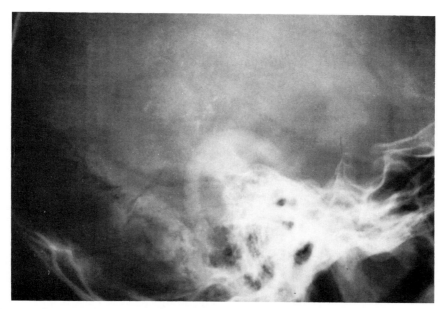

FIGURE 2–84. *Calcified Arteriovenous Malformation:* Multiple small speckled areas of calcifications project superior and posterior to the mastoid air cells. Curvilinear areas of arterial or venous calcification also may be seen.

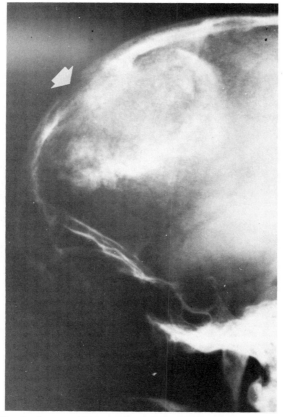

FIGURE 2–85. *Calcified Meningioma with Invasion of the Calvaria:* There is invasion of the frontal bone at the point of attachment of the meningioma, without evidence of reactive bone formation. This bony invasion occurs in a small percentage of cases. (Case courtesy of Drs. O. Sugar and G. Dobben.)

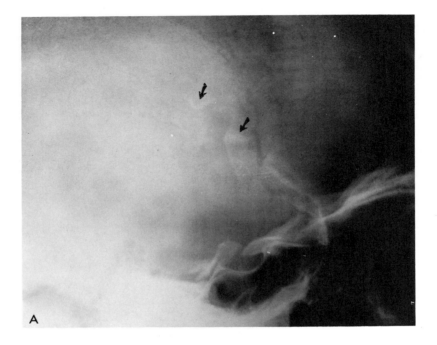

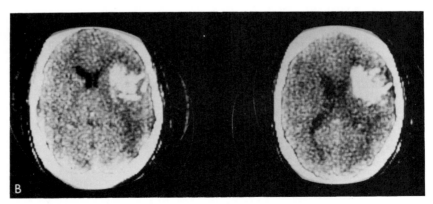

FIGURE 2–86. *Oligodendroglioma: A,* The plain film shows multiple curvilinear areas of calcification (*arrows*); a 3-mm shift of the pineal gland to the contralateral side also was present. The CT scan (*B*) demonstrates extensive areas of apparent dense calcification deep in the right hemisphere, associated with moderate compression of the frontal horn of the right lateral ventricle. A postinfusion scan was not performed. This is a surgically proved oligodendroglioma. (Skull film courtesy of the Carle Clinic Radiology Group.)

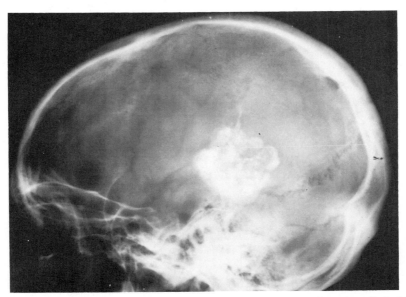

FIGURE 2–87. *Oligodendroglioma:* The plain skull demonstrates a large, densely calcified lobulated mass. This is a spectacular case of a calcified oligodendroglioma. The pneumoencephalogram also demonstrated a cystic component to the tumor. This case was studied before the discovery of CT scanning; however, the CT scan would have beautifully demonstrated both the calcified and cystic components of the tumor.

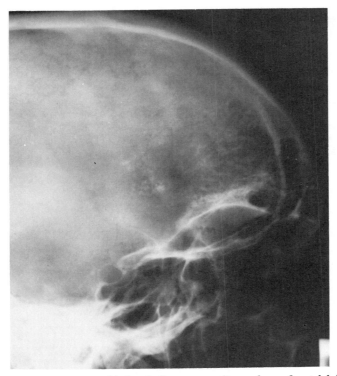

FIGURE 2–88. *Astrocytoma:* Small, speckled calcifications outline a large frontal lobe astrocytoma. It has been stated that as many as 20 per cent of astrocytomas demonstrate calcifications that are visible on plain skull films. However, since the development of new diagnostic techniques, it appears that only a very small percentage of astrocytomas contain radiographically visible calcification. Indeed, we only occasionally see a calcified astrocytoma on CT scans.

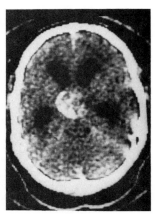

postinfusion

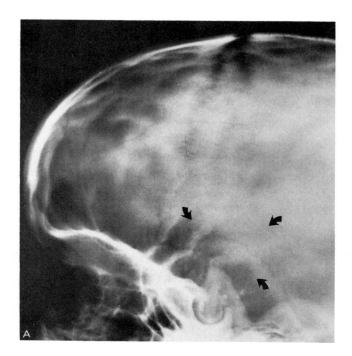

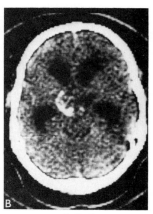

preinfusion

FIGURE 2–89. *Craniopharyngioma:* Craniopharyngiomas arise in the suprasellar area from remnants of Rathke's pouch, producing an enlargement of the sella with their intrasellar extension. There are two age group peaks for craniopharyngiomas. The lower age group ranges through the first three decades; the second is patients over the age of 50. In the younger group, approximately 60 per cent of the tumors are calcified; in the older group, only 20 per cent are calcified. These tumors are often cystic, calcifying around the periphery of the tumor (A). The calcification may not outline the entire tumor mass. These calcifications are often apparent on plain skull examination but are much more readily apparent on the CT scan. They may be scattered and punctate or curvilinear in configuration. Note widened coronal suture.

In the case shown, the full extent of the suprasellar calcification cannot be appreciated, but the process extends into the suprasellar cistern. The pituitary gland demonstrates extensive peripheral calcifications.

Hypervascularity of the tumor may not be apparent on the arteriogram but will be readily visualized on the CT scan (B) as a rim of enhancement that outlines the tumor to best advantage.

The craniopharyngiomas may not calcify at all. If this is the case, there will be simply a cystic mass in the suprasellar cistern that extends into the sella. The fluid within the cyst is of higher density than cerebrospinal fluid and reflects the fluid that has been described as "crank-case oil" when surgically removed. These craniopharyngiomas may enlarge sufficiently to produce hydrocephalus secondary to obstruction at the level of the foramen of Monro.

It should be noted that, if hydrocephalus of this type is present, it may be necessary to shunt both ventricles so that the decompression of one ventricle does not lead to herniation of the opposite ventricle under the falx cerebri secondary to the ventricle's behaving as a mass lesion.

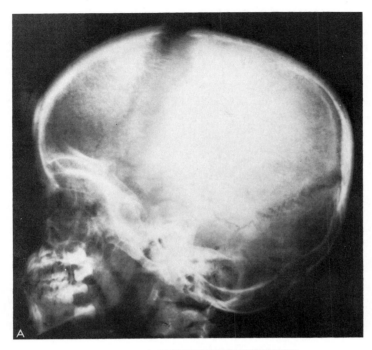

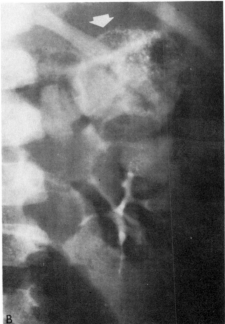

FIGURE 2–90. *Neuroblastoma:* A, The skull film demonstrates scattered areas of lucency throughout the calvaria secondary to osteolytic metastatic deposits of neuroblastoma in the calvarial bones. In addition, there is wide separation of the coronal suture because of spread of the tumor cells into the meninges.

B, The intravenous pyelogram reveals a left suprarenal mass that is rounded and contains diffuse areas of calcification. The left kidney is displaced inferiorly. This is a primary neuroblastoma arising in the left adrenal gland. (Case courtesy of Dr. John Fennessy.)

Metastatic leukemic infiltrates may produce changes in the skull similar to those seen with neuroblastoma.

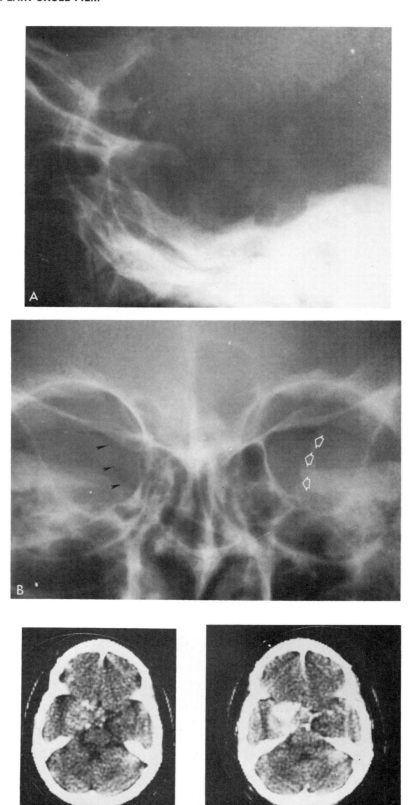

FIGURE 2–91. *See legend on the opposite page.*

FIGURE 2–91. *Aneurysm:* Giant aneurysms are described as those greater than 2.5 cm in size.

Aneurysm of the cavernous portion of the internal carotid artery may cause unilateral sellar enlargement if the aneurysm reaches a sufficient size. Most commonly, the changes in the sella will be unilateral and will consist of erosion of the anterior clinoid process and dorsum sellae and floor of the sella on the side of the aneurysm (A). In addition, there may be an associated curvilinear calcification adjacent to the sella, which substantiates the diagnosis of a vascular mass. Besides the changes in the sella, there may be erosion of the superior orbital fissure secondary to mass effect and pressure erosion of the aneurysm (B). Tomograms of the sella will help to confirm the configuration of the sellar erosion; in addition they may reveal areas of curvilinear calcification not apparent on the plain films.

The CT scans (C) of these large aneurysms have rather characteristic appearances. The preinfusion scan reveals a large area of increased density in the parasellar area. These large aneurysms may also have areas of calcification in their walls; these are readily apparent on the CT scan. After infusion of contrast material there will be enhancement of all or a portion of the aneurysm. The area of enhancement will vary with the size of the aneurysm; also, it should be noted that frequently there is only a small area of enhancement because the rest of the aneurysm is filled with clotted blood.

The increased density on the preinfusion scan is secondary to both flowing and clotted blood in the aneurysm. In fact, the pattern of enhancement may be somewhat unusual because of this fact. At times, one may mistakenly think of other pathologic entities, e.g., parasellar meningiomas, because of the high density on the preinfusion scan and the marked and often homogeneous enhancement. It would appear that a correct diagnosis is not always possible in these cases, but the possibility of an aneurysm should be strongly suggested—especially since the wall of the aneurysm tends to calcify, resulting in peripheral calcification rather than homogeneous calcification. Arteriography will, of course, be necessary to confirm the diagnosis and also to evaluate the full extent of the disease.

Clinically, these giant aneurysms often present as a partial or complete "cavernous sinus syndrome" with involvement of cranial nerves II, III, IV, V, and VI. Patients will complain of the gradual progression of blindness and varying degrees of extraocular muscle paralysis. There may also be retro-orbital pain with these large aneurysms. (Case courtesy of Dr. John Fennessy.)

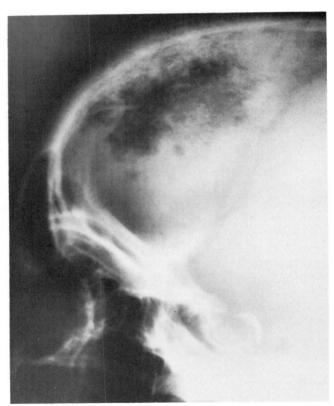

FIGURE 2–92. This patient demonstrates a large, poorly marginated osteolytic metastatic deposit in the frontal bone. The patient is known to have breast cancer.

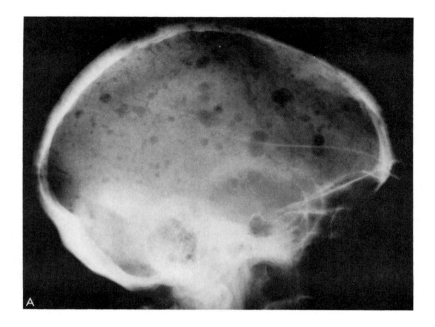

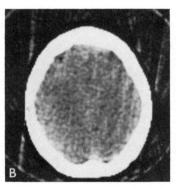
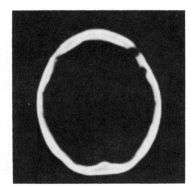

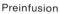
Preinfusion   Preinfusion

FIGURE 2–93. *Multiple Myeloma:* The skull lesions seen with multiple myeloma (A) are scattered radiolucent areas with poorly defined margins that give the appearance of "droplets of oil on brown paper." Absolute differentiation from mulitple metastases is impossible, and diagnosis rests on results of laboratory data.

Multiple myeloma may involve the mandible, whereas other types of metastases rarely do. This finding may help in differential diagnosis.

CT scans of the head (B) reveal that the bony calvaria appears to be normal at standard window widths and window levels, whereas on higher window widths and levels the metastatic lesions can readily be identified in the diploë of the skull. It is important to view the CT scan of the skull on high window width and window levels whenever bony metastases are suspected.

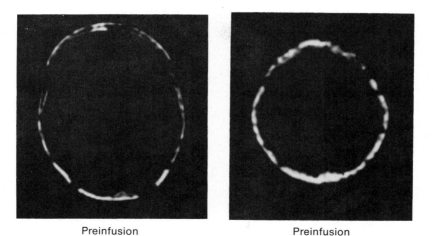

Preinfusion   Preinfusion

FIGURE 2–94. *CT Scan of Multiple Myeloma:* The CT scan of the bony calvaria, using high window widths and window levels, reveals innumerable osteolytic metastatic deposits throughout the calvaria secondary to multiple myeloma.

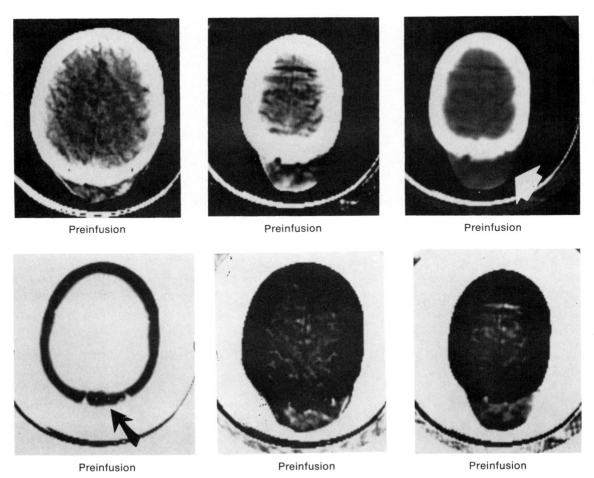

Preinfusion   Preinfusion   Preinfusion

Preinfusion   Preinfusion   Preinfusion

FIGURE 2–95. *Soft Tissue Metastasis with Minimal Bony Involvement:* The CT scans reveal a large extracranial soft tissue mass in the occipital region. Alteration of the window width and window level allows the invasion of the bony calvaria beneath the soft tissue metastasis to be seen to better advantage (*arrows*). The patient had a primary lung cancer.

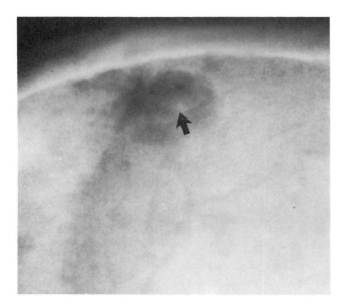

FIGURE 2–96. Target Lesion, Metastatic Breast Carcinoma: In the center of this osteolytic metastatic disease process there is an area of increased bone density (*arrow*). The appearance is that of a target—hence the name "target lesions" of the skull. This appearance is most common with metastatic breast carcinoma that has been treated and is in the healing phase. A similar phenomenon can be seen with healing eosinophilic granuloma and other less common disease processes.

FIGURE 2–97. Osteolytic Metastases Involving the Bony Calvaria and the Sella Turcica: *A*, The lateral radiograph of the skull reveals several rounded metastatic deposits in the frontal area of the bony calvaria. In addition, there is massive bone destruction involving the entire base of the skull surrounding the sella turcica.

B, The two low cuts of the CT scan through the region of the sella turcica reveal a large area of bone destruction. The entire sphenoid sinus is destroyed by the metastatic tumor, and there is encroachment on the ethmoid sinuses, the anterior clinoid processes, and the clivus and petrous apices, both of which are amputated. The CT scan demonstrates beautifully the exact extent of involvement of the bony structures. (Case courtesy of Dr. David Neer.)

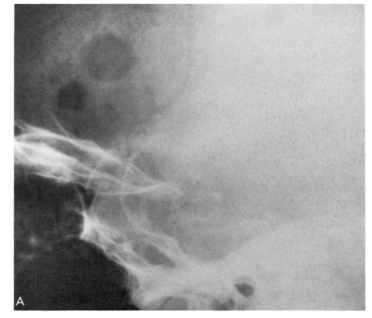

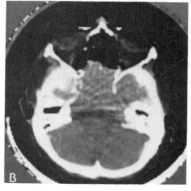

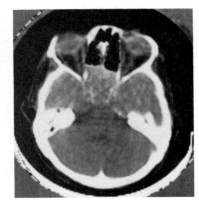

Preinfusion   Preinfusion

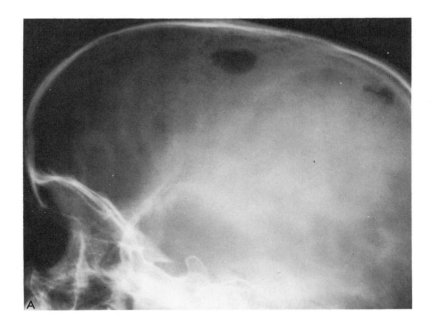

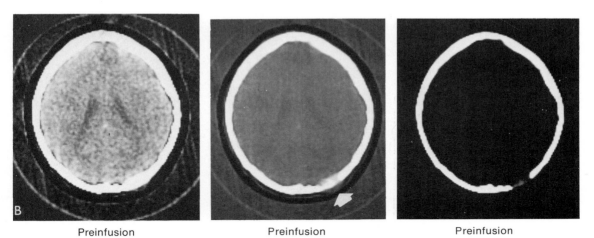

Preinfusion   Preinfusion   Preinfusion

FIGURE 2–98. *Eosinophilic Granuloma:* The skull lesion (*A*) is an area of lucent destructive change with a clear, slightly irregular border. In the healing phase, a sclerotic border may develop. The granulomas often are solitary but may be multiple and may present as part of a syndrome of histiocytosis. These lesions may be seen in adults but are more common in young individuals.

The lesions respond well to radiation therapy and may develop a "target" appearance.

B, CT scans of another patient reveal a well-defined area of bony destructive change associated with a small soft tissue component (*arrowhead*). Note that on the standard viewing levels the bony involvement cannot be readily appreciated. It could have been overlooked if views at higher window widths and levels had not also been obtained.

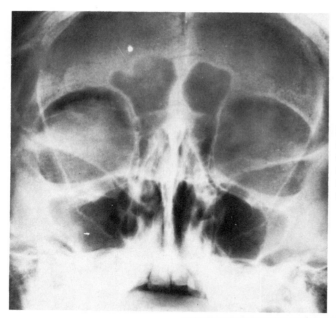

FIGURE 2–99. *Traumatic Orbital Emphysema:* The bony defect in the lamina papyracea cannot be seen with this medial wall blowout fracture; however, its presence can be suspected when the air is identified around the globe of the right eye.

FIGURE 2–100. *Air Under Eyelids:* In patients with deepset globes, air may be trapped over the lid, giving a false impression of orbital emphysema. This change is usually bilateral, which aids in differentiation from orbital emphysema, which usually is unilateral.

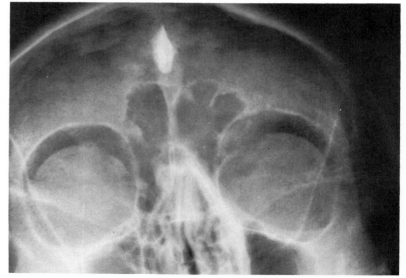

FIGURE 2–101. *Calcified Subdural Hematoma:* A chronic subdural hematoma may be suspected when plain film radiography demonstrates a shift of the pineal gland. An appropriate history may or may not be available in these patients.

These extracerebral accumulations of blood may very rarely calcify. At times, differentiation by plain skull examination from the reactive bone formation secondary to meningioma may be difficult.

A, The plain skull films in this patient demonstrate a well-defined calcified lentiform mass adjacent to the inner table in the left frontal region (*arrows*). This was proved surgically to be a chronic subdural hematoma that had calcified.

B, The CT scans demonstrate a large, chronic calcified subdural hematoma in the right temporal and parietal areas. The preinfusion scan reveals a low-density lentiform accumulation with central and peripheral calcification. There is marked shift of the midline from right to left. An engorged straight sinus and vein of Galen appear posteriorly on the lowest cut, and these can be seen to enhance on the postinfusion scan. The patient developed the subdural accumulation following the placement of a shunt tubing device in the left lateral ventricle. There is also marked enhancement of the membrane of the subdural hematoma on the postinfusion scan.

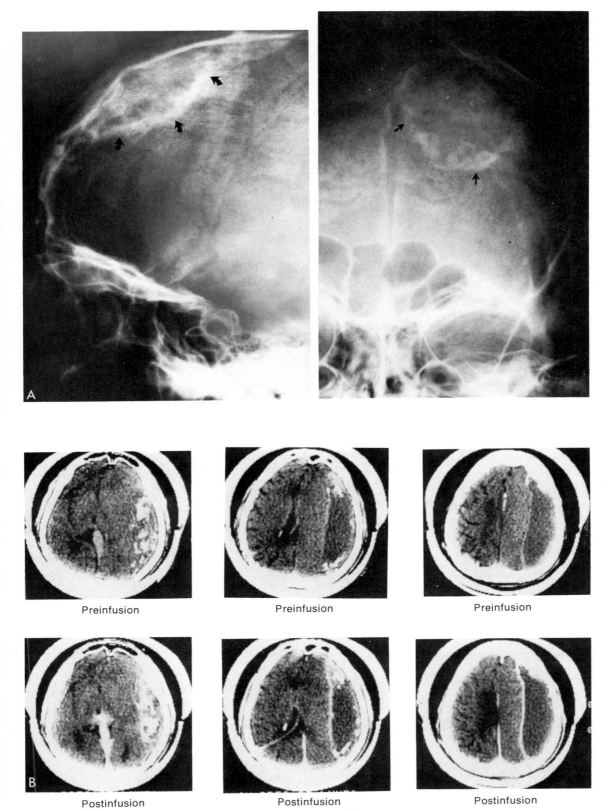

Preinfusion   Preinfusion   Preinfusion

Postinfusion   Postinfusion   Postinfusion

FIGURE 2–101. *See legend on the opposite page.*

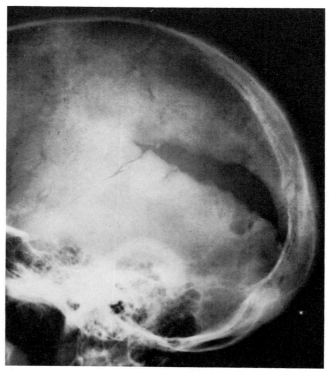

FIGURE 2–102. *Leptomeningeal Cyst:* Leptomeningeal cysts may occur following a linear skull fracture. If the leptomeninges protrude through an associated tear in the dura and are trapped in the linear skull fracture, the continued transmitted pulsations of heart beat and respiration may result in gradual smoothing and expansion of the fracture line—a leptomeningeal cyst. This cyst may be associated with a palpable soft tissue mass. Underlying brain damage may also be present in these cases.

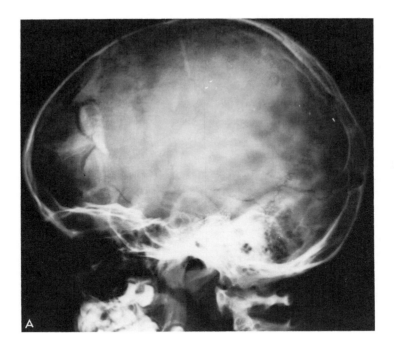

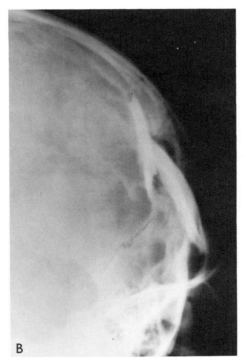

FIGURE 2–103. *Depressed Skull Fracture:* Following a direct blow to the frontal region, this patient developed a depressed comminuted fracture of the skull (A). The amount of depression is best demonstrated on the tangential view (B) (see also Chapter 11). These depressed skull fractures are readily demonstrated on CT scans.

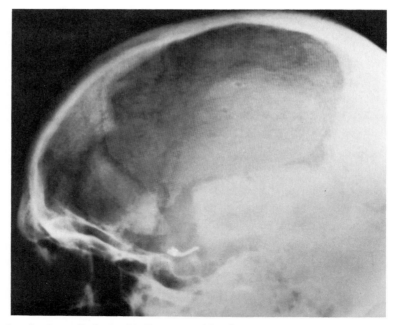

FIGURE 2–104. *Craniectomy Defect with Tantalum Wire in Place:* Because of osteomyelitis involving the bony flap, the entire flap was removed and replaced with tantalum wire mesh. This wire has a cross-hatch appearance similar to wire used for commercial purposes. The aneurysm clip is in place. Because these metallic devices interfere with CT scans they are rarely used today, and their use is strongly discouraged. Insertion of solid metallic plates is also discouraged. Magnetic resonance of patients with aneurysm clips is not possible because studies have shown that the magnetic field may cause rotation of ferromagnetic clips. Obviously this could result in torsion of the clip off of the neck of the aneurysm.

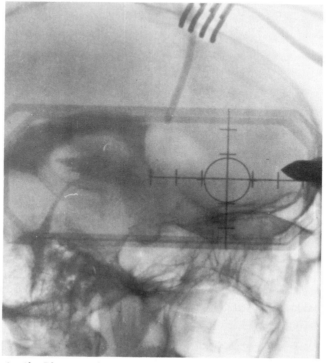

FIGURE 2–105. *Stereotactic Biopsy using X-ray Control:* A metallic device holds the patient immobile. After an air and metrizamide ventriculogram, the biopsy is identified in two planes, and a small needle biopsy is made. The localizing device is projected over the frontal region on this view.

3

COMPUTED TOMOGRAPHY AND MAGNETIC RESONANCE

_____ Introduction and Normal Anatomy

COMPUTED TOMOGRAPHY

The technique of computed tomography (CT) was the concept of Mr. Godfrey Hounsfield, scientist, EMI Ltd., Middlesex, England. The technique was introduced into clinical practice in England in 1972, but its use has expanded rapidly since then. The CT scan is not a direct x-ray of the brain, but rather a mathematical reconstruction of the tissue densities of the brain. The method requires the use of a computer as well as sophisticated scanning equipment.

Since the development of the original instruments there have been significant advances in the field of CT scanners. The translate/rotate scanners have been modified so that scans can now be performed more rapidly, with a slice scanning time of less than 20 seconds. This, of course, has greatly enhanced our ability to obtain accurate scans, and now the scan can be done with less risk of patient-motion artifact. Further, the ability to scan faster has made it possible to examine a larger number of patients in the same amount of time.

The first scanners used a water bag that surrounded the patient's head and a thin x-ray beam with a single detector for each slice. Simply stated, in the first generation scanner, the x-ray tube moved back and forth on a rail at the side of the patient's head. Two hundred and forty density measurements were made during each traverse of the tube by detectors placed at the side of the patient's head opposite the x-ray tube. In the example shown in Figure 3–1 (p. 113), a "mass lesion" has been placed in the left hemisphere. Two sodium iodide crystal detectors, which are closely aligned with the x-ray tube, simultaneously record the finely collimated beam, resulting in two cuts per scan, with a thickness of 1.3 cm per cut. After each traverse the scanning device rotates 1 degree until the unit has rotated 180 degrees; at the completion of 180 degrees of rotation the unit pauses, and in 30 seconds the computer solves 43,200 equations of the tissue density measurements. The scan itself takes 4½ minutes. The result is a 160 × 160 dot matrix of tissue absorption density measurements of the brain, the skull, and the surrounding water bag. The A and B cuts of each level are obtained simultaneously with each 180-degree rotation of the unit. The dot matrix is made up of 25,600 points, each of which represents a column of tissue 13 mm tall and 1.5 × 1.5 mm square. The information is presented in three different ways—on the cathode x-ray tube, where density measurements can be made; on an x-ray, which can be used for permanent reference; and on the number print-out sheet.

Second-generation scanners are based on the same principle as the original water-bag scanners, but eliminate the water-bag and replace it with a bolus that surrounds the patient's head with a material that approximates more closely the density of the intracranial contents. These scanners also use a fan beam x-ray source and multiple detectors.

Third-generation scanners are based on the rotation of both the tube and the detector or detectors around the patient's head. These scanners are exceptionally fast—some requiring less than 5 seconds of actual scanning time. Fourth-generation scanners use a moving source but multiple stationary detectors.

The matrix size varies from manufacturer to manufacturer; the initial 80 × 80 dot matrix has now increased to a matrix as large as 512 × 512 dots. There is a trade-off with increasing matrix size because more time is necessary to present the larger computed density matrix for viewing.

Figure 3–2 (p. 114) demonstrates a routine "topogram" with the scan slices superimposed upon the skull. Each numbered slice is also annotated on the scan image so that the levels of the various anatomic structures or abnormalities can be easily identified. With the Siemens Somotome II and the Siemens DR 3, each slice is 8 mm thick for a routine examination. Slices can also be routinely obtained at 4-mm or 2-mm thickness. This "topogram" image is actually a digital radiograph and has a good contrast. The author suggests that this type of image be obtained on each patient, both for localization purposes and because metastatic disease is not uncommon in the bony calvaria and is easily appreciated on the topogram image.

Figure 3–3 (p. 114) demonstrates a typical topogram image of a patient who is having an examination of the orbit. The scan slices are 4 mm thick for the orbit scans rather than 8 mm thick for the routine brain scans. For better resolution the 4-mm thick slices can be overlapped by 2 mm. This latter technique also allows excellent quality coronal, sagittal, or oblique images to be generated using reconstruction techniques. Direct coronal images can also be obtained with the patient in the prone or supine position.

Computed tomography of the brain has revolutionized our approach to the diagnosis of intracranial abnormalities. The CT scan demonstrates such abnormalities with an exactness and precision that never before had been possible. The technique is noninvasive, provides better definition of the extent of intracranial lesions than other methods, and is especially useful in defining midline lesions and abnormalities of the posterior fossa. With proper training, the CT scan is easily performed, with essentially no discomfort to the patient, and may be done on either an outpatient or inpatient basis.

The newer rapid speed scanners allow an entire examination—including both the pre- and postinfusion portions—to be done in less than 45 minutes in the cooperative patient. Furthermore, the newer scanners also allow for alterations in the standard positioning of the head, making it possible to obtain views in the coronal and other projections.

The author recommends a standard patient positioning for every new case, regardless of the clinical presentation, because the physical signs and the patient's symptoms frequently do not accurately reflect the position of the intracranial pathology. Furthermore, when the patient returns for a follow-up examination, the study can be repeated and the views compared without a great deal of difficulty. If a suspicious area is seen but the standard views are not satisfactory, or if an additional view is desired, the position of the patient's head can be changed and additional cuts can be obtained.

The patients are scanned at an angle of approximately 20 to 25 degrees to the orbital meatal line. Twelve to 14 slices, each 8 mm thick, are obtained on each patient, although the number of slices obtained necessarily varies with the patient's head size. The lowest slice is positioned so that the upper cervical region or the foramen magnum is visible; with this slice angle, the roof of the orbit, or even the orbit itself, should be visible. The slices are then positioned so that each is contiguous with the next until the entire cranial contents, up to and including the high convexities, have been visualized. The angle of the slices is such that the higher cuts demonstrate the parietal rather than the frontal lobes—a source of confusion to those who are being initiated into the technique. This is particularly important to remember when a surgical approach is being planned.

Figures 3–4 through 3–10 (pp. 115 to 121)

demonstrate normal anatomic sections of the brain correlated with the appropriate CT scans. Anatomic structures are labeled both on the specimen and the CT scan slice. Note that there is some variation in the CT scan appearance from patient to patient. As in any biologic study, there is a good deal of variation even among normal patients, and no two scans are identical. In addition there is always some variation whenever the patient is positioned in the scanning unit.

The sella turcica is best studied using direct coronal images and 4-mm slices (see Chapter 9). These scans should be obtained postinfusion only or pre- and postinfusion, depending upon the clinical presentation. If the patient cannot obtain the coronal position, then 4-mm slices overlapped by 2-mm can be obtained in the axial plane, with the plane of examination parallel to the base of the skull. This will allow for excellent reconstruction images in the coronal and sagittal planes. Magnetic resonance will probably replace CT for imaging of the sella and parasellar regions.

The scans presented in this text were obtained on a variety of scanners. Some of the older scans were obtained on an EMI 1010 model and have been preserved for their teaching value. Many of the newer scanners have a standard 5-cm line incorporated into each image that is always in proportion to the image and thus facilitates the evaluation of the size of each lesion.

After the completion of each standard preinfusion scan, a repeat scan may be performed following the intravenous administration of contrast material. For adults, I use 300 cc of Conray 30 per cent in an infusion set; the first 150 cc is infused before beginning the scan; the remainder is infused slowly throughout the duration of the scan. For pediatric patients we use 4.4 cc/kg (2 cc/lb). It would appear that the type of contrast medium used is not critical, but that the amount of iodine necessary is 40 gm in the adult to ensure an adequate load of contrast material. There is a very real although rare possibility of an anaphylactoid reaction to the contrast medium as well as emesis with aspiration of gastric contents. For these reasons the use of contrast infusion should not be undertaken without some consideration.

All the scans throughout this volume are labeled so that the right hand side of the picture represents the left hemisphere—i.e., as if one is looking up at the patient's head.

Although some examiners favor a postinfusion scan on each individual, the potential danger of an adverse affect on the kidneys—even including renal shut-down—precludes this approach to computed tomography. The author recommends a cautious, rather than blanket, approach to the use of contrast infusion. Those patients who should have contrast enhancement are listed below. In addition, for an initial examination, I *STRONGLY* recommend a preinfusion scan before the study following contrast infusion. Some argue convincingly that only a postinfusion scan should be performed. However, those cases in which the diagnosis is obscured—e.g., the differentiation between basal ganglia hemorrhage and enhancing infarct, or obscuring of an infarct by the infusion—make this method less desirable than the conservative approach of a preinfusion scan followed by a postinfusion study. Perhaps the use of "postinfusion only" scans should be limited to patients with a tumor diagnosis who are returning for follow-up. There is no doubt that additional information not appreciable on the preinfusion scan is gained on the postinfusion scan. Those patients who should have a postinfusion study in addition to the preinfusion are:

1. All patients with suspected metastases.
2. All patients with evidence of a space-occupying lesion on the preinfusion scan.
3. Postoperative brain tumor patients.
4. Patients with suspected arteriovenous malformations.
5. Individuals with demyelinating diseases or seizure disorders who are being worked-up for the first time.
6. Patients with suspected chronic bilateral isodense subdural hematomas.
7. Patients undergoing initial work-up for hydrocephalus.

Those patients who need a routine preinfusion CT scan only:

1. Patients with dementia.
2. Patients with acute head trauma.
3. Follow-up of change in size of lateral ventricles post-shunting.
4. Follow-up after evacuation of a hematoma.

POSTERIOR FOSSA

The posterior fossa is best examined using 4-mm slices angled at 20 to 25 degrees to the skull base. Studies are performed pre- and postinfusion. Coronal scans may also be helpful for further evaluation. Newer scanners allow images to be reconstructed in the coronal, sagittal, and oblique planes. Direct coronal images can also be obtained. In some scanners 2- or even 1-mm slices are helpful for evaluation of the temporal bones and particularly for evaluation of the internal auditory canal. If available, magnetic resonance is the procedure of choice for patients with posterior fossa abnormalities (see Chapter 13).

The quality of the image depends on the patient's remaining relatively immobile throughout the scan. This can prove particularly troublesome in children, and the author recommends adequate sedation before the scan. The standard dosage schedule for pediatric neuroradiologic procedures is recommended, with the amount of sedation used on the low end of the schedule. The sedative is administered intramuscularly 45 to 60 minutes before the procedure. These patients must be observed closely for any depression of vital signs. In some patients, both children and adults, it will be necessary to perform the scan under general anesthesia.

WINDOW WIDTH AND WINDOW LEVEL

Although it has been found that certain types of intracranial abnormalities measure a specific density on the CT scan, there is a good deal of "overlap" between the lesions (see Chart 3–1). The various scanning units are equipped with devices that measure the density of the structures visualized. These numerical measurements may be helpful to determine the histologic nature of the abnormality being viewed. During the course of reviewing intracranial findings, the bony calvaria is often examined in only a cursory fashion. It may become apparent after manipulation of the "measuring" device that more information can be gained only if a more thorough examination of the cranial contents and the bony calvaria is performed.

A description of the method of examination of the bony calvaria will serve as a basis for discussion of these methods of measurement. These methods require a review of some very

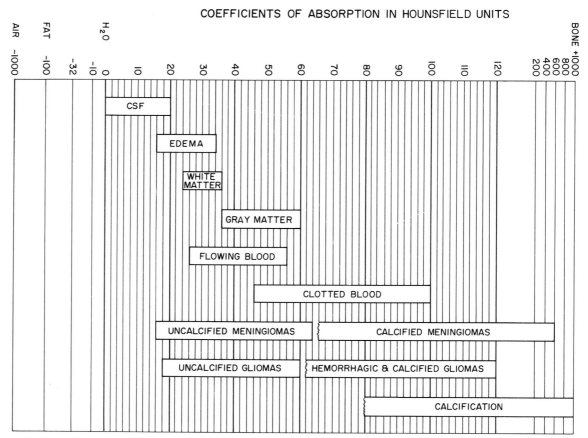

COEFFICIENTS OF ABSORPTION IN HOUNSFIELD UNITS

CHART 3–1

basic radiologic concepts, including the topics of *window width* and *window level*. The measuring devices on these scanners employ an arbitrary numerical scale that places the density of water at 0, the density of bone at +1000 and the density of air at −1000. These density units are called "Hounsfield units" after Mr. Godfrey Hounsfield, the developer of the CT scanner.

Contrast. Radiographic contrast may be considered as the difference between the blackest black and the whitest white. *High* contrast means that there is a large difference between the shades of gray, black, and white. With maximum contrast, the densities on the radiograph are either black or white, and there are no shades of gray. On most scanners this contrast level is obtained by placing the unit in the "measure mode." On the measure mode the image is either black or white at a given window density level (L) expressed in Hounsfield units (u). The level can be moved up or down to obtain the density range of an abnormal area. Certain abnormalities tend to fall within a certain density range, and at times a diagnosis can be made with a fair degree of certainty. This is especially true when there is clotted blood secondary to an intra- or extracerebral hematoma.

The latitude, on the other hand, is the number of shades of gray that may be seen on the photograph or radiograph. When there is a wide latitude, large numbers of shades of gray can be seen. When using the scanner, latitude can be altered by changing the *window width*. The viewing system can readily be changed from a very high contrast system to a very low contrast system in which the difference between densities becomes less in the shades between black and white.

The significance of these alterations becomes of practical importance when certain intracranial and calvarial changes can be appreciated only by altering the window width and window level. This is especially true of bony lesions, where abnormalities become apparent only after thorough inspection on the oscilloscope screen, examining each slice at varying window widths and window levels. For comparison purposes, an identical window width and window level should be used from time to time and from case to case.

The abnormalities of the bony calvaria usually are more readily apparent on the plain skull examination; however, the skull radiographs are not always available for examination at the time of the CT study. Conversely, it has been stated that after a CT scan there is no need for a routine skull series. As discussed in Chapter 2, neither view is entirely correct. In most cases, skull radiographs provide information not available from the CT scan or that is more readily apparent on the skull film than on the scan. However, when skull radiographs are not available, examination of the bony calvaria by CT scan is very helpful.

Throughout this text are examples that demonstrate the changes that become apparent when one examines the brain or calvaria by other than standard measurements. On a daily basis, one should develop a standard method of recording each case. The best window width, window level, and image size will vary with each scanning unit.

RECONSTRUCTION TOMOGRAPHY

By utilizing advanced computer techniques, a CT image can be manipulated to provide a view in a plane other than the initial scanning plane. This is accomplished by first performing multiple overlapping cuts in a single plane and then "feeding" the density readings in the overlapping sections into a computer, which "rearranges" the data so that a scan originally performed in the axial projection can be viewed in the sagittal plane.

This can be done for any plane desired. To be successful, the method does require a cooperative, immobile patient. The overlapping cuts also result in a significant increase in radiation dose to the patient.

The method is especially useful for studies of the sella and is also helpful in diagnosing lesions of the lumbar spine.

ARTIFACTS

A variety of artifacts or false images may be produced by the CT scanners. They are generated by many different phenomena. All artifacts degrade or alter the CT image; therefore, it is helpful to understand their origins. If the origin can be determined, artifacts can at times be altered or eliminated.

The various scanners available have different scanning speeds. With the older models and with slower scanning speeds, there is a greater chance of artifact secondary to patient motion. Such motion can degrade the image to such a great extent that the study becomes uninterpretable.

Metallic surgical clips are also a significant

cause of artifacts, and their use should be discouraged.

Metallic plates interfere with scanning so greatly that CT examinations usually cannot be performed in such patients. The metal connecting portions of shunt tube devices also degrade scan images. This degradation usually occurs only on the scan slice at the level of the metallic device and so may not interfere with interpretation.

Various other electrical and mechanical problems also may alter the images—e.g., weak or defective photomultiplier tubes, alteration of the kilovoltage during scanning, or mechanical interference with the scanner motion.

Air in the lateral ventricles causes a specific artifact. The scan will demonstrate a white line surrounding the peripheral margin of the retained air. This artifact is computer generated because of the very great density change between the air in the ventricle and the surrounding brain tissue.

Pantopaque in large quantities also can degrade the image.

MAGNETIC RESONANCE IMAGING

The recent addition of magnetic resonance (MR) has added a new dimension to our diagnostic armamentarium. The method is noninvasive, has excellent patient tolerance, and is easily performed as an outpatient procedure. It has no known biologic effects and is accurate and more sensitive than CT scanning, providing multiplanar images without the use of ionizing radiation. It is doubtful that MR will replace CT entirely, but there are certain classes of patients that will be better and more accurately evaluated by MR than by CT. The following is a list of disease entities that can be best evaluated by these two methods:

INDICATIONS FOR MAGNETIC RESONANCE	INDICATIONS FOR COMPUTED TOMOGRAPHY
• Demyelinating disease	• Known enhancing tumor
• Contrast allergy	• Suspected meningioma
• Posterior fossa tumors	• Orbital tumor
• Subdural hematomas (subacute or chronic)	• Osseous temporal bone abnormality
• Acoustic neuromas	• Acute hemorrhage
• Pituitary tumors	• Uncooperative patient
	• Aneurysm clips or pacemaker

Magnetic resonance imaging is one of the newest scientific tools to become available for clinical investigation. At this early stage in its clinical application this imaging technique is particularly effective for evaluation of the central nervous system. The method is sensitive to motion, which may degrade the image, and therefore has proven to be less useful in the chest and abdomen, where heart, respiratory, and bowel motion all tend to degrade the image. Advances in cardiac and respiratory gating have circumvented some of these problems, but this also results in increased examination times (see Figs. 3–18 to 3–25, pp. 124 to 129).

Clinical Magnetic Resonance Is Hydrogen Proton Imaging. At the present time the method involves the examination of hydrogen nuclear protons within the various tissues. Since hydrogen makes up a significant portion of most body tissues and has native magnetic properties, it is most suitable for MRI. In addition, the hydrogen proton responds well to perturbation when subject to a radiofrequency (RF) pulse. In the future other nuclei such as ^{13}C, ^{15}N, ^{17}O, ^{23}Na, and others that have magnetic properties may also be used for magnetic resonance imaging.

Magnets

There are three types of magnets: (1) permanent magnets, (2) resistive electromagnets, and (3) superconductive electromagnets. Permanent magnets are simply large magnets that are used in a similar manner to the resistive and superconductive magnets. They do not require the use of electricity or liquid helium and nitrogen.

The superconductive electromagnets differ from the resistive electromagnets in that they require cooling by liquid helium and nitrogen. Resistive magnets can produce field strengths of up to 0.2 Tesla maximum. Superconductive magnets can produce field strengths of up to 2.0 Tesla. It currently appears that the 1.5 Tesla field strength *may* be the ideal field strength for neuroradiologic imaging, although excellent images can also be obtained at lower field strengths.

The superconductive systems provide greater stability of the magnetic field and will be able to scan faster and may produce better images. The liquid gases, helium and nitrogen, that are consumed for cooling, cost approximately $35,000 per year. Electricity costs for the superconductive systems are negligible. On the other hand, resistive magnets have relatively poor stability of the magnetic field, and electricity, or "current," costs approximate the cost of the liquid cooling agents.

The total cost for the site preparation and purchase and installation of a magnetic resonance apparatus varies. The permanent magnets are the least expensive and the superconductive magnets most expensive. A *general* range of total cost is between one and three million dollars.

Technical Factors of MR Using a Teslacon 0.5T (5 Kilogauss) Superconductive Magnet*

The majority of images in this text are from the Technicare 5-kilogauss (0.5 Tesla) superconductive magnet. This instrument demonstrates the following characteristics:

- With each scan multiple slices can be obtained simultaneously.
- MR scan slices can be varied from several millimeters to several centimeters.
- The usual slice thickness is 1 cm for the brain. These slices are contiguous.
- The matrix size can be varied from 128 × 256 to 256 × 256. The pixel size for the head coil is approximately 1 × 2 mm. The pixel size for the body coil is approximately 1.6 × 3.2 mm.
- Images can be readily obtained in axial, coronal, and sagittal planes.
- A typical T-1 weighted multislice image takes approximately 5 minutes of scanning time.
- A typical T-2 weighted multislice image takes approximately 10 to 14 minutes of scanning time.
- A *two-echo multislice* series of images can be obtained using such imaging factors as TR3120/TE60-120 spin-echo (SE) technique. In other words, it is possible to obtain a multislice image while simultaneously using two different echoes and one long TR interval.
- A *single slice* can be obtained using *multiple echoes* such as TR2240/TE 30, 60, 90, 120, 150, 180, 210, 240. In other words, a single slice centered on an area of interest can be obtained using eight separate echoes simultaneously with one long TR interval.
- At this writing a variety of coils are available: head coil, body coil, surface coil, breast coil.

The surface "coils" are actually made up of coiled wire and look similar to a heating pad. These coils allow a "close-up" view of the area of interest and are simply placed over that area for examination. The coils have a variety of depth capabilities; the surface coil allows excellent visualization of the spine. In the future, coils will become available to visualize the orbit, the temporomandibular joints, the neck to evaluate carotid artery flow, and additional areas. These coils may act as both transmitters and receivers of radiofrequency waves or may provide only one of these functions.

MR Images

Images of MR are presented on an arbitrary gray scale. By convention, tissues with a short T-1 and a long T-2 are bright (whiter) on short or T-1 weighted images. Materials such as liquids and CSF have a long T-2 and are bright on T-2 weighted images. As a general rule, magnetic resonance is more sensitive than CT for the diagnosis of CNS pathology. However, the question of specificity is yet to be answered. As a general statement regarding the comparison between CT and MR, one can state the following:

- Everything that is *black* on CT is *white* on T-2 weighted images
- Everything that is *white* on CT is *dark* on MR images
  Except for subacute (greater than 48 hours old) blood collections (such as intracerebral or subdural hematomas) and fat (such as lipomas), which are bright or increased in signal intensity with *both* the T-1 and T-2 weighted images.

Technical Considerations

One can think of the MR scanner as a series of very large magnets similar to the small circular magnets that are used to hold reminder notes on the refrigerator door. The scanner magnets are large enough to allow the body to fit in the center ring. These magnets generate a magnetic field. The magnets are used clinically to image the hydrogen nuclei in the various body tissues. As the body slides into the magnet a small number—perhaps millions—of the hydrogen protons or nuclei in the body, which total in the multibillions, line up in the magnetic field that is generated. The patients do not have any abnormal feeling as they are placed into the magnetic field, and there is no sensation of heating or pain. After the patient is positioned in the magnetic field, a radiofrequency pulse is applied to the field. This causes a small number of the hydrogen nuclear protons to tip off their alignment in the field. The radiofrequency (RF) pulse can be applied in such a way as to tip the protons off-axis at a 90- to 180-degree tilt. Following this excitation by the application of a RF pulse, the hydrogen protons emit energy that is detected as a radiofrequency signal as they return to their equilibrium state. The RF pulse is then turned off and the amount of energy given off by these

---

*Technicare Corporation, Solon, Ohio.

protons is measured. This energy is also related to the "proton density," or number of hydrogen protons that are present in various visualized structures. Normal tissues give off one signal, while abnormal structures or tissues give off another signal. This obviously allows differentiation between the various normal and pathologic tissues. Unfortunately, these alterations are not absolute, and so tissue specificity cannot be achieved with certainty. The tissue densities are presented on an arbitrary density scale, which is a gray scale similar to that used for CT scanning.

Gray Scale Presentation

In addition, with this technique, structures with a bright appearance on one spin-echo sequence will appear dark on a different spin-echo sequence. Therefore, one cannot speak in terms of a certain gray scale density appearance—this is dissimilar to CT scanning. A variety of techniques can be used to tilt the protons off their axes. The sequences most commonly used are spin-echo sequences. Some other sequences are the inversion recovery, proton density, and partial saturation.

Spatial Encoding

The application of a gradient or a gradually increasing field strength to the main magnetic field produces spatial encoding of the protons, since each proton emits a radiofrequency signal that corresponds to a specific position in the gradient field. Therefore one can "find" the location of the protons and determine the anatomic location of the various normal as well as pathologic signals.

Definitions

TE. Time to echo: expressed in milliseconds, this is the time between radiofrequency excitation of the nuclei and the receipt of a signal or "spin echo" from the nuclei. The source of the radiofrequency waves usually acts as both a transmitter and receiver of the RF signals.

TR. Time to repetition: expressed in milliseconds, this is the amount of time one waits between the application of radiofrequency pulses.

T-1. (1) Time for protons to align in a magnetic field—an exponential process—time constant T-1. (2) Time constant to return to equilibrium (relaxation) following a radiofrequency disturbance.

Physical characteristics of the sample such as temperature, viscosity, and molecular structure of solutes all affect T-1. In general, solids and pure liquids such as CSF have a long T-1 and are of low signal intensity on T-1 weighted spin-echo images; hemorrhage and fat have a short T-1 and are bright on T-1 weighted images. This is also known as spin-lattice, or longitudinal, relaxation time. Increased field strength also results in an increase in T-1; this may result in longer scanning times at higher field strengths.

T-1 Weighted Image. This general term is used for short spin-echo sequences. Generally speaking, this is a spin-echo sequence of TR530/TE30. This sequence is a standard pulse sequence used for most studies. It is an ideal sequence to evaluate the "anatomy" because the various anatomic structures are well visualized.

T-2 Relaxation Time. The time it takes the nuclei to reach equilibrium with each other. This is also known as the spin-spin or transverse relaxation time. It is the time expressed in milliseconds it takes for the nuclei (nuclear magnets) or protons to return to an equilibrium distribution in which there is no transverse magnetization; i.e., the energy of the system cancels itself out. T-2 is related to the loss of nuclear spin coherence, and the net magnetization in the XY plane converges to zero. T-2 is the exponential loss of signal. Solids have a short T-2, the protons rapidly desynchronize, and their signal decays very rapidly. Liquids have a long T-2.

T-2 Weighted Image. In general terms, this is used for spin-echo sequences in which the TE is greater than 90 milliseconds and the TR is greater than 2,000 milliseconds (2 seconds).

Scanning Sequences. Typical spin-echo (SE) sequences are TR530/TE30 and TR3120/TE120. TR530/TE30 is a short SE sequence and is referred to as a T-1 weighted image; the TR3120/TE120 is a long SE sequence and is referred to as a T-2 weighted image (see Table 3–1).

As a general rule of thumb, one can remember that everything that is black or low density on the CT images is white on the T-2 weighted SE MR images. The reverse is also true except in the case of fat and "subacute" blood, which demonstrate increased signal intensity—appear white or bright—on both the T-1 and T-2 weighted images. Therefore, while MR is more sensitive than CT in many cases, the fact is that MR is not (as yet) more specific than CT.

Scanning Times. Scanning times are signifi-

Table 3–1. Standard Spin-Echo Sequences for Clinical Evaluation

CATEGORY	TR530/TE30	TR3120/ TE60-120	PLANES
Brain tumor	X		Axial and coronal or sagittal
Demyelinating disease	X		Axial
		X	Axial and coronal
Seizure disorder	X		Axial
		X	Axial and coronal or sagittal
Infarct	X		Axial
		X	Axial and coronal or sagittal
Metastases	X		Axial
		X	Axial and coronal or sagittal
Posterior fossa	X	X	Sagittal and axial or coronal
Trauma (subdural or epidural)	X		Axial and coronal
		X	Axial and coronal
Pituitary tumor	X	X	Coronal and sagittal
Degenerated discs	X		Sagittal, 5 slices and axial through abnormal discs
		X	Sagittal
Spine metastases	X	X	Sagittal and axial or coronal

cantly longer with MR than CT. A typical T-1 weighted scan may take approximately 5 minutes, while a typical T-2 weighted scan may take up to 15 minutes. This is contrasted to newer CT scanners, which may take less than 5 seconds to produce a single image. One benefit of MR is the fact that it is a multislice technique in which a large number of slices (approximately 10 to 15 contiguous 1-cm slices include the entire brain) are generated simultaneously in one scanning time. As with CT, motion at any time during the scan will degrade the entire examination. This is obviously critical at the longer scanning times. A typical routine MR scan of the brain performed in two planes takes approximately one hour.

Gauss. A unit of magnetic field strength. One gauss is the approximate strength of the earth's magnetic field at the surface. 1 kilogauss = 1000 gauss.

Gradient Magnetic Field. A magnetic field that increases in strength in a certain given direction. The patient is placed into the magnetic field, and a certain number of nuclear protons (nuclear magnets) of the billions of hydrogen protons in the body align themselves in a magnetic or antimagnetic direction. A net magnetization in the direction of the field results.

Negative Flow Defect. Flowing blood appears as an area of low signal intensity, or negative flow defect. This occurs because as blood flows through the section of image plane the hydrogen protons in the flowing blood align in the gradient field. Those aligned protons are then "hit" with a RF wave, which causes them to tilt off alignment. However, before the tilted protons can realign in the field they have moved—by virtue of normal blood flow—out of the section of image. The application of the RF pulses only lasts for a short period, as does the time for receipt of the signal; however, this is sufficient time to allow the protons to move out of the image plane and prevents a signal from returning: thus a negative flow signal or defect.

Occasionally the aligned, and subsequently "tilted," protons will flow into another adjacent slice in the multislice image. Therefore the protons "activated" in one slice will actually *return* the signal in a *different* slice, of variable strength and brightness depending upon the number of "activated" protons. This situation is commonly seen on the axial images of the abdominal aorta, and has been termed a paradoxic effect of blood flow imaging. Areas of slow or turbulent flow, such as the jugular veins or cortical veins of the brain, may also give a bright signal. Therefore a single blood vessel may theoretically give any number of signal intensities depending upon a number of factors, including speed of flow and position in the multislice image.

Radiofrequency (RF) Pulse. A short pulse or radiofrequency wave that is in the megahertz frequency range. The Teslacon 0.5T superconductive unit transmits at approximately 20.9 MHz.

Tesla. 10 kilogauss = 1 Tesla.

Cross-over Point. When using spin-echo sequences, the various structures change in signal intensity when changing from short to long sequences. The references to the "cross-over point" are to the appearance of cerebrospinal fluid, which changes from dark (short SE) to bright (long SE) (Fig. 3–26, p. 129). In this text "cross-over point" is generally used to describe CSF. With spin-echo imaging and an increasing TE and TR, CSF has low signal intensity with a TE less than 90 msec, is isodense with the brain at a TE of 90 msec, and has high signal intensity with a TE longer than 90 msec. This varies with field strength.

The Future of Magnetic Resonance

Magnetic resonance has already proved itself to be a reliable clinical diagnostic tool. It is unlikely that MR will replace CT in the near future; however, there is likewise no doubt that MR is a better imaging method for many abnormalities, particularly for demyelinating disease and for posterior fossa tumors. There is great promise, and hope, that the availability of gadolinium-DTPA for use as a contrast agent will improve the diagnostic capabilities and specificity of MR. The exact time frame for the availability of gadolinium-DTPA is not yet known. At this time it appears that a magnet strength of 1.0 to 1.5 Tesla will be ideal for clinical use. (Magnets of 4 to 5 Tesla will be necessary for spectroscopy, a topic that is beyond the scope of this book.) While a 1.0 to 1.5 Tesla magnet can be operated at 0.5 Tesla, the converse is not true. A magnet that is 0.5 or 0.6 Tesla in strength cannot be upgraded to a 1.0 or 1.5 Tesla magnet. Therefore, it would appear prudent to purchase at least a 1.0 or 1.5 Tesla magnet so that one may operate at the higher field strength if desired.

The higher field strength magnets can also obtain thinner slices than are possible with the lower strength magnets. This will be particularly advantageous when one is examining the pituitary fossa and internal auditory canals. There is an increase in the time of the T-1 with the higher field strength magnets, which does slow scanning time but not sufficiently to overcome the faster scans that are generally available with the higher field strength magnets. With such magnets, there are additional cost and shielding considerations; however, it would appear that the advantages outweigh the disadvantages. At this time it does not appear that there is an absolute "ideal field strength," but only additional clinical experience will allow us to make that determination with certainty.

In a practical sense, it appears advisable to have both CT and MR available. It does not seem advisable to have only MR available without CT; therefore, if only one instrument is possible, then CT is the machine of choice at this time.

Additional "software" capabilities that will be added to MR scanners in the near future but are not universally available now include the following:

- Angled cuts
- Readily variable slice thickness
- A field enlargement option for region of interest
- "Push-button" T-1 and T-2 measurement availability
- Surface coils
- Automatic scan sequence modes with push-button control

Table 3–1 outlines a method of spin-echo sequences that can be used as a general guide and altered to suit the physician's needs and preferences.

The great advantages of MR can be readily appreciated simply by examining the images. The exact relationship of the soft tissue structures to the surrounding bony structures is readily demonstrated by MR, particularly when one is examining the spinal cord. This makes accurate evaluation of the spinal column and its contents extraordinarily easy and convenient. This feature is exceptionally attractive, since it does not require the injection of contrast material. For examination of the intracranial contents MR again demonstrates definite advantages when performed for the presence of demyelinating disease. At times the increased sensitivity for the detection of brain tumors is also very impressive. The evaluation by MR represents a convenient, safe, noninvasive, reproducible, and accurate examination for clinical diagnoses.

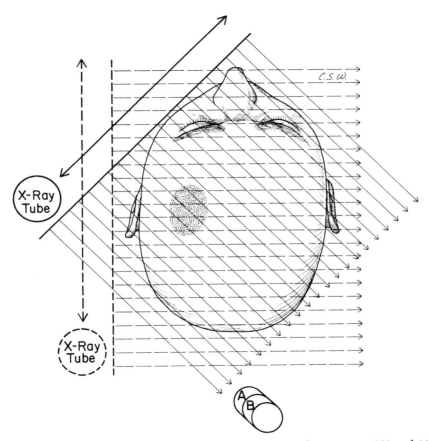

FIGURE 3–1. Schematic drawing of first-generation scanner (see text pp. 103 and 104).

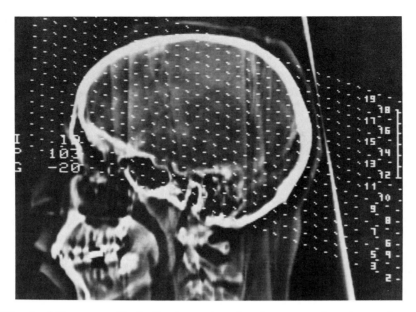

FIGURE 3–2. *Standard Topogram.* Each slice is numbered and corresponds to image slice numbers. Slices are 8 mm thick.

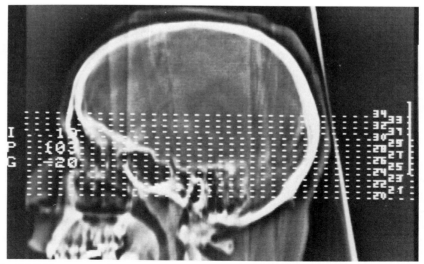

FIGURE 3–3. *Orbit Topogram* Slices are 4 mm thick and are obtained parallel to the plane of the globe.

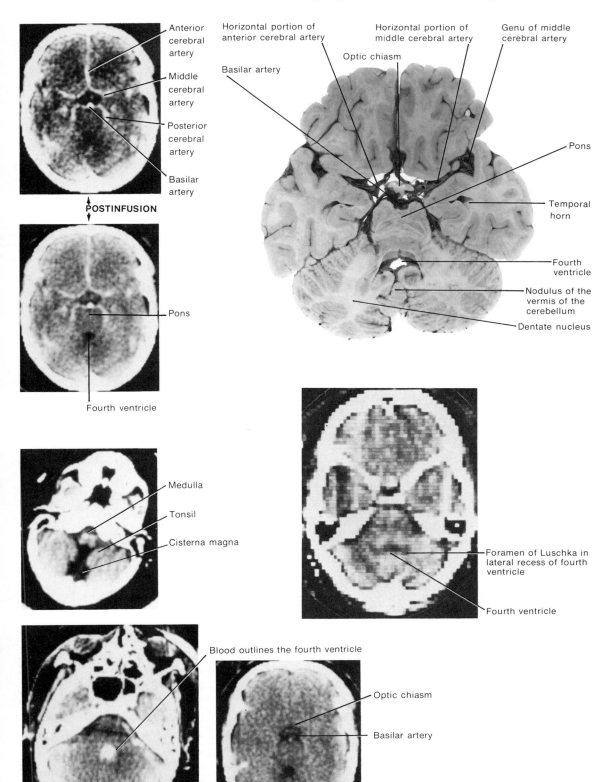

FIGURE 3-4

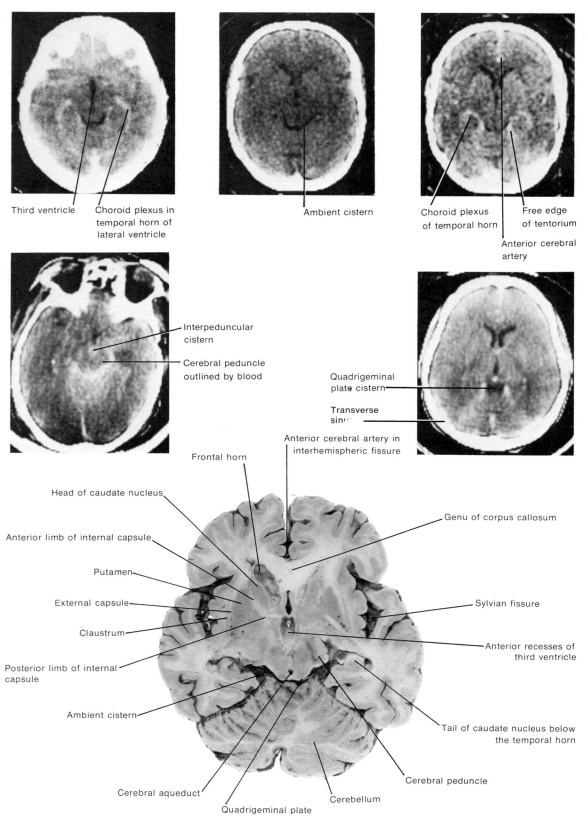

FIGURE 3—5. Normal gross neuroanatomy and corresponding CT slices.

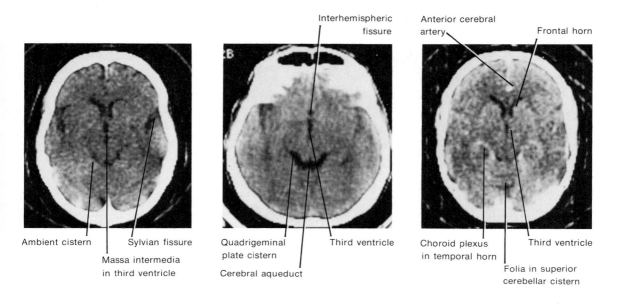

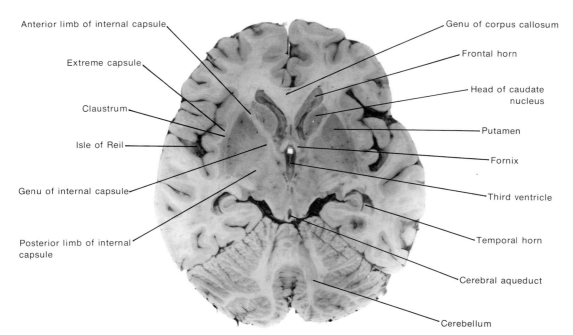

FIGURE 3–6. Normal gross neuroanatomy and corresponding CT slices.

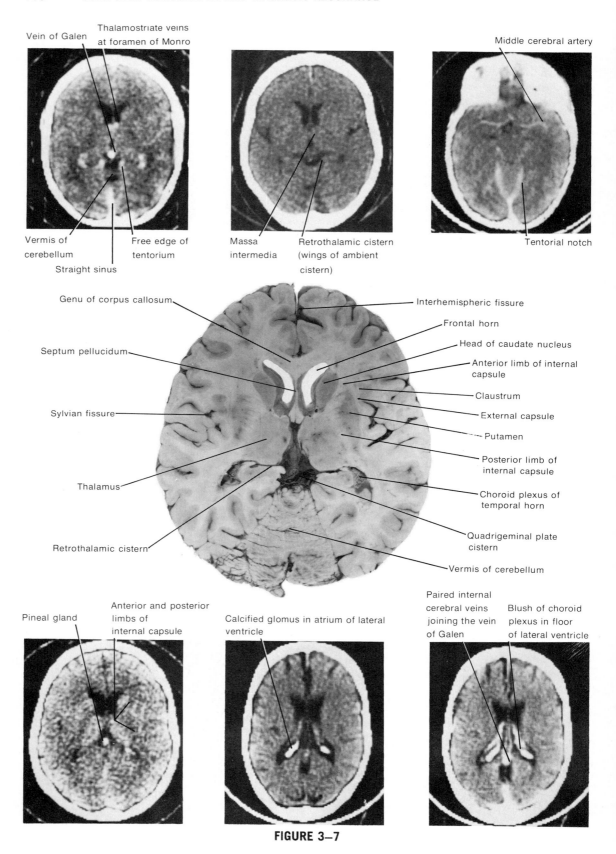

Vein of Galen

Thalamostriate veins at foramen of Monro

Middle cerebral artery

Vermis of cerebellum

Straight sinus

Free edge of tentorium

Massa intermedia

Retrothalamic cistern (wings of ambient cistern)

Tentorial notch

Genu of corpus callosum

Septum pellucidum

Sylvian fissure

Thalamus

Retrothalamic cistern

Interhemispheric fissure

Frontal horn

Head of caudate nucleus

Anterior limb of internal capsule

Claustrum

External capsule

Putamen

Posterior limb of internal capsule

Choroid plexus of temporal horn

Quadrigeminal plate cistern

Vermis of cerebellum

Pineal gland

Anterior and posterior limbs of internal capsule

Calcified glomus in atrium of lateral ventricle

Paired internal cerebral veins joining the vein of Galen

Blush of choroid plexus in floor of lateral ventricle

FIGURE 3–7

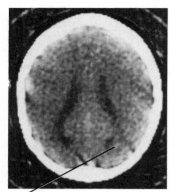

Posterior extent of occipital horn
of lateral ventricle

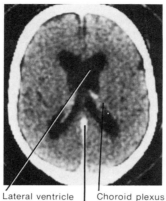

Lateral ventricle   Choroid plexus
                     postinfusion

Straight sinus

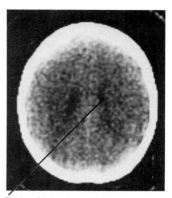

Body of lateral ventricle

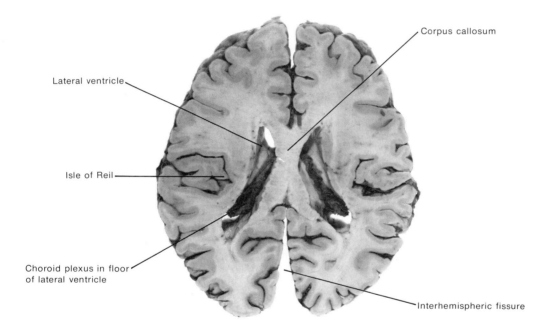

Corpus callosum

Lateral ventricle

Isle of Reil

Choroid plexus in floor
of lateral ventricle

Interhemispheric fissure

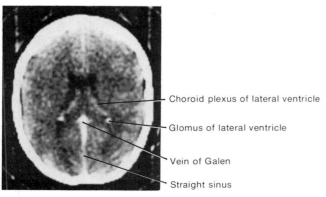

Choroid plexus of lateral ventricle

Glomus of lateral ventricle

Vein of Galen

Straight sinus

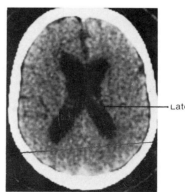

Lateral ventricle

FIGURE 3–8

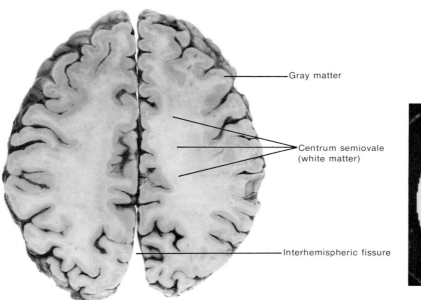

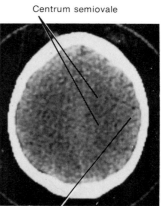

FIGURE 3-9

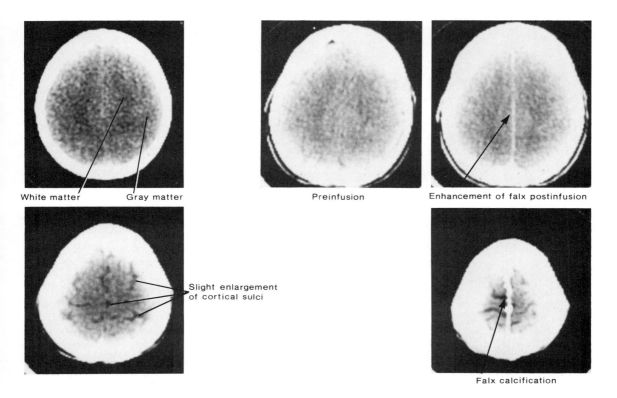

White matter   Gray matter

Preinfusion

Enhancement of falx postinfusion

Slight enlargement of cortical sulci

Falx calcification

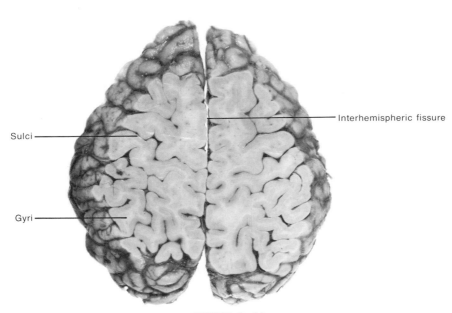

Sulci

Gyri

Interhemispheric fissure

FIGURE 3–10

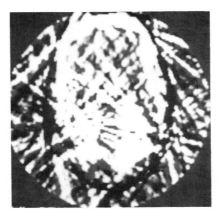

Preinfusion

FIGURE 3–11. Motion artifact.

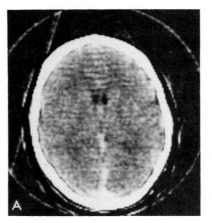

Postinfusion

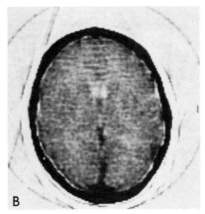

Postinfusion

FIGURE 3–12. Reduced tube output (caused by poor beam quality) leads to a "noisy" picture.

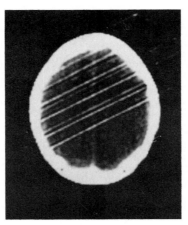

Preinfusion

FIGURE 3–13. Changing detector sensitivity during scan.

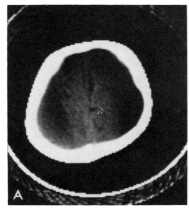

Preinfusion   Preinfusion

FIGURE 3–14. Shading artifacts secondary to saturation of detectors.

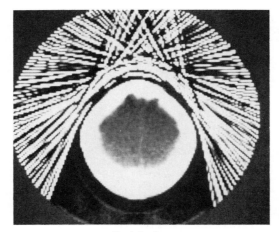

Preinfusion

FIGURE 3–15. Artifact secondary to air around calvaria. This can be seen in patients with bouffant or Afro hair-styles.

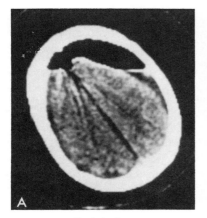
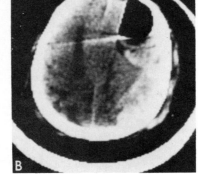

Preinfusion   Preinfusion

FIGURE 3–16. A white line computer overswing artifact caused by air within the calvaria.

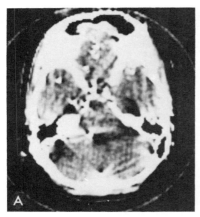 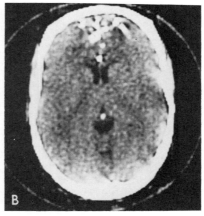

Preinfusion   Preinfusion

FIGURE 3–17. Pantopaque droplets.

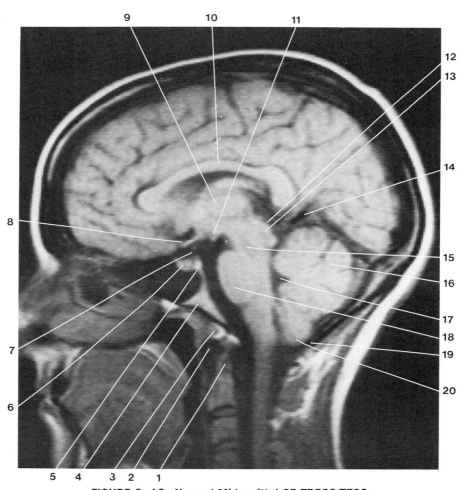

FIGURE 3–18. *Normal Midsagittal SE TR530/TE30.*

1 Odontoid.
2 Anterior arch of C_1.
3 Fat pad between odontoid and clivus.
4 Clivus.
5 Fat in posterior sella turcica.
6 Pituitary gland.
7 Pituitary stalk (infundibulum).

8 Optic chiasm/optic tract.
9 Massa intermedia.
10 Corpus callosum.
11 Mammillary body.
12 Quadrigeminal plate.
13 Cerebral aqueduct.
14 Vein of Galen.

15 Red nucleus.
16 Cerebellar vermis.
17 Fourth ventricle.
18 Pons.
19 Posterior margin of foramen magnum.
20 Cerebellar tonsil.

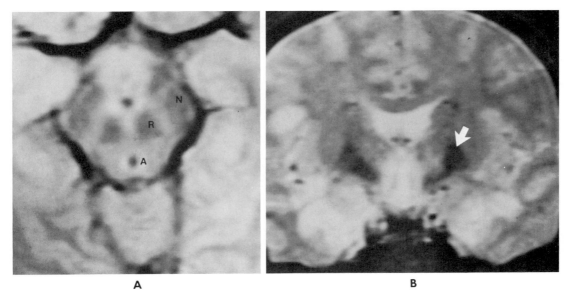

A   B

FIGURE 3–19. *Normal Midbrain and Basal Ganglia by MR:* *A,* Axial SE TR2120/TE120 image with a 1.5 Tesla magnet reveals the red nucleus (R), the substantia nigra (N), and the Sylvian aqueduct (A). The vessels of the circle of Willis appear as areas of negative flow.

B, Axial SE TR2120/TE120 image reveals that the globus pallidus of the basal ganglia (*arrow*) exhibits low signal intensity. The red nucleus, the substantia nigra, and the globus pallidus all reveal low signal intensity because they contain an increased amount of iron. (Case courtesy of Dr. Brent Greenberg.)

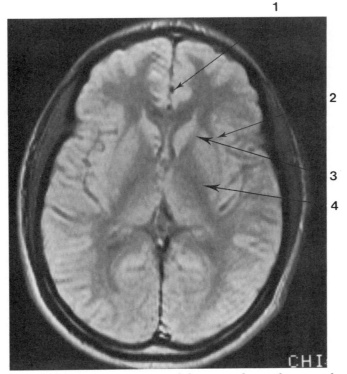

FIGURE 3–20. Normal SE TR2120/TE60 at the level of the internal capsule. Note the excellent gray/white differentiation. The white matter appears lower in signal intensity than the gray matter with this imaging technique.

1 Negative flow defect of the anterior cerebral artery.
2 External capsule.
3 Anterior limb of internal capsule.
4 Posterior limb of internal capsule.

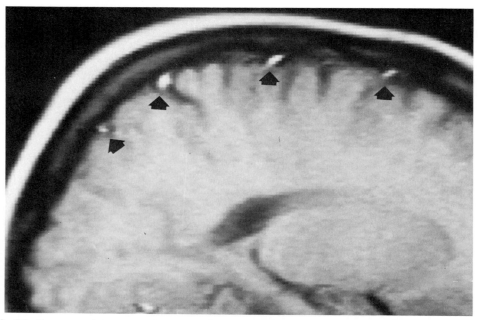

FIGURE 3–21. Parasagittal SE TR530/TE30 reveals high signal intensity in the cortical veins because of slow flow.

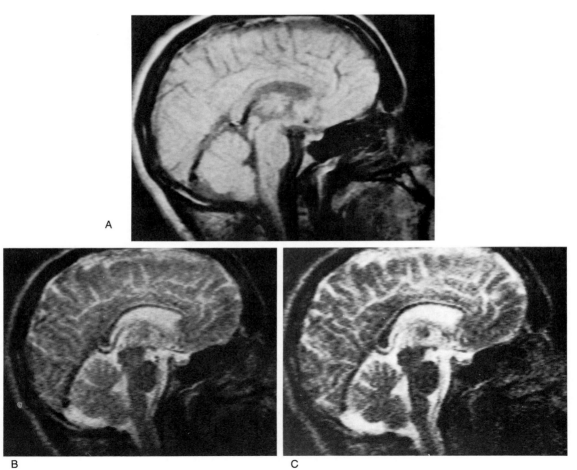

FIGURE 3–22. These images represent a single midsagittal slice using a variety of SE techniques. This series reflects the changes in signal intensity of the normal structures with a single long TR internal of 2240 milliseconds and a changing TE. A = TE60, B = TE150, C = TE240. Note that the CSF changes from black to white, and the normal brain substance changes from relatively high signal intensity to relatively low signal intensity. The basilar artery, vein of Galen, and straight sinus are seen as negative flow defects on the last two SE sequences. (See Figure 3–26.)

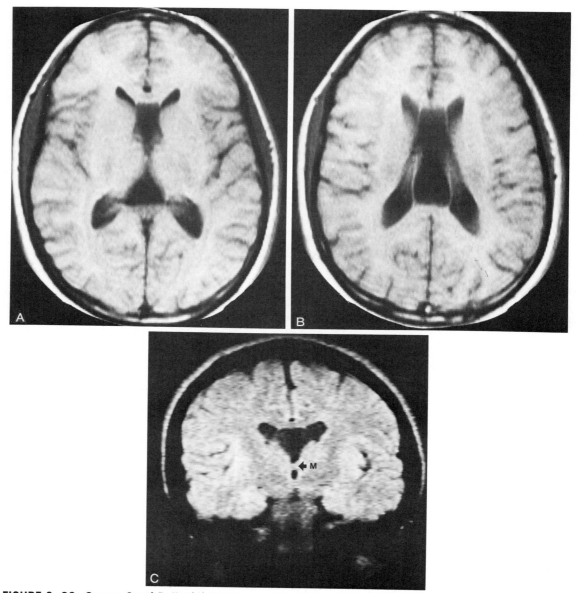

FIGURE 3–23. *Cavum Septi Pellucidi and Cavum Vergae:* *A* and *B*, SE TR530/TE30 images reveal a cavum septi pellucidi between the frontal horns of the lateral ventricles. The posterior extension of the cavum septum pellucioum is the cavum vergae. The cavum vergae separates the bodies of the lateral ventricles and is separated from the ventricles by a thin membrane.

C, The direct coronal SE TR530/TE30 at the level of the massa intermedia (M) also demonstrates the cavum vergae and the separation of the ventricles.

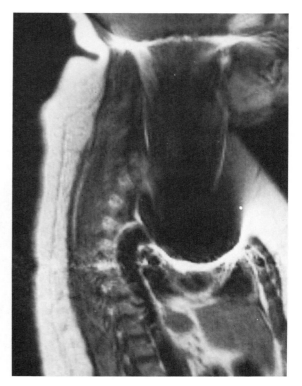

FIGURE 3–24. *Safety Pin Artifact:* The mid-sagittal, T-1 weighted image is greatly degraded by artifact from a safety pin attached to the patient's clothing.

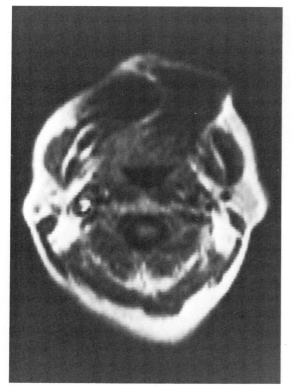

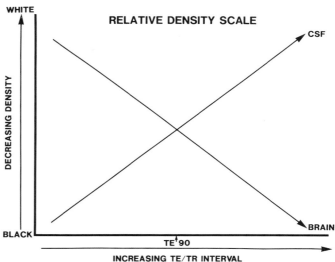

FIGURE 3–25. *Dental Bridge Artifact:* The T-1 weighted slice obtained at the level of the patient's dental bridge reveals "warping" of the field at that level. Usually this type of artifact is confined to the slice that contains the dental device, but occasionally, the device causes distortion of the field even beyond the level of the slice in which the device is located.

FIGURE 3–26. *Cross-over Point:* On a relative density scale, with a TR interval of 1500 milliseconds or greater, one can see that CSF is approximately equal to brain density at a TE interval of 90 milliseconds. This point will be considered the "cross-over" point in discussions in this text; it is at this point that CSF changes from dark or low signal intensity to bright or high signal intensity. Spin echo studies with TR/TE intervals to the left of the cross-over point will be considered "T-1 weighted," while spin-echo studies with TR/TE intervals to the right of the cross-over point will be considered "T-2 weighted." (Teslacon, 0.5 Tesla.)

RELATIVE DENSITY SCALE

WHITE

CSF

DECREASING DENSITY

BRAIN

BLACK

TE 90

INCREASING TE/TR INTERVAL

4

ANGIOGRAPHIC TECHNIQUE AND APPLIED CEREBROVASCULAR EMBRYOLOGY AND NORMAL ANATOMY

Angiographic Technique

SPECIAL PROCEDURE ROOM

Few hospitals have the luxury of a special procedure room devoted solely to neuroradiologic studies. More commonly, the special procedure room is used for GI studies in the morning and for the arteriographic studies in the afternoon, and often these facilities must be shared with others performing arteriography of the abdomen and lower extremities. Not uncommonly these rooms are not designed for biplane arteriography, making it necessary to use two separate injections to obtain a biplane study. This is suboptimal but can be made to work if necessary.

Under ideal circumstances, a neuroradiologic suite should be set up such that it is equipped for biplane arteriography, including an image intensifier, so that both fluoroscopy and biplane arteriography can be performed without difficulty. The biplane technique can be either simultaneous or—if possible, and preferably—using alternating exposure technique. The table should have a free floating top and be movable in the up-down direction. A sliding top above a fixed top is helpful for patient positioning (Figs. 4–1 and 4–2, p. 155). The focal spot size should be 1.3 mm or less, and a small focal spot (0.3 mm or less) should also be available for selection so that magnification technique can be utilized conveniently. A high-quality image intensifier should be situated so that catheter placement is possible with a minimum of patient movement and that filming can proceed with a minimum of patient motion after the catheter is in place.

A large, esthetically pleasing room away from main traffic areas is ideal and should allow access only to those involved in the procedures. The room should be quiet and set up so that the surroundings do not frighten the patient. Excess "clutter" should be eliminated, and the

130

room should be well-lighted and quiet. Large leaded windows should be available for patient monitoring, and remote monitors also may facilitate examination. The theory of a "place for everything and everything in its place" should certainly be practiced in this setting. This is particularly true in those rare emergency conditions when equipment should be available quickly and conveniently.

An emergency cart with the necessary equipment for possible emergency and resuscitative procedures also should be readily available to be pushed to the bedside should the need arise. This emergency cart is stocked with all emergency drugs that might be needed. Any drugs used should be replaced immediately.

X-RAY EQUIPMENT

In general, the type of equipment is a matter of personal choice. Many manufacturers have equipment available for purchase that will produce a satisfactory series of radiographs. It is the author's opinion that a 1,000 MA generator with three-phase equipment is preferable because it allows a wider range of technique choices and results in films with better contrast. In addition, it is helpful to have the capability of simultaneous biplane filming for adequate study of intracranial abnormalities. Magnification techniques are also necessary if an optimal study is to be performed. In general, the large focal spot for routine filming should be 1.3 to 1.2 mm in size. The small focal spot is then 0.2 to 0.3 mm in size.

INJECTORS

Manual Injections. Contrast material can be injected by hand when small amounts of contrast material are to be injected, when the vessel to be injected is very small, or when it is desirable to remove the catheter from the vessel as soon as the injection is completed. On the other hand, this procedure results in excessive radiation exposure to the operating physician. In the author's opinion, injection by hand is undesirable except in unusual circumstances. The modern automatic injectors allow the injection of even small amounts of contrast material and—again in my opinion—all injections, with rare exceptions, should be made with the automatic injector.

Automatic Injectors. Injectors are available that can inject a bolus of contrast material at a pre-set pressure or at a rate of a pre-set volume per unit time. The pressure injectors reflect the pressure of the fluid at the hub of the catheter—not at its tip—making their desirability questionable. Volume injectors deliver a preset volume of contrast material in a predetermined period of time. For example, the volume injector can be set to deliver 10 cc per second for 2 seconds: a total dose of 20 cc. The settings of amount and time of delivery can be made at the time of injection.

The author has had many years of excellent and dependable service from the Viamonte-Hobbs injector. This unit has a built-in voltage ground to safeguard against an electric current passing through the patient. The Viamonte-Hobbs injector operates on the principle of a metered delivery rate; this can be set accurately and conveniently at the tableside just before injection. One dial is used to select the duration of the injection (variable from 1 to 4 seconds); a second dial is used to set the delivery rate (variable from 2 to 60 cc per second). There is also a back-up device, set before each injection, that prevents the delivery of more contrast material than desired. This is a mechanical stop device that also can be used to control the amount of contrast material injected. It can be set if the injection is to continue longer than 4 seconds—and at the maximum setting of the dial. Thus, if one would like to inject 6 cc per second for 8 seconds, the injector time button is switched to "off." The volume per second is set on one dial and the total volume is set by using the back-up device. When the predetermined volume has been delivered, the mechanical device will stop the injector.

The Viamonte-Hobbs injector also has a dial that can be set to delay either the injector or the filming if desired. This is helpful when one needs a "blank" film at the beginning of the run to use for subtraction techniques. In this case, the unit is placed on an "injector delay" of one tenth of one second; i.e., the injection of contrast material occurs one tenth of one second after radiographic filming begins. This produces one exposed film without contrast before contrast material arrives at the area of interest. The unit also can be set for "x-ray delay" if that is desired.

FILM CHANGERS

Hand-Pulled Cassettes. After the injection of contrast material, the exposures are made, and each individual cassette is pulled out of the line of x-rays. This was the original method of filming, and it is still used today by some institutions. The films obtained with this technique are of good quality because the film screen contact is excellent, and a relatively rapid sequence of films can be obtained. The method is undesirable, however, because the firing rates are slow and inaccurate and because the scatter of radiation to the personnel increases individual exposure. Separate injections also must be made for biplane filming.

Automatic Cassette Changers. The Sanchez-Perez film changing unit uses automatically advanced cassettes and produces films of excellent quality. However, the units are noisy and are cumbersome because of the weight of the cassettes. They also are limited to the number of films that can be obtained.

Cut Film Changers. The Elema-Schonander film changing unit is the most popular of the cut film changers. The AOT changers are available for use with two film sizes—14 × 14 inch (35 × 35 cm) or 10 × 12 inch. The 14 × 14 inch size is more desirable because it has wider uses than do the smaller film sizes, which are limited for the most part to use in studies of intracranial pathology. Departments that perform only studies of intracranial pathology also may find the small size a limitation, because it is difficult to visualize the extracranial vessels and nearly impossible to perform an arch angiogram without multiple injections. It is the rare institution that has the luxury of a room used solely for intracranial pathology studies. The 14 × 14 film changer also can be used for abdominal arteriography, and it seems wise to have a capability for both. The Schonander-AOT cut film changers are dependable and versatile and withstand years of hard use and abuse without malfunction. The receivers can easily be transported to the dark room for film processing.

The film carriers are heavy and awkward to load, but do allow easy filming in both single and series films. There is minimal film wastage if the equipment is used properly, and unexposed films can be reloaded and used. The film carriers can be loaded with up to 30 films, and filming can be performed at a rate of up to 6 films per second. The filming program can be pre-selected so that almost any series can be obtained. Films can be exposed simultaneously in biplane projection; to prevent cross-fogging, the films can be loaded in the carriers alternately for single plane filming. At our institution we have an electronic system that allows for alternating filming without cross-fogging and without alternating film loading. This has resulted in increased film quality.

Puck. Elema-Schonander manufactures a lightweight movable unit that also uses 14 × 14 inch cut films. Films are limited to two per second, and the carrier is limited to 20 films. This is inadequate for use in a neuroradiology section where more rapid filming is desired. Computer cards are used to program the units, but this method does not seem advantageous. Motion artifacts may occur with these lightweight units.

Roll Film Changers. *Franklin Changer.* This is the best known of the roll film units. It can be used with the biplane technique, and the dimensions of the units allow for an area 11 × 14 inches.

Alternating exposures results in single plane filming—but also in a waste of film. Films may be exposed at a rate of up to 6 per second.

Roll film changers waste more film than do cut film changers. A single test film requires one exposure on a large sheet of film. The last length of film often is too short for a full run, resulting in excessive wastage.

SUMMARY

Although each injector and film changer has its advantages and disadvantages, the author has found the Elema-Schonander 14 × 14 AOT changers and the Viamonte-Hobbs injector to be safe, versatile, dependable, and efficient for use in our neuroradiology procedures.

TECHNICAL COMPLICATIONS

It is clear that the inexperienced operator will have greater difficulty performing angiographic procedures, leading to a greater complication rate. It is imperative that the angiographer be given a basic introduction to standard angiographic methods and techniques—preferably an introduction to angiography using the Seldinger technique for the femoral approach. A sound knowledge of the fundamentals will facilitate the technique of angiography. For neurosurgery residents, who must, by necessity, learn cerebral angiography without the benefit of prior angiography experience, close monitoring of these procedures—preferably by a neuroradiologist—is necessary. The neuroradiologist is versed in film technique and the proper use of equipment as well as in angiographic techniques.

The first introduction to cerebral angiography following thorough verbal instructions should be observation of an experienced operator.

There are some basic techniques that should be followed and certain precautions always to be taken; however, each operator soon develops his or her own techniques. These include minor personal variations on the basic technique.

PREMEDICATION

For adults the author recommends 100 mg Nembutal and 0.4 mg of atropine IM before angiography. For children, I recommend the dosage originally suggested by Taveras as shown at the bottom of this page.

ARTERIOGRAPHY

Definition. *Arteriography* is the visualization of an artery or arteries by x-ray after injection of a radiopaque contrast material. *Angiography* is the radiography of vessels after the injection of a radiopaque material.

History

Cerebral arteriography was first introduced by Egazs Moniz in 1927. The procedure at first employed Thorotrast as a contrast material. It was found later that Thorotrast, because of its properties as both a B⁻ emitter and an alpha particle emitter and because it was taken up by the reticuloendothelial system and not excreted, caused the development of certain types of tumors. The alpha particles are especially implicated because of their short tissue penetration and the great ionization of the tissues through which they pass. Therefore, Thorotrast is no longer used as a contrast material. Through the years many materials have been developed that provide excellent visualization and have only slight toxicity. At the present time, Conray 60 per cent is used most commonly for study of the intracranial vessels. It appears that the meglumine salt of Conray is less toxic to the nervous system than is the sodium salt of other contrast materials. However, many other contrast materials have been and continue to be used for cerebral angiography.

Informed Consent

Before angiography, it is wise for the individual who will be performing the examination to discuss the procedure with the patient, explaining in some detail what will be done. Without going into excessive detail, one must explain both the procedure itself and the possible complications in such a fashion that the patient will readily understand. At the present time the public is well aware of the "informed consent"; because of this, the patient should be told of possible complications, including the possibility of a "stroke." In order to avoid frightening the patient away from a needed procedure, it is wise to use a good deal of discretion when explaining such possibilities to the individual or the family. Such possible difficulties as soreness of the neck, arm, or leg for several days following the procedure and "black and blue" marks at the puncture sites will be readily accepted as normal consequences if the patient is told about them well in advance. Fear of the unknown often frightens the patient most, and any information about the procedure that will alleviate such fears not only will help the patient, but will most certainly be to the operator's advantage.

Anesthesia

As a general rule, all our angiograms are done with the patients awake. General anesthesia can be used and may be necessary in certain cases. It is often used in the pediatric age group.

Filming Technique

Routine filming technique for carotid angiograms is 2 films per second for 3 seconds, and 1 film per second for 6 seconds. We inject 10 cc for a routine common carotid arteriogram, 7 cc for an internal carotid arteriogram, and 3 to 7 cc for an external carotid angiogram, depending on the size of the external carotid or branch vessel being studied. By knowing the timing of the filming sequence, one can evaluate the circulation time in the intracranial system.

AGE (yrs)	SECOBARBITAL (mg/kg)	MEPERIDINE (mg/kg)	ATROPINE, TOTAL DOSE (mg)	CHLORPROMAZINE (mg/kg)
1–4	8–10	1–1.5	0.1–0.2	1.5
5–8	5–7	1–1.5	0.3	1.0
9–12	3–4	1.0	0.4	0.75

Arteriovenous Circulation Time

The period from the greatest beginning concentration of contrast material in the carotid siphon to the maximum concentration in the parietal veins is called the "arteriovenous circulation time." According to various authors, the average time is 4.13 seconds to 4.37 seconds. The circulation time is normally faster in children, and a circulation time greater than 6 seconds is definitely prolonged.

The time can be determined by knowing the timing of the filming sequence, i.e., 2 films per second for 3 seconds and then 1 film per second for 6 seconds. Therefore, one can determine the various circulation times simply by counting the number of films.

In brain death the circulation time is markedly prolonged, and the contrast material does not proceed above the supraclinoid portion of the internal carotid artery. Other causes of a prolonged circulation time are marked increased intracranial pressure, arterial thromboses, diffuse arteriosclerosis, and arterial spasm.

A shortened circulation time is seen with arteriovenous malformations and arteriovenous fistula; it also may be seen with any process that results in early venous drainage, such as infarcts, glioblastoma multiforme, metastases, and brain abscesses.

The author recommends that one should not inject more than 7 or 8 cc into the vertebral artery, except in the presence of an arteriovenous malformation or a very vascular tumor, where a higher volume injection is necessary for visualization of the abnormality.

Puncture Needles

A variety of different needles may be used for cerebral angiography. Figures 4–3 to 4–6 (pp. 156 to 157) illustrate the various needles and guidewires that the author has found satisfactory in daily use.

Cournand-Potts Needle. This needle has a beveled tip and a matching beveled needle hub. In Figure 4–4 (p. 156) it is shown locked into position on the Davis rake. The needle is correctly positioned with the bevel down. The metallic needle extends out beyond the hub of the needle to eliminate "dead space" and to avoid the risk of clot formation within the lumen. The Luer-Lok fitting fastens tightly over the needle hub.

The Davis rake helps to immobilize the needle while it is in the vessel.

Davis Needle. The Davis needle is a long, firm plastic needle with a slight curve at its distal end. The needle has a blunt plastic cannula that occludes the needle between injections. The needle–catheter is placed into the carotid artery using the Seldinger technique. Under fluoroscopic control, the catheter can be manipulated selectively into the internal and external carotid arteries by taking advantage of the distal curve and using the guidewire if necessary.

Brachial Angiography

The brachial angiogram is one of our safest and most frequently performed procedures and usually can be done rapidly and with minimal patient morbidity. As with carotid angiography, the procedure should be discussed at length with the patient. It should be stated that the needle puncture will be in the arm—right or left—and that the injection itself will be quite painful, causing a stinging and burning sensation that will last approximately 10 to 15 seconds. If the injection is into the right arm, pain will be felt in the right elbow, the right shoulder, the right side of the face and neck, in the teeth and behind the eye. If the right brachial injection fills the left carotid these sensations also will be felt in the left carotid distribution. In addition, a less strong sensation will be felt in the rectum and lower extremities caused by the contrast material that enters the arch of the aorta and the descending aorta. The injector and the film changer will create a certain amount of noise while the film series is generated. All these things ideally should be explained to the patient before the examination, and a brief description of the events that will occur during the study should help greatly in allaying the patient's fears.

Technique

The patient should be positioned on the table as comfortably as possible so that the area of interest can be filmed without moving the patient after the needle is in place. The arm is then placed palm up in a 30- to 45-degree abducted position on a firm armboard. A blood pressure cuff is positioned on the lower portion of the forearm. A rolled towel is placed below the distal humerus just above the elbow. This serves to hyperextend the arm and allows for easier puncture of the brachial artery by making the pulse more readily palpable. The arm is then fixed to the armboard by two strips of adhesive tape that circle the arm and attach to the armboard in the upper humeral region and at the level of the wrist.

The brachial artery is palpated and an antiseptic solution applied to the area surrounding the puncture site. A bleb of local anesthetic is then introduced into the skin just over the brachial artery. The artery should be punctured just above the elbow skin crease, where it is most readily palpable. A tiny nick is then made in the anesthetized skin over the brachial artery. The skin nick is made with a surgical blade and prevents dulling of the needle tip by the strong layer of skin. The puncture is then made by piercing the brachial artery. The author prefers a through-and-through puncture of the vessel followed by slow withdrawal of the needle after the inner cannula has been removed. As the needle enters the lumen of the vessel there will be free flow of pulsating blood from the hub of the needle. A flexible guidewire is then introduced and the needle is advanced over the guidewire until it is positioned well in the vessel.

At times the brachial vein will be entered and only venous blood will exit from the hub of the needle. The needle puncture should then be made slightly more laterally, as the brachial artery is lateral to the vein with the patient in the anatomic position.

Steps in Needle Puncture

1. The pulse is palpated by the free hand, and the needle is then passed through the skin nick and soft tissues until its tip rests on the brachial artery and a transmitted pulse can be felt through the needle.

2. The brachial artery is then punctured just above the elbow crease with a sharp forward thrust.

3. The needle should pass through-and-through the vessel; the inner metal cannula is then removed and the plastic sheath slowly withdrawn until there is free flow of pulsating arterial blood.

4. The soft-tipped guidewire is then advanced through the plastic sheath until the tip of the guidewire extends beyond the tip of the needle. The plastic needle is then advanced over the guidewire to the hub of the needle so that its entire length rests in the vessel.

5. The guidewire is then removed and the plastic needle is occluded with the obturator.

6. If there is difficulty advancing the needle—because of an area of narrowing from arteriosclerosis or previous arterial cutdown—

the vessel may then be punctured at a more proximal point. If the puncture is performed at a higher than usual level, great care must be taken to be certain that the vessel is firmly compressed at the puncture site when the needle is removed.

7. At the termination of the procedure, the needle is removed. Firm pressure is applied at the puncture site for 10 minutes.

Occasionally both the brachial artery and vein will be entered simultaneously. Initially one obtains venous blood, followed by pulsating arterial blood. If this is the case, after the needle has been advanced into the artery, pressure should be applied to the puncture site for several minutes to prevent the occurrence of a hematoma.

Volume of Injection

The injections are made using a volume injector. The injector is connected to the needle with a high-pressure clear plastic tubing with an intervening stopcock that allows removal of air bubbles without disconnecting the tubing device. *45 cc of Conray 60 per cent is injected at a rate of 25 cc/second for 1.8 seconds.*

Technique of Filming

If examination of the vessels of the neck is desired, 0.5 second of x-ray delay is recommended, and films are obtained at a rate of 4 films per second for 2 seconds. For the intracranial series, a similar injection is made with 0.7 to 1.0 second of x-ray delay, and filming is done at a standard rate of 2 films per second for the first 3 seconds and 1 film per second for the next 6 seconds. At the time of the injections, the cuff is inflated at the wrist to promote retrograde flow of the contrast material and to prevent antegrade flow of the contrast down to the hand, which is quite painful. All filming is done using a biplane technique.

Some operators perform a single test radiograph of the brachial artery at the puncture site, using a small amount of contrast material. Using our present needle puncture technique, we have found this unnecessary, except in rare cases.

Following the injection, the cuff is deflated at the wrist and the obturator is replaced in the needle. For more exact timing on the intracranial series, the operator should inspect the films to determine how many seconds or what fraction of a second will be required in order to set

Table 4–1. Filming Technique and Contrast Amounts—Conray 60 Per Cent

PROCEDURE	CONTRAST MATERIAL AMOUNTS	TOTAL
Common carotid arteriogram	10 cc/sec for 1 sec	10 cc
Internal carotid arteriogram	10 cc/sec for 0.7 sec	7 cc
External carotid arteriogram	10 cc/sec for 0.3 to 0.7 sec	3–7 cc
	or	
	0.3 to 0.7 cc/sec for 1 sec	3–7 cc
Brachial arteriogram	25 cc/sec for 1.8 sec	45 cc
Arch arteriogram	25 cc/sec for 2 sec	50 cc
	(Renografin-76)	
Innominate or subclavian arteriogram for visualization of vertebral artery when selective catheterization cannot be performed	10 to 14 cc/sec for 2 to 3 sec	20–40 cc
Vertebral arteriogram	10 cc/sec for 0.3–0.7 sec	3–7 cc
	or	
	0.3 to 0.7 cc/sec for 1 sec	

an appropriate "x-ray delay." Thus, there will be one blank film followed by films with contrast material in the intracranial circulation.

This method of filming allows for adequate visualization of the intracranial circulation in nearly all cases. Slower and more prolonged filming may be needed when there is slow circulation of contrast material owing to elevated intracranial pressure.

Complications

Occasionally contrast material will extravasate from the vessel into the muscle of the arm. This is very painful for the patient, and a film will reveal the radiodense contrast in the soft tissues. When this occurs the needle should be removed and compression applied. No further puncture attempt should be made until 48 hours have passed.

A subintimal injection also may occur that dissects the vessel over a variable length. Figure 4–7 (p. 158) demonstrates the intimal flap.

Because of the force of the injection, the needle rarely may be pushed backward out of the vessel; for this reason, precautions should be taken that the needle is secured in place before injection.

Anatomic Variations

In approximately 1 per cent of patients one will encounter an aberrant right subclavian artery. In such a case, only the vertebral artery will fill from the brachial injection, and right carotid arteriography will have to be performed. In 20 to 25 per cent of cases, the left carotid artery arises as a common trunk with the right innominate vessel. This normal anatomic variation may or may not be of help. If one does not wish to fill the left carotid circulation, the left carotid vessel can be compressed during the time of the injection and into the early venous phase. This will prevent contrast from entering the left carotid artery, allowing visualization of only the right carotid artery and the right carotid and right vertebral circulation. Obviously, a second injection without left carotid compression will allow comparison between the two sides (see Fig. 4–20, p. 167). On the other hand, compression of the left carotid artery may cause the contrast material to cross over to the left side via the anterior communicating artery—again filling the left internal carotid system.

The left vertebral artery arises as a separate trunk from the aortic arch in approximately 5 per cent of cases. In the vast majority of patients, the left vertebral circulation will be visualized by left brachial injection. In the majority of cases the left vertebral artery is the dominant supplying vessel to the vertebralbasilar system. It should be noted that, in 5 per cent of cases, the vertebral artery will end in the posterior inferior cerebellar artery, and there will be no visualization of the remainder of the posterior fossa. In such instances, contralateral brachial arteriography will be needed.

Percutaneous Carotid Arteriogram

This procedure should be discussed with the patient before it is undertaken. It is important that both the procedure itself and its risks should be discussed at sufficient length to ensure informed consent. The more a patient knows about the procedure, the better. The fear element is reduced, and, in general, the patient is able to co-operate better. The physician who is to perform the procedure should visit the patient in the hospital room.

Puncture Technique

Individual angiographers soon develop a personal technique that is satisfactory and comfortable for them. However, while learning the methods, the beginning angiographer will be assisted by these guidelines for puncture technique:

1. Extend the neck by elevating the table and allowing the head to fall over the end of the table or by inflating a balloon under the patient's shoulders. These steps result in extension of the neck.

2. The area is then cleaned widely with three washes of antiseptic solution, the last an application of alcohol.

3. The carotid artery is then palpated in the neck with the hand that will not hold the puncture needle.

4. When the pulse is well localized, a local anesthetic is injected into the skin at the anticipated point of puncture. The author recommends puncturing the vessel two finger-breadths above the clavicle. This way, the puncture should always be well below the bifurcation. A second injection of local anesthetic is then introduced between the trachea and carotid artery and beneath the carotid artery. This second bolus should be approximately 5 to 6 cc and it serves several purposes.

   a. It anesthetizes the local area in the neck where the puncture needle will be thrust when the puncture attempts are made.

   b. The bolus serves to immobilize the vessel, therefore allowing an easier puncture.

   c. If the carotid artery is situated too far medially and under the trachea, this bolus of local anesthetic will move the vessel laterally and forward into a more accessible position. This bolus of anesthetic should be injected deep enough so that it is *below* the vessel. Putting the local anesthetic in the tissues between the skin and the vessel only serves to obscure the pulse and make the puncture more difficult.

5. A small nick is then made in the skin with a scalpel blade so that the tip of the puncture needle is not dulled while entering through the skin.

6. The vessel is then palpated and immobi-

lized by the free hand. This can be done by reaching lateral to the vessel with the fingertips and pulling the vessel medially, thus trapping the vessel between the fingers and the bolus of local anesthetic. Or the vessel can be immobilized by trapping it between the tips of the index and middle finger—one finger on either side of the vessel.

7. The puncture needle is then advanced through the skin nick and soft tissues until the tip of the needle rests directly on the carotid artery and the pulsations transmitted from the vessel can be felt in the needle.

8. The vessel is then impaled by a single forward thrust of the needle or by multiple short forward thrusts.

9. If a Cournand-Potts needle (see Fig. 4–4, p. 156) is used, the needle puncture is performed with the bevel up.

10. I recommend through-and-through puncture of the vessel, although some operators prefer to puncture only the anterior wall.

11. The needle is then rotated 180 degrees so that the bevel is down and is slowly withdrawn, holding the hub close to the patient's neck and chest, until bright red pulsating blood appears from the hub of the needle.

12. The soft-tipped guidewire is then advanced through the needle until the tip of the wire is well beyond the tip of the needle. The needle is then advanced over the guidewire approximately 1 cm. The guidewire is then withdrawn, the obturator is placed in the needle, and the needle is immobilized with a Davis rake (see Figs. 4–3 and 4–8, pp. 156 and 159).

13. The patient is then placed in position for filming. If desired, a short run of films or even a single film may be exposed following the injection of contrast material to rule out the presence of a subintimal injection.

There should be free flow of blood from the needle at all times and easy flushing of the vessel with nonheparinized saline throughout the procedure. The absence of a free flow of blood or easy flushing may mean that the needle tip is subintimal or has become dislodged from the vessel lumen. *NEVER* inject contrast if these criteria are not met. The injection of contrast under less than optimal conditions presents significant danger to the patient. Complete occlusion of a vessel could prevent flow to the hemisphere, possibly resulting in a stroke or even death.

The author recommends the use of the obturator between injections rather than continuous or intermittent flushing. At the time of injection, a short, flexible connecting tube is attached to a syringe filled with saline. A stopcock is placed between the saline-filled tube and the syringe. The tubing is connected to the hub of the needle after the obturator is removed; then the closed stopcock is opened, and blood is allowed to fill the clear plastic tubing. If no bubbles of air are present, the tube is flushed with saline. Then the patient may be asked whether there is a cold, salty taste in his mouth from the flushing solution (confirming injection into the carotid system) or whether he feels pain in his neck (possibly implying a subintimal or extravascular injection). If all is well, the syringe is disconnected, the tubing is connected to the tubing on the injector, and the study is performed. I recommend the use of a volume injector and a dose of 10 cc/second over a 1-second period. The injection can be made by hand, but this is less readily reproducible and results in needless radiation exposure to the operator. There is no advantage to hand injection of contrast, and I do *not* recommend it.

Film exposure should begin with the contrast injection. This will ensure a blank film followed by films showing contrast material in the circulation.

The normal carotid bifurcation is at the level of C_4. At the time of intravascular injection, the contrast material will be seen as a "jet stream" (Fig. 4–8, p. 159); later films demonstrate the normal carotid bifurcation. A slight dilatation of the proximal internal carotid artery is normal; this is the carotid sinus.

The location of the bifurcation can vary, and it may be seen either above (Fig. 4–9, p. 160) or below (Fig. 4–10, p. 160) the C_4 level.

Occasionally an enlarged superior thyroid artery will be punctured in the mistaken belief that it is the carotid artery. A successful examination is unlikely if this occurs.

If a clamp has been placed on the common carotid artery that partially occludes the vessel, puncture can be performed above the clamp.

The carotid artery occasionally may exhibit a "buckle" along its course. This may vary in size or position.

Complications

If there is a *subintimal injection* demonstrated on the neck series, or if there is some other technical difficulty with the procedure, the needle should be removed and 10 minutes of compression applied to the puncture site. It should be remembered that, even with a subintimal injection, there may be excellent flow from the needle—apparently because the intimal flap "holds" the cephalad flow of blood and actually directs the blood to the tip of the needle. The author has noted that patients frequently complain of pain in the ear or in the angle of the jaw when there is a subintimal injection. This pain also occurs occasionally without a subintimal injection; thus it should not be used as a definite sign of this complication (Figs. 4–11 and 4–12, p. 161).

Injection into the soft tissues of the neck is very painful for the patient and results in an amorphous collection of contrast in the patient's neck on the radiographs. If injection is subintimal or extravascular, the needle should be removed and compression applied for 10 minutes. The procedure is then delayed for 48 hours.

Occasionally a hematoma will develop in the neck during the procedure. If this occurs, pressure should be applied locally. If a hematoma develops while the needle is in place, gentle but firm pressure should be applied over the needle and the study performed and completed without further delay. In this situation, it may be necessary to remove the needle before viewing the films. It appears that these hematomas occur from bleeding from small muscular branches or from the back wall puncture site in the common carotid artery. This may occur because of a coagulopathy secondary to anticoagulation therapy or liver disease, or a hematoma may develop secondary to bleeding from the back wall puncture site when the needle has gone through-and-through the vessel. If the hematoma becomes so large that it compromises the airway, the study should be terminated.

At the time of administration of the local anesthetic, *great* care should be taken to prevent the intra-arterial injection of xylocaine, since this leads to grand mal seizures. If this should occur, the study should be terminated and undertaken at another time.

Percutaneous vertebral artery puncture was first performed in 1940. With the use of femoral artery catheterization and selective study of the intracranial vessels, this method is no longer in popular use. The author has had no experience with this technique and does not recommend its use. The vertebral artery arises from the subclavian vessels and enters into the foramina transversaria at the level of the sixth cervical vertebra in most of the cases. There is some variation in the level of entrance into the foramina transversaria, however, and the vessel may enter at any level (Fig. 4–13, p. 162). The vessel is probed and punctured as it travels in the foramina transversaria. Following the procedure, there is no way to apply adequate pressure to the puncture site, and conceivably excess bleeding could lead to a hematoma and occlusion of the vertebral artery. At the present time, vertebral angiotherapy is performed using direct catheterization. Approximately 4 to 7 cc of contrast material is used with either percutaneous angiography or the catheterization technique.

The catheterization technique can provoke arterial spasm. An example is shown in Figure 4–14, p. 163.

Occasionally at the time of carotid angiography, the vertebral artery will be entered inadvertently. In this case, the puncture needle is usually found to be quite deep in the soft tissues of the neck. In addition, it will be noted that while the guidewire may thread up the vessel, the puncture needle will not follow because the vessel is within the foramina transversaria. This is particularly common when the metallic puncture needle is used; the plastic needle occasionally will thread without difficulty.

The true nature of the puncture site may not become apparent until the films are processed. Fairly commonly both the vertebral and carotid arteries will be entered simultaneously. If this is suspected, the puncture needle should be withdrawn slowly and correctly positioned when there is pulsating flow from the carotid artery after the needle has been removed from the vertebral vessel.

Femoral Artery Catheterization

History and Complications

Femoral artery catheterization and selective injection of the visceral vessels was first described by Seldinger in the 1950s. This method has increased greatly in popularity since its discovery and is now used quite commonly in most centers. It has greatly facilitated the evaluation of those patients requiring study of multiple vessels. With this method, multiple vessel studies can be accomplished without a great deal of difficulty or trauma to the patient. There are, of course, certain dangers.

The limitations are obvious in older patients who have significant peripheral vascular disease and interruption of the vascular supply to the legs. The placement of the femoral catheter may compromise blood flow to such a degree that the leg may become cold and pulseless. If

there is any possibility that this may occur, another approach should be used. In addition, in the older age groups, the femoral vessels may have become so tortuous that retrograde catheterization is impossible. In addition to the arteriosclerotic changes that occur in the lower limbs and the tortuosity of the vessels, one must also contend with similar changes in the great vessels as they arise from the arch of the aorta. It has been shown by pathologic studies that the great vessels tend to be spared from arteriosclerotic change from their point of origin at the arch to the levels of the carotid artery bifurcations. While there is little arteriosclerotic change, there is often a good deal of tortuosity, making the catheterization of the vessels difficult. The changes secondary to aging appear to become much more pronounced in hypertensive patients.

Axillary Artery Catheterization

If femoral catheterization is not possible, one can use the axillary approach. The axilla is prepped and draped in the same fashion as is used for the femoral approach. The axillary artery, preferably on the right side, is punctured high in the axilla, and after guidewire placement the catheter is placed in the arch and then selectively placed into the great vessels as they arise from the arch, using fluoroscopic guidance. The same catheters that are used for the femoral approach are used for the axillary studies. Because atherosclerotic changes may also affect the subclavian arteries, care must be taken with manipulation in the subclavian arteries so that inadvertent embolization of atherosclerotic debris does not occur. Because of these severe atherosclerotic changes, axillary catheterization may sometimes be impossible. If this is the case, then percutaneous studies can be performed.

In busy departments there are occasional patients who will need percutaneous examination; although this event is uncommon, a discussion of the percutaneous approach is included in this text. In those departments where invasive studies are performed by the neurosurgeon or neurologist, the radiologist should be aware of the uses and hazards of these various techniques.

Catheters Available

Various types of catheters have been used, and each has advantages in certain situations. In the very young age groups, and in the absence of anomalous vessels, a straight or gently curved catheter may be all that is necessary to selectively catheterize all the cerebral vessels. The order of study would appear to be in part arbitrary. However, if there is a particular area of interest, it would seem prudent to review the circulation in this vessel distribution first. If the study should be ended prematurely, the area of interest will be visualized. In patients in their second and third decades, the gently curved catheter may be used with a good deal of success. In most instances, the left carotid artery is the most difficult vessel to visualize, and, anticipating this, one might proceed directly to the catheterization of this artery. An argument can be made in favor of this approach, since the catheter loses its rigidity while it remains in the body heat. In anticipation of these various vascular patterns, some operators do not use standard manufactured catheters but choose to create their own from basic materials. In this way the curve of the catheter can be formed to meet the needs of each case. This works well for some; however, I have found that the standard, preformed manufactured catheters have served our purposes well.

With the development of newer catheters it has become possible to perform catheterization studies in older individuals. Patients with iliofemoral vascular occlusive disease cannot, of course, undergo femoral catheterization.

A variety of standard-shaped catheters are now available from multiple manufacturers. The individual operator will discover, through trial and error, which catheters best suit his or her needs. A straight or pigtail multiple-end and side-hold catheter is necessary for arch angiography except when digital angiographic techniques are used.

In older patients, I have found the "Sidewinder-Femoral Cerebral #III" catheter manufactured by the Cordis company to be especially satisfactory. In more difficult cases, the right carotid and either the left or right vertebral artery are catheterized with the "Femoral-Cerebral I" with the gentle curve. The catheter is then changed to the "Sidewinder" for catheterization of the left carotid artery.

This "S"-shaped catheter is unique, but with experience the individual angiographer can become accustomed to its use. The manufacturer recommends forming a loop with the catheter so that the large curve of the catheter rests in the ascending aorta, the distal part of the catheter curls back upon itself, and the small curve is directed cephalad. The tip of the catheter is then manipulated until it rests in the origin of the vessel to be catheterized. A small amount of injected contrast ensures that the proper vessel has been catheterized. At times it is necessary to perform the study by injection from this point. If this is the case, 12 cc of Conray 60 per cent should be injected rather than the usual 10 cc. To position the catheter tip higher in the vessel, it is necessary to pull *back* on the catheter at the puncture site. This will cause the catheter to unroll and advance up into the vessel. The author has found this catheter unsatisfactory for catheterization of the vertebral arteries.

For any catheter and catheterization technique, liberal use of the guidewire is recommended to facilitate both catheter placement and advancement. At our institution the guidewires and catheters are used once and then discarded.

Injections in the common carotid artery should be 1.5 cm below the carotid bifurcation. Intermittent flushing should be done with saline containing 1 cc of 1000 units/cc of heparin/500 cc of saline.

With experience and practice each operator develops an individual technique for both puncture and catheter placement.

Complications of Cerebral Angiography

Complications that may occur with any type of arteriographic study are:

1. hematoma
2. subintimal injection
3. hypotension or hypertension
4. allergic reaction
5. femoral embolus
6. cerebral embolus
7. angina
8. emesis
9. nausea
10. change in mentation
11. monoparesis
12. hemiparesis
13. aphasia
14. visual disturbance
15. seizure
16. vertigo
17. numb fingers
18. headache
19. global amnesia
20. death

During the course of the study, it is wise to converse with the patient so that any change in the mental status will be readily appreciated. If such a change does occur, the study should be stopped and performed at another time.

General Guidelines for Post-Angiogram Orders

Post-Angiogram Orders

For brachial angiogram:
1. Bed rest for 4 hours
2. Keep arm straight for 1 hour
3. Vital signs every 15 minutes for 2 hours, every 30 minutes for 2 hours, every 60 minutes for 2 hours and until stable
4. Resume previous diet and orders
5. IV orders as needed
6. Cold packs to puncture site for pain

For carotid angiogram:
1. Bed rest for 8 hours
2. Vital signs every 15 minutes for 2 hours, every 30 minutes for 2 hours, every 60 minutes for 2 hours and until stable
3. Resume previous diet and orders
4. Cold packs to puncture site for pain
5. IV orders as needed

For femoral angiogram:
1. Flat in bed for 8 hours and complete bed rest for 24 hours
2. Vital signs every 15 minutes for 2 hours, every 30 minutes for 2 hours, every 60 minutes for 2 hours and until stable
3. Check peripheral pulses and puncture site when taking vital signs
4. IV orders as needed
5. Cold packs to puncture site as needed for pain
6. Resume previous diet and orders

Knotted Catheter

It should be mentioned that certain catheters with multiple loops at the end sometimes tie in a knot (Fig. 4–15, p. 163). In addition to the hazard of knot formation, the catheter may loop back upon itself and form a functional knot. Various methods have been described to remove these knots or untie them without operative intervention. If this unfortunate event should occur, *DO NOT* remove the catheter from the aortic arch, which provides sufficient room for catheter manipulation.

Most frequently, knotting occurs when the catheter is being torqued rapidly in 360-degree circles in an attempt to enter a vessel; with multiple-end curved catheters, however, this rapid torquing should *not* be used for just this reason. The steps described below should be followed when attempting to unknot the catheter:

1. Pass a guidewire through the catheter, using the firm end in the hope of loosening the knot.
2. Inject the maximum amount of contrast material in an attempt to open or loosen the knot and to provide space for a guidewire to open the catheter.
3. The opposite femoral artery can be punctured and a straight catheter passed through the loop in the knot. The knotted catheter is then pulled against this to open the knot.
4. If the catheter is kinked upon itself but is not knotted, firm pressure over the groin while the catheter is pulled down and removed will forcibly open the catheter as it exits from the vessel. With such traumatic removal of the catheter, the limb should be observed very carefully for compromise of the circulation.
5. If all attempts fail, the catheter will have to be removed surgically.

The long multicurved catheters should be manipulated gently and never "twirled" in an attempt to achieve placement. Indeed, because of the possibility of complications, a vascular surgeon should be available for consultation and emergency procedures if needed.

Subtraction

The technique of subtraction was originally described by Ziedses des Plantes in 1935. The purpose of "subtraction" is to remove or "subtract" the image of the bony structures from the radiograph by using various photographic techniques. This allows visualization of the normal vasculature, but, more important, exposes areas of abnormal vascularity which are seen only faintly or not at all without the use of subtraction. The technique is especially helpful when studying the vessels at the base of the brain and in the study of the posterior fossa anatomy, where there are dense overlying bony structures.

We use a subtraction unit that has a timer that allows for fixed exposure times. Times can be varied from one tenth of a second through 15 seconds. This type of unit makes possible dependable reproduction and repetition of the desired exposure times. In addition, the unit can function as a view-box for continuous viewing. There is also a variety of light bulbs of varying intensity that have independent switches for alteration of the light exposure level. The unit has the appearance of a view-box with a glass top; the lights of varying intensity are positioned below the viewing area and the exposure timer. The technique requires the use of a darkroom.

Although many different methods for performing the subtraction have been worked out using a variety of films, at our institution we use Kodak subtraction masking film and Du Pont Cronex subtraction print film.

The technique requires the use of a "blank" film of a standard serial run of films plus a film taken after contrast material has been introduced into the vessels. It is important that the patient remain motionless during the serial run of films.

The first step is making of the subtraction mask film. The blank film of the run is placed in the view-box of the unit. A single sheet of Kodak subtraction masking film is placed emulsion side down over the area to be subtracted. The unit's lid is closed, and an exposure is made using a 7-watt bulb for 3 seconds. When this mask film is processed it will be a very dark reversal image of the original blank film.

The mask film is then placed on the view-box and taped in position. A film from the serial run demonstrating contrast material within the vessels is then exactly superimposed on the subtraction mask. Exact superimposition will be impossible if the patient moved during the film run. This second film is taped in place so that it too is immobile. The films are superimposed while the unit is on continuous view, and the operator will be able to see the "subtraction" of the bones and the exposure of the previously unvisualized portions of the vascular system.

A single sheet of Du Pont subtraction print film is then placed over the area of interest (emulsion down), and the lid of the unit is closed so that good film contact is obtained. The final exposure is then made, using a 40-watt bulb and an exposure time of 0.5 second. When this film is processed, the final image will demonstrate the vessels without the overlying bony structures.

One may choose to subtract only one film of a series, or the entire film run can be subtracted. The technique of making the mask or final print can be varied from case to case, depending on the exposure of the films. In general, however, the method described will prove satisfactory for most cases.

Tips for Use

1. Either the arterial or venous phase may be subtracted.

2. The exposure times may be varied to obtain a more precise technique in an individual case.

3. If the patient moved during the filming, the final print film may still prove satisfactory if an attempt is made to subtract the image in a small area of interest. The remainder of the image may be blurred, but that is of no consequence.

4. If several areas must be viewed, subtractions can be made individually in the areas of interest.

5. If no blank films are obtained at the start of a serial run, the late venous phase or last film of the run sometimes can be used as the "blank."

Applied Cerebrovascular Embryology and Normal Anatomy

EMBRYOLOGY

During the course of embryologic development there are six brachial arches and clefts. A number of these disappear entirely; however, some remain to form the brachiocephalic system as we know it. Figure 4–16 (p. 164) demonstrates the origin of the various segments of the cleft and arches and the vessels that are present in the normal adult. These development changes need not be committed to memory but do aid in achieving an understanding of the anatomy of the great vessels.

Aberrant Right Subclavian Artery. This anomaly is of some significance to the angiographer. The aberrant right subclavian artery arises distal to the origin of the left subclavian artery. This occurs because the stem of the right subclavian artery originates from the right dorsal arch and the seventh intersegmental artery. With shortening of the aorta between the left common carotid artery and the left subclavian artery, the abnormal right subclavian artery is found below the left subclavian. Because its origin is from the right side, it must cross the midline to reach the right arm.

When this happens, the right common carotid artery arises directly from the arch as an independent branch, and only the right vertebral artery arises from the right subclavian. Therefore, a right brachial arteriogram demonstrates only the vertebral circulation; the right carotid circulation must be studied separately. Catheterization of these vessels will also need to be adapted to the anatomic variations.

ANASTOMOSES

Primitive Internal Carotid— Vertebrobasilar

Three main vessels connect the internal carotid with the vertebrobasilar system. They are, in order of occurrence, the persistent trigeminal artery, the primitive acoustic artery and the primitive hypoglossal artery. The possibility of one of these persistent primitive communications should come to mind when a common carotid injection also fills in a large part of the anatomic distribution of the vertebrobasilar system. However, with advanced arteriosclerotic occlusive vascular disease there may be filling of the vertebrobasilar system via collateral circulation from the external carotid artery. In such patients, close examination is required to be certain that indeed a primitive communication is present between the internal carotid artery and the basilar artery.

Persistent Trigeminal Artery. Of the three persistent primitive communications between the internal carotid and vertebrobasilar system, the persistent trigeminal artery is the most common (Fig. 4–17, p. 165).

The trigeminal artery originates from the internal carotid artery just proximal to the intracavernous portion of the carotid artery and follows a tortuous curvilinear course posteriorly to join the basilar artery. Without proper attention, this vessel may be mistaken for a large posterior communicating artery; however, the point of origin is different. The posterior communicating artery arises from the supraclinoid portion of the internal carotid artery.

The persistent trigeminal artery is associated with an increased incidence of aneurysms.

Primitive Acoustic Artery. The second most common primitive communicating vessel is the acoustic artery. This vessel connects the petrous portion of the internal carotid artery with the basilar artery.

Primitive Hypoglossal Artery. This rare persistent communication (Fig. 4–18, p. 166) connects the cervical portion of the internal carotid artery with the basilar artery via the hypoglossal canal.

NORMAL ANATOMY

The right carotid artery arises from the innominate artery shortly after its take-off from the arch of the aorta. The left common carotid artery arises as a separate trunk from the arch of the aorta (Figs. 4–19 to 4–22, pp. 167 and 168). The left subclavian artery arises just distal to the left carotid artery.

The bifurcations of the carotid arteries into the internal and external carotid arteries occur at the level of the fourth cervical vertebra. The bifurcation level varies from individual to individual, but the bifurcations usually are at the same level on each side. At the level of the bifurcation in the neck, the internal carotid artery usually courses lateral and posterior to the external carotid artery. The artery runs in the carotid sheath, and is medial to the internal jugular vein. The vagus nerve runs posteriorly between the two vessels. The internal carotid artery then courses cephalad until it enters the carotid canal at the base of the skull. The internal carotid artery may have kinks or tortuous loops in the neck. These are normal anatomic variations (see illustration). There are four divisions of the internal carotid artery. They are the (1) cervical portion, (2) petrous portion, (3) cavernous portion, and (4) supraclinoid, or intradural, portion. There are no branches of the cervical portion of the internal carotid artery. The other three segments have various branches—only some of which are of consequence to the neuroradiologist. The petrous portion: caroticotympanic, artery of the pterygoid canal (vidian artery). The cavernous portion: cavernous branches, hypophyseal branches, semilunar branches, meningeal branches, ophthalmic artery. The supraclinoid portion: posterior communicating artery, anterior choroidal artery, anterior cerebral artery, middle cerebral artery.

After its entrance into the carotid canal, the internal carotid artery courses anteromedially until it lies adjacent and just lateral to the sella turcica. As the internal carotid artery courses in the carotid canal it passes endocranially past the foramen lacerum. Indeed, as viewed from below, the internal carotid artery can be seen in the foramen lacerum, but the artery does not pass "through-and-through" the foramen lacerum. As the carotid enters into the cavernous portion of its course, it turns to course superiorly toward the posterior clinoid process; it then turns to course first anteriorly and then superiorly on the medial side of the anterior clinoid process and perforates the dura mater. In the cavernous portion, the internal carotid artery lies in close relationship to the third, fourth, sixth, and ophthalmic and the maxillary branches of the fifth cranial nerves. Because of the close relationship of these nerves at the level of the cavernous sinus, a cavernous sinus thrombosis may be diagnosed clinically by pareses of these nerve branches. Beneath the anterior clinoid process the internal carotid artery turns to course first superiorly and then posteriorly. Because of this "S"-shaped course, this is called the carotid siphon. Just at the level of the exit of the internal carotid artery as it pierces the dura to become intracranial, the ophthalmic artery arises and courses anteriorly to supply the globe.

At its origin, the ophthalmic artery lies lateral to the optic nerve. More distally, the artery will be seen to cross superiorly over the optic nerve and then to lie on the medial side of the optic nerve. The ophthalmic artery then gives off multiple retinal arteries, ethmoidal branches, and may give rise to an angiographically visible anterior meningeal artery. The terminal branches of the ophthalmic artery exit through the supraorbital foramen and distribute themselves over a small patch of skin covering the medial end of the eyebrow and forehead on each side. It is the branches of the external carotid feeding the teeth, tongue, cheek, and the soft tissues of the neck and scalp that cause the stinging and burning sensations felt when contrast material is injected. By avoiding injection of contrast material into the external carotid system, one can prevent considerable discomfort to the patient. Also, in a combative patient, if an internal carotid angiogram is performed rather than a common carotid artery angiogram, there is less likely to be motion artifact on the study. This is, of course, in the absence of a tumor (e.g., a meningioma), where the external carotid feeders may supply vital information concerning vascular supply to the tumor.

As the carotid artery makes its final bend superiorly above the anterior clinoid process, the posterior communicating artery arises. The posterior communicating artery is one portion of the circle of Willis. It courses posteromedially to join with the posterior cerebral artery on the same side. This vessel does not fill on each arteriogram. Indeed, it may vary greatly in size from individual to individual, and may even be hypoplastic and nonfunctioning in some cases. There is sometimes a junctional dilatation at the level of the vessel's origin. This is called an *infundibulum*. If the junctional dilatation measures more than 3 mm, it may be considered an aneurysm. If the posterior cerebral artery arises directly from the internal carotid artery, as it does occasionally, it is considered a primitive posterior cerebral artery.

Just above the origin of the posterior communicating artery the anterior choroidal artery arises (Fig. 4–28, p. 174). This vessel may also have a junctional dilatation. On the anterior view, this vessel will be seen to course laterally in a curvilinear fashion. The anterior choroidal artery also simultaneously courses posteriorly until it enters the anterior tip of the temporal horn, where it feeds the choroid plexus in the roof of the temporal horn. Occasionally, on the lateral view one may see the blush of the choroid plexus in the temporal horn as it feeds the very vascular capillary plexus of the choroid.

Vascular Alterations with Transtentorial Herniation

One should remember that there is a choroid plexus in all of the ventricles. The choroid plexus of the lateral ventricle lies in the floor of the ventricle; it then follows around to the atrium of the lateral ventricle and then continues to the roof of the temporal horn. The hippocampal gyrus of the temporal horn runs in the floor of the temporal horn; thus, when transtentorial herniation is present, the anterior choroidal vessel will be seen to have a more medial position than normal.

The posterior cerebral artery and the basal vein of Rosenthal also follow a similar course. Therefore, with transtentorial herniation, it will be seen that these vessels are displaced medially. One must remember that the free edge of the tentorium extends forward from the level of the attachment of the falx and the straight sinus up to the posterior clinoids; its most anterior extent is up to the anterior clinoids. Through this tentorial notch extends the midbrain. The midbrain itself consists of the cerebral peduncles, the collicular plate, and a portion of the cerebral aqueduct.

Correlation with Midbrain Anatomy

All the descending tracts from the cerebral hemispheres descend and coalesce at the level of the cerebral peduncles. At this level, all these tracts pass from the supratentorial to the infratentorial areas through the tentorial notch or "slit," as it is sometimes called. Because all the tracts are confined to a small area at this level, even a small lesion will produce considerable neurologic damage. For a lesion on the cerebral cortex to produce the same amount of damage, the affected area would have to be quite large.

The third cranial nerve arises along the inferior portion of the belly of the pons and also courses forward along the free edge of the tentorium. Because of this anatomic proximity, the third nerve is also affected when there is temporal lobe herniation, and the third nerve is trapped by the free edge of the tentorium as the uncus of the hippocampal gyrus is forced over and below the free edge of the tentorium. This will be reflected by physical examination as a third nerve palsy on the affected side.

Anterior Cerebral Artery

Above the origin of the anterior choroidal artery, the supraclinoid internal carotid artery divides into the anterior and middle cerebral arteries. The anterior cerebral artery courses anterior and medially, lying along and supplying the medial surface of the cerebral hemisphere.

Anterior Communicating Artery

Just anterior to the lamina terminalis, the anterior cerebral arteries are very close together and are connected by the anterior communicating artery. This also is a portion of the circle of Willis. Proximal to the anterior communicating artery, the horizontal portion of the anterior cerebral artery gives rise to the medial group of lenticulostriate arteries (Fig. 4–29, p. 174).

The anterior cerebral artery then gives rise to the frontopolar artery, which supplies the frontal lobe along its medial surface and laps over the anterior inferior surface to become visible on the lateral view. The anterior cerebral trunk then gives rise to the pericallosal artery, which roughly parallels the course of the callosal artery but is more superiorly placed. The callosal marginal artery and its branches also supply the frontal lobe; it extends up and over the medial surface of the frontal lobe to become visible on the lateral surface of the brain (see Fig. 4–26, p. 172).

The pericallosal artery follows along the edge of the corpus callosum, although it is not closely applied to it in the normal state. This pericallosal artery then breaks up posteriorly into a small but vascular capillary plexus that lies on top of the corpus callosum and appears as a tiny "moustache" on the arteriogram (see Fig. 4–38, p. 181). The position of the pericallosal plexus can give an important clue about the presence of a tumor or space-occupying lesion when there is a tilting of the "moustache" on the AP view. This pericallosal plexus is not readily seen on the lateral view. In addition, there are potential collateral anastomoses with the posterior pericallosal branches of the posterior cerebral artery. These anastomoses may open if there is a block of the more proximal pericallosal artery.

Recurrent Artery of Heubner

The recurrent artery of Heubner arises from the anterior cerebral artery distal to the anterior communicating artery. The artery then courses laterally behind the anterior cerebral artery. Its position is approximately horizontal to the horizontal portion of the anterior cerebral artery. The artery then enters the medial portion of the anterior perforated substance, where it supplies the anterior limits of the internal capsule, the rostral and medial aspects of the putamen, and the head of the caudate nucleus. In standard angiographic projections this vessel is obscured by the horizontal portion of the anterior cerebral artery.

Middle Cerebral Artery

The middle cerebral artery runs anteromedially in the sylvian fissure between the frontal lobes and the anterior tip of the temporal lobe. Along its horizontal portion, the middle cerebral artery gives rise to the orbital frontal branch, which feeds the inferior portion of the frontal lobe over the roofs of the orbits. Also along its horizontal portion, the middle cerebral artery gives rise to the lateral lenticulostriate vessels, which pierce the anterior perforated substance and supply the basal ganglia. (*Stria* is another term for basal ganglia; *lentiform* nucleus means the putamen, the internal capsule, and the globus pallidus.) The middle cerebral artery branches in its more lateral extent in a rapid series of bifurcations or into a single trifurcation (see Fig. 4–31, p. 176). This region of the middle cerebral artery is known as the genu (or knee) of the middle cerebral artery, or, more generally, as the region of the "trifurcation" of the middle cerebral artery. The middle cerebral artery then enters the region of the isle of Reil. This island of tissue develops as the brain enlarges, and the temporal and parietal lobes grow over this area of tissue. Indeed, in the anatomic specimen, if one pulls open the sylvian fissure by pulling the parietal lobe up and the temporal lobe down, the isle of Reil is visible. The main branches of the middle cerebral artery are contained in this isle before they exit and distribute themselves over the convexities of the brain.

It is at this point that the branches of the middle cerebral artery in the isle of Reil course posteriorly and superiorly. Each branch of the middle cerebral artery courses superiorly in the sylvian fissure until it reaches the isle of Reil; the branches then turn inferiorly and then laterally along the operculum (lid) of the isle until they reach the opening of the sylvian fissure, where they exit, turn superiorly or inferiorly, and then distribute themselves over the cerebral convexities.

As a rule, each of these branches is named after the area it supplies: e.g., the frontoparietal opercular branches, the parieto-opercular branches, etc. Meticulous anatomic studies have been performed to provide individual labels for each of the branches of the middle cerebral artery, but such detail is beyond the scope of this book. The branches that supply the temporal lobe course inferiorly and are named the temporal opercular branches.

It can be seen that the isle of Reil is triangular, with one limb along the upper portion of this area of tissue. This part is known as the roof of the sylvian triangle. A line can be drawn along the tops of the middle cerebral branches as they rise to the top of the isle of Reil and then turn down and laterally to exit. This line connecting the upper portions of the loops of the middle cerebral artery, from the most anterior to the most posterior branch, forms the angiographic roof of the sylvian triangle. Normally, four to six loops form the roof of the triangle. The other two sides of the sylvian triangle are established by connecting a point placed at the level of the genu of the middle cerebral artery (as seen on the lateral view) with the most anterior and most posterior points of the roof (see Fig. 4–23, p. 169).

The Sylvian Triangle

The sylvian triangle is one of our most useful angiographic landmarks. Each time an angiogram is reviewed, the sylvian triangle should be identified and its position checked relative to the anticipated normal. The beginning angiographer should *measure* the position of the triangle after identifying it. According to Traveras, in the normal individual the sylvian point—which is the last branch to exit from the sylvian triangle—should be 30 to 43 mm from the inner table of the skull in its side-to-side position, as measured on the AP film. The sylvian point should lie approximately midway, ± 1 cm, between a line drawn tangent to the inner table of the skull and the top of the petrous bone or the orbital roof, whichever is lower. Any displacement from this anticipated normal position should be noted (Fig. 4–25, p. 171).

On the lateral view, the top of the sylvian triangle is identified by drawing a line connecting the tops of the four to six loops of the middle cerebral artery branches as they rise to the upper limit of the isle of Reil (Fig. 4–24, p. 170). As previously noted, this line represents the "roof" of the sylvian triangle, and normally should be straight, although one of the loops may be displaced above or below the line without definitely suggesting the presence of pathology. The anterior inferior limit of the sylvian triangle is the genu of the middle cerebral artery, and the floor of the triangle is determined by connecting the genu of the middle cerebral artery to the sylvian point. The anterior limb is a line connecting the anterior loop to the genu of the middle cerebral artery. These three lines thus make the sylvian triangle. Normally, the position of the triangle is such that the main middle cerebral artery branch along the floor of the triangle lies above the clinoparietal line (Fig. 4–24, p. 170). The position of this line is determined by drawing a line 9 cm up from the internal occipital protuberance to the inner table of the skull in the parietal region. A line is then drawn from this point on the parietal bone to the anterior clinoid process—hence the *clinoparietal* line. The main middle cerebral artery branch should be within 1 cm above or below this line. In the normal individual, the middle cerebral artery branch generally is above this line. In children, the middle cerebral artery branches ride even higher than in the adult. Any deviation from this anticipated normal position should be noted.

The author has also found that the horizontal portions of the anterior and middle cerebral arteries usually are superimposed upon each other in the normal individual. Although there can be normal variations in position of the initial segments of these vessels, if they are readily visible as separate vessels on the lateral view one should anticipate that there *may* be displacement of these vessels from their normal position.

Similarly, in the normal individual only the first or possibly the first two branches of the middle cerebral artery should project anterior to a line drawn superiorly from the internal carotid artery at the level of its bifurcation into the anterior and middle cerebral arteries. If more branches are anterior to the internal carotid artery bifurcation, one should consider the possibility of forward displacement of the sylvian triangle. Conversely, if no loops are anterior to the internal carotid artery bifurcation, there may be posterior displacement of the sylvian triangle. In addition, one may see a telescoping together of the various branches of the middle cerebral artery when a mass lesion is present. The telescoping may be either anterior or posterior in direction, depending on the position of the mass lesion. There may also be superior or inferior displacement of the sylvian triangle—or any combination of these changes—depending on the position of the mass and on whether multiple lesions are present.

Because of the standard angiographic projection, which is 12 degrees toward the feet in the AP projection, a forward displacement of the sylvian triangle may give the impression that the sylvian point is being displaced inferiorly. On the other hand, a posterior displacement of the sylvian point may translate to a superior displacement of the sylvian triangle on the AP view. These changes should be kept in mind when reviewing an angiogram. No final opinion should be made on an angiogram without thorough examination of both the AP and lateral views.

It is sometimes difficult for the beginning angiographer to identify the sylvian triangle. If there is such difficulty, the very early films should be reviewed in the lateral projection, where the early filling of the middle cerebral artery branches in the sylvian triangle are not obscured by the contrast-filled opercular branches of these vessels. The sylvian triangle can then be identified and any changes in the anticipated normal position of the vessels noted.

On some occasions, a very large mass lesion of the temporal lobe will cause such marked elevation of the sylvian triangle that, on the lateral view, it takes on the anatomic appearance of the anterior cerebral artery. Only comparison with the AP view will reveal the true nature of the angiographic changes. On the other hand, occlusion of the middle cerebral artery may be mistaken for gross distortion of this vessel. Again, comparison with the AP view will reveal the true nature of the abnormality.

The triangle is of great angiographic significance because it lies roughly in the midportion of the brain, deep in the cerebral hemisphere. It is therefore affected by most mass lesions. In fact, many lesions are named by their position relative to the triangle, e.g., presylvian, suprasylvian, infrasylvian, or retrosylvian. When interpreting arteriograms it is important to attempt to visualize the triangle *in each instance* because of its critical anatomic position. The branches of the middle cerebral artery form a "candelabra" appearance on the lateral view.

Each vessel is a named branch, but as noted earlier they are grouped according to the anatomic area they supply. The last branch out of the triangle is called the angular branch. This last branch courses posteriorly and is the middle cerebral artery's contribution to the visual cortex, supplying the area of macular vision. The remainder of the visual cortex is supplied by the calcarine branch of the posterior cerebral artery.

Inspection of the cerebral cortex from the lateral view reveals that the middle cerebral artery and its branches supply the bulk of the visible cerebral cortex. The anterior cerebral artery extends up and over from the medial side to supply a small peripheral area of the cortex; the posterior cerebral artery supplies a similar territory posteriorly.

Anatomic/Neurologic Correlation

Thinking back to basic neurology, one remembers that the homunculus is placed over the cerebral cortex so that its foot is at the high convexity while the trunk, chest, arm and face are placed low over the convexity—the homunculus being upside down on the cerebral convexity. In addition, one will remember that the tongue and fingers are disproportionately enlarged, with the thumb even more so to reflect its large representation on the cerebral cortex.

These relative sizes and positions are important in the presence of occlusive cerebrovascular disease. When the middle cerebral artery is occluded, the face and arm will be affected much more than the leg because of the blood supply to the cortex. Conversely, in the presence of a high-convexity meningioma, the foot and leg will be much more affected—not only because of the blood supply, but because of the pressure on the cerebral cortex represented by the foot and leg in the high-convexity region.

In addition to major vascular occlusions, one can also see branch occlusions in any vascular distribution. In many cases, retrograde collateral flow from other vessels will attempt to fill these branches. Without adequate collateral flow, occlusion of these vessels usually results in permanent neurologic damage.

Posterior Cerebral Artery

The basilar artery is formed by the joining of the two vertebral arteries. It courses up in the prepontine cistern just posterior to the clivus until it reaches the interpeduncular fossa. Here the terminal bifurcation of the basilar artery becomes the posterior cerebral arteries. From their bifurcation in the interpeduncular cistern, the posterior cerebral arteries must course first laterally, under the cerebral peduncles, and then posterosuperiorly to the level of the quadrigeminal plate. On the AP view this course is readily apparent (see Chapter 13); indeed, they often outline the cerebral peduncles very well. On the lateral view, however, the horizontal portion of the posterior cerebral arteries is not appreciated because we are seeing the vessels "end-on." This results in a telescoping of the vessels and a failure to appreciate their initial lateral course.

The posterior cerebral arteries then course around the brain stem in the perimesencephalic cistern, which makes up only a small portion of the ambient cistern. More posteriorly and superiorly, the perimesencephalic cistern and the quadrigeminal plate cistern converge. At the quadrigeminal plate cistern, the posterior cerebral arteries nearly meet at the midline. In the region of the quadrigeminal plate, the posterior cerebral arteries are closely related to the pineal gland and the vein of Galen. The superior cerebellar arteries arise just inferior to the posterior cerebral arteries, also in the interpeduncular cistern. The posterior cerebral and superior cerebellar arteries are separated from each other by the tentorium, which extends forward at this point and divides the supratentorial compartment from the infratentorial compartment. In the presence of a tentorial meningioma that arises along the free edge of the tentorium, the posterior cerebral and superior cerebellar arteries will be splayed apart from each other by the tumor mass.

The posterior communicating artery arises from the horizontal portion of the posterior cerebral artery, a short distance from the midline (see Chapter 13). The posterior communicating artery then courses anteriorly and slightly laterally to join with the internal carotid artery in its supraclinoid portion. One may see this posterior communicating artery fill retrograde when contrast material is injected into the vertebral artery. On the other hand, if the posterior communicating vessel does not fill retrograde, one may see a filling "defect" in the posterior cerebral artery from "washout" of unopacified blood from the posterior communicating artery, which fills from the carotid artery system. This area of "washout" should not be mistaken for an area of vascular spasm or arteriosclerotic narrowing.

In some cases, the posterior cerebral artery does not fill from the vertebrobasilar system, but arises directly from the internal carotid artery—a variation known as a "primitive posterior cerebral artery" (see Fig. 4–37, p. 180). The significance of this anatomic finding becomes most apparent when one wishes to examine the left posterior cerebral artery distribution and finds that neither right nor left brachial arteriography is helpful. Percutaneous left carotid arteriography will then be required. If catheterization is performed, an additional injection will be needed.

The anterior and posterior thalamoperforating arteries arise from the posterior communicating artery and the proximal portions of the posterior cerebral arteries, respectively. The posterior pericallosal artery then arises, followed by the medial and lateral posterior choroidal arteries (see Chapter 13). These later branches are not well seen in the AP view. The posterior pericallosal artery supplies the posterior portion of the corpus callosum and has the potential to provide collateral flow to the distribution of the pericallosal artery. The medial posterior choroidal arteries project anteriorly on the lateral view, have a "reverse three" configuration in many cases, and supply the choroid plexus of the third ventricle as it runs in the roof of the third ventricle. The lateral posterior choroidal vessels project more posteriorly on the lateral view; they supply the choroid plexus of the lateral ventricles in the region of the atrium of the lateral ventricle. The posterior cerebral artery then gives rise to the posterior temporal branch, which supplies all of the medial and undersurface of the temporal lobe, with a small portion of its distribution over the convexities of the temporal lobe. Coursing further posteriorly, the posterior cerebral then becomes the internal occipital artery; this branches into the calcarine artery, which supplies the visual cortex, in the region of the calcarine fissure along the medial surface of the occipital lobe. The other branch is the parieto-occipital artery, which supplies the bulk of the occipital lobe and a portion of the posterior aspect of the parietal lobe.

The branches of the posterior cerebral artery are:

1. Posterior communicating a.
2. Thalamoperforating a.
3. Posterior pericallosal a.
4. Medial posterior choroidal a.
5. Lateral posterior choroidal a.
6. Posterior temporal a.
7. Internal occipital a.
   a. parieto-occipital a.
   b. calcarine a.

External Carotid Artery

The external carotid artery (Fig. 4–32, p. 177) is the smaller of the two vessels at the level of the bifurcation of the common carotid artery in the neck. External carotid angiography is of particular importance in the study of a meningioma because these tumors obtain the bulk of their blood supply from the external carotid system via the internal maxillary artery, which gives rise to the middle meningeal artery. At the level of the carotid bifurcation in the neck, in most cases, the external carotid artery courses medial and anterior relative to the internal carotid artery. The external carotid artery then gives rise to eight main branches:

1. Superior thyroid artery; supplies the thyroid gland.
2. Lingual artery; supplies the tongue.
3. Facial artery (often arises in common with the lingual artery); supplies the face.
4. Occipital artery; supplies the muscles of the neck and the scalp over the occipital portion of the skull.
5. Posterior auricular artery; supplies the ear and the scalp above and behind the ear.
6. Ascending pharyngeal artery; may give rise to various inconstant branches, including pharyngeal and meningeal branches.
7. Superficial temporal artery; supplies mainly the scalp over the parietal region.
8. Internal maxillary artery.

Of all the branches, the internal maxillary artery gives rise to the artery that most concerns us from an arteriographic and diagnostic point of view, for it gives rise to the middle meningeal. When a meningioma is present, the internal maxillary artery may be greatly enlarged, and the middle meningeal branch is also enlarged on the arteriogram. Indeed, if one suspects a meningioma, a common carotid angiogram and/or selective internal and external carotid angiograms should be done.

Examination of the external carotid distribution will reveal that the middle meningeal artery is visualized in almost all cases as a small vessel that originates from the internal maxillary artery and courses superiorly and medially. This middle meningeal vessel enters the bony calvaria via the foramen spinosum and supplies the meningeal coverings of the brain. The vessel will be seen to travel in the meningeal artery groove in the inner table of the skull in the adult. The foramen spinosum will be enlarged in some cases of meningioma, as will the meningeal artery groove. However, normal variations occur in the size of both the foramen spinosum and the meningeal artery groove, so this finding is certainly not pathognomonic. It merely serves to substantiate other findings (see Chapter 8).

External Carotid Angiography. In the presence of such meningeal supply to a brain tumor, selective catheterization of the external carotid artery and a selective external carotid artery angiogram can be performed (Fig. 4–32, p. 177). Depending on the size of the vessel, one may inject from 3 to 8 cc of contrast material. If superselective catheterization of the vessel of interest is possible, this is also advantageous. By test injections under fluoroscopic control, the size of the vessel can be determined so that an appropriate amount of contrast material can be injected. This must be balanced against the amount of contrast material that may represent excessive filling, consequently resulting in overfilling of the external carotid system and retrograde flow into the internal carotid system. In addition to the mechanical and technical difficulties of this type of injection, the patient will feel considerable discomfort from injection into the external carotid system. The patient should be forewarned about this. Both the presence of the catheter in the vessel and the injection of contrast material into the vessel irritate the vessel wall. This may result in spasm of the vessel, which will also promote retrograde flow into the internal carotid system. This spasm of the external carotid artery often will be visible fluoroscopically at the time the catheter is placed. The author has seen one case of this type of vascular spasm that resulted in a remote spasm involving one major branch of the middle cerebral artery group.

Anatomic Dissection and Correlation

During the course of each resident group rotation on the neuroradiology service, we dissect a preserved brain in order to gain a greater appreciation of the intracerebral structures in their three-dimensional positions. This anatomic dissection is carried out by very loosely structured groups of three to five residents. Axial sections are dissected to establish correlation with the CT scan findings. The standard coronal sections are also done. A single brain cut in two through the corpus callosum will serve both purposes. Initially, a superficial inspection of the brain is made, noting the positions of the falx cerebri and the tentorium cerebelli, and making particular note of the free edge of the tentorium and the dural sinuses and arachnoid villi. Following this, the parietal and temporal lobes are opened, and the isle of Reil or insula is inspected. Thus, the course of the cerebral arteries can be visualized: the pattern of rising to the highest portion of the isle of Reil by the middle cerebral artery branches, followed by the descent of each branch until it reaches the operculum of the isle of Reil and then turns either superiorly to course over the frontal and parietal lobes or inferiorly to distribute over the temporal bone. This visual reinforcement of understanding the distribution of the middle cerebral vessels serves to crystalize in the student's mind the anatomic course and position of these branches in the isle of Reil. Further dissection of the brain can proceed in a random fashion at the discretion of the neuroanatomy students or the instructor. Often, following the course of individual vessels is quite helpful. Certainly the position of the ventricles relative to the other structures of the brain should be noted. The identification of as many landmarks as possible is very useful for review and helps the uninitiated student to learn more about the normal anatomy. The quadrigeminal plate cistern with the pineal, internal cerebral veins, vein of Galen, and posterior continuation into the superior cerebellar cistern certainly should be pointed out. The close relationship to the splenium of the corpus callosum, and the pulvinar of the thalamus (most posterior nucleus of the thalamus) also should be noted.

In many cases, the veil-like membrane of the cisternae magna will be seen as it extends posteriorly from the lobes of the cerebellum as a fold of the arachnoid membrane of the lepto-meninges. Close inspection of this area will also reveal the normal pathways of the posterior inferior cerebellar artery (PICA) and anterior inferior cerebellar artery (AICA) as well as the vertebrobasilar system itself. It also will show the multiple small pontine perforating vessels, which are not seen on angiograms. In addition, of course, with review of a large number of specimens, one begins to get a feel for the many normal anatomic variations that may be seen. This is particularly noteworthy when one compares the various sizes of the cisternae magna and the inverse relationship between the size of the PICA and the size of the AICA.

JUGULAR VENOGAPHY

Indications. Jugular venography may be used to outline the cavernous sinus—for example, to determine the lateral extension of a pituitary tumor. It also may be used to demonstrate invasion of the internal jugular vein by a glomus jugulare tumor.

Technique. The internal jugular vein lies lateral to the internal carotid artery in the carotid sheath. The neck is prepared and draped in a fashion similar to the procedure followed for carotid puncture. A local anesthetic should be injected around the puncture site. Since the internal jugular vein is lateral to the carotid in the neck, the needle should be directed lateral to the carotid artery for the puncture. Suction should be applied to the hub of the needle as it is being withdrawn. When free flow of venous blood is obtained, a guidewire is threaded through the needle and a polyethylene catheter or Davis needle is placed into the internal jugular vein, using the Seldinger technique. The needle is advanced until its tip is at the jugular bulb. Contrast material is injected at a rate of 8 cc per second for 2 to 2.5 seconds to visualize the jugular vein. To visualize the cavernous sinus, pressure should be applied at the time of injection to the jugular vein below the injection site; it may be necessary to compress both internal jugular veins during injection.

The jugular vein can also be catheterized using the Seldinger technique and puncture of the femoral vein in the groin. The catheter is then advanced in a retrograde fashion under fluoroscopy and positioned in the jugular vein.

EMBOLIZATION

With advances in techniques, invasive radiology has become a part of many neuroradiologic practices. Catheters are used to introduce small spheres or particles of occlusive materials in order to decrease the blood supply to arteriovenous malformations and certain types of vascular tumors. This method may be the definitive treatment for arteriovenous malformations: it also decreases the vascularity of tumors, making them more readily amenable to surgical removal. Meningiomas and glomus jugulare tumors in particular may benefit from embolization.

The technique of embolization is beyond the scope of this book. It is enough to say that great care is needed to prevent the embolic materials from entering the internal carotid system and causing a stroke (Fig. 4–39, p. 181).

NORMAL VENOUS ANATOMY

Falx Cerebri and Tentorium Cerebelli

For a full understanding of the venous drainage of the cerebrum, one must know the structure of the falx cerebri and the tentorium cerebelli.

The brain is enclosed in three meningeal layers:

The *pia mater* is a thin, delicate connective tissue closely applied to the brain and spinal cord that carries the rich network of blood vessels that supply the brain and cord. The pia dips into each fissure and sulcus and forms the choroid plexuses of the lateral, third and fourth ventricles.

The *arachnoid layer* is a delicate, avascular membrane lying between the dura mater and the pia mater. The subarachnoid space contains the arteries, the veins, and the cerebrospinal fluid.

The *dura mater* is a dual-layered membrane that is composed of dense fibrous connective tissue and collagen. The outer periosteal layer forms the periosteum of the inner table of the skull. The inner meningeal layer is smooth and forms the various partitions of the brain. The falx cerebri is a thin dural reflection of the *meningeal* layer, which extends down between the cerebral hemispheres. This inner layer also forms the tentorium cerebelli and the falx cerebelli, which separates the two cerebellar hemispheres.

The falx cerebri is attached anteriorly at the crista galli. At its anterior extent, the falx is not very wide, but it widens progressively as it extends from front to back. The straight sinus is the posterior point of attachment of the falx, and the length of the straight sinus reflects the width of the falx posteriorly. The superior sagittal sinus is formed by the dural reflection; it is triangular in shape. The inferior sagittal sinus runs along the inferior margin of the falx cerebri to enter the straight sinus at the level of the vein of Galen posteriorly. The straight sinus then courses posteroinferiorly to the level of the torcular Herophili, or confluence of sinuses. This confluence of sinuses is at the level of the internal occipital protuberance, which is opposite the external occipital protuberance. Extending laterally from the confluence of sinuses are the right and left transverse or lateral sinuses. The transverse sinuses drain into the sigmoid sinuses just posterior to the petrous bones bilaterally and from there into the internal jugular veins bilaterally. In most cases, the right transverse sinus is larger than the left. It has been shown that most of the blood from the superior sagittal sinus drains into the right transverse sinus, whereas most of the blood from the inferior sagittal sinus drains into the left transverse sinus. There is a great deal of anatomic variation in the position of the superior sagittal sinus as it drains into the transverse sinus; in some cases, the superior sagittal sinus may enter the transverse sinus far lateral to the midline (see Fig. 4–45, p. 186).

The transverse sinuses follow the tentorium at the level of its attachment to the occipital bone. The transverse sinuses also are triangular, and they lie just below the tentorium. The straight sinus, at the level of its junction with the inferior sagittal sinus and the vein of Galen, is superior to the transverse sinuses. The middle of the tentorium is then also in a higher position than the lateral portions of the tentorium; indeed, from the level of the straight sinus, the tentorium slants downward and forward to cover the cerebellum. The tentorium is attached bilaterally to the petrous bones along their upper margins; the free edge of the tentorium slants forward from the tentorial notch around the midbrain and extends anteriorly to attach as far forward as the anterior clinoid processes bilaterally. The tentorium is then "tent-shaped," as its name would suggest. The top peak is at the level of the junction with the inferior sagittal sinus and the vein of Galen. The straight sinus then forms the roof, and the remainder of the tentorium slants downward and forward to cover the posterior fossa structures (see Fig. 4–47, p. 188). Because the dural structures are enhanced by contrast infusion, they are visualized readily on the postinfusion scan. The superior sagittal sinus, the inferior sagittal sinus, and the falx are readily visualized on the CT scan (see Chapter 3).

Because it is in the same plane, or nearly the same plane, as the standard CT scan cut, the tentorium may be seen as a sheet-like area of enhancement rather than a linear structure. Depending on the angle of the cut, one may visualize much or little of the tentorium on a single scan slice.

The tentorial notch is formed by the anteriorly sloping free edges of the tentorium as they slope down and forward from the straight sinus. This notch appears as a V-shaped area on the postinfusion scan. In addition to the notch, one sees a contiguous portion of the straight sinus posterior to the notch as the straight sinus drains toward the torcular Herophili, or confluence of sinuses. The visualization of this notch and the blush of the tentorium are helpful when one is attempting to decide whether a lesion is above or below the tentorium. Obviously, the vermis and midportion of the cerebellum extend higher than the rest of the cerebellar structures; therefore, on an individual CT scan cut, a more medially placed lesion is likely to be in the vermis of the cerebellum, whereas a more laterally placed lesion is more likely to be in the occipital lobes. Coronal CT, reconstruction views, or magnetic resonance scans can readily demonstrate the anatomic location of the mass.

The main diagnostic difficulty is the question of an occipital pole versus a cerebellar lesion. If one remembers basic neurology, it will be recalled that a *left* homonymous hemianopsia is consistent with a *right* occipital pole lesion and that a *right* homonymous hemianopsia is consistent with a *left* occipital pole lesion. The presence of a visual field defect therefore is quite suggestive of an occipital pole lesion. Ataxia is more suggestive of a cerebellar mass lesion, particularly in the presence of obstructive hydrocephalus or displacement of the fourth ventricle.

Supratentorial Venous System

The venous drainage of the supratentorial system can be roughly divided into superficial and deep venous systems. The deep venous system is of the greatest clinical importance because of the displacements that are caused by mass lesions in various positions in the brain. On the other hand, there are many superficial veins that can be of some assistance in diagnosing abnormalities within the cranial vault.

Superficial Veins

Close inspection of any angiogram will show that the superficial cortical veins drain upward for the most part and enter the superior sagittal sinus. In addition to draining in an upward direction, the veins will be seen to enter the superior sagittal sinus in such a fashion that the flow will be against the normal front-to-back flow in the sinus. This pattern of venous drainage occurs because the normal growth and development of the cerebral cortex draws the veins forward. Only two of the superficial veins are of any real consequence: (1) The vein of Trolard is a large superficial cortical vein in the parietal region. It will be seen to drain upward and then forward into the superior sagittal sinus. (2) The vein of Labbé is a superficial cortical vein that drains from the parietal region inferiorly and posteriorly to enter the transverse sinus. To commit the two to memory, one must only recall that "Trolard" begins with a "T," and the vein drains to the *Top*; whereas Labbé begins with "L," and the vein drains to the *Lateral* sinus (transverse sinus) over the *Lateral* aspect of the brain and is *Lower* over the cortex.

The middle cerebral vein, as its name suggests, is formed by a group of superficial tributary veins that drain the middle cerebral artery distribution and course anteriorly and inferiorly to enter the cavernous sinus. Gross vascular displacements are unusual in the superficial venous system, so these veins do not often provide significant diagnostic value. On the other hand, the neurosurgeon uses these cortical veins as a guide to the position of an underlying mass lesion. These cortical veins provide landmarks for the neurosurgical approach to the area of abnormality.

It will be noted also that the normal sequence of filling of the cortical veins is from the frontal region initially, then progressing posteriorly. When reviewing a serial run of films, this does not mean that the frontal veins will be filled on the first film, the parietal veins on the second film, and so on—but it does mean that the occipital veins should not be filled before the frontal veins. Review of the serial film run may reveal that the cortical veins fill simultaneously. This finding may be normal, or it may imply some slowing of filling in the frontal region. Slow filling of the cortical venous system is a reflection of a localized increase in intracranial pressure that prevents blood from entering the cortical veins. With some mass lesions there will be a total absence of filling of the veins. Such absence of venous filling provides further confirmatory evidence of the presence of a mass lesion.

If the anterior cerebral artery on the side of the injection is occluded, or, more commonly, if an anterior cerebral artery fills from the contralateral carotid artery as a normal variation, there will be poor arterial flow to the frontal region. This poor flow will appear as slow or even absent venous filling in the frontal region. If this is the case, the condition should not be mistaken for evidence of a frontal mass lesion. Because of poor arterial opacification of the frontal region, there will be poor venous opacification—even in the absence of a mass lesion. In these cases, there generally are other signs, such as the presence or absence of a midline shift, that will help one decide whether a mass lesion is present or absent.

Deep Veins

Not many of the deep veins are of major significance in the diagnosis of mass lesions. The internal cerebral veins are of major importance and command our greatest attention. These veins are paired and lie just on either side of the midline. They begin anteriorly at the level of the foramen of Monro and travel in the roof of the third ventricle posteriorly until they terminate in the vein of Galen. The internal cerebral veins are enclosed in the velum interpositum. This is a thin, veil-like membrane that envelops the veins and is of no real significance except that air or CSF may sometimes enter between the leaves of the velum interpositum and form what is called a "cavum velum interpositum." On the lateral view it will be seen that the internal cerebral veins will form a gentle hump in the midportion of its course (see Fig. 4–43, p. 184). Anteriorly, the internal cerebral vein is joined at the level of the foramen of Monro by the thalamostriate vein and the septal vein.

The angiographically visible portion of the thalamostriate vein runs in the floor of the lateral ventricle and courses gently forward to join the internal cerebral vein at the level of the foramen of Monro. On the anteroposterior view, the thalamostriate vein will be seen to form a curvilinear outline of the body of the lateral ventricle as it curves inferiorly to join the internal cerebral vein. In fact, when one compares the normal brow-up view of a pneumoencephalogram with the anteroposterior view of the angiogram, the correlation between the two is easy to appreciate. The body of the lateral ventricle as it is outlined by air will be seen to correspond with the position of the thalmostriate vein, thus providing the arteriographic and pneumoencephalographic correlation (see Chapter 15).

Also joining the internal cerebral vein at the level of the foramen of Monro is the septal vein. This vein originates in the septum pellucidum and follows a curvilinear course posteriorly to enter the internal cerebral vein. At the level of the junction between the internal cerebral vein and the thalamostriate vein is the anatomic position of the foramen of Monro. This junction and the angle that is formed are known as the "venous angle" (see Fig. 4–41, p. 183). If the thalamostriate vein enters the internal cerebral vein posterior to the foramen of Monro so that the internal cerebral vein is divided into two segments, making the upward hump smaller than the descending hump, one has a "false venous angle." The significance of the false venous angle is that it no longer marks the foramen of Monro; additionally, the evaluation of hydrocephalus on the anteroposterior venous angiogram can no longer be made. In other words, when judging the presence of hydrocephalus angiographically, one must first rule out the presence of a false venous angle.

The paired internal cerebral veins course posteriorly until they join the vein of Galen at the level of the quadrigeminal plate cistern. The unpaired vein of Galen then enters into the straight sinus in the tentorium of the cerebellum at the level of its attachment with the falx cerebri. The straight sinus is also joined by the inferior sagittal sinus at the level of the junction with the vein of Galen.

The internal cerebral vein may be up to 2 mm in diameter. Therefore, when the internal cerebral vein is measured to determine whether there is or is not a shift, the point of measurement should be to the medial side of the vein. The medial side theoretically should lie just lateral to the midline. Up to 2 mm of shift of the internal cerebral vein are accepted as within normal limits.

In addition to the thalamostriate vein, multiple small veins also lie in the floor of the lateral ventricle at different levels. These veins run in the subependymal layer and will, on close inspection, reveal a "Y" shape at their superior margin as they follow the roof of the lateral ventricle. By measuring the height of these subependymal veins as they form the "Y" shape at the top of the ventricle down to the level of the internal cerebral veins, one can obtain an accurate measurement of the size of the lateral ventricle (see Fig. 4–40; p. 182). The normal ventricular size appears to increase with age. By comparing the anticipated normal size and the measured size one can evaluate the presence of abnormal ventricular enlargement. The lateral vein of the atrium drains the lateral ventricle and enters the internal cerebral vein at the level of the vein of Galen. Since the development of CT scanning these measurements have been de-emphasized, and the reader is referred elsewhere for precise measurements.

The basal vein of Rosenthal (Fig. 4–44, p. 185) drains the posterior portion of the frontal lobe and the anterior tip of the temporal lobe. The basal vein of Rosenthal is seen arteriographically in both the anteroposterior and lateral projections. The basal vein of Rosenthal is seen to begin deep in the hemisphere at the anatomic level of the anterior perforated substance. This is the same point where the lenticulostriate arteries perforate into the region of the basal ganglia. The vein then courses posteriorly along the medial edge of the hippocampal gyrus of the temporal lobe, where it then follows the free edge of the tentorium and curves around the midbrain in the perimesencephalic (ambient) cistern to enter the vein of Galen. Most of its course is similar to that followed by the posterior cerebral artery; thus, changes in the position of the posterior cerebral artery are also reflected in changes in the position of the basal vein of Rosenthal. It should also be noted that the third nerve, which arises from the pons and passes forward between the posterior cerebral arteries and the superior cerebellar arteries, follows a similar course. It also is affected in the presence of other mass lesions that affect the adjacent artery and vein. The basal vein lies medial to the temporal horns of the lateral ventricles.

The veins just described represent the major veins that concern us. The deep veins—particularly the midline veins—are of great importance in the diagnosis of mass lesions in the supratentorial region.

Medullary Veins

Medullary veins normally are present but usually are not seen on the normal angiogram except by magnification techniques. They are abnormal if greater than 1.5 cm in length. They are seen with glioblastomas, arteriovenous malformations, and infarcts (Fig. 4–47, p. 188).

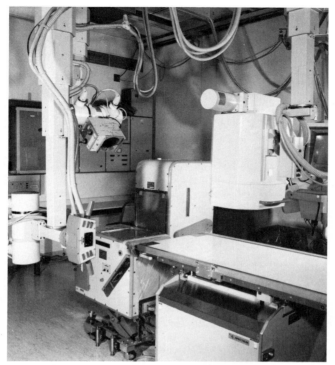

FIGURE 4–1. *Angiography Equipment:* The AP and lateral tubes are in place and are aligned with the film-changing units. The floating top table rests against the film-changing device. The image-intensifying unit rests above the table and can be seen in the right of the picture. The room is large and well-lighted.

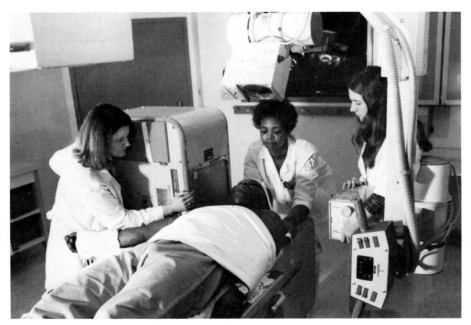

FIGURE 4–2. *Biplane Filming:* The patient is being positioned for simultaneous filming in the AP and lateral projections. Note that the patient is positioned as close to the lateral film changer as possible. This is done to eliminate magnification. The AP grid is a focused grid and is "off-centered" to one side of the 14 × 14 grid. This grid is rotated, and the film changer is switched, depending on which side of the patient is being studied, so that the lateral film changer is always closest to the side injected.

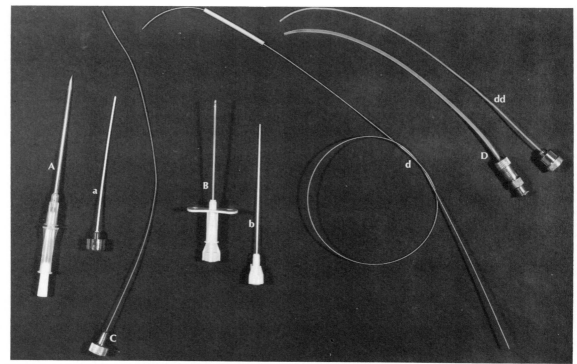

FIGURE 4–3. *Typical Angiogram Needles:* A, Brachial angiogram needle. The needle is metal and has an outer plastic sheath. The solid plastic obturator (*a*) occludes the needle between injections.

B, Cournand-Potts needle. This metal needle is used for carotid angiography and has a beveled tip and a hub with a matching bevel. The metallic obturator (*b*) occludes the needle between injections.

C, The soft-tipped metal guidewire is used to position both the brachial and carotid needles.

D, Davis needle. This short catheter needle can be used for selective internal and external carotid angiography. The short guidewire (*d*) is passed through the puncture; then, using the Seldinger technique, the Davis needle is advanced over the guidewire and into the carotid artery. The plastic obturator (*dd*) occludes the needle between injections. The Davis needle also can be used for jugular venography.

FIGURE 4–4. *Cournand-Potts Needle:* A, The needle is held immobile by the Davis rake. The inner core of the needle extends beyond the hub of the needle so that, when connected to the tubing for contrast injection with a Luer-Lock fitting, all dead space is eliminated.

B, The bevel of the needle faces down and corresponds to the bevel at the tip of the needle.

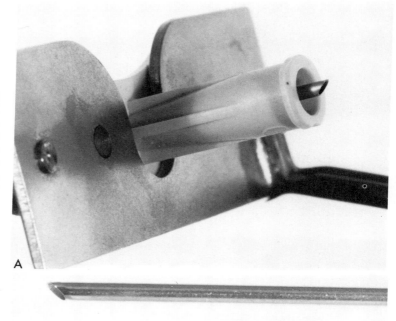

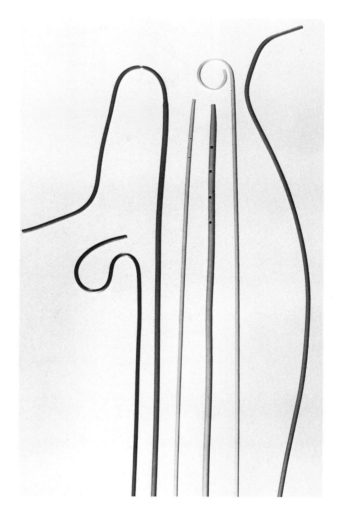

FIGURE 4–5. *Catheters for Cerebral Angiography:* This selection of catheters includes single end-hole catheters for selective catheterization as well as multiple side- and end-hole catheters that are used for arch studies. There are a large number of other catheters commercially available in addition to those illustrated here.

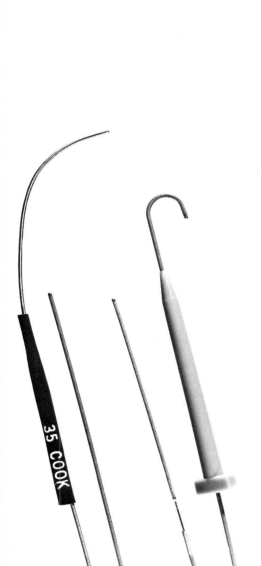

FIGURE 4–6. *Guidewires:* This selection of guidewires illustrates a small number of the large selection of guidewires which is available. The wire second from the right illustrates the movable core of the guidewire. Each wire may be used for a number of different catheters, and it is not uncommon for a variety of guidewires to be used to aid catheterization in a difficult case. The tips of the guidewires have a variable amount of firmness, softness, or "floppiness," and the movable-core guidewires can be changed from a firm to a floppy guidewire by insertion or removal of the movable core.

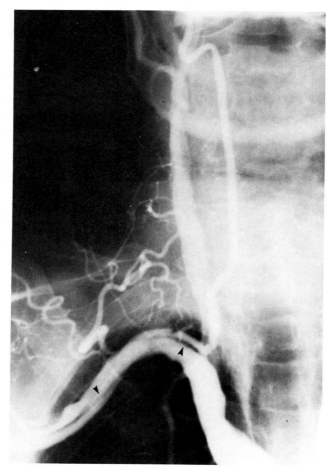

FIGURE 4–7. *Subintimal Injection:* A large subintimal flap has been raised in this patient secondary to the brachial arteriogram. The arrows mark the flap of the intima, which extends to the level of the origin of the vertebral artery.

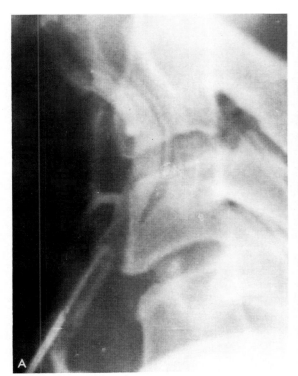

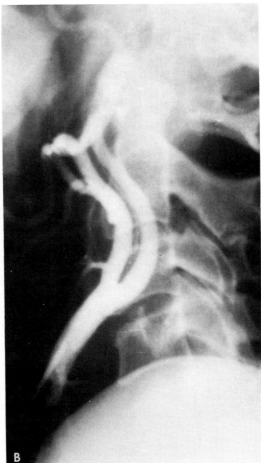

FIGURE 4–8. *Normal Carotid Bifurcation:* *A,* The needle is in place in the carotid artery, and the bevel of the needle is directed downward. A jet stream of contrast material is visible exiting the tip of the needle.

B, The carotid bifurcation is visualized and is normal. The internal carotid artery is posterior to the external carotid artery, and the slight dilatation of the internal carotid artery is the carotid sinus.

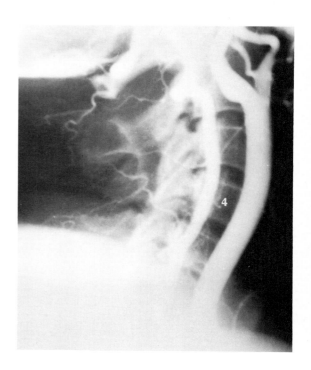

FIGURE 4–9. *High Carotid Bifurcation:* The carotid bifurcation is at the level of C_2; the normal level is C_4.

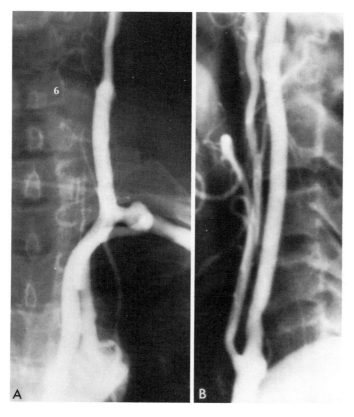

FIGURE 4–10. *Low Carotid Bifurcation:* The carotid bifurcation is at the level of C_6. In this case it was visualized via a left brachial angiogram because there a surgical anastomosis had been made between the left subclavian and the left common carotid artery to prevent a "steal" down the left vertebral artery secondary to stenosis of the proximal left subclavian artery.

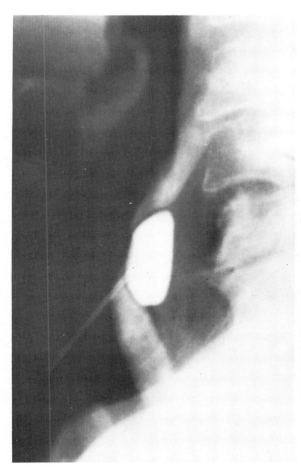

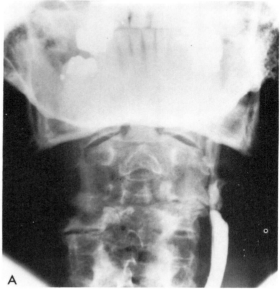

FIGURE 4–11. *Subintimal Injection:* A large subintimal accumulation of contrast material has almost completely blocked the antegrade flow of contrast material.

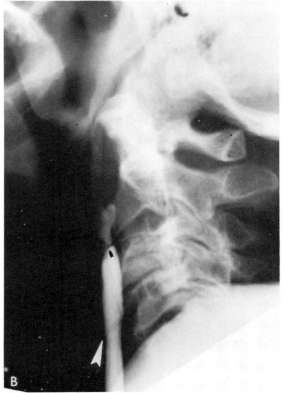

FIGURE 4–12. *Subintimal Injection: A,* The use of a soft plastic catheter has resulted in a large subintimal flap that has completely blocked the antegrade flow of contrast material through the internal carotid artery. The internal carotid artery was subsequently shown to be widely patent.

B, The small black arrow indicates the intimal flap; the white arrow shows the point of entry of the needle into the carotid artery.

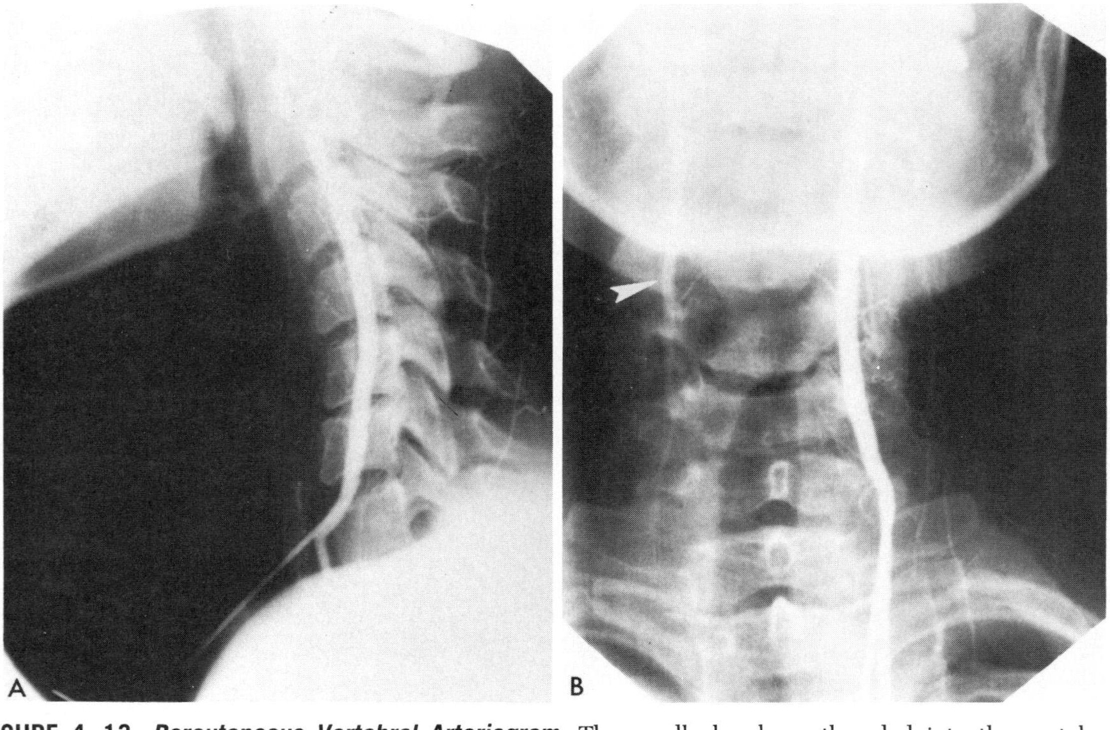

FIGURE 4–13. *Percutaneous Vertebral Arteriogram:* The needle has been threaded into the vertebral artery. With the injection of contrast material the flow is also noted to go retrograde down the contralateral vertebral artery (*arrow*) because of the force of the injection.

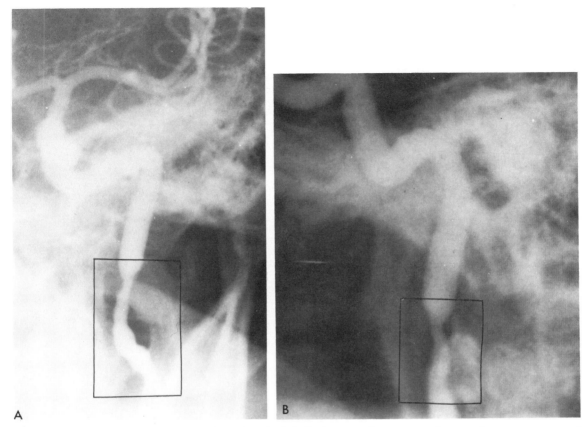

FIGURE 4–14. *Spasm Associated with a Cerebral Catheter:* A catheter is in place in the common carotid artery. With the injection of contrast material, the AP (A) and lateral (B) views demonstrate marked spasm of the proximal portion of the internal carotid artery. Subsequent injections showed the vessel to be normal. This spasm may be remote from the injection site and may even be seen in the cranial vault in the cerebral circulation.

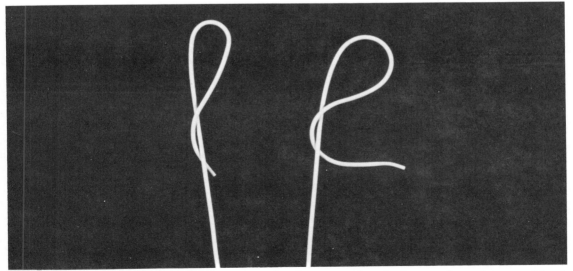

FIGURE 4–15. *Knotted Catheters:* The long curved catheters may loop back upon themselves, resulting in a functional knot. At times the tip of the catheter may even pass through the loop, resulting in a true knot. Great caution should be exercised to avoid this complication. These catheters should not be twirled, but should always be moved slowly and deliberately.

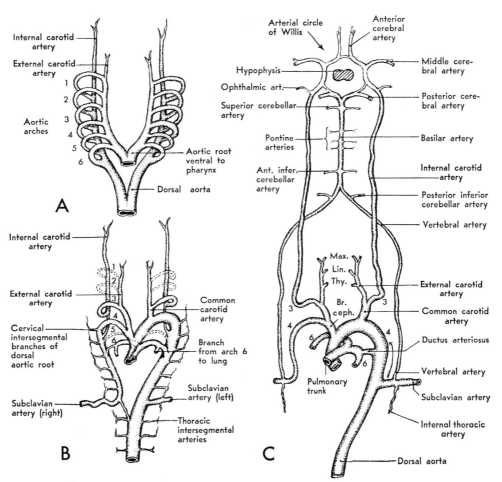

FIGURE 4–16. The primitive brachial arches and clefts are variously resorbed and persist to form the brachiocephalic vessels as we know them in the normal individual. These diagrams illustrate the major changes that occur in the aortic arches of mammalian embryos. *A,* Ground plan of complete set of aortic arches. *B,* Early stage in modification of arches. *C,* Adult derivatives of the aortic arches. *Abbreviations:* Br. ceph. = brachiocephalic (innominate) artery; Lin. = lingual artery; Max. = maxillary artery; Thy. = thyroid artery. The arrow in *C* indicates the change in position of origin of left subclavian artery that occurs in the later stages of development. (Reproduced, by permission, from Carlson, B. M.: Foundations of Embryology. 3rd ed. New York, McGraw-Hill, 1974.)

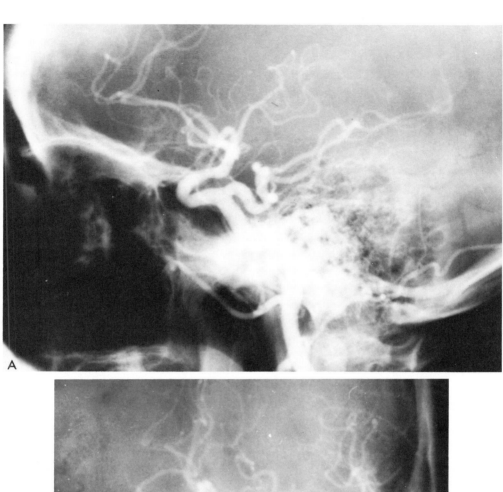

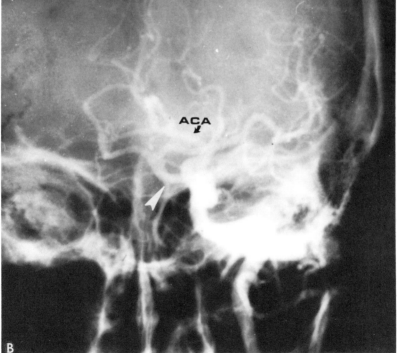

FIGURE 4–17. *Persistent Trigeminal Artery:* *A*, The lateral view demonstrates a large trigeminal artery coursing posteriorly to fill both posterior cerebral arteries.

B, The AP view demonstrates the trigeminal artery, which courses posteromedially (*arrow*) to fill the posterior cerebral arteries. The anterior cerebral artery (*ACA*) projects just above the trigeminal artery.

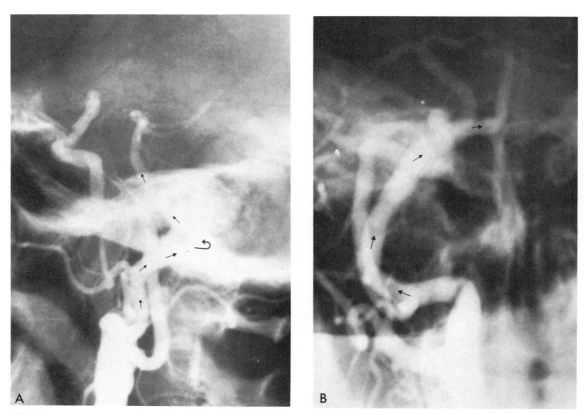

FIGURE 4–18. *Primitive Hypoglossal Artery:* The hypoglossal artery arises from the internal carotid artery in its cervical portion. As seen in these lateral (*A*) and AP (*B*) views, the vessel then courses through the hypoglossal canal to join with the basilar artery (*arrows*). The carotid artery overlies the hypoglossal artery on the AP view.

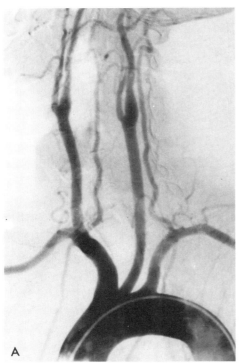
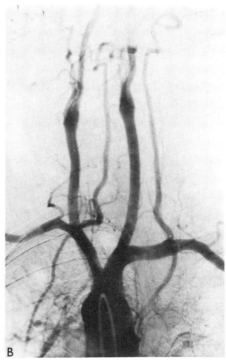

FIGURE 4–19. *Normal Arch Angiogram:* The catheter is in place, with the tip of the multiple-end and side-hole catheter in the ascending aorta approximately 2 cm above the aortic valve. Films obtained in (A) the right posterior oblique (RPO) and (B) left posterior oblique (LPO) projections demonstrate good antegrade flow through the normal great vessels. Both carotid and both vertebral arteries are demonstrated and appear normal.

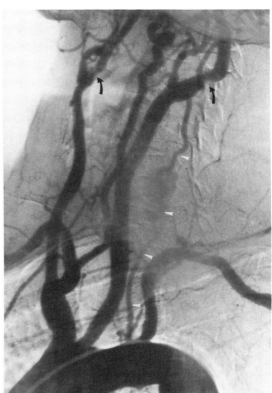

FIGURE 4–20. *Abnormal Arch Angiogram:* The arch angiogram in the RPO projection demonstrates bilateral carotid stenosis (*black arrows*) and a left vertebral artery that arises directly from the arch of the aorta (*white arrows*).

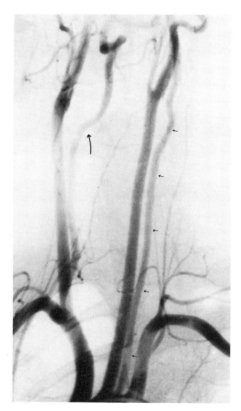

FIGURE 4–21. *Arch Angiogram—Anatomic Variations:* The arch angiogram in the RPO projection demonstrates that the left vertebral artery arises directly from the arch of the aorta (*small arrows*) and that both vertebral arteries enter into the foramina transversaria of the cervical vertebrae at the C_4 level rather than the normal C_6 level. This is a normal anatomic variation and should not be mistaken for a mass displacing the vessels. A separate origin of the left vertebral artery occurs in 5 to 6 per cent of individuals.

FIGURE 4–22. *Aberrant Subclavian Artery:* The right subclavian artery arises distal to the left subclavian artery. In this case the right common carotid artery arises directly from the arch of the aorta; therefore, only the right vertebral artery fills from the right brachial injection.

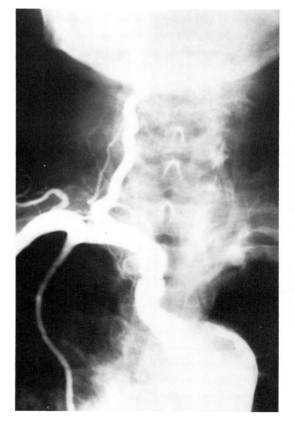

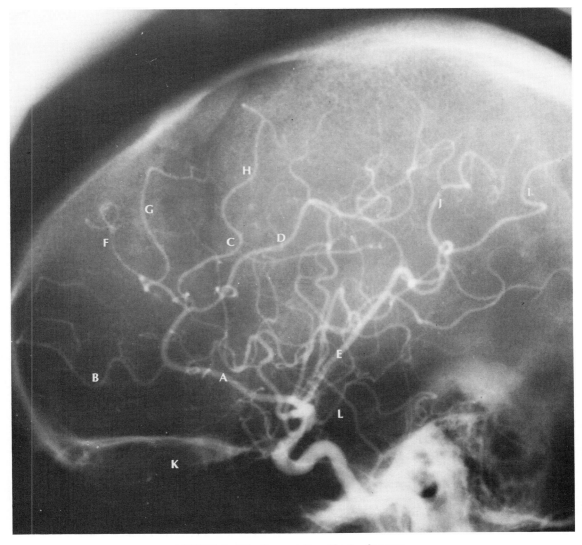

FIGURE 4–23. *Normal Carotid Angiogram:*

A, Anterior cerebral artery.
B, Frontal polar a.
C, Callosal marginal a.
D, Pericallosal a.
E, Middle cerebral artery branch.
F, Anterior internal frontal a.

G, Middle internal frontal a.
H, Posterior internal frontal a.
I, Angular a.
J, Anterior parietal a.
K, Ophthalmic a.
L, Anterior choroidal a.

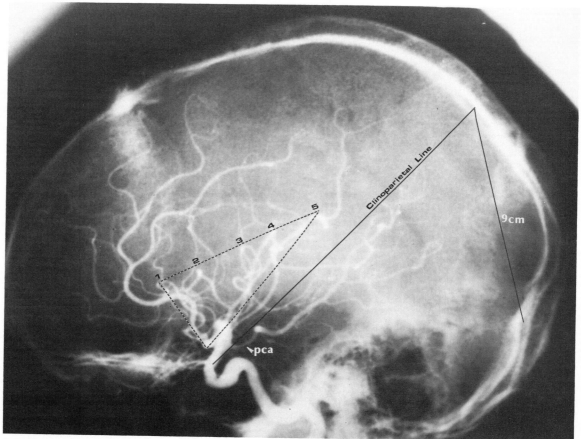

FIGURE 4–24. *Clinoparietal Line:* To determine the anticipated normal position of the sylvian triangle, a line is drawn from the internal occipital protuberance 9 cm up to the inner table of the skull in the parietal region. A line is then constructed from this point to the anterior clinoid process—the *clinoparietal line*. The main middle cerebral artery branch should fall within 1 cm above or below this line.

The dotted lines demonstrate the sylvian triangle. The tops of the loops of the middle cerebral artery branches are numbered 1 to 5 as they rise to the top of the sylvian fissure. Point 5 is the *sylvian point*—the last branch of the middle cerebral artery to exit from the sylvian fissure.

The posterior communicating artery (*pca*) and posterior cerebral artery project below the clinoparietal line. The origin of the anterior choroidal artery projects above the clinoparietal line just distal to the posterior communicating artery.

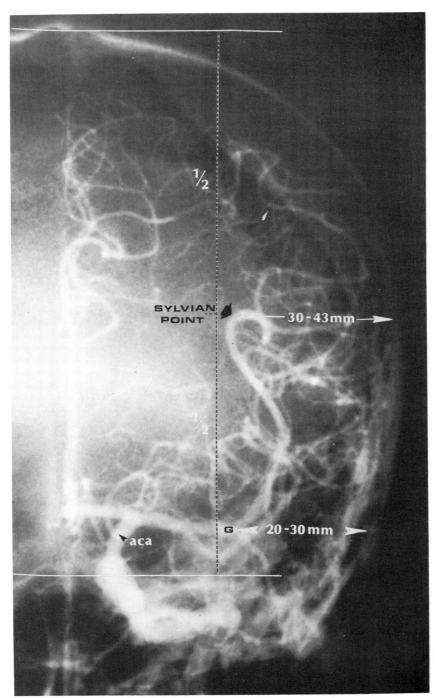

FIGURE 4–25. *AP View of Normal Sylvian Point:* The sylvian point normally projects 30 to 43 mm from the inner table of the skull. The point normally lies half way along a line (*dotted line*) perpendicular to a tangent to the inner table in the high convexity area and the orbital roof or the petrous pyramid, whichever is lower. There is a ± 1 cm range of normal.

The genu (*G*) of the middle cerebral artery normally measures 20 to 30 mm from the inner table of the skull.

The anterior choroidal artery (*aca*) can be seen as it arises from the internal carotid artery.

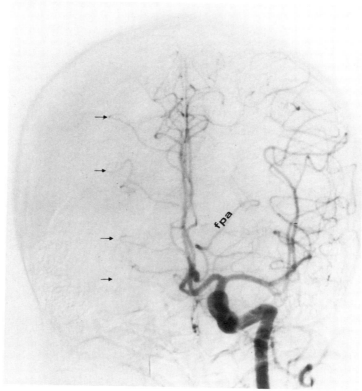

FIGURE 4–26. *Normal AP View of Left Carotid Arteriogram:* Both pericallosal arteries fill from the left carotid artery. The normal distribution of the anterior cerebral artery and its branches as they distribute over the cerebral convexity are well demonstrated on the right side (*small arrows*). The frontal polar artery is well seen (*fpa*).

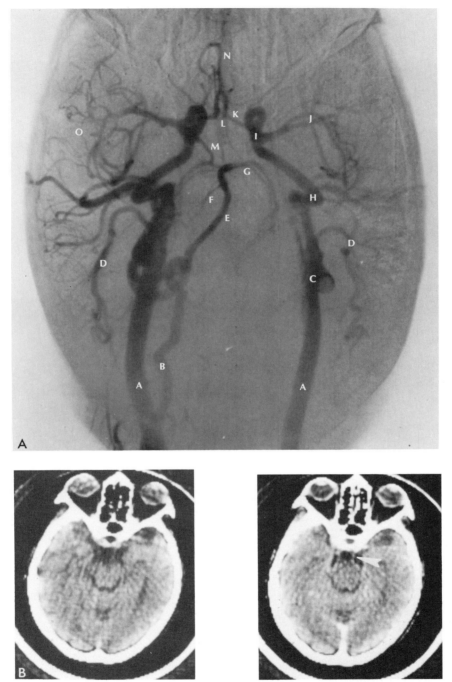

FIGURE 4–27. *Submentovertex View of Right Brachial Angiogram with Filling of Left Carotid Artery:* The right brachial arteriogram (*A*) demonstrates filling also of the left common carotid circulation, providing an excellent demonstration of the anatomic structures in the circle of Willis, and throughout the normal circulation. (*A*, Common carotid artery. *B*, Vertebral artery. *C*, Carotid bifurcation. *D*, External carotid artery. *E*, Basilar artery. *F*, Anterior superior cerebellar artery. *G*, Posterior cerebral arteries. *H*, Internal carotid artery in the carotid canal. *I*, Bifurcation of internal carotid artery. *J*, Genu of middle cerebral artery. *K*, Horizontal portion of anterior cerebral artery. *L*, Anterior communicating artery. *M*, Posterior communicating artery. *N*, Anterior cerebral arteries. *O*, Middle cerebral artery branches in the isle of Reil.)

The CT scans (*B*) also demonstrate the posterior communicating arteries as they are bathed in the cerebrospinal fluid in the suprasellar cistern (*arrow*). They are faintly seen on the preinfusion scan.

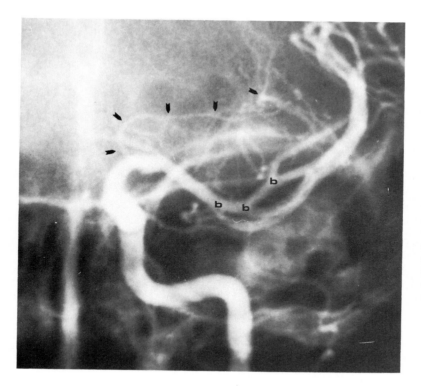

FIGURE 4–28. *Anterior Choroidal Artery:* The anterior choroidal artery arises from the carotid artery and courses posteriorly. It then curves laterally, continuing in a lateral course until the vessel enters the choroid plexus of the temporal horn of the lateral ventricle (*black arrows*). It is said that a dime will fit beneath the first curve of the anterior choroidal artery. The multiple bifurcations (*b*) of the middle cerebral artery were well demonstrated on this examination.

FIGURE 4–29. *Lenticulostriate Arteries:* The multiple small vessels that arise from the horizontal portions of the anterior and middle cerebral arteries and supply the lentiform nucleus are the lenticulostriate arteries. The medial lenticulostriate arteries from the anterior cerebral artery; the lateral lenticulostriate arteries arise from the middle cerebral artery.

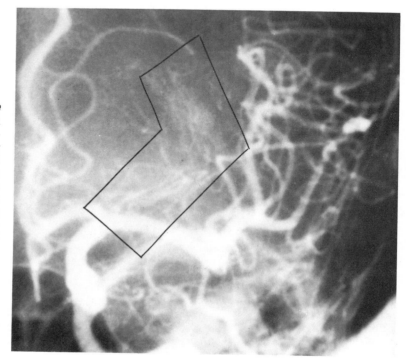

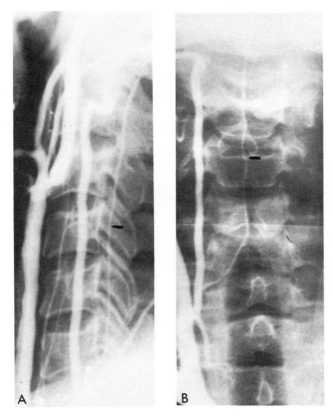

FIGURE 4–30. *Anterior Spinal Artery:* The anterior spinal artery is greatly enlarged in this patient because it is used as a source of collateral blood supply. Note its position in the midline along the anterior margin of the cervical spinal cord (*arrows*).

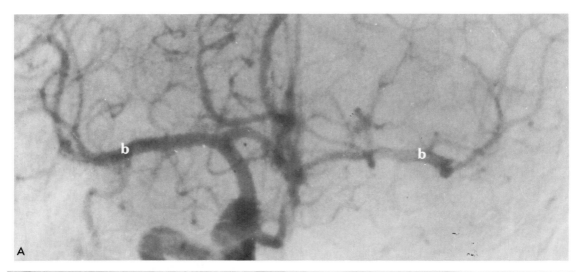

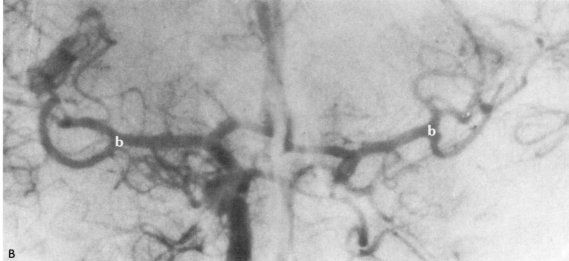

FIGURE 4–31. *Cross Compression:* This RBA was performed with cross compression of the contralateral carotid artery in the neck. This causes the blood to cross over to the opposite hemisphere via the anterior communicating artery. The (*b*) marks the bifurcations of the middle cerebral arteries.

B, The patient is positioned with the chin elevated so that the region of the middle cerebral artery projects through the orbit, providing an excellent demonstration of the region of the middle cerebral bifurcation. This view is especially useful in patients with an aneurysm at this level.

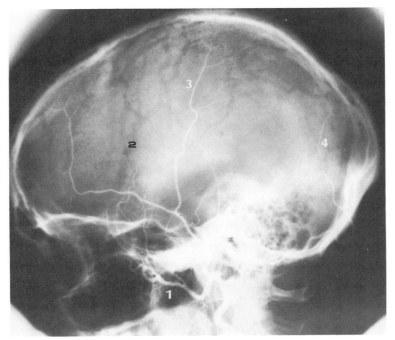

FIGURE 4–32. *External Carotid Arteriogram:* This normal external carotid arteriogram demonstrates (*1*) the internal maxillary branch, (*2*) the middle meningeal artery, which arises from the internal maxillary artery, (*3*) the superficial temporal artery, and (*4*) the occipital branch of the external carotid artery.

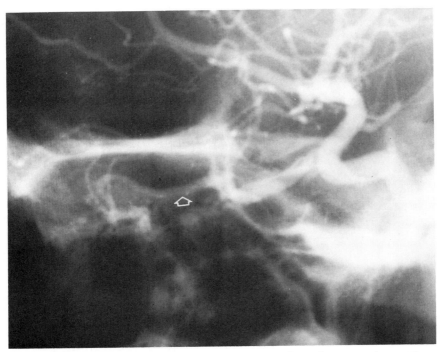

FIGURE 4–33. *Ophthalmic Artery:* The ophthalmic artery arises from the internal carotid artery and then passes through the optic canal lateral to the optic nerve. The artery then courses superiorly and medially, up and over the optic nerve, and then anteriorly, where it gives rise to the retinal branches, the ethmoidal branches, and the supraorbital artery. The vessel is greatly enlarged in this case because the terminal branches supplied a hemangioma of the face.

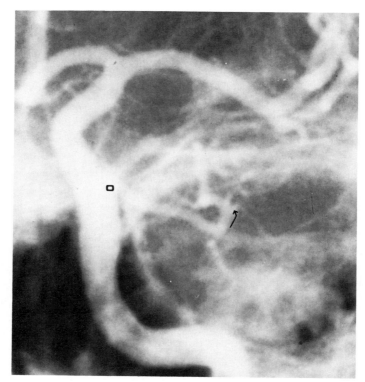

FIGURE 4–34. *AP View of the Ophthalmic Artery:* The artery can be seen from its point of origin from the internal carotid artery (☐). It then courses anterolaterally, following the lateral aspect of the optic nerve. The vessel then crosses superomedially to rest medial to the optic nerve (*curved arrow*) and then anteriorly to give its terminal branches.

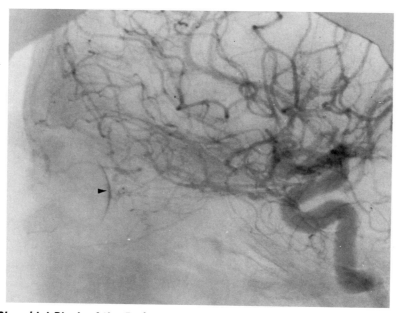

FIGURE 4–35. *Choroidal Blush of the Retina:* The blush of the retina can be seen in most cases. It is best demonstrated with subtraction techniques (*arrow*), as in this case. It is a curved line that follows the posterior margin of the globe of the eye.

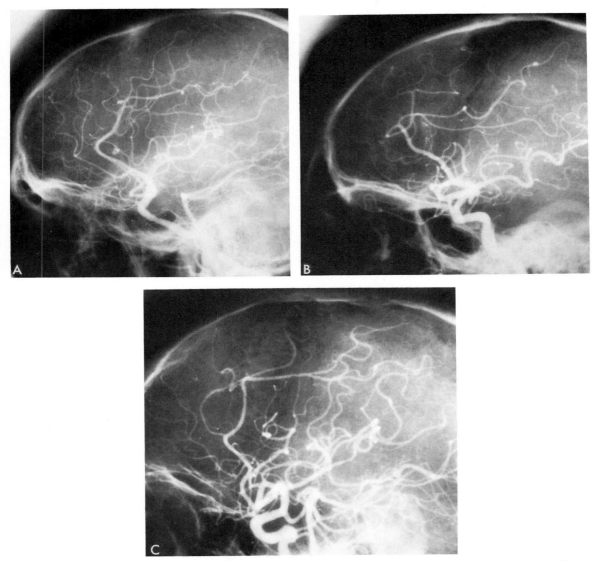

FIGURE 4–36. *Normal Anatomic Variations of the Pericallosal Artery:* The normal course of the pericallosal artery can vary greatly and should not be mistaken for displacement secondary to a mass lesion.

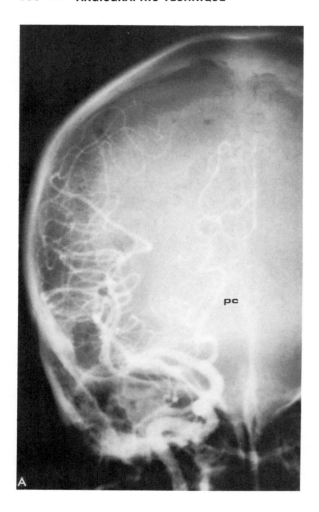

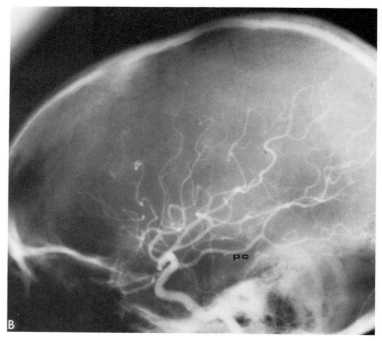

FIGURE 4–37. *Absent Filling of the Anterior Cerebral Artery: A,* The internal carotid injection in this case demonstrates filling only of the middle and posterior cerebral arteries.

B, The posterior cerebral artery is readily demonstrated on the lateral view *(pc)*. This appearance should not be mistaken for a shift of the anterior cerebral artery on the AP view. The anterior cerebral artery filled when an injection was made on the opposite side.

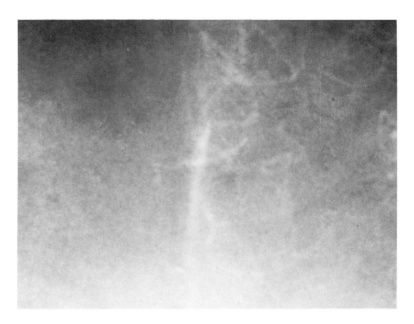

FIGURE 4–38. *Pericallosal Plexus:* The pericallosal artery breaks up into a capillary plexus—the pericallosal plexus —that has the appearance of a "moustache." On the right the pericallosal plexus is normal in position, but on the left it is tilted upward. This "tilting" of the pericallosal plexus may be either upward or downward when a mass lesion is present. This sign may help to delineate the position of the mass.

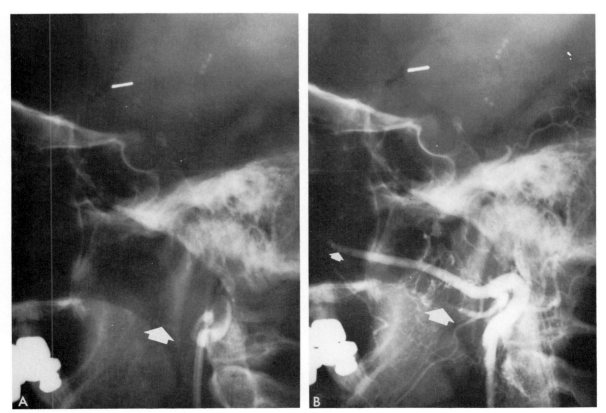

FIGURE 4–39. *Embolization:* The preliminary film (*A*) demonstrates multiple small Silastic balls in the terminal branches of the external carotid artery. Some are in the superficial temporal artery over the bony calvaria; others are in branches of the internal maxillary artery (*arrow*). Following the injection of contrast material (*B*), there is interruption of the flow of the contrast material through these branches because of the mechanical obstruction.

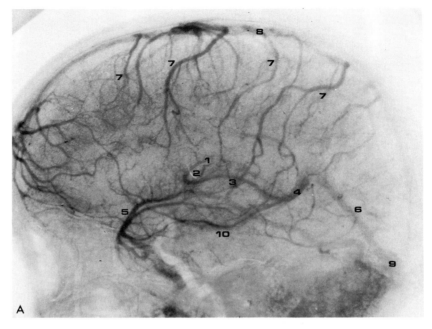

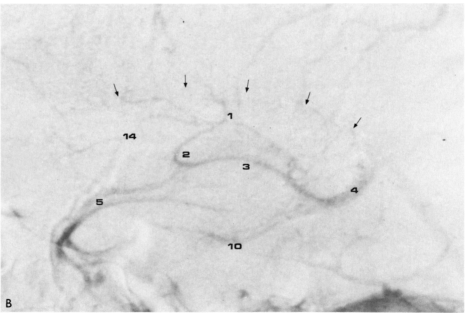

FIGURE 4–40. *Normal Venous Anatomy:* The deep and superficial venous structures are readily identified in most cases.

1 Thalamostriate vein.	6 Straight sinus.
2 Venous angle.	7 Superficial cortical veins.
3 Internal cerebral vein.	8 Superior sagittal sinus.
4 Vein of Galen.	9 Torcular Herophili.
5 Middle cerebral vein.	10 Basal vein of Rosenthal.

In *B* the small arrows demonstrate the subependymal course of the veins. A linear measurement made from one of the small veins to the internal cerebral vein reflects the height of the lateral ventricle. 14 is an anomalous course of the septal vein.

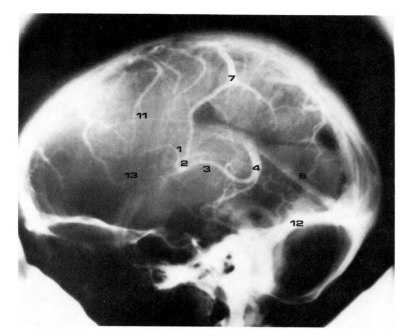

FIGURE 4–41. *Normal Superficial and Deep Venous Anatomy:*

1 Thalamostriate vein.	8 Superior sagittal sinus.
2 Venous angle.	9 Torcular Herophili.
3 Internal cerebral vein.	10 Basal vein of Rosenthal.
4 Vein of Galen.	11 Inferior sagittal sinus.
5 Middle cerebral vein.	12 Transverse sinus.
6 Straight sinus.	13 Septal vein.
7 Vein of Trolard.	

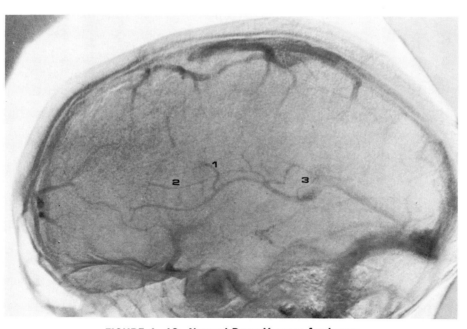

FIGURE 4–42. *Normal Deep Venous Anatomy:*
1 Thalamostriate vein.
2 Middle terminal vein.
3 Common atrial veins.

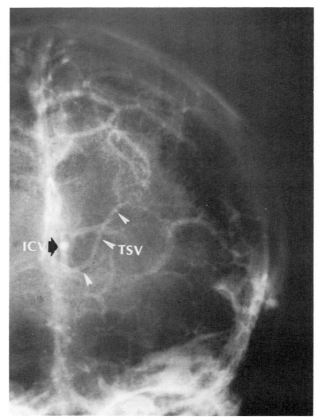

FIGURE 4–43. Normal AP view of the deep venous system, showing the internal cerebral vein (*ICU*) and the thalamostriate vein (*TSV*).

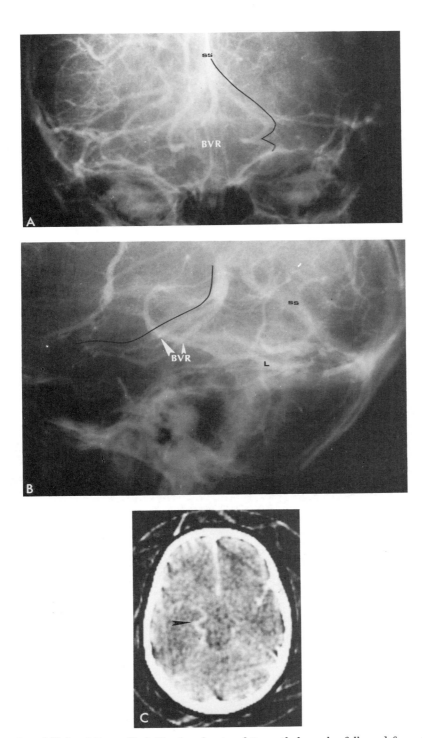

FIGURE 4–44. *Basal Vein of Rosenthal:* The basal vein of Rosenthal can be followed from its origin at the anterior perforated substance posteriorly and around the brain stem, where it joins with the vein of Galen and then drains into the straight sinus (*SS*). The course of this vein is demonstrated on one side in both the AP (*A*) and the lateral (*B*) views (*black line*). In *B*, *L* is the vein of Labbé, which drains into the transverse sinus.

C, The CT scan also demonstrates the course of the basal vein in the axial projection.

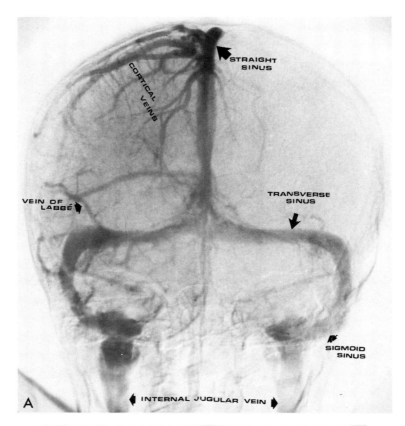

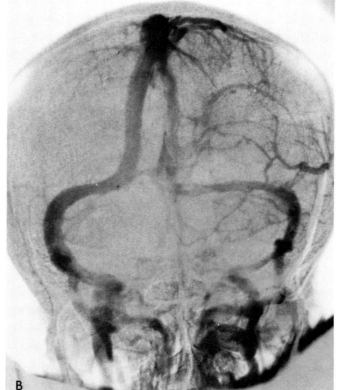

FIGURE 4–45. *Superior Sagittal Sinus:* The superior sagittal sinus normally lies at the midline but can drain in an off-centered manner and still be considered entirely normal. The sinus may be placed to the right or the left of the midline.

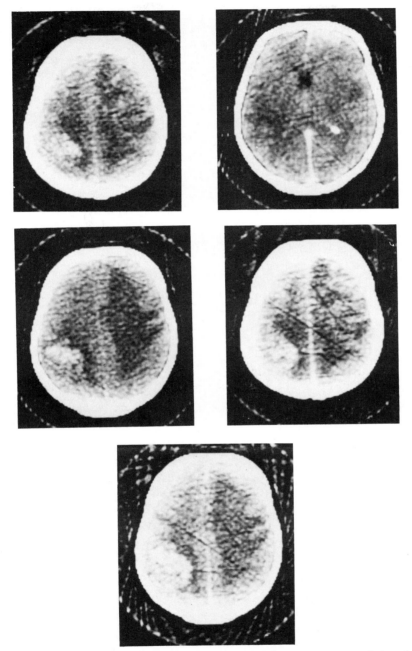

FIGURE 4–46. *Superior Sagittal Thrombosis:* With occlusion of the superior sagittal sinus by clot, there are infarcts in the areas of distribution of the superficial cortical veins. In many cases, hemorrhagic infarcts may develop, as are present in this patient.

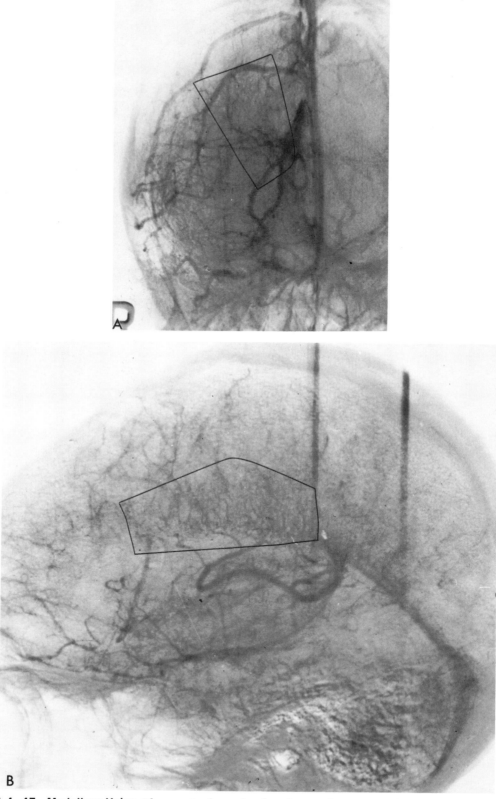

FIGURE 4–47. Medullary Veins: These veins have developed secondary to an infarct deep in the cerebral hemisphere. The veins are longer than 1.5 cm and can be seen draining into the deep venous system on both the AP (*A*) and lateral (*B*) views.

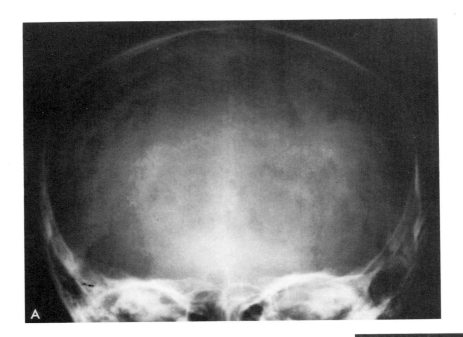

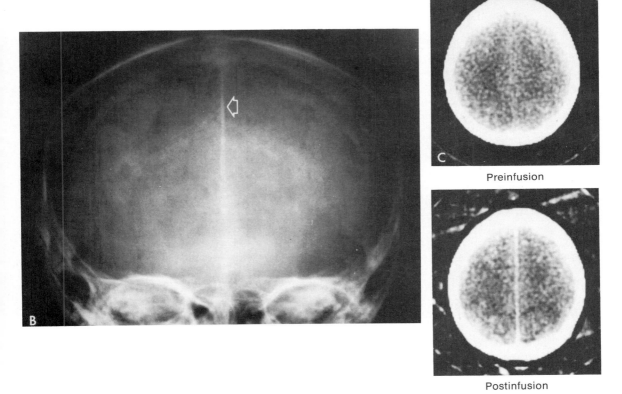

Preinfusion

Postinfusion

FIGURE 4–48. *Blush of the Falx:* The falx cerebri normally concentrates the contrast material. This is demonstrated on this patient, where the falx is seen on the postinjection film (*arrowhead*). This phenomenon is also seen on the CT scans.

5

THE ABNORMAL ANGIOGRAM

VASCULAR DISPLACEMENTS SECONDARY TO MASS LESIONS

Intracranial mass lesions can cause a variety of abnormal angiographic appearances. In some instances, particularly that of meningiomas, the pattern is quite typical, and the diagnosis can be made with a high degree of certainty from the angiographic appearance alone. For this reason, Chapter 8 has been devoted entirely to meningiomas. Some other tumors also have a relatively characteristic angiographic appearance—particularly the malignant glioblastoma multiforme, which presents with a host of abnormal vessels, early draining veins, and marked mass effect. Rarely, however, is it possible to make an unequivocal statement about the histology of a specific mass from the angiogram alone. The development of computed tomography has added greatly to our ability to diagnose the nature of a mass; in certain entities the CT scan has decreased or eliminated the need for angiography. This is especially true in patients who have had cerebral trauma or have suffered an intracerebral hemorrhage. In these, the need for angiography has been nearly eliminated. On the other hand, in other disease entities angiography and computed tomography are complementary techniques.

The present chapter on the abnormal angiogram first offers a general overview of the various disease processes and their anticipated histologic, plain skull, angiographic, CT, and MR findings. Then, illustrations are provided to demonstrate the variety of vascular displacement patterns seen with mass lesions in several supratentorial anatomic locations. Mass lesions in these various locations tend to provoke typical patterns of shift of arterial and venous structures. The author has attempted to correlate the angiograms with corresponding CT or MR scans whenever possible. The CT and MR scans usually follow the angiograms so that the reader can "test" his or her diagnostic acumen before correlation with the CT scan. Because a variety of lesions can be seen in a given anatomic site, these cases have been grouped by location rather than by disease process.

Typical or classic cases have been chosen whenever possible. The angiogram and CT and MR scans are from the same patient when possible, and from a very similar patient when corresponding studies were not available.

MAGNETIC RESONANCE OF BRAIN TUMORS

Magnetic resonance has aided our ability to diagnose brain tumors because of its increased sensitivity as compared to CT scanning and other diagnostic tests. For the patient with an enhancing lesion, CT is probably the procedure of choice. The reason is that while MR is more sensitive in diagnosing an abnormality, it is not necessarily more specific. The greater value of MR is its ability to identify an abnormality when the CT scan is normal or demonstrates only a minimal abnormality. Clinically, this has been helpful in those patients who have a history of a long-term seizure disorder or abnormal clinical signs and symptoms, but no definite abnormality on other diagnostic tests. In those cases, MR may identify a process such as a glioma, arachnoid cyst, or other type of focal lesion. The multiplanar imaging capability of MR has been particularly helpful in the temporal lobe region (see Chapter 13 on posterior fossa tumors) where artifact frequently interferes with excellent evaluation by CT. On the other hand, as the examples illustrate, MR may identify the abnormality in the face of a normal CT.

For routine screening of any patient in whom the order is "rule out brain tumor," the author recommends the following as a standard screening examination:

Axial: SE TR530/TE30
           SE TR3120 or 2120/TE60-120
Coronal: SE TR3120 or 2120/TE60-120

If there is any question of the possibility of a midline type of tumor such as a pinealoma or hypothalamic glioma, then images should also be obtained in the sagittal plane. If that is the case, then either the axial or coronal images can be omitted and replaced by sagittal plane images. Because these patients frequently have had a CT scan in the axial plane, an MR scan in a similar plane is helpful for additional evaluation and correlation.

The future availability of gadolinium-DTPA will be helpful in the evaluation and localization of brain tumors. The gadolinium-DTPA given intravenously in appropriate concentrations causes the tumors to be "bright" or increased in signal intensity on the T-1 weighted images and therefore results in demonstration of the tumor on the shorter scanning sequences. It remains to be seen if this will add to our ability to make a histologic diagnosis of the abnormality.

The T-1 weighted or SE TR530/TE30 images demonstrate the "anatomy" and any shift in the midline or alteration in the normal position of the various structures. The signal-to-noise ratio is also greater with the T-1 weighted images, so the overall image is better. It is the T-2 weighted images using TR3120 or 2120 and TE120 that best demonstrate the pathology. If possible, it is best to use a two-echo, multislice sequence, such as the TR3120/TE60-120 SE. This allows one to obtain one echo to the left of the cross-over point and one echo to the right of it. The T-2 weighted image causes both the tumor and the surrounding area to become "bright," or increased in signal intensity. The use of the two-echo sequence sometimes causes the tumor to respond in one way and the surrounding edema to respond in another. This, of course, allows the examiner to differentiate the tumor from the surrounding edema. Unfortunately, this is not always the case even with the two-echo, multislice technique; thus one of the "deficiencies" of MR is the inability to differentiate between tumor mass and surrounding edema. In this regard, CT has an advantage over MR because the postinfusion CT does help to differentiate the edema from the tumor, since the tumor demonstrates enhancement while the surrounding edema does not. Because of this, if a patient is known to have an enhancing tumor, then CT is the procedure of choice rather than MR.

The multiplanar capability of MR is an advantage that allows one to demonstrate the exact location of the tumor in various planes and also to determine its relationship to the surrounding structures. This three-dimensional examination of the brain is a great asset. While theoretically possible with CT, often, in fact, it is compromised by the patient's inability to maintain the sometimes awkward positions necessary. In addition, the CT scans also suffer from motion artifact, from the "Hounsfield" artifact in the temporal lobes, and from dental fillings and various dental artifacts.

Glioblastoma Multiforme

Glioblastomas are malignant tumors of astrocytic origin. The tumors usually have a rapidly progressive course, leading to death. They are encountered in all age groups, but their incidence decreases after the age of 40. After surgical removal, glioblastomas recur in the bed of the surgical site, and have rapid local extension. These tumors may rarely metastasize outside the central nervous system. Not infrequently the patients present with the adult onset of a seizure disorder; a progressive hemiparesis is fairly common. If located in a relatively "silent" area, such as the frontal lobes, the tumor may become quite large before there is any apparent problem. In point of fact, however, it seems that glioblastomas commonly are quite large at the time of initial presentation.

Pathology. These tumors are highly pleomorphic. There are polygonal cells with mitotic figures, some with multinucleated giant cells, fusiform cells with pseudopalisades and areas of necrosis, astroblasts in perivascular pseudorosettes, and a variety of astrocytes. The tumors invade the corpus callosum and grow across the midline to the opposite side, demonstrating a "butterfly" pattern of growth. Areas of necrosis are also commonly seen in these tumors as their rapid growth exceeds the blood supply.

Plain Skull. There may be a shift of the pineal gland to the contralateral side. Usually the growth of the tumor is so fast that the patient becomes clinically symptomatic before the secondary changes of increased intracranial pressure can develop. Rarely, areas of calcification may be seen.

Computed Tomography. The preinfusion scan usually demonstrates a poorly defined low-density area of varying size associated with shift of the midline to the contralateral side. There may rarely be scattered areas of calcification and/or hemorrhage. The area of involvement often is surprisingly large, even in a patient with minimal symptomatology. On the other hand, it is not uncommon to have a patient who is symptomatic demonstrate a normal CT scan initially—only to return in six weeks to six months with a spectacularly abnormal scan.

After the infusion of contrast material there is commonly an irregular ring of enhancement with a lucent center—apparently secondary to tumor necrosis in some cases—and a varying amount of surrounding edema. Less commonly, there is homogeneous enhancement of the tumor mass, also with varying degrees of surrounding edema. Rarely there will be no demonstrable areas of enhancement on the postinfusion scan.

Magnetic Resonance. MR is sensitive to the presence of an abnormality and may demonstrate a low-grade glioma or infiltrating, non-enhancing glioblastoma even when the CT scan is normal or shows only a minimal abnormality. The SE TR530/TE30 sequences demonstrate the distortion of the anatomy, while the SE TR3120/TE120 image reveals that the tumor and the surrounding edema are increased in signal intensity. The SE TR3120/TE60-120 is recommended because it may show the tumor as separate from the surrounding edema. At times the tumor responds in one way, while the edema responds in another, or the "rim" of the tumor may appear lower in signal intensity than either the center of the tumor or the surrounding edema. This low signal intensity appears to be the enhancing rim that is identified on the postinfusion CT scan.

MR is particularly helpful in evaluation of temporal lobe tumors, both because MR does not exhibit artifacts found in CT and because of its multiplanar capability. If the tumor is calcified, such as might be seen with an astrocytoma or oligodendroglioma, the MR scan may identify the tumor and surrounding edema but will be unable to identify the calcification. CT is particularly sensitive to calcification. Calcification has few "mobile" protons and therefore is poorly visualized by MR because it does not become increased in signal intensity on the T-2 weighted images.

One of the unique properties of MR is that it may identify an area of abnormal signal intensity in a patient with positive signs and symptoms but no other abnormality identified by various tests, including CT. Because of this increased sensitivity in a patient with symptoms or signs or a long-term seizure disorder and an otherwise normal work-up, an MR scan is suggested prior to considering the work-up complete.

Angiography. These tumors usually are supplied by branches of the internal carotid artery. Rarely they may demonstrate blood supply from the external carotid system. They may present as avascular masses or very vascular tumors with large feeding arteries and early draining veins. The presence of neovascularity and early draining veins, particularly with drainage into the deep venous system, usually correlates with a high degree of malignancy. Frequently the size of the tumor mass as reflected by the abnormal vessels is much smaller than the mass effect, reflecting a large amount of surrounding edema.

If there is no neovascularity to demonstrate the true position of the tumor, one of the great benefits of the CT scan is that it can show the true anatomic location of the tumor relative to the surrounding edema, which not uncommonly is asymmetric in its distribution around the tumor. In demonstrating the anatomic location more accurately, the CT scan aids in treatment planning, whether it be surgery or radiation therapy.

Oligodendroglioma

These tumors are rare, usually occur in adults, and, of all brain tumor types, are reported to be calcified in the highest percentage of cases. Oligodendrogliomas not uncommonly contain areas of calcification which can be seen by plain skull radiography and are readily demonstrated by CT scanning. In addition, oligodendrogliomas may also contain areas of hemorrhage—again readily demonstrable by CT scan.

Magnetic resonance of an oligodendroglioma will demonstrate any mass effect on the T-1 weighted images and increased signal intensity on the T-2 weighted images. Areas of calcification may be demonstrated as amorphous areas of low signal intensity, although they are frequently identified only poorly or not at all because of the low number of mobile protons.

Astrocytomas

These are tumors of astrocytes—the supporting cells of the brain. They are seen at all ages but are less common after 40. Astrocytomas are relatively benign brain tumors and are found in all parts of the central nervous system. They can rarely be removed entirely at surgery and frequently undergo malignant transformation.

Histology. These tumors are made up of astrocytes: frequently they demonstrate either gross or microscopic evidence of cyst formation. There may also be perivascular cuffs of lymphocytes. It is important to remember that astrocytomas lack (1) areas of necrosis and hemorrhage; (2) capillary endothelial proliferation; (3) cellular pleomorphism; (4) mitotic figures. Evidence of any of these four characteristics may signify the presence of a glioblastoma. Therefore, a limited surgical biopsy might not include a more abnormal area and would not reflect the true nature of the tumor.

Computed Tomography. These tumors may demonstrate areas of calcification and not uncommonly are cystic. Areas of either central or peripheral calcification may be seen.

Magnetic Resonance. MR is very sensitive to areas of abnormality and is therefore particularly useful for the diagnosis of low-grade astrocytoma. On the other hand, the calcified portion of the tumor will be visualized poorly or not at all. Because low-grade astrocytomas may be found in patients with idiopathic seizure disorders, MR is suggested for complete evaluation because of its increased sensitivity.

Ependymomas

These tumors arise from ependymal cells and may occur in any part of the ventricular system. They also sometimes develop from the ependymal lining of the central canal of the spinal cord. They may contain areas of calcification.

Choroid Plexus Papillomas

These tumors, which arise from the normal choroid plexus, are very similar in histologic appearance to normal tissue. They are rare and usually are found in children. Positional headaches may be the presenting complaint if a tumor blocks the foramen of Monro and causes obstructive hydrocephalus when the head is in a certain position. They may be associated with an excessive production of cerebrospinal fluid.

Colloid Cysts

These cystic tumors arise from the anterior part of the third ventricle and frequently cause obstructive hydrocephalus because of obstruction of the foramen of Monro. They are rounded and isodense or demonstrate increased density on the preinfusion CT scan. However, they enhance homogeneously on the postinfusion scan.

Magnetic Resonance. The author has had the opportunity to examine two patients with colloid cyst of the third ventricle. In one the CT was abnormal; in the other, the CT was normal except for enlargement of the lateral ventricles. The MR in both these cases revealed that the cyst was of low signal intensity on the T-1 weighted image and became increased in signal intensity on the T-2 weighted image, with a low signal intensity center.

Metastases

Patients of any age group may present with cerebral metastases. The finding of multiple lesions supports the diagnosis of metastases, although it is not uncommon to see a solitary metastatic lesion. On the other hand, some primary brain tumors such as the microglioma may develop from multiple sites. In an active clinical practice there is rarely a day that passes that one does not see an example of multiple brain metastases. This is the most common type of brain tumor that is seen (see section on Metastases).

Plain Skull. The routine skull series usually is normal. There may be a shift of the pineal gland, but if the metastases are multiple and "balancing," there will be no shift of the midline structures. Multiple metastatic deposits also may be found in the bony calvaria.

Computed Tomography. The CT scan with infusion is the most efficient and accurate method of demonstrating the presence of metastatic lesions. The CT scan should be performed both with and without the infusion of contrast material, although after the diagnosis is established the patient's response to treatment may be followed with a postinfusion scan only. Lesions may be seen on the postinfusion scan that cannot be identified on the preinfusion scan. In such patients the preinfusion scan may be normal, or there may be an increased number of metastatic lesions demonstrated on the postinfusion scan. This finding may alter the approach to treatment.

Metastatic nodules may be isodense, lucent, or of greater density than the normal brain. They may even present a combination of these findings. Metastatic squamous cell carcinoma tends to be of lower than normal brain density, whereas metastatic adenocarcinoma shows higher than normal density. These lesions may or may not be space-occupying; there may be no edema or spectacular surrounding edema. They usually enhance homogeneously, but may be of a "ring" type. At times differentiation from a primary brain tumor is impossible—especially when only a solitary metastatic deposit is present.

The bony calvaria may be evaluated for metastases by reviewing the standard cuts at high window width and window level. The skull film is more accurate for diagnosis of metastases.

Magnetic Resonance. MR is very helpful for the evaluation of metastatic disease because of its sensitivity. It is unclear at the time of this writing whether MR will replace CT for the evaluation of metastatic disease. The SE TR3120/TE60-120 images are most helpful for evaluation and reveal that the metastatic deposits become increased in signal intensity. Metastatic deposits in the posterior fossa, involving the brain stem or cerebellum, are particularly well evaluated by MR (see Chapter 13). The metastatic deposits demonstrate increased signal intensity on the T-2 weighted images. Both the mass and the surrounding edema demonstrate increased signal intensity, although at times the SE TR3120/TE60-120 sequence reveals the mass to be of a different signal intensity than the surrounding edema, or the rim of a cystic or necrotic deposit to be lower in signal intensity than the solid portion or surrounding edema.

A solitary metastatic deposit cannot be differentiated from a primary brain tumor or abscess.

Angiography. Multiple lesions may be demonstrated angiographically, but far less accurately than by CT scan. The lesions may be avascular, or they may demonstrate abnormal vascularity with early draining views. Generally speaking, if multiple lesions consistent with metastases are demonstrated by other means, angiography is not performed as part of the work-up. However, with a solitary lesion, or when the diagnosis is in doubt, angiography may be performed to aid in diagnosis. The mass or masses may be avascular, demonstrating only vessel displacement and a shift to the contralateral side. On the other hand, metastatic lesions may demonstrate neovascularity, with an abnormal accumulation of vessels and early draining veins. At times, differentiation from a glioma may be difficult—especially with a solitary mass—regardless of whether it is avascular or demonstrates abnormal vessels. With balancing lesions, there may be little or no shift of the midline structures.

Abscess

Abscesses usually are caused by pyogenic bacteria, which may spread from middle ear infections, sinusitis, or mastoiditis or from hematogenous spread. The latter occurs most often with endocarditis or intravenous drug abuse. A history of recent dental manipulation is not uncommon. Brain abscesses may act as a mass lesion in the same way as any other mass. Rupture into the ventricular system may cause death. Multiple abscesses are occasionally seen—especially in association with bacterial endocarditis.

Plain Skull. The plain skull examination usually is normal, but it may show a shift of the pineal gland if there is sufficient mass effect. The source of infection, e.g., sinus or ear, may be visible by plain film examination.

Actually, it is impossible to differentiate with absolute certainty between an abscess and a glioblastoma in most cases. A high index of suspicion is helpful in diagnosis.

Arteriography. Most commonly there is an avascular mass; however, a capsular stain may be seen, and rarely a thick-walled, prolonged capsular stain may be visualized that persists into the venous phase. With multiple abscesses the arteriogram will reflect this finding, showing stretching of vessels in separate areas and scattered areas of capsular stain—a sign typical of abscess formation. Early-draining veins also may be seen.

Computed Tomography. Typically, there is a large irregular area of radiolucency associated with a shift of the ventricular system to the contralateral side. In the rare case of multiple abscesses, scattered low-density areas are seen. The areas of lucency have irregular margins; rarely, the higher density rim of the actual abscess may be visible within the area of radiolucency, even on the preinfusion scan. Postinfusion, there is enhancement in a ring pattern that usually demonstrates a thick-walled rim of enhancement surrounded by edema. Occasionally, there is a multilobulated pattern of enhancement in one area or multiple separate rings of enhancement.

If there is a cerebritis without actual abscess formation, there may not be any evidence of enhancement—only an area of radiolucency that may or may not demonstrate mass effect.

Magnetic Resonance. MR reveals increased signal intensity areas in the region of an area of cerebritis or abscess formation on the T-2 weighted SE images. There is no unique appearance with MR, and a solitary abscess could mimic the appearance of a primary or secondary brain tumor.

Medullary Veins

These veins, which drain the white matter, are normally present but usually are not visible at arteriography. With magnification and subtraction techniques, it is sometimes possible to demonstrate the medullary veins, even in the normal individual. In the normal state, these very numerous veins are less than 1.5 cm long and are very fine vascular structures that run parallel to each other. They drain into the deep veins around the walls of the lateral ventricles. At times, these veins will outline the position of the lateral ventricle.

The medullary veins become enlarged in the presence of arteriovenous malformations, glioblastoma multiforme, or infarction. Abnormal medullary veins can be seen on routine arteriography because they are enlarged and longer than 1.5 cm.

The Abnormal Angiogram

Each mass lesion in the various lobes of the brain and in the region of the basal ganglia, the pituitary, and the midline structures demonstrates a relatively typical pattern of vascular displacement. The following pages offer discussions and summaries of the types of arterial and venous displacement that may be seen with a space-occupying lesion in these various positions. The reader must remember that it is not uncommon for a mass to cross over these boundaries; thus, each angiographic appearance usually cannot be absolutely categorized into an individual lobar position. However, an attempt has been made in the following illustrations to categorize these lesions by anatomic location and to demonstrate the "classic" vascular dislocations that occur. The section on mass lesions

has been divided into anatomic locations without regard to histologic type. Whenever possible, each case is correlated with the corresponding CT scan or with a scan from a similar patient.

If the reader commits to memory the anticipated vascular dislocations caused by the various space-occupying lesions, an individual angiogram can be evaluated and interpreted without a great deal of difficulty. One must keep in mind that it is a rare lesion that can be diagnosed with certainty by its angiographic appearance alone. The differential diagnosis should be an important part of the interpretation of each angiogram, even when a CT or MR scan is also available.

FRONTAL LOBE MASS LESIONS

When a mass is present in the frontal lobe, there is displacement of the anterior cerebral artery to the contralateral side. Because the mass is anteriorly placed, most of the effect on the anterior cerebral artery will be on its proximal portion. This results in a rounded appearance of the vessel as it is displaced across the midline on the AP arteriographic views. This has been called "round shift of the anterior cerebral artery" but could also be called a "proximal shift" of the artery. Before the vessel returns to the ipsilateral side of the falx, the pericallosal artery returns to a more normal position, so that there is not an abrupt shift under the falx. An anteriorly placed mass lesion also creates little or no displacement of the internal cerebral vein because it is remote from the anatomic position of the vein. If there is any shift of the internal cerebral vein, it will certainly be less than the shift of the anterior cerebral artery.

By using this approach to diagnosis of the position of the mass, the observer should be able to determine the position of the mass, before proceeding to the lateral view. In other words, if the pericallosal artery is shifted more than the internal cerebral vein, the mass is anterior in position.

The lateral view will not reveal the normal undulations of the anterior cerebral artery because the vessel is stretched as it is displaced from its normal plane toward the contralateral side. Depending on the intrinsic vascularity of the mass, one will find an avascular area in the frontal lobe region with stretching of the vessels in the frontal region together with evidence of poor or delayed venous filling secondary to localized increased intracranial pressure. Depending on the size of the mass, there may or may not be posterior displacement of the branches of the middle cerebral artery group. Most frequently, if there is any change it will be seen at the anterior portion of the sylvian triangle, leading to posterior displacement and posterior telescoping of the triangle.

The venous phase of the lateral view reveals that there is closing of the venous angle—i.e., the thalamostriate vein is displaced posteriorly and downward closer to the internal cerebral vein, making a more acute or "closed" venous angle. There is also posterior displacement of the venous angle and poor venous filling in the frontal region.

In summary, the angiographic findings with a frontal lobe mass lesion are:

AP View

1. Proximal shift of the anterior cerebral artery.
2. Less shift of the internal cerebral vein.

Lateral View

3. Disruption of the anterior portion of the sylvian triangle.
4. Posterior displacement of the sylvian point and posterior telescoping of the sylvian triangle.
5. Posterior displacement of the venous angle and a closed venous angle.
6. An area of avascularity in the frontal region.
7. Delayed filling of the frontal veins.

Subfrontal mass lesions and their pattern of vascular displacement are discussed in Chapter 8.

PARIETAL LOBE MASS LESIONS

Mass lesions in the parietal lobe cause a distal shift of the anterior cerebral artery to the contralateral side. Because the mass is situated adjacent to the more distal portion of the vessel, there is a rather abrupt return of the pericallosal artery to its own side of the falx. This results in a rather sharp angle of the pericallosal artery just at its point of return under the falx. This point of shift under the falx is readily identifiable on the AP view; it often can be identified on the lateral view as well. There is inferior displacement of the sylvian point. If the mass is in a parasagittal position, there will be lateral displacement of the sylvian point; if the mass is low over the convexity, there will be medial displacement of the sylvian point.

The internal cerebral vein will be shifted to the contralateral side. The degree of shift is approximately equal to the shift of the pericallosal artery.

The lateral view reveals downward displacement of the sylvian triangle and stretching of the anterior and middle cerebral artery branches around the mass lesion. Depending on the intrinsic vascularity of the mass, there is an area of avascularity. There may be delayed venous filling. The sylvian point will be inferiorly displaced.

The venous phase of the lateral view will reveal that there is an "open" venous angle, and downward displacement of the internal cerebral vein may be seen.

In summary, the angiographic findings with a parietal lobe mass lesion are:

AP View

1. Distal shift of the pericallosal artery.
2. An approximately equal shift of the internal cerebral vein.

AP and Lateral View

3. Downward displacement of the sylvian triangle.
4. Downward displacement of the sylvian point.

Lateral View

5. Stretched vessels in the parietal region, arterial phase.
6. An "open" venous angle.
7. An area of avascularity or neovascularity in the parietal region.

OCCIPITAL LOBE MASS LESIONS

Mass lesions in the occipital lobe may or may not produce a shift of the anterior cerebral artery. If a shift is detected, there will be slight posterior shift of the pericallosal artery under the falx cerebri. In rare instances there may be a shift of the more proximal anterior cerebral artery. There is a greater shift in the internal cerebral vein; indeed, this may be the only arteriographic finding in some cases. The sylvian point may be displaced anteriorly; because of the angiographic projection, this will give the appearance of superior displacement on the AP view. Superior and anterior displacement also may occur.

The lateral view may appear to be within normal limits. A relatively normal appearance is seen especially when the posterior cerebral artery does not fill from the internal carotid. Then one normally can anticipate an area of relative avascularity in the occipital region on the lateral view. If the mass is sufficiently large, there is stretching of the vessels in the parietal as well as the occipital region. Depending on the intrinsic vascularity of the mass, an area of avascularity associated with delayed venous filling may be noted.

The lateral view of the venous phase reveals an open venous angle.

The sylvian triangle will be displaced anteriorly, with telescoping of the branches of the middle cerebral artery group. The sylvian point will be displaced anteriorly and, on occasion, superiorly.

In summary the angiographic findings with an occipital lobe mass lesion are:

AP View

1. Slight or no distal shift of the anterior cerebral artery.
2. A greater shift of the internal cerebral vein.

Lateral View

3. Anterior telescoping of the sylvian triangle.
4. There may be superior and/or anterior displacement of the sylvian point.
5. An "open" venous angle.
6. An area of avascularity or neovascularity in the occipital region.

TEMPORAL LOBE MASS LESIONS

Large temporal lobe mass lesions cause both superior and medial displacement of the sylvian point. The branches of the middle cerebral artery will be displaced medially, and the genu of the middle cerebral artery, which normally is 20 to 30 mm from the inner table of the skull, also will be displaced medially. (This latter measurement is one of the least reliable of the angiographic measurements.) The anterior cerebral artery usually demonstrates an equal proximal and distal shift under the falx cerebri. There is a greater shift of the internal cerebral vein. The thalamostriate vein is medially displaced. The lenticulostriate vessels are medially displaced, as is the anterior choroidal artery.

The lateral view reveals superior displacement of the sylvian point and the entire sylvian triangle. If the mass is sufficiently large, the main branch of the middle cerebral artery will simulate the normal anatomy of the anterior cerebral artery; on the lateral view this may be mistaken for occlusion of the middle cerebral artery rather than the marked distortion that is really present. The temporal opercular branches will be markedly stretched.

If the mass is intrinsic within the temporal lobe, the branches of the middle cerebral artery will be "draped" over the mass. This draping sign is helpful when there is difficulty in differentiating an intrinsic from an extrinsic mass of the temporal lobe. An extrinsic mass, such as a sphenoid wing meningioma, may have a similar pattern of vessel dislocation but will not demonstrate the draped appearance of the temporal opercular branches.

Depending on the intrinsic vascularity of the mass, there may be an avascular region in the temporal lobe.

In summary, the angiographic findings with a temporal lobe mass lesion are:

AP View

1. Varying shift of the pericallosal artery, which may be equal proximally and distally or have only distal shift.
2. A greater shift of the internal cerebral vein.
3. Superior displacement of the sylvian point and medial displacement of the middle cerebral vessels.

Lateral View

4. Superior displacement of the sylvian point and the sylvian triangle.
5. Stretching of the vessels in the temporal lobe region.

BASAL GANGLIA MASS LESIONS

Mass lesions in the region of the basal ganglia may be very subtle; not uncommonly there are no abnormal arteriographic findings. In many cases the arteriogram is normal, except for a slight or moderate shift of the internal cerebral vein to the contralateral side. With a mass of sufficient size there is a proximal and distal shift of the anterior cerebral artery of varying degree and a greater shift of the internal cerebral vein. The sylvian point and the other branches of the middle cerebral artery are displaced laterally. Depending on the exact position of the mass there may be an alteration of the position of the lenticulostriate arteries as they feed the region of the basal ganglia. If the mass—usually a hemorrhage—involves the globus pallidus and the medial portions of the basal ganglia, there will be lateral displacement of the lenticulostriate vessels and the anterior choroidal artery. If hemorrhage into the putamen has occurred—and this is by far the most common location—there will be medial displacement of the lenticulostriate and anterior choroidal arteries associated with lateral displacement of the middle cerebral artery branches. The latter pattern is the most common and occurs secondary to hypertensive hemorrhage into the putamen of the basal ganglia; it is secondary to rupture of small aneurysms that involve the lenticulostriate vessels.

If the hemorrhage has ruptured into the lateral vesicles, a resulting ventricular dilatation may displace the thalamostriate laterally and bow the thalamostriate vein in a manner similar to that seen with any other cause of hydrocephalus.

The lateral view usually is normal, but may show stretching of the branches of the middle cerebral artery in the region of the basal ganglia; or, if the hemorrhage extends superiorly, stretching of the opercular branches of the middle cerebral artery in the posterior frontal and anterior parietal regions will be seen.

Included with the section on hypertensive basal ganglionic hemorrhages are several examples of hypertensive brain stem and cerebellar hemorrhages. These cerebellar hemorrhages are not uncommon. Computed tomography is the diagnostic procedure of choice, and early surgical evaluation may be life-saving.

Magnetic Resonance of Hemorrhage

Computed tomography is the procedure of choice for the evaluation of acute hemorrhage. With MR of acute hemorrhage, the area of hemorrhage appears to be of low signal intensity during the first 48 hours following hemorrhage. This low signal intensity is thought to be secondary to a paramagnetic effect of the iron in the hemoglobin molecule. With the passage of time—approximately 48 hours—there is metabolism of the hemoglobin molecule to methemoglobin, resulting in a shortening of the T-1 of the blood and the appearance of an area of increased signal intensity. Because it is important to differentiate ischemic from hemorrhagic areas of infarction, MR is not the procedure of choice for the acutely ill patient. In addition, the patient with basal ganglia hemorrhage is often acutely ill, requiring various life-support systems that cannot be used in the scanning room because the magnetic field will interfere with their function. After the first 48 hours the blood appears increased in signal intensity and is easily diagnosed and evaluated. MR may be

especially helpful in those patients with a small area of increased density on the CT scan which, because of the partial volume effect, cannot be differentiated from an area of calcification. MR reveals increased signal intensity if this is hemorrhage and decreased signal intensity if this is an area of calcification.

Acutely, within the first 48 hours, an intracerebral hematoma will appear as an area of low signal intensity on T-1 weighted images when studied with a 5 kilogauss, 0.5 Tesla MR scanner. Therefore, differentiation between hematoma and other processes such as brain tumor or space-occupying infarct cannot be made. Consequently, if an acute hemorrhage is a diagnostic consideration, then CT scanning, which is exquisitely sensitive to hemorrhage, is the procedure of choice. Studies have shown that the decreased signal intensity is caused by deoxyhemoglobin in the hematoma. After approximately 48 hours the deoxyhemoglobin is metabolized to methemoglobin, which has a higher signal intensity. Typically, this change in signal intensity commences at the periphery of the hematoma, so that the MR appearance is that of a peripheral margin of increased signal intensity surrounding the decreased signal intensity intracerebral hematoma (Fig. 5–30, p. 248). Further metabolism and evolution of the intracerebral hematoma result in an appearance of homogeneous increased signal intensity throughout the hematoma. This probably takes a varying period of time depending upon the size of the hematoma.

With the further passage of time, the hematoma resolves and frequently leaves a deposit of hemosiderin in the bed of the hematoma. Because hemosiderin is strongly paramagnetic, this material shortens both the T-1 and T-2 measurements and produces an area of markedly decreased signal. This finding of a decreased signal area is not uncommonly seen in association with processes such as occult arteriovenous malformations or even true arteriovenous malformations that have hemorrhaged. Another process that exhibits a similar appearance is basal ganglia hematoma, such as that associated with hypertensive hemorrhage.

In summary, the angiographic findings with mass lesions in the basal ganglia area are:

AP View

1. The angiogram may be entirely normal.
2. There may be a proximal and distal shift of the pericallosal artery to the contralateral side.
3. There may be lateral displacement of the middle cerebral artery vessels.

4. The lenticulostriate vessels will be displaced medially or laterally, depending on the position of the hemorrhage.

5. There may be hydrocephalus secondary to rupture of the hemorrhage into the lateral ventricle.

Lateral View

6. The lateral view is usually normal, but may show stretching of the vessels in the suprasylvian region.

On the venous phase of the angiogram a mass in the region of the thalamus may demonstrate elevation and displacement of the internal cerebral vein and curvilinear displacement of the basal vein of Rosenthal in a posterior and lateral direction. This latter finding may be the only detectable abnormality.

The region of the basal ganglia and thalamus are well demonstrated on the CT scans, and CT is the procedure of choice. Angiography is usually not necessary.

MIDLINE MASS LESIONS

Mass lesions in the midline of the cerebrum are very difficult to detect angiographically. They are best studied by CT scanning, and, in fact, the CT scan has proved to be an ideal method for examining these patients. Angiography of the midline structures requires study of both the carotid and the vertebrobasilar systems.

Hypothalamic lesions provide a "normal" angiogram in most cases. If the mass is of sufficient size, there may be obstruction of the foramen of Monro and resulting hydrocephalus. The vertebral angiogram may demonstrate abnormal vessels supplying the tumor, but this is uncommon.

Pineal tumors demonstrate hydrocephalus because of obstruction of the outlet of the third ventricle and the aqueduct of Sylvius. The hydrocephalus may be the only discernible abnormality seen on the carotid arteriogram. The venous phase at times reveals localized curvilinear elevation of the internal cerebral vein and the vein of Galen as it is displaced around the tumor mass. This finding should be looked for. The vertebral angiogram is more likely to demonstrate abnormal vessels supplying the region of the tumor. The vessels are derived from the medial and lateral posterior choroidal vessels and supply the region of the pineal; in some cases they supply a very vascular area with abnormal vessels and early draining veins, best seen on the lateral view. Even this finding of abnormal vascular supply from the vertebro-

basilar system is unusual. In most cases no abnormal vessels can be seen, and the only really abnormal finding is the hydrocephalus.

The CT scan is the ideal method to evaluate midline tumors. With tumors of pineal origin there is evidence of a midline mass lesion, usually of higher density than that of normal brain substance; very commonly, areas of amorphous calcification also are seen. It is of particular interest to note that the normal pineal gland may be calcified and positioned at the midline while an abnormal mass surrounds the pineal and allows the gland to occupy its normal midline position. Therefore, a midline position of the pineal gland on the plain skull films certainly does not rule out the possibility of a pineal tumor. On the other hand, the size of the calcification does not correlate with the size of the pineal tumor because the calcification often either does not occupy the entire bulk of the tumor or is subradiographic. At times the tumor may be asymmetrically calcified, and the calcification may, indeed, lie off the midline. The calcification of the tumor, which is readily demonstrated on the CT scan, is usually *subradiographic.*

Computed Tomography of Pinealomas

A pineal tumor creates distortion of the posterior portion of the third ventricle, and the anterior portion of the ventricle is also distorted in a curvilinear fashion around the mass. There is encroachment upon the wings of the ambient cistern (retrothalamic cistern) and a mass of varying size, which may or may not contain areas of calcification. The postinfusion CT scan demonstrates marked enhancement of the tumor—usually in a homogeneous fashion, although occasional tumors enhance in an irregular fashion. In addition, these pineal tumors are known to spread through the central nervous system axis, and at times the "drop metastasis" to the region of the pituitary may be demonstrated on the postinfusion scan. These metastatic lesions apparently occur from abnormal deposits of cells that travel around the midbrain and proliferate in the suprasellar cistern. These deposits may be asymptomatic; their presence is discovered only by demonstration on the CT postinfusion scan. Spread also may occur to the region of the spinal cord secondary to drop metastases.

Classification of Pineal Tumors. Three histologic tumor types arise from the region of the pineal gland:

1. Pinealomas: either pineoblastoma or pineocytoma

2. Gliomas
3. Teratomas
   a. Typical and teratoid
   b. Germinoma (most common) or atypical teratoma

Ectopic pinealomas are similar to the germinomas and occur in the pituitary region.

Pituitary Tumors

Plain skull radiographs may reveal enlargement of the sella turcica in the presence of a pituitary tumor. In most cases with clinical evidence of bitemporal hemianopia there will be sellar enlargement and thinning and posterior displacement of the dorsum sellae and the posterior clinoids. (See Chapter 2 for a more thorough discussion.)

The angiogram may be normal if the tumor is small. In fact, one of the primary reasons for performing an angiogram on these patients is to rule out an internal carotid artery aneurysm as a cause of the symptoms. If the tumor is of sufficient size and extends into the suprasellar cisterns, there will be lateral displacement of the cavernous portions of the internal carotid arteries and elevation of the horizontal portions of the anterior and middle cerebral arteries. If the suprasellar extension is only in the midline, there will be elevation only of the horizontal segment of the anterior cerebral artery. Care must be taken in the interpretation of this finding because in the normal individual the horizontal portion of this vessel may be elevated even in the absence of a pituitary tumor.

Lateral magnification views may demonstrate hypertrophy of multiple small branches of the cavernous internal carotid artery supplying the tumor. There may be enlargement of the meningiohypophyseal trunk as well.

When it is of sufficient size to obstruct the foramen of Monro, a pituitary tumor causes obstructive hydrocephalus.

The venous phase demonstrates elevation of the venous angle, the septal vein, and the internal cerebral vein if the tumor is of sufficient size. With lateral extension of the tumor into the medial cranial fossa, there is lateral displacement and superior elevation of the anterior portion of the basal vein of Rosenthal. Often this can be readily demonstrated in the lateral view, where the basal vein of Rosenthal is displaced superiorly in a curvilinear fashion as it courses around the lateral extension of the pituitary mass.

With large mass lesions associated with destruction of the dorsum sellae and posterior clinoids, there is posterior displacement of the basilar artery; and, if the mass is of sufficient bulk, the lesion may create superior elevation of the proximal portions of the posterior cerebral arteries in a curvilinear fashion as they course over the posterior-superior portion of the tumor. Posterior displacement of the anterior pontomesencephalic vein is also associated with this change, reflecting posterior displacement of the pons.

COMPUTED TOMOGRAPHY OF THE SELLA

If magnetic resonance is unavailable, then CT is the method of choice for the evaluation of the sella turcica. The base cuts in the axial projection reflect the enlargement of the bony margins of the sella turcica as well as the extension of the mass into the sphenoid sinus. The more superior cuts demonstrate the suprasellar cistern and any evidence of obliteration of either the cistern or the anterior recesses of the third ventricle. The examination of the region of the sella can also be performed in the coronal plane. If a calcified tumor is suspected, then a preinfusion scan should be performed followed by the postinfusion portion of the examination. With the newer high-resolution scanners, this technique, particularly with 2- or 4-mm cuts through the sella, should allow adequate evaluation of the pituitary fossa. The postinfusion scan usually demonstrates enhancement of the mass in the sella (except for microadenoma of the pituitary) and any suprasellar extension. Pituitary tumors may be cystic and the thin rim of tumor may be difficult to demonstrate, even with the high-resolution scanners, and impossile to visualize with the first- and second-generation scanners. Therefore, in a patient who is losing vision it is necessary to pursue the evaluation with metrizamide cisternography if MR is not available. The metrizamide cisternogram will establish the presence or absence of a mass or an empty sella. This latter condition can also be suspected if the fluid within the sella is of CSF density and does not change in density after the infusion of contrast material (see Chapter 9).

MAGNETIC RESONANCE OF PITUITARY TUMORS

Magnetic resonance has proved to be particularly helpful in the diagnosis of pituitary tumors. The region of the sella can be readily demonstrated, and the multiplanar capability of MR makes it an ideal method for evaluation of the region around the sella. The short or T-1 weighted sequences nicely demonstrate the anatomy around the sella as well as any compromise of the sphenoid sinus. The longer spin-echo sequences or T-2 weighted images demonstrate areas of high signal intensity in the region of the tumor. Any cystic or hemorrhagic portions of the tumor are readily demonstrated. One of the nice benefits of MR scanning is the fact that the flowing blood within the blood vessels around the sella turcica produces a "negative flow defect," which allows for ready demonstration of the blood vessels. This is particularly helpful when the tumor is quite large and has grown around the blood vessels. Each vessel can be individually visualized and separated from the tumor mass by virtue of the negative flow defect. MR is superior to CT in this regard because after the infusion of contrast material there is enhancement of the tumor, the cavernous sinus, and the carotid arteries—these often all appear to enhance homogeneously, and exact localization of the vessels is obviously impossible. Again, the multiplanar capability is very helpful for evaluation. It appears that MR will become the procedure of choice for evaluation of the pituitary gland.

In the normal individual the anterior and posterior lobes of the pituitary may be visualized and this is best demonstrated in the midsagittal plane. Microadenomas of the pituitary gland are readily demonstrated and show areas of altered signal intensity when compared to the normal gland. These are areas of high signal intensity. Again, multiplanar imaging is excellent for demonstration.

METRIZAMIDE CISTERNOGRAPHY

Metrizamide (Amipaque, Winthrop Co.) introduced in 1978, is a water-soluble myelographic contrast material that also may be used for cisternography in conjunction with computed tomography. Evaluations of the sella and suprasellar cisterns are possible after the introduction of this water-soluble contrast material into the lumbar subarachnoid space and manipulation of the contrast material into the suprasellar cisterns.

Craniopharyngioma. The vascular displacements seen with a craniopharyngioma are similar to those seen with a pituitary tumor with suprasellar extension, except that the craniopharyngioma may demonstrate abnormal vessels. In addition, craniopharyngiomas frequently are calcified. These calcifications can be demonstrated on plain skull radiographs.

Computed tomography of a craniopharyngioma reveals a cystic lesion in the region of the suprasellar cistern that extends into the sella. The fluid within the cyst is of higher density than CSF fluid and reflects the density of the abnormal material within the cystic tumor. The areas of calcification are within the walls of the craniopharyngioma and are readily detected on the CT scan, even when they are subradiographic.

"PITFALLS" OF ANGIOGRAPHY

Not all masses fit precisely into the categories that have been defined. Masses that are small but occupy two lobes of the brain, or masses that are very large and thus affect multiple areas of the brain, will produce vascular displacements that include changes seen in more than one category of lesion. In fact, a combination of changes will be seen rather than a classic pattern of displacement. By the same token, multiple lesions will also alter the appearance of the angiogram and result in a combination of changes that includes patterns of vascular displacements from two different groups.

The beginning angiographer should commit to memory the various normal positions of the anatomic structures that have standard measurements. Thus, deviations from the normal can be readily evaluated by actual linear measurement. It should be kept in mind, however, that no single measurement should be clung to tenaciously, because a variety of changes may come to play upon the actual vessel displacements. Most important, balancing lesions may be present in both hemispheres, or there may be two separate lesions in the same hemisphere that will alter anticipated vascular displacements.

Initially, when reviewing an angiogram all pertinent information should be at hand to provide help in arriving at an accurate diagnosis. The chart, clinical history, and pertinent physical findings should be well known to the angiographer. Any other positive or significant negative test results also should be available for comparison or correlation with the angiographic study. This is true, after all, for the clinician who sees the patient in consultation; and it is of vital importance when evaluating the clinical condition and the angiographic findings. With increasing experience, the clinical history and physical findings may be all one needs to arrive successfully at the correct diagnosis. This knowledge of the clinical situation will also help the angiographer choose an approach to the procedure and decide which vessels are to be studied. For example, if a meningioma of the posterior fossa is suspected, a vertebral angiogram for the posterior fossa must be performed—but it is also important to study the carotid circulation to determine whether there is vascular supply to the tumor from the tentorial artery.

Angiography of Multiple Lesions. With multiple lesions the angiographic picture is not as straightforward as when there is a solitary mass. If multiple lesions are present, there may be a balancing or nearly balancing effect of the masses, and thus no shift of the midline struc-

tures. In such a case the mass will be localized by evaluation of the intrinsic displacement of various intracranial vessels and of the displacement of vessels from their anticipated normal position, even in the absence of midline shift. When multiple lesions are present, the CT scan has proved invaluable in demonstrating abnormal areas. Indeed, it is the ideal method for diagnosis of multiple lesions.

Because there is definite morbidity and risk of mortality from angiography, there is little or no room for error. It is important that the *appropriate* angiogram be performed. Great care should be taken to obtain excellent film studies so that an accurate diagnosis can be made and therapy instituted (see Chapter 10).

FIGURE 5–1. *Frontal Lobe Abscess:* A, The AP view demonstrates a greater shift of the proximal than the distal portion of the anterior cerebral artery. Note that the falx cerebri is displaced to the contralateral side. The anticipated normal position is marked by the dotted line.

B, The early arterial lateral view shows posterior displacement of the anterior cerebral artery (*arrows*), which also demonstrates some areas of narrowing. There is an avascular area in the frontal region. The anterior meningeal artery as it arises from the ophthalmic artery is also enlarged (*white arrowheads*).

C, The capillary phase of the angiogram demonstrates a capsular blush (*arrowheads*) with a lucent center.

D, CT scans from a different patient demonstrate a thick-walled, rounded mass in the frontal region which has a radiolucent center and is surrounded by edema. The edema is quite marked and has an irregular distribution. There is marked shift to the contralateral side. There is distortion of the left frontal horn and dilatation of the right lateral ventricle. The postinfusion scan demonstrates marked enhancement of the thick rim of the abscess.

Differential diagnosis includes primary glioma and metastatic tumor.

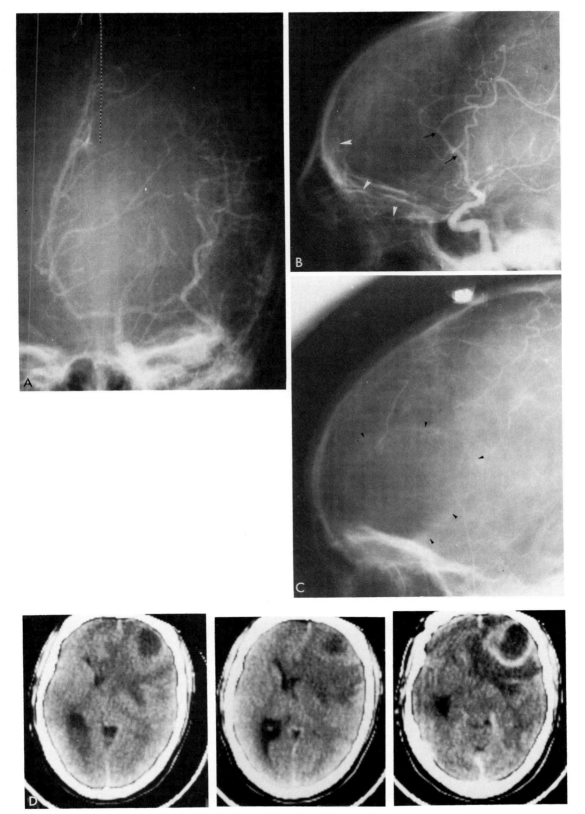

FIGURE 5–1. *See legend on the opposite page.*

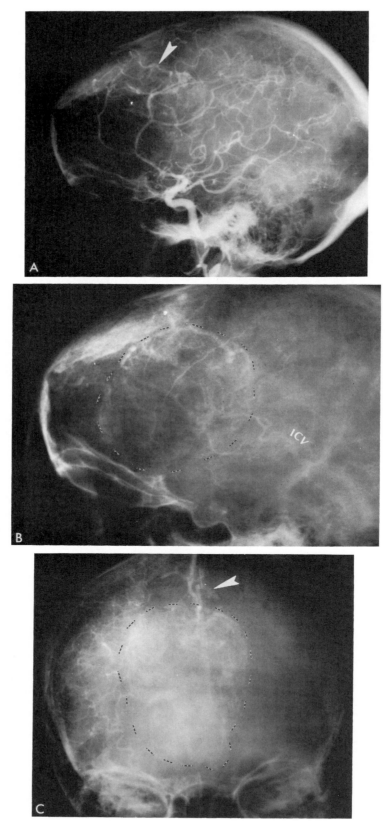

FIGURE 5–2. *See legend on the opposite page.*

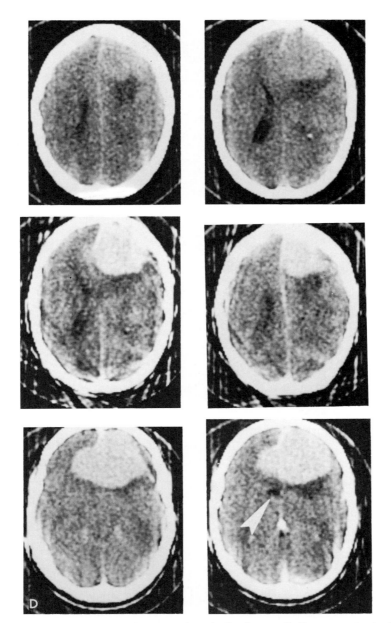

FIGURE 5–2. *Glioblastoma Multiforme with Extension via the Corpus Callosum: A,* In the lateral arteriogram there is evidence of neovascularity in the midfrontal region. Irregularity of the branches of the callosal marginal and pericallosal arteries also is evident in this region. There is downward displacement of the pericallosal artery. An early draining vein is seen in the high parasagittal region (*white arrowhead*).

B, The late capillary phase demonstrates a large tumor mass with a diffuse tumor stain (*dotted lines*) and multiple draining veins. The internal cerebral vein is displaced and buckled posteriorly (*ICV*).

C, The AP view demonstrates the deep blush (*dotted lines*) and the early draining vein in the high parasagittal region (*white arrowhead*). Note that the tumor extends contralaterally across the midline.

D, CT scans reveal a large tumor of slightly higher density than normal brain tissue in the frontal region. The mass extends across the midline. An area of edema extends around the tumor posteriorly. There is compression of the body of the ipsilateral ventricle and distortion of the frontal horns of the ventricular system. The postinfusion scan shows marked homogeneous enhancement of the tumor mass, which can be seen to extend across the midline. The frontal horns are displaced far posteriorly (*white arrowhead*). The true extent of the tumor and its extension across the midline via the corpus callosum can be readily demonstrated on the CT scan.

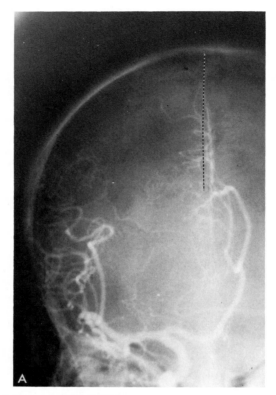

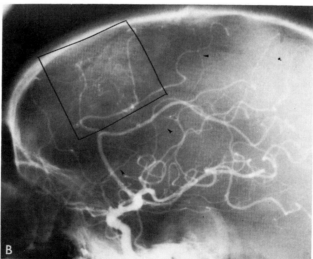

FIGURE 5–3. *Frontal Glioblastoma Multiforme:* A, In the AP view a shift of the pericallosal artery is more marked distally than in its proximal portion. The pericallosal artery demonstrates a sharp angulation under the falx (*dotted line*), which is displaced to the left of the midline.

B, The lateral view reveals an area of neovascularity (*black lines*) with inferior displacement of the pericallosal artery and sylvian triangle. There is posterior displacement of the sylvian triangle. The middle meningeal artery is prominent (*black arrowheads*) because of increased flow into the external carotid system due to increased intracranial pressure.

In addition to glioblastoma, the differential diagnosis includes metastasis.

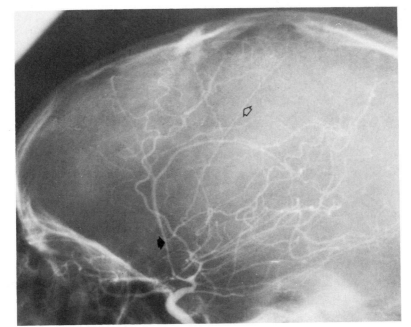

FIGURE 5–4. *Bifrontal Intracerebral Hematoma:* This angiogram demonstrates both straightening and posterior displacement of the pericallosal artery, as well as spasm of the proximal position of the vessel (*closed arrow*). There is a large avascular area in the frontal region. The sylvian triangle is telescoped posteriorly. The spasm of the vessel is caused by blood in the subarachnoid space, which may be secondary to the intracerebral hematoma or may occur independently. Note also the excessive filling of the middle meningeal artery (*open arrow*) and the superficial temporal branch of the external carotid artery. This filling is secondary to the increased intracranial pressure, which does not allow filling of the internal carotid circulation. The AP view (not shown) demonstrated no shift of the midline because the hematoma is bilateral and symmetrical.

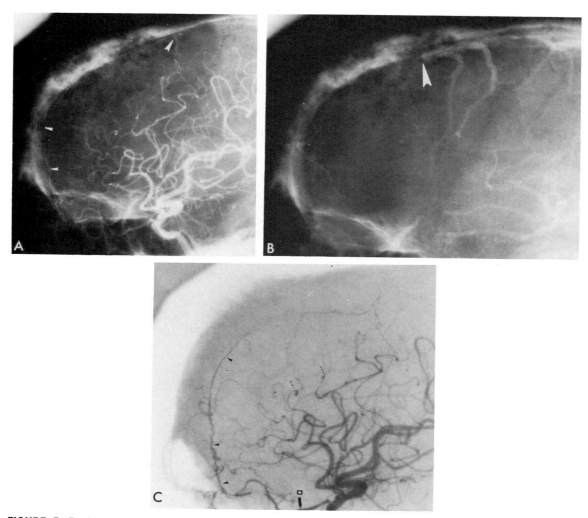

FIGURE 5–5. *Metastases to the Calvaria and Frontal Region:* An irregular lytic and blastic metastatic process involves the frontal bone of this skull. *A,* The angiogram demonstrates both an enlarged middle meningeal artery (*large arrowhead*) and an enlarged anterior meningeal artery, which arises from the ophthalmic artery (*small arrowheads*). These vessels supply the tumor, which involves the meninges in the frontal region.

B, The venous phase demonstrates invasion of the superior sagittal sinus (*arrowhead*) and a large avascular area, both in the frontal region. The pericallosal artery fills from the opposite carotid artery.

C, The subtraction view better demonstrates the enlarged anterior meningeal artery (*black arrowheads*), which is dilated and tortuous and arises from the ophthalmic artery (*O*). The frontal opercular branches of the middle cerebral artery are attenuated and displaced inferiorly by the tumor in the frontal region (*dashed lines*).

Illustration continued on the following page

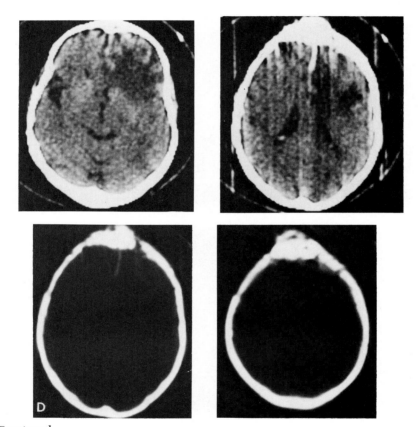

FIGURE 5–5 *Continued.*

D, The CT scans reveal the irregular metastatic deposit involving the frontal bone bilaterally. They also demonstrate the edema in the frontal region, mainly on the right side, which is secondary to intracranial tumor extension. There is posterior displacement of the right frontal horn, compression of the body of the right lateral ventricle, and minimal shift of the midline to the contralateral side.

The CT scan at high window widths and window levels demonstrates the involvement by the metastatic tumor, which is both osteoblastic and osteolytic.

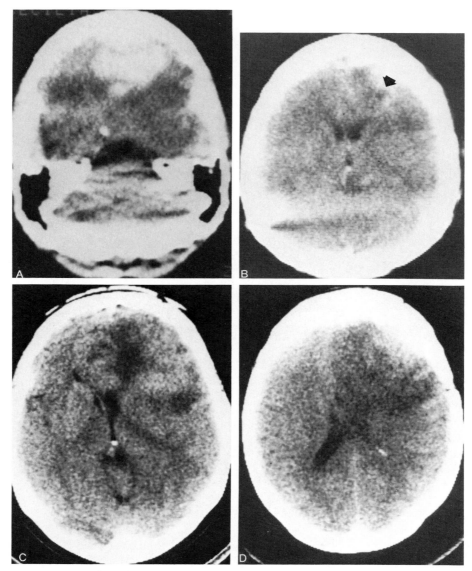

FIGURE 5–6. *Hemorrhagic Glioblastoma:* Thirty-seven–year–old female with sudden onset of severe headache.

A and *B*, Preinfusion CT demonstrates a large irregular area of hemorrhage in the left frontal lobe and extending across the midline. In *B* a small lucent area is identified at the periphery of the hemorrhage (*arrow*). There is a slight mass effect with posterior displacement of the frontal horn of the lateral ventricle. Angiography and surgical removal of the hemorrhage did not reveal tumor at this time. The patient continued to have headache, and approximately three months later the repeat CT was grossly abnormal.

C and *D*, The preinfusion CT scan demonstrates a large, irregular, mottled, low-density mass in the left frontal regions, now with marked shift to the contralateral side and compression of the ipsilateral lateral ventricle.

Illustration continued on the following page

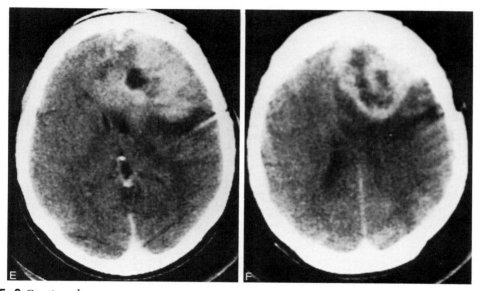

FIGURE 5–6 *Continued.*

E and *F*, The postinfusion scan demonstrates irregular, cystic, and solid areas of enhancement. The enhancing margin is poorly defined and extends across the midline.

Illustration continued on the following page

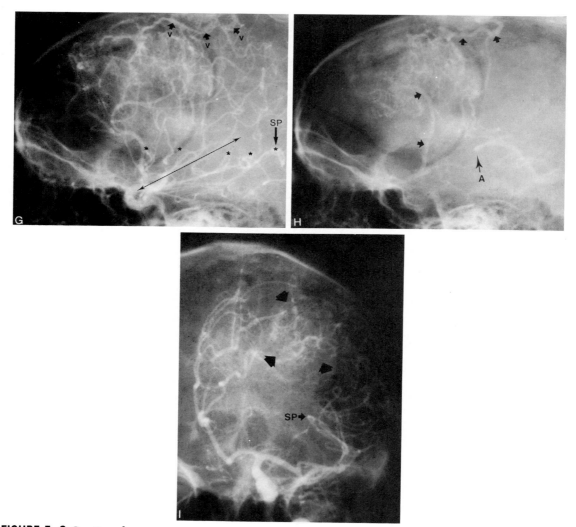

FIGURE 5–6 *Continued.*

G, Lateral view of the carotid angiogram reveals the large area of neovascularity (tumor vessels) in the frontal region. Several early draining veins are identified along the superior margin of the tumor (*V*). There is marked depression of the tops of the loops of the sylvian triangle (*asterisks*), and posterior and inferior displacement of the sylvian point (*SP*). There is splaying of the opercular branches of the middle cerebral artery because of tumor and surrounding edema. Surgery after the second angiogram revealed glioblastoma multiforme.

H, The venous phase of the LCA reveals a tumor blush and several prominent draining veins (*arrows*). The venous angle is closed (*A*).

I, The AP view demonstrates proximal and distal shift of the anterior cerebral artery in a curvilinear fashion across the midline. The sylvian point is markedly depressed (*SP*). The early tumor blush is also seen (*arrows*). This appearance is very typical of glioblastoma multiforme. It is also noted that the original location of hemorrhage is very atypical for a hypertensive etiology or secondary to an aneurysm, and so the possibility of hemorrhage into a tumor should be a strong consideration in cases such as this.

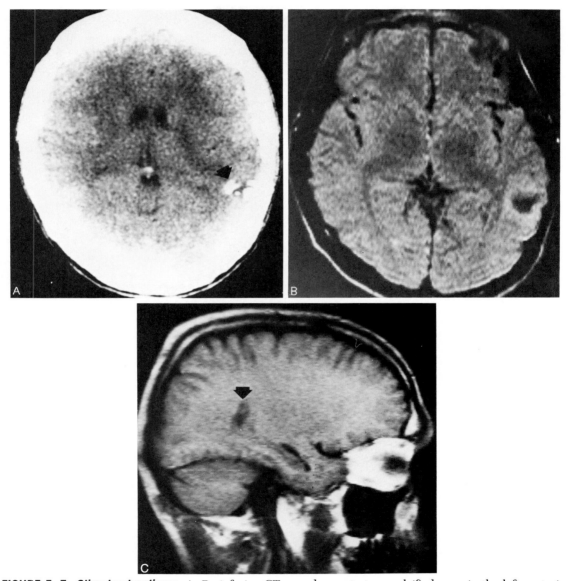

FIGURE 5–7. *Oligodendroglioma:* *A,* Preinfusion CT scan demonstrates a calcified mass in the left posterior temporal lobe (*arrow*). There is no mass effect, and there was no enhancement on the postinfusion scan.

B, SE TR530/TE30 demonstrates the area of decreased signal intensity but does not otherwise aid in characterizing the lesion.

C, Sagittal SE TR530/TE30 provides convenient anatomic localization of the calcified mass in the posterior temporal region (*arrow*). SE TR3120/TE120 images added no additional information (not shown). Surgically proved oligodendroglioma. An astrocytoma, parasitic infection, calcified vascular malformation, and tuberculoma could all have this appearance.

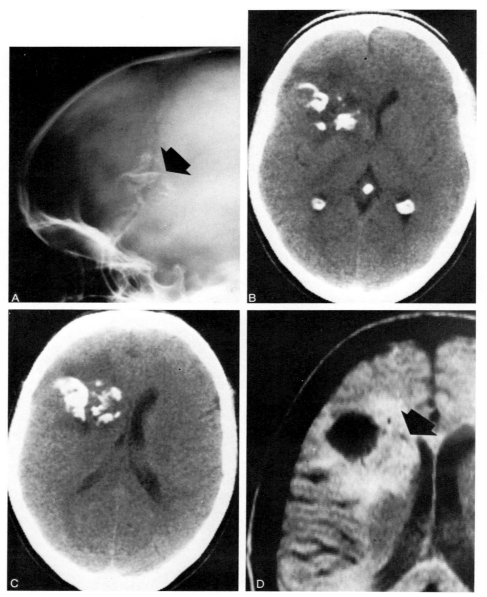

FIGURE 5–8. *Oligodendroglioma:* *A–G,* Thirty-seven–year–old female with headaches. *A,* The lateral skull radiograph reveals linear and amorphous calcification deep in the frontal region (*arrow*).

B and *C,* Preinfusion CT scan demonstrates the area of calcification, slight surrounding edema, and mass effect with compression of the frontal horn and anterior body of the lateral ventricle. The appearance is typical of oligodendroglioma. There was no enhancement on the postinfusion portion of the examination (not shown), and there had been no change in five years.

D, SE TR530/TE30 reveals the decreased signal intensity of amorphous calcification (*arrow*) and the compression of the frontal horn. Lateral to the calcification there is a postsurgical area of porencephaly surrounded by an asymmetric area of increased signal intensity, probably secondary to surrounding edema.

Illustration continued on the following page

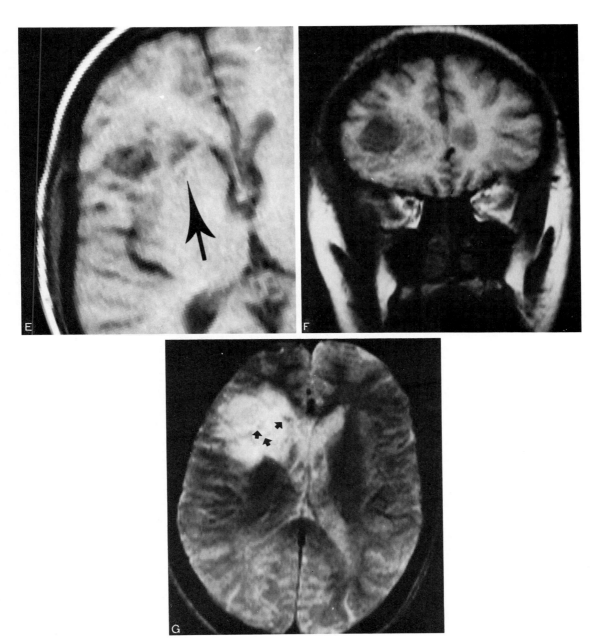

FIGURE 5–8 *Continued.*

E, A slightly lower SE TR530/TE30 slice demonstrates the decreased signal intensity of the areas of calcification (*arrow*) to better advantage.

F, Coronal SE TR530/TE30 reveals the postsurgical area of porencephaly and the areas of calcification that project just medially. The postoperative changes of the bony calvaria are less well seen with MR than with CT.

G, The SE TR3120/TE120 demonstrates the area of increased signal intensity that reflects both tumor and postsurgical edema. The areas of calcification are only faintly seen (*arrows*). The appearance is very typical of oligodendroglioma, although in the majority of cases the calcification cannot be demonstrated on the MR scan because of the poor signal. Therefore, as a general statement, if a calcified tumor such as meningioma or oligodendroglioma is suspected, then CT is the examination of choice.

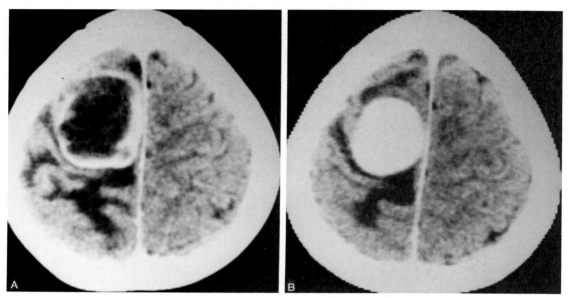

FIGURE 5–9. *Glioblastoma Multiforme:* A, Postinfusion CT scan demonstrates a slightly irregular rim of enhancement with a low-density central portion and irregular surrounding edema.

B, Following a one-half hour delay the repeat CT scan demonstrates the appearance of homogeneous enhancement of the tumor. This change in appearance following a delay has been identified by other observers, and a ring of enhancement does not necessarily imply a necrotic central portion of the tumor.

C, SE TR530/TE30 reveals a low signal intensity mass in the posterior frontal–anterior parietal region. There is obliteration of the cortical sulci on the side of the abnormality, but the edema is otherwise not appreciated.

D, The SE TR3120/TE120 reveals as a low signal intensity margin the rim of tumor that was demonstrated as the enhancing margin on the CT scan, and the surrounding edema appears as an irregular area of increased signal intensity surrounding the mass.

E, The sagittal SE TR3120/TE120 again reveals the tumor rim as a low signal intensity area (*arrows*) and nicely illustrates its relationship to the surrounding edema. The exact anatomic location of the tumor is readily identified, which facilitates surgical planning.

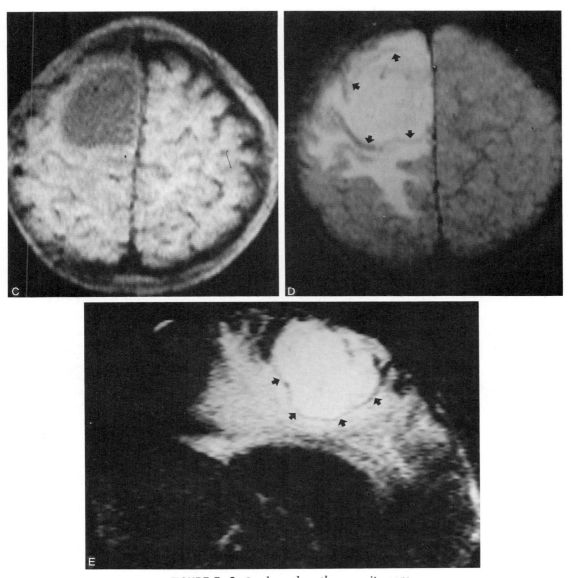

FIGURE 5–9. *See legend on the opposite page.*

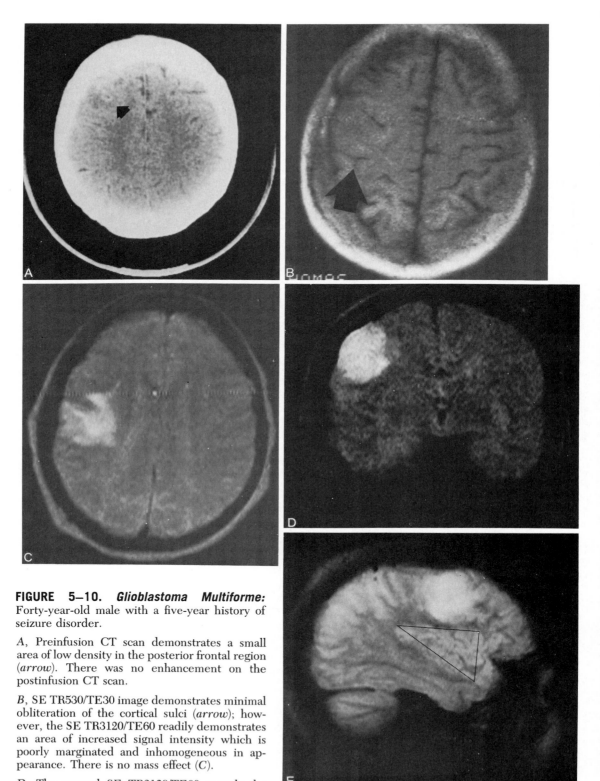

FIGURE 5–10. *Glioblastoma Multiforme:*
Forty-year-old male with a five-year history of seizure disorder.

A, Preinfusion CT scan demonstrates a small area of low density in the posterior frontal region (*arrow*). There was no enhancement on the postinfusion CT scan.

B, SE TR530/TE30 image demonstrates minimal obliteration of the cortical sulci (*arrow*); however, the SE TR3120/TE60 readily demonstrates an area of increased signal intensity which is poorly marginated and inhomogeneous in appearance. There is no mass effect (*C*).

D, The coronal SE TR3120/TE60 reveals the location of the tumor to better advantage. There is slight prominence of the cerebral cortex in the area of the abnormality.

E, Parasagittal SE TR3120/TE60 demonstrates the posterior frontal location of this poorly marginated tumor. Its suprasylvian position is also readily appreciated (sylvian triangle outlined with black lines). Surgically proved infiltrating glioblastoma multiforme. This patient illustrates the increased sensitivity of MR as compared to CT. However, the specificity of MR remains to be determined.

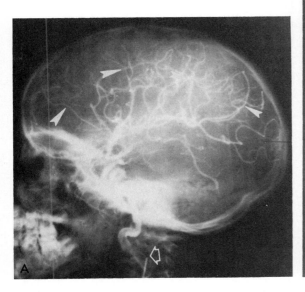

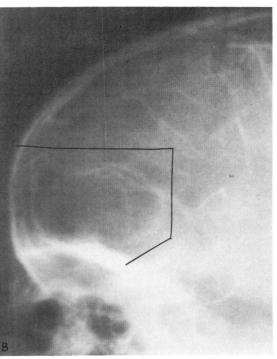

FIGURE 5–11. *Frontal Abscess and Parietal Abscess:* *A*, The arterial phase of the angiogram demonstrates stretching of the vessels in the frontal region and curvilinear displacement of the distal branches of the middle cerebral artery in the posterior parietal region (*white arrowheads*). Note the improper needle placement (*open arrow*) with the tip of the needle high in the internal carotid artery just below the base of the vault.

B, The venous phase reveals a faint rim of enhancement around the frontal abscess. This patient has cyanotic congenital heart disease and has developed two brain abscesses (*black lines*).

C, CT scans from a different patient with a similar history show a large, low-density lesion in the right frontal region, which also has surrounding edema. A thick wall of enhancement is seen on the postinfusion scan. The lesion continues to have a lucent center.

In a different clinical setting the presence of multiple lesions should suggest the possibility of multiple metastases.

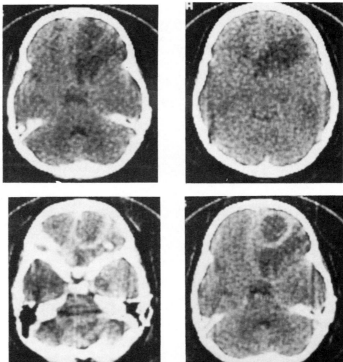

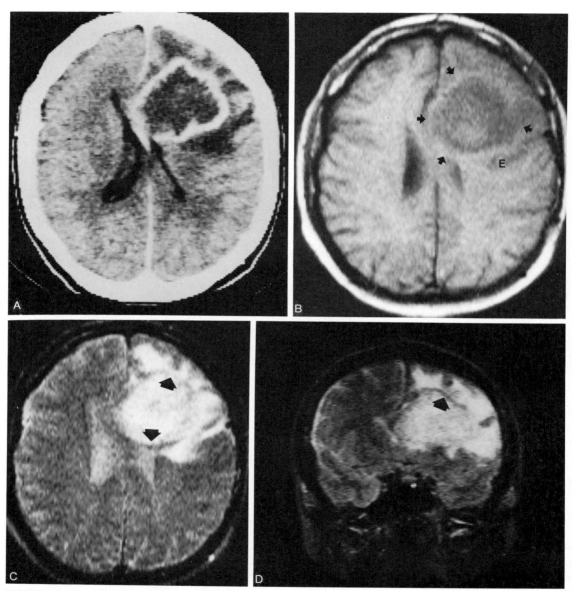

FIGURE 5–12. *Glioblastoma Multiforme:* Forty-seven–year–old female with headaches and a mild right hemiparesis. *A*, Postinfusion CT scan demonstrates an irregular rim of enhancement of a large frontal mass. There is extension of the tumor across the midline via the anterior corpus callosum—an appearance typical of glioblastoma. There is asymmetric surrounding edema and compression of the ipsilateral lateral ventricle and shift to the contralateral side.

B, SE TR530/TE30 reveals the tumor as a low signal intensity area. There is compression of the lateral ventricle, and, although the appearance is similar to the CT scan, the edema is poorly demonstrated. It appears that the enhancing rim of the mass is isodense on the T-1 weighted MR scan (*arrows*), and the surrounding edema is seen posteriorly (*E*).

C, SE TR3120/TE120 reveals the high signal intensity of the mass and the surrounding edema. The rim of tumor is of low signal intensity (*arrows*).

D, Coronal T-2 weighted image nicely demonstrates the deep frontal location of the tumor (*arrow*) as well as the extension across the midline via the corpus callosum. Surgically proved glioblastoma multiforme.

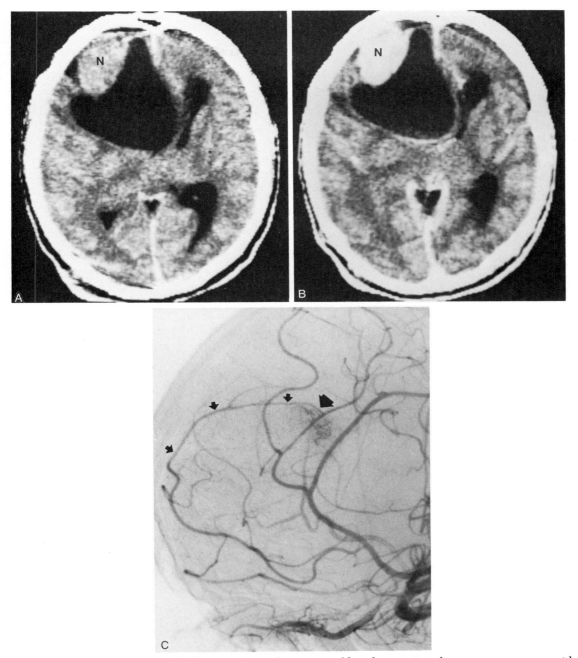

FIGURE 5–13. *Glioblastoma Multiforme:* Thirty-three–year–old male entering the emergency room with headache. *A,* Preinfusion CT scan shows a cystic mass in the right frontal region with a nodule of slightly higher than normal brain density in the periphery of the cyst (*N*). There is marked shift to the contralateral side and subfalcian herniation.

B, Postinfusion CT scan demonstrates dense enhancement of the nodule (*N*) and a thin rim of enhancement involving the cystic position of the tumor.

C, Subtraction view of the internal carotid angiogram shows enhancement of the nodule of tumor with an area of neovascularity (*large arrow*) supplied by a branch of the frontal polar artery (*small arrows*). Surgery revealed a cystic glioblastoma multiforme.

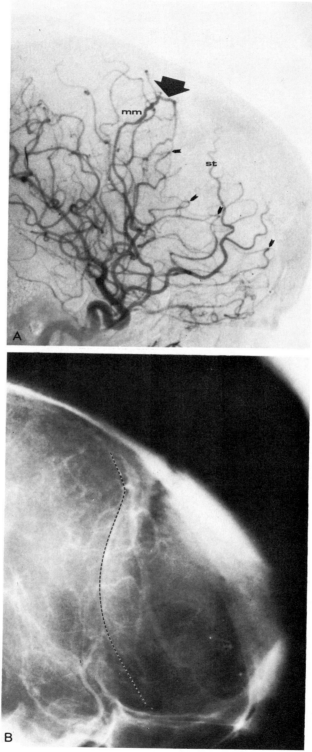

FIGURE 5–14. *See legend on the opposite page.*

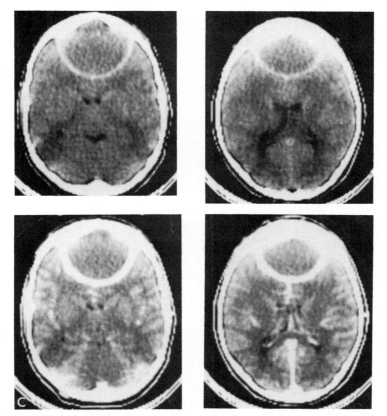

FIGURE 5–14. *Bifrontal Chronic Epidural Empyema: A,* The left lateral arteriographic view of the left carotid shows that all the distal branches of the middle cerebral artery are displaced posteriorly and inferiorly (*arrowheads*) and that there is a large avascular area in the frontal region. The middle meningeal artery (*mm*) is greatly enlarged to supply the inflamed and thickened meninges. The superficial temporal artery (*st*) also is very prominent.

B, The lateral view of the venous phase of the right carotid angiogram demonstrates that the superior sagittal sinus is displaced posteriorly away from the inner table of the skull by the large epidural collection (*dotted line*). The cortical veins that are more laterally positioned reach more anteriorly but never approximate the inner table of the skull. Note that the skull is thickened and sclerotic but that there is an area of thinning in the low frontal region. These findings are consistent with a chronic osteomyelitis.

C, The CT scans are spectacularly abnormal. There is a large rounded mass in the frontal region bilaterally, causing massive posterior displacement of the frontal horns of the lateral ventricles. The contents of the mass are isodense with the normal brain, but its wall is dense and well-defined. The postinfusion scan provides marked enhancement of the wall of the mass as well as marked vascular prominence of the remainder of the cerebral vessels.

At surgery the lesion proved to be a large epidural abscess secondary to chronic frontal sinusitis and associated with chronic osteomyelitis of the frontal bone.

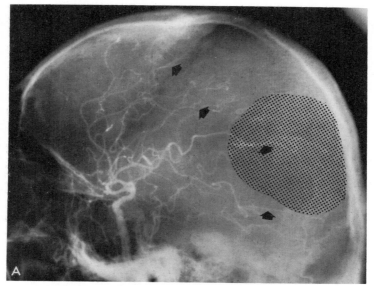

FIGURE 5–15. *Parieto-occipital Glioblastoma:* *A*, The lateral view demonstrates marked forward telescoping of the entire sylvian triangle. At least half the loops of the middle cerebral artery vessels (*arrows*) are anterior to the level of the internal carotid artery bifurcation. There is stretching of all the branches of the middle cerebral artery, even in the posterior frontal region. The most marked stretching of the vessels occurs in the posterior parietal region, where the approximate location of the mass is marked by the dotted area.

B, The AP view of the arterial phase reveals a greater shift of the distal portion of the pericallosal artery than of the proximal portion. There is a relatively sharp angular deformity as the vessel crosses beneath the falx cerebri. Because of the angle of the projection used for the angiogram, the sylvian point appears to be displaced downward.

C, There is a greater shift of the internal cerebral vein than of the artery, indicating a more posteriorly placed mass (*arrowhead*).

D, The CT scans disclose a poorly defined lesion in the right hemisphere with areas of increased and decreased density. The abnormal area involves the right temporal, parietal, and occipital lobes. There is shift of the frontal horns to the contralateral side and compression of the body of the right lateral ventricle. The postinfusion scan demonstrates an irregular pattern of enhancement in the tumor bed and a small amount of edema anterior to the tumor itself. On the highest cut there is evidence of extension of the tumor through the corpus callosum to involve the opposite hemisphere.

Differential diagnosis includes a primary or secondary brain tumor.

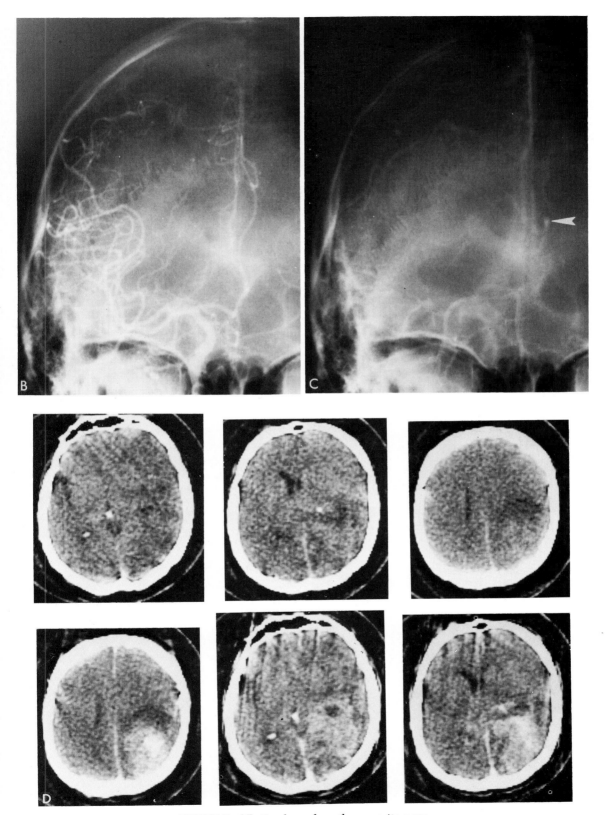

FIGURE 5–15. *See legend on the opposite page.*

FIGURE 5–16. *Parietal Glioblastoma:* A, The lateral view demonstrates forward telescoping of the sylvian triangle (*long arrow*) and stretching of all the vessels in the frontal, parietal, and occipital regions (*small arrows*).

B, The late arterial view (using magnification technique) reveals multiple small irregular "tumor" vessels in the midparietal and posterior temporal regions (*black lines*). The surrounding vessels are displaced around the tumor mass.

C, The AP view shows that the very proximal portion of the anterior cerebral artery meanders across the midline but then returns to the midline and remains there for the rest of its course. The sylvian point (*SP*) is displaced both inferiorly and medially by the convex tumor. There was a mild to moderate shift of the internal cerebral vein (not shown).

The CT scans originally obtained seven months before angiography were within normal limits—even in retrospect. The present CT scans (*D*), obtained at the same time as the angiogram, demonstrate an abnormal area of mixed high and low density in the left parietal convexity region. The higher density portion of the tumor seems to be central and surrounded by an area of edema. There is compression of the left frontal horn but no real evidence of shift of the frontal horns—confirming the angiographic findings. There is a slight shift of the third ventricle that correlates with the shift of the internal cerebral vein.

Because of the rather superficial location, differential diagnosis includes meningioma as well as glioma and/or metastatic tumor.

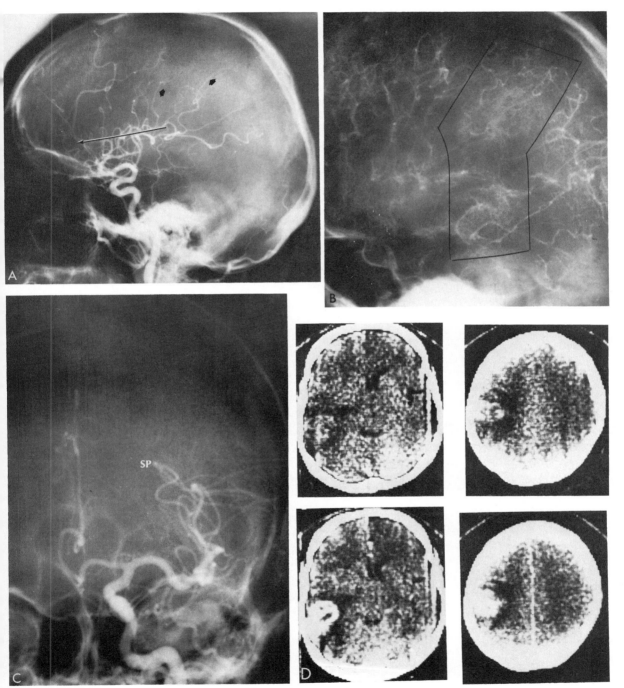

FIGURE 5–16. *See legend on the opposite page.*

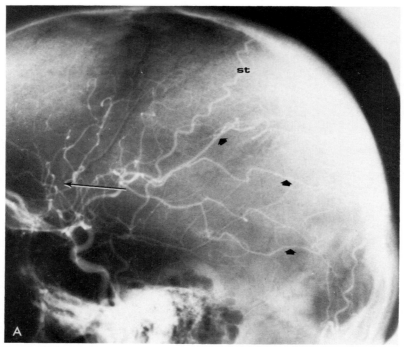

FIGURE 5–17. *Parietal Glioblastoma: A*, The angiogram reveals forward telescoping of the sylvian triangle (*long arrow*) and marked stretching of the vessels in the parietal and occipital regions (*arrows*). There is no evidence of neovascularity. There is increased filling of the superficial temporal artery (*st*) because of the increased intracranial pressure.

B, The initial CT scans demonstrate an area of radiolucency in the right parietal region that extends deep into the hemisphere in the region of the centrum ovale. There is shift of the midline to the contralateral side and compression of the body of the right lateral ventricle. The postinfusion scan demonstrates an irregular lobulated area of enhancement around the periphery of the radiolucent area.

Differential diagnosis includes abscess formation as well as glioma and/or metastatic brain tumor.

C, A follow-up scan following both surgical and radiation treatment demonstrates that the area of radiolucency and enhancement has enlarged over a three-month period. This follow-up scan was degraded by patient motion artifact.

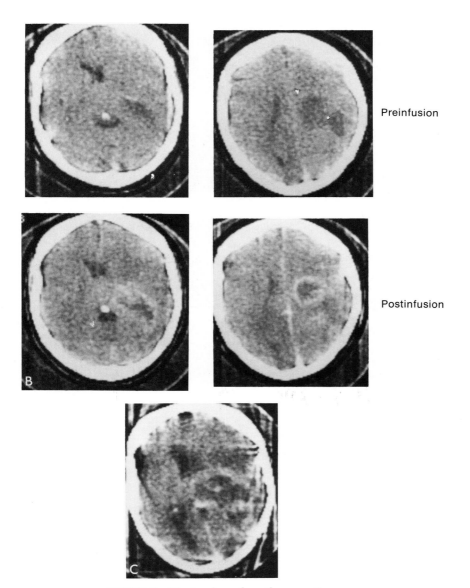

Preinfusion

Postinfusion

FIGURE 5–17. *See legend on the opposite page.*

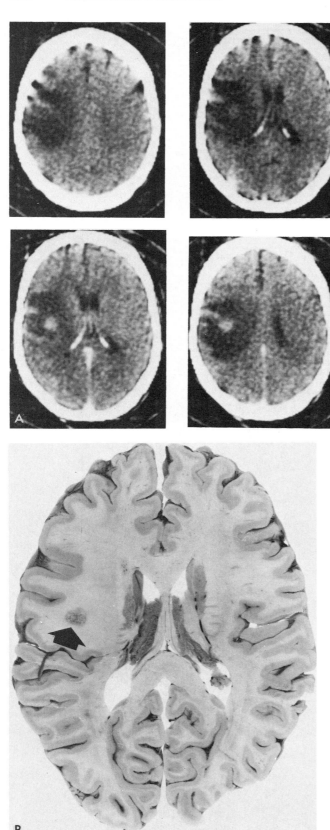

FIGURE 5–18. *Solitary Metastasis: A,* The CT scans demonstrate a single enhancing lesion deep in the hemisphere surrounded by a marked amount of symmetrical edema. There is only slight compression of the body of the lateral ventricle.

B, The postmortem pathologic specimen demonstrates the solitary metastatic lesion deep in the hemisphere (*arrow*) which is surrounded by marked swelling of the cerebral tissues.

A solitary metastatic nodule is the most likely diagnosis, although a small early primary brain tumor is a possibility.

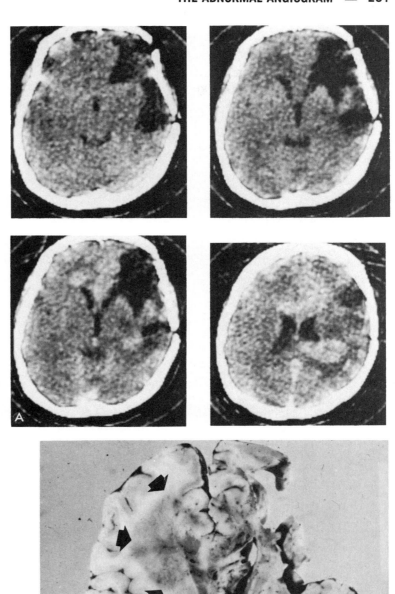

FIGURE 5–19. *Frontoparietal Tumor with Extension across the Corpus Callosum:* *A,* The preinfusion CT scans reveal postoperative changes in the right frontal and parietal regions with large irregular areas of radiolucency in the obvious bony defects. There is no shift of the midline structures. The postinfusion scans demonstrate poorly visualized areas of enhancing tumor deep in the frontal region which extend across the midline in the region of the genu of the corpus callosum. The frontal horns of the lateral ventricles are splayed apart by the tumor. In addition, there is evidence of enhancing tumor in the right hemisphere posterior to the area of surgery and deep in the right hemisphere. On the highest cut the tumor extends almost to the splenium of the corpus callosum.

B, The pathologic specimen shows that the growth of the tumor to the contralateral side (*arrows*) has progressed beyond that demonstrated on the CT scan. The postsurgical change is present in the right frontal region. The tumor growth has a "butterfly" distribution typical of glioblastoma.

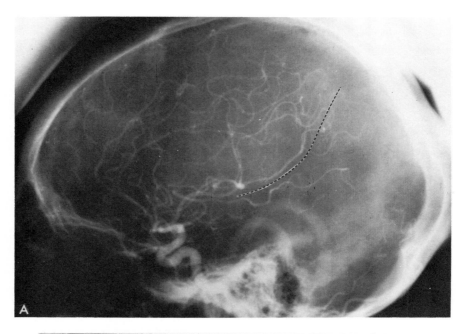

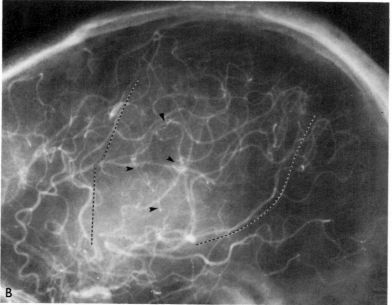

FIGURE 5–20. *Parietal Glioblastoma:* *A,* The lateral angiographic view reveals downward displacement and some forward telescoping of the sylvian triangle. The posterior branches of the middle cerebral artery are displaced in a curvilinear fashion around the mass (*dashed line*).

B, A magnified view of the same area demonstrates multiple, small abnormal "tumor" vessels in the parietal region which could not be visualized in the standard angiogram (*arrowheads*). The curvilinear displacement of the vessels around the abnormal area is again demonstrated (*dashed line*).

Illustration continued on the following page

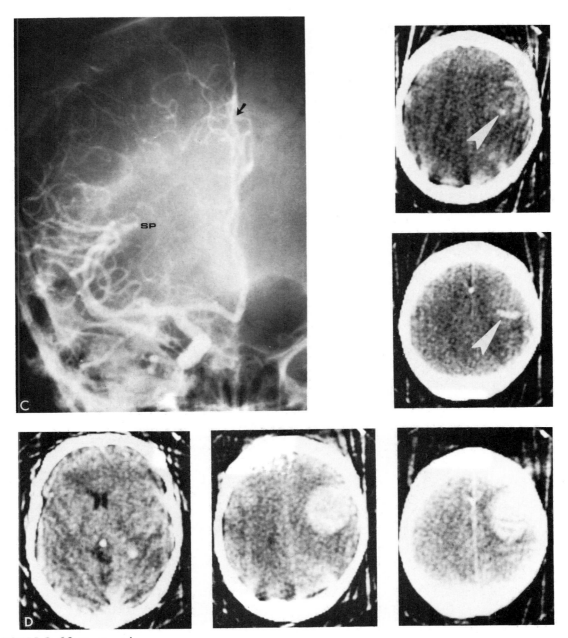

FIGURE 5–20 *Continued.*

C, The AP view shows a distal shift of the pericallosal artery with a right-angle turn at the point of shift under the falx cerebri (*arrow*). The sylvian point (*SP*) is displaced inferiorly and medially.

D, CT scans demonstrate a calcified mass high in the right parietal convexity region (*arrowheads*). The mass is of higher density than normal brain tissue and contains multiple small areas of curvilinear calcification. On the postinfusion scan there is marked homogeneous enhancement of the tumor.

Surgically, this proved to be a glioblastoma, although differential diagnosis includes meningioma, oligodendroglioma, and astrocytoma.

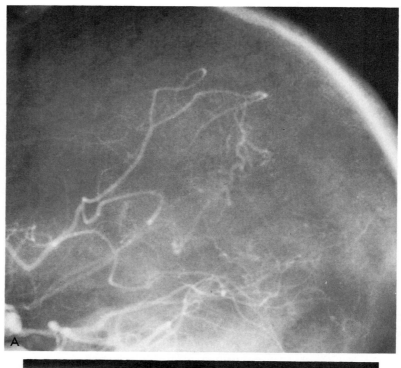

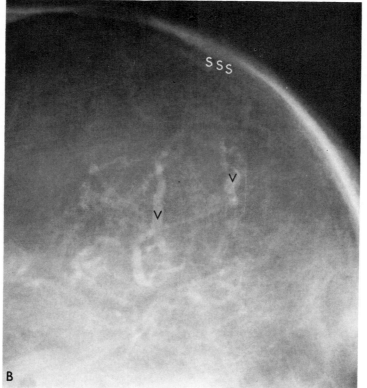

FIGURE 5–21. *See legend on the opposite page.*

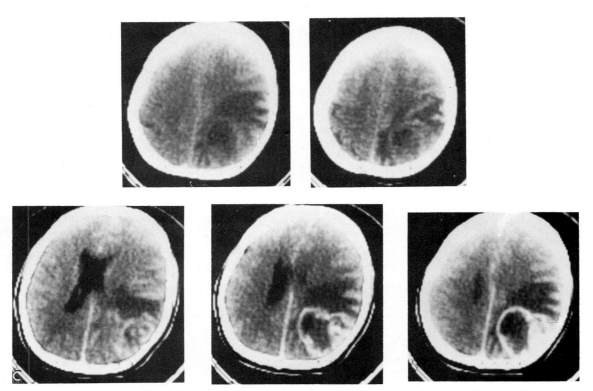

FIGURE 5–21. *Parietal Glioblastoma: A,* The angiogram reveals a large area of neovascularity in the parietal region that is supplied by enlarged branches of the middle cerebral artery. The supplying branches also demonstrate curvilinear displacement around the area of neovascularity.

B, The capillary phase shows a large area of stain with multiple early draining veins (V) that drain to the superior sagittal sinus (SSS).

C, CT scans from a different patient with a similar tumor demonstrate a large irregular area of radiolucency in the right parietal region. There is a surrounding area of scalloped edema. On the postinfusion scan, an irregular ring of enhancement is seen—also a solid portion of the tumor that is positioned posteriorly and is superficial. There is compression of the body of the right lateral ventricle.

This appearance is quite typical of glioblastoma, although a metastatic tumor could look this way.

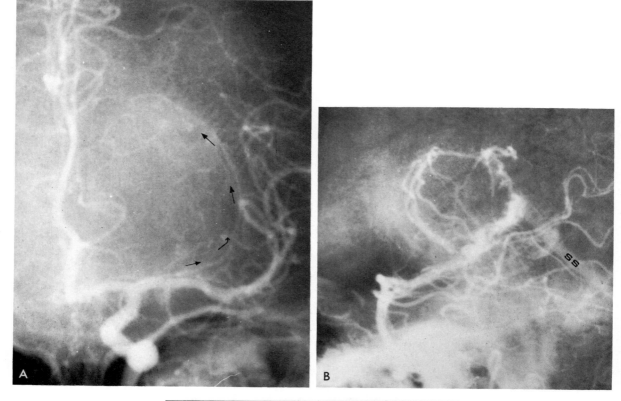

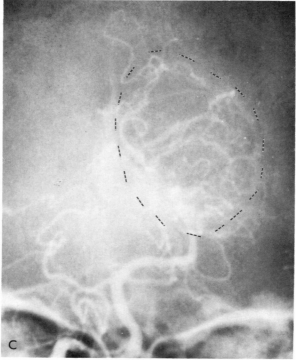

FIGURE 5–22. *See legend on the opposite page.*

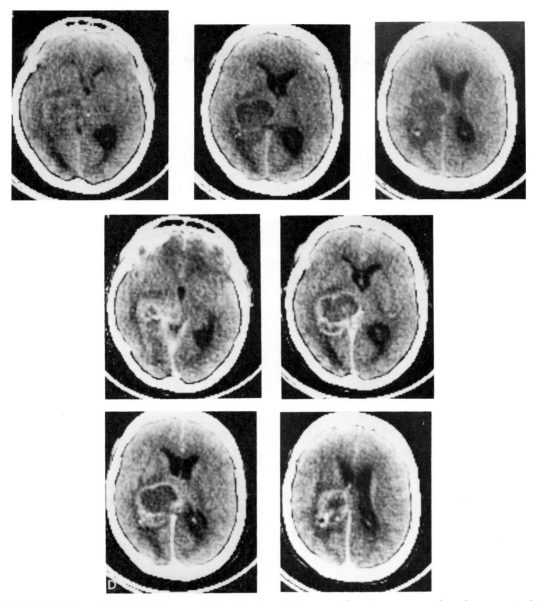

FIGURE 5–22. *Deep Parietal Glioma: A,* The AP view of the carotid angiogram reveals enlargement of the anterior choroidal artery (*arrows*), which courses posteriorly and then medially to supply a large, deep-seated tumor in the left hemisphere. There is lateral displacement of the middle cerebral vessels secondary to the mass.

B, The lateral view of the vertebral angiogram shows marked hypertrophy of the medial and lateral posterior choroidal arteries that supply the tumor. There are also anomalous vessels that arise from the posterior cerebral artery to supply the area of neovascularity. There is evidence of early venous drainage with filling of the straight sinus (*SS*) on this early arterial film. On the AP view of the vertebral angiogram (*C*), the large area of neovascularity is seen deep in the left hemisphere (*dashed lines*).

D, The preinfusion CT scans demonstrate a large radiolucent area deep in the left hemisphere with an irregular ring of higher density that enhances markedly on the postinfusion scan. There is also a moderate amount of irregular surrounding edema. There is distortion of the left lateral ventricle and shift of the midline to the contralateral side.

Surgically proved glioblastoma multiforme.

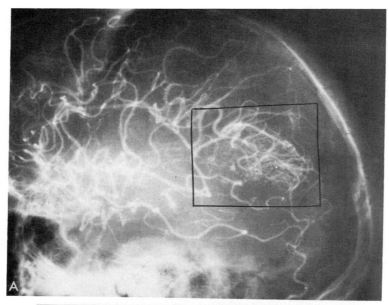

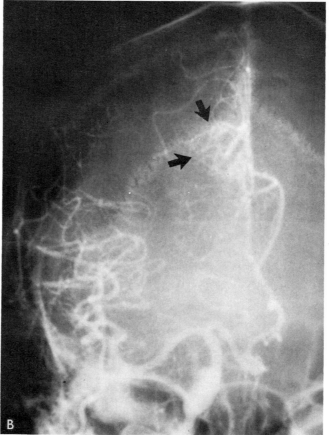

FIGURE 5–23. *Solitary Metastasis:* *A*, The lateral view reveals a large vascular tumor that exhibits evidence of neovascularity (*black lines*) as well as a larger area of mass effect with stretching of the vessels secondary to surrounding edema. There is forward telescoping of the entire sylvian triangle.

B, The AP view demonstrates that the area of neovascularity lies just adjacent to the falx cerebri (*arrows*). There is a distal shift of the anterior cerebral artery under the falx. The sylvian point appears to be displaced inferiorly.

At surgery this proved to be a solitary metastatic deposit from primary renal carcinoma. Differential diagnosis includes glioblastoma multiforme.

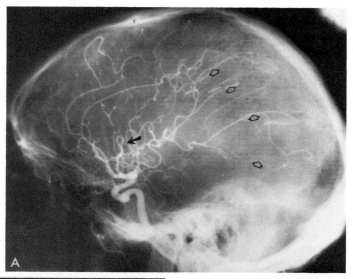

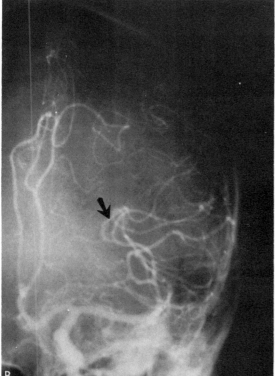
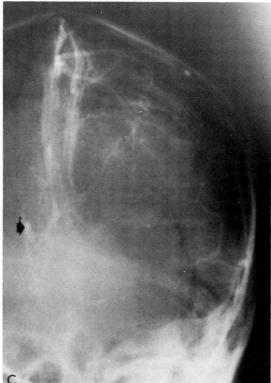

FIGURE 5–24. *Occipital Lobe Abscess:* *A,* The lateral angiographic view reveals forward telescoping of the sylvian triangle (*large arrow*) and stretching of the distal branches of the middle cerebral artery group in the posterior parietal and occipital regions (*open arrows*). The mass is avascular.

B, The AP arterial view demonstrates downward and medial displacement of the sylvian point (*arrow*) and a distal shift of the pericallosal artery under the falx cerebri.

C, The venous phase shows a shift of the internal cerebral vein that is equal to or slightly greater than the arterial shift (*arrow*).

This was proved surgically to be an occipital abscess.

Differential diagnosis includes a primary or secondary brain tumor, an intracerebral hematoma, or even a porencephalic cyst.

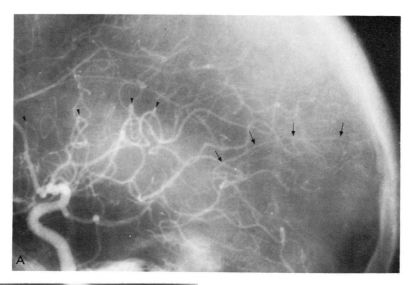

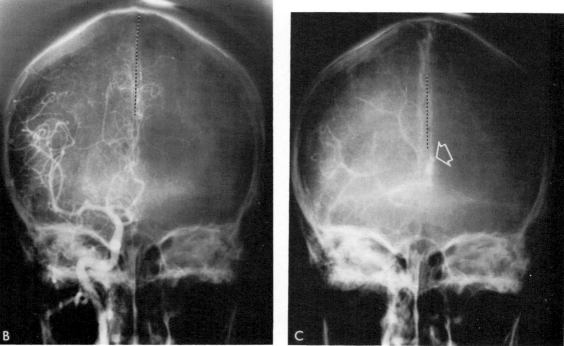

FIGURE 5–25. *Occipital Glioblastoma:* *A,* The lateral angiographic view shows stretching of a single branch of the posterior cerebral artery in the occipital region (*long arrows*). The sylvian triangle (*arrowheads*) is in normal position. There is no evidence of either neovascularity or a capsular stain.

B and *C,* The AP arterial phase is entirely within normal limits (the dotted line indicates the falx), and there is only a very slight shift of the internal cerebral vein (*arrow*), which still measures within normal limits.

Illustration continued on the following page

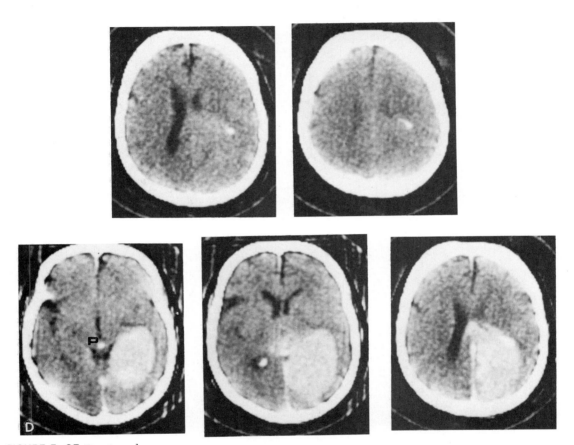

FIGURE 5–25 *Continued.*

D, CT scans from another patient reveal a slight increase in the density of the brain tissue in the left occipital region on the preinfusion scan with anterior displacement of the choroid plexus calcification in the atrium of the lateral ventricle. Forward displacment of the body of the left lateral ventricle is also seen. The postinfusion scan reveals homogeneous enhancement of a large mass in the left parietal and occipital regions that extends into the posterior aspect of the corpus callosum. The pineal *(P)* is in the midline.

This was proved surgically to be a glioblastoma.

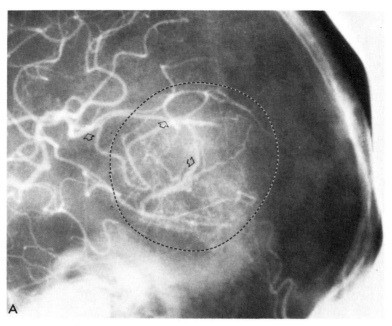

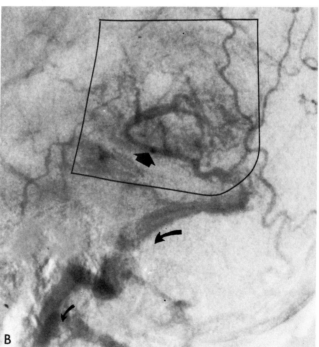

FIGURE 5–26. *Occipital Lobe Glioblastoma:* A, The lateral magnification view of the occipital region shows multiple branches of the middle cerebral artery; these follow an abnormal and tortuous course (*arrows*) and supply a large area of neovascularity (*dotted lines*).

B, The capillary phase demonstrates the large abnormal stain (*black lines*) and a large early-draining vein, which drains directly into the lateral sinus and then into the sigmoid sinus and the internal jugular vein (*curved arrows*).

Illustration continued on the following page

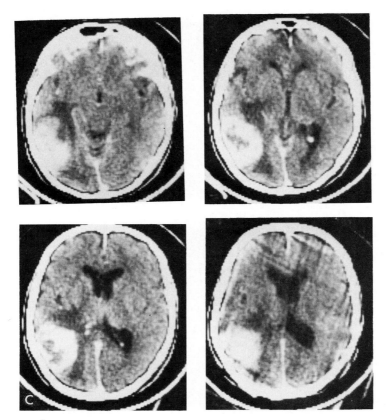

FIGURE 5–26 *Continued.*

C, The CT scans (postinfusion only) reveal a large, thick-rimmed enhancing lesion with a radiolucent center in the right occipital lobe. The lesion has poorly defined outer margins and exhibits an irregular area of surrounding edema. There is minimal mass effect with little shift of the midline.

Surgically proved glioblastoma. Differential diagnosis also includes a vascular metastasis.

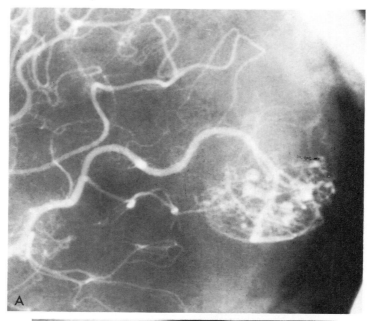

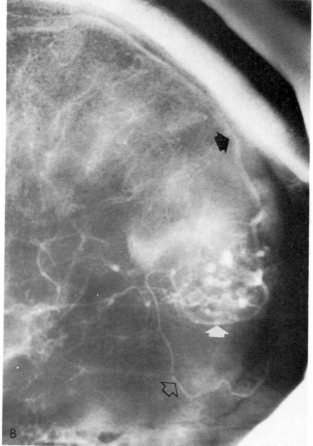

FIGURE 5–27. *See legend on the opposite page.*

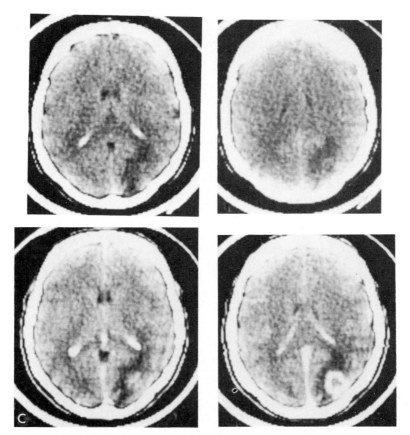

FIGURE 5–27. *Occipital Glioblastoma: A,* The lateral view of the selective internal carotid angiogram demonstrates an enlarged branch of the middle cerebral artery, which courses posteriorly to supply an area of abnormal vascularity in the occipital region. There are multiple abnormal vessels and puddling of the contrast material in multiple scattered abnormal accumulations. There is a surrounding area of avascularity secondary to the surrounding edema.

B, The capillary phase shows the abnormal area (*white arrow*) with a tumor stain and multiple early draining veins—one that drains inferiorly (*open arrow*) and another that drains superiorly into the superior sagittal sinus (*black arrow*).

C, CT scans reveal an area of radiolucency in the occipital region that surrounds an enhancing lesion with a lucent center in the left occipital pole. There is slight anterior displacement of the choroid plexus of the left lateral ventricle.

Surgically proved glioblastoma multiforme.

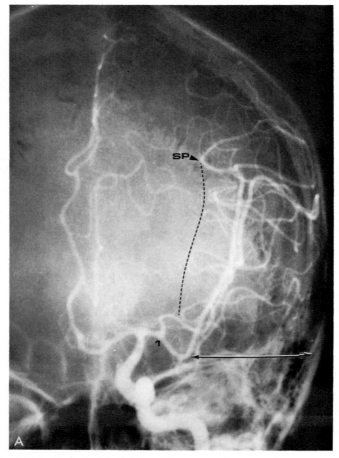

FIGURE 5–28. *Temporal Lobe Hematoma:* *A*, The AP angiographic view shows superior displacement of the sylvian point (*SP*) and medial displacement of all the branches of the middle cerebral artery. The genu of the middle cerebral artery is displaced medially (*doubleheaded arrow*). The middle cerebral artery bifurcation is well demonstrated (*1*). There is proximal and distal shift of the anterior cerebral artery.

B, The lateral view demonstrates that there is marked superior displacement of the entire sylvian triangle and the sylvian point (*arrows* and *sp*). In fact, the sylvian triangle is so elevated that the main branches of the middle cerebral artery appear to follow the course of the anterior cerebral artery. The bifurcation of the middle cerebral artery is well seen (*1*) because of the distortion of the middle cerebral artery group.

C, The CT scans (viewed from above) reveal a large intracerebral hematoma in the right temporal lobe. There is marked shift to the contralateral side. There is an area of radiolucency posterior to the hematoma in the low temporal region; there is also obliteration of the cortical sulci on the side of the hematoma.

IMP: Giant temporal lobe hematoma.

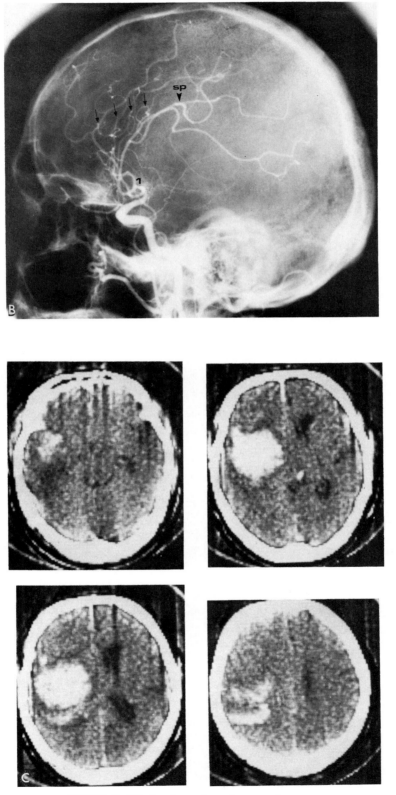

FIGURE 5–28. *See legend on the opposite page.*

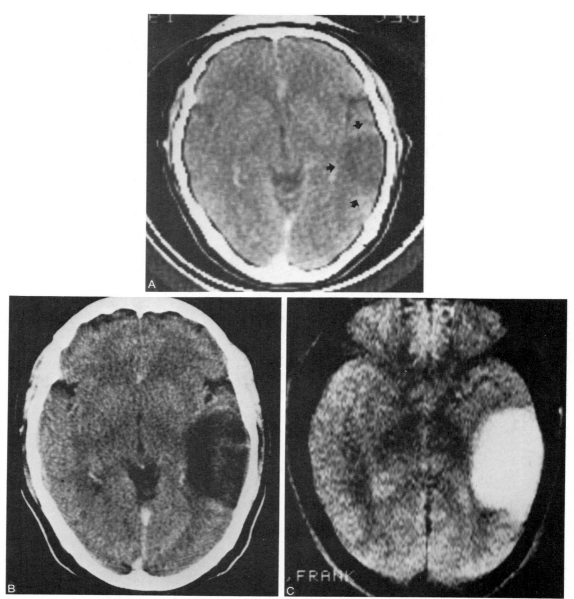

FIGURE 5–29. Glioblastoma: *A*, Postinfusion CT scan demonstrates a poorly visualized area of low density in the left temporal lobe (*arrows*).

B, Three years later the CT continues to demonstrate a nonenhancing mass in the temporal lobe. The mass is slightly larger and more visible than on the initial scan.

C, MR inversion recovery sequence readily demonstrates the mass as an area of increased signal intensity. The tumor is better visualized on the MR scan because of its increased sensitivity, but the MR is not more specific. Surgically proved glioblastoma multiforme.

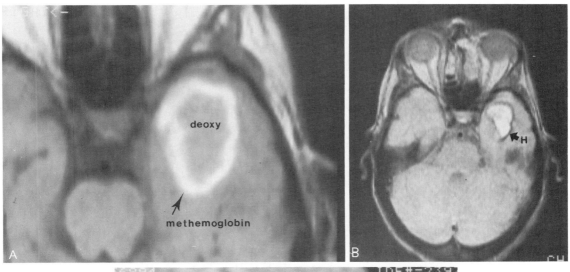

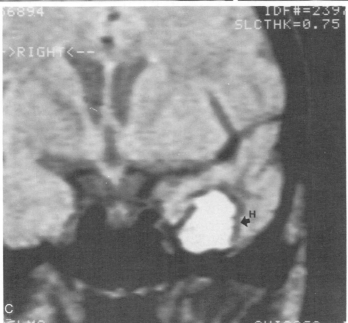

FIGURE 5–30. *Intracerebral Hematoma: Four days old:* *A*, T-1 weighted image reveals that the peripheral margin of the hematoma is increased signal intensity because the blood has metabolized to methemoglobin. The central portion of the hematoma is decreased in signal intensity because it is composed of deoxyhemoglobin. At this time the CT scan revealed a high-density left temporal lobe intracerebral hematoma.

B, Approximately six weeks later the entire hematoma is increased in signal intensity on the T-1 weighted image, with a peripheral margin of decreased signal intensity secondary to breakdown of blood to hemosiderin, a strongly paramagnetic substance.

C, The T-2 weighted image obtained at the same time as *B* reveals that the center of the hematoma increases in signal intensity, and the peripheral margin of decreased signal, secondary to hemosiderin (H), is better demonstrated.

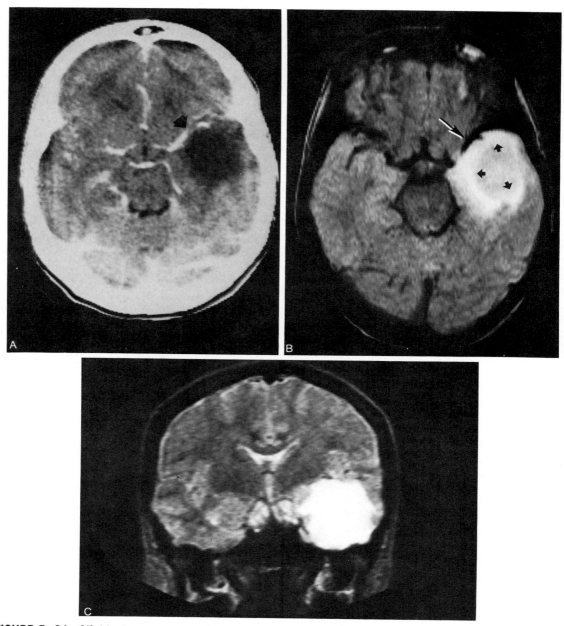

FIGURE 5–31. *Glioblastoma: A,* Postinfusion CT scan demonstrates a nonenhancing, cystic-appearing mass in the temporal lobe in this 36-year-old female with only headaches and no abnormal physical findings. There is mass effect with foreward displacement of the genu of the middle cerebral artery (*arrow*).

B, SE TR3120/TE60 demonstrates the tumor in the left temporal lobe. The mass is slightly lower in signal intensity than the surrounding edema (*arrows*). Therefore, there is an advantage of MR over CT in this case because the location of the tumor relative to the surrounding edema is easily seen. The displaced genu of the middle cerebral artery now appears as a negative flow defect (*black and white arrow*).

C, The longer, SE TR3120/TE120 sequence causes the tumor and the surrounding edema to appear of the same signal intensity. The irregular margin of the surrounding edema is easily appreciated. Surgically proved glioblastoma multiforme. This example illustrates the value of a variety of pulse sequences for complete evaluation.

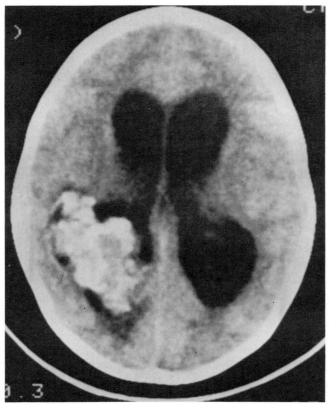

FIGURE 5–32. *Choroid Plexus Papilloma:* The CT scan is from a newborn baby with a large head size. The study reveals a very large, higher than normal brain density mass arising within the ventricle. There is marked ventricular enlargement. The appearance is very typical of choroid plexus papilloma. They are very vascular, which results in their increased density on the preinfusion scan, and they produce an excessive amount of CSF, which results in enlargement of the ventricular system. (Case courtesy of Antonio D. Zelaya, M.D.)

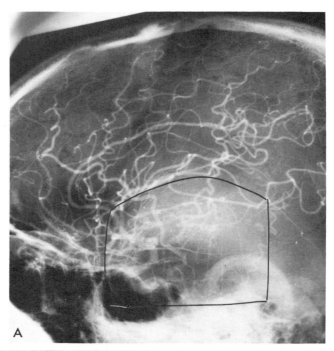

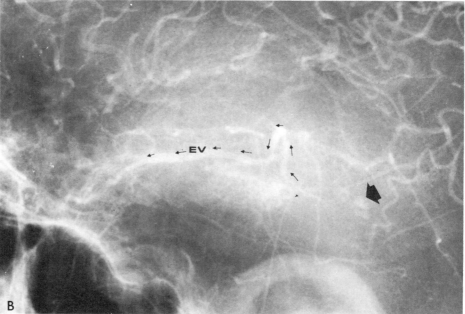

FIGURE 5–33. *Temporal Lobe Glioma:* The early arterial view (A) reveals elevation of the sylvian triangle and multiple, small, abnormal-appearing vessels in the temporal region (*black lines*).

B and C, The lateral magnification views of the posterior temporal region show the abnormal vessels to better advantage and also demonstrate an early vein (*small arrows*), which drains into the middle cerebral vein (*EV*). There is also an abnormal area of puddling of the contrast material in the posterior temporal region (*large arrow*). This puddling of contrast material persists well into the venous phase (*black arrow* in C).

Illustration continued on the following page

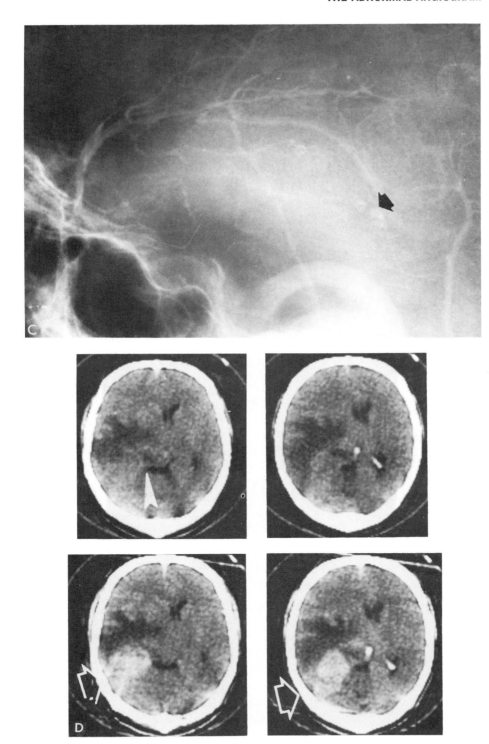

FIGURE 5–33 *Continued.*

D, CT scans from another patient with a similar process demonstrate an enhancing lesion (*open arrowhead*) in the posterior portion of the left temporal lobe. There is a large amount of irregular edema anterior to the mass, and there is distortion of the retrothalamic cistern (*closed arrowhead*). There is marked shift to the contralateral side.

Surgery revealed a glioblastoma in both cases.

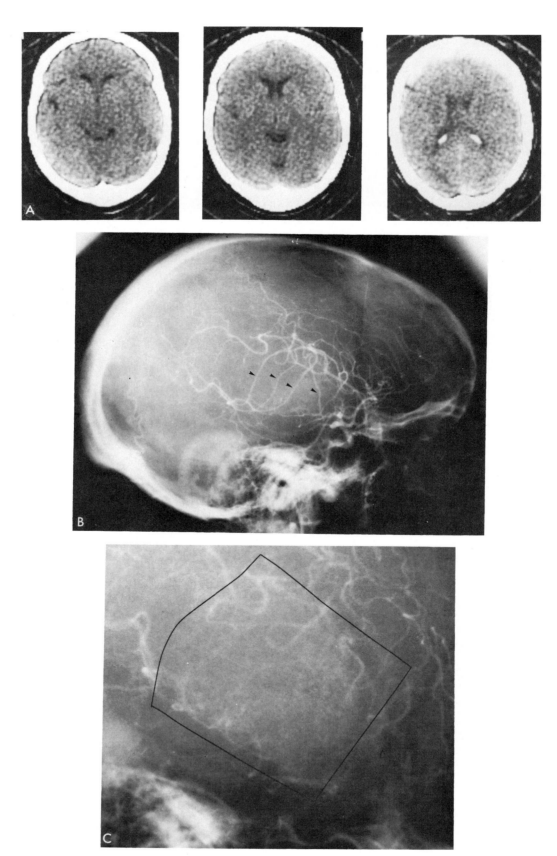

FIGURE 5–34. *See legend on the opposite page.*

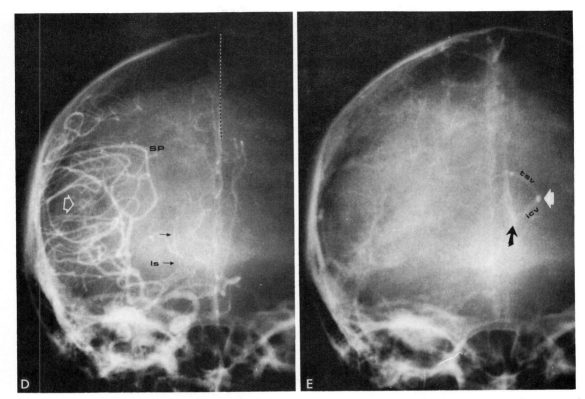

FIGURE 5–34. *Temporal Lobe Glioblastoma:* This patient presented with signs and symptoms of a temporal lobe mass; however, the initial CT scan (A) appeared to be within normal limits. A postinfusion scan was not performed at that time, but the angiogram (not shown) was normal.

Two months after the initial study, the patient returned, and a second angiogram was performed. B, The lateral view demonstrates stretching of all the vessels in the temporal lobe region (*arrowheads*). The opercular vessels are draped over the enlarged temporal lobe, which now contains a mass. The late arterial view (C) reveals an area of neovascularity in the temporal region (*black lines*), and the findings are very typical of glioblastoma.

The AP view (D) reveals elevation and medial displacement of the sylvian point (SP). There is a distal shift of the anterior cerebral artery, and medial displacement of the lenticulostriate vessels (*ls*) is evident. The area of abnormal vascularity can be seen in the temporal region on the AP view as well (*open white arrow*).

The AP venous phase (E) reveals that the thalamostriate vein is displaced to the contralateral side (*tsv*), joins the internal cerebral vein (*white arrow*), and then courses inferiorly and posteriorly to join the vein of Galen in the midline (*large black arrow*).

Illustration continued on the following page

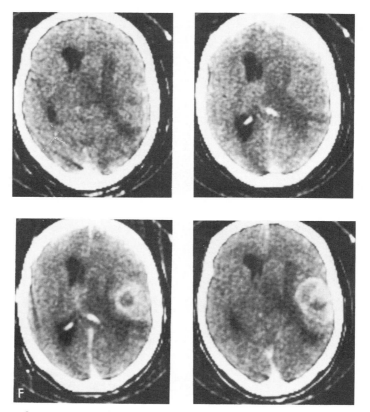

FIGURE 5–34 *Continued.*

F, CT scans (viewed from above) taken at this time show a large, thick-walled ring of enhancement in the right temporal region. The tumor has a lobulated appearance and a radiolucent center—consistent with necrosis of the inner portion of the mass. There is a large amount of irregular surrounding edema and a marked shift to the contralateral side.

Illustration continued on the following page

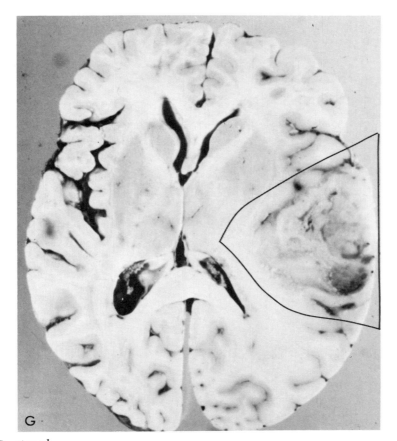

FIGURE 5–34 *Continued.*
G, The pathologic specimen correlates well with the CT scan, demonstrating the tumor with central necrosis in the temporal lobe (*black lines*).

Diagnosis: Glioblastoma multiforme.

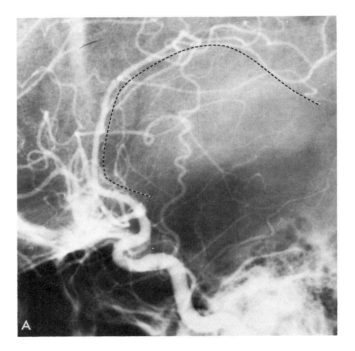

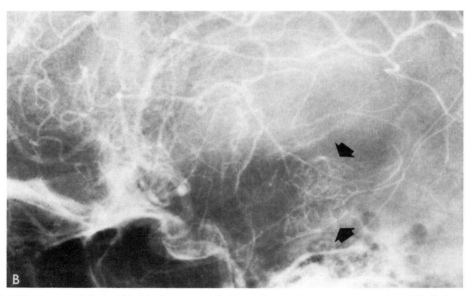

FIGURE 5–35. *Temporal Lobe Glioblastoma: A*, The lateral view demonstrates such marked elevation of the middle cerebral branches that they appear to be the anterior cerebral artery (*dotted line*).

B, The lateral arterial phase shows multiple small tumor vessels and a small separate collection of neovascularity in the posterior temporal region (*arrows*) that almost appears to be separated from the rest of the tumor.

C, The AP view of the vertebral angiogram reveals medial displacement of the posterior cerebral artery (*dashed line*) on the left side. The right posterior cerebral artery follows a normal course.

D, CT scans (viewed from above) demonstrate a large radiolucent mass with a well-defined margin in the left temporal lobe. There is shift to the contralateral side. The middle cut shows a nodule of tumor projecting into the cystic portion of the tumor, which demonstrates enhancement on the postinfusion scan (*arrowhead*) and is apparently the separate area of neovascularity seen on the angiogram. The postinfusion scan also reveals a solid area of homogeneous enhancement (*wide arrow*) low in the temporal region and a ring of enhancement around the partially cystic and partially solid glioblastoma.

Illustration continued on the following page

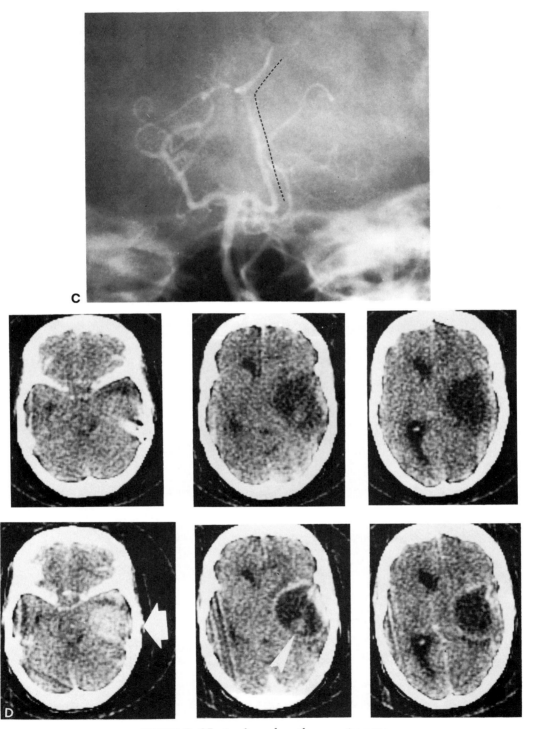

FIGURE 5–35. *See legend on the opposite page.*

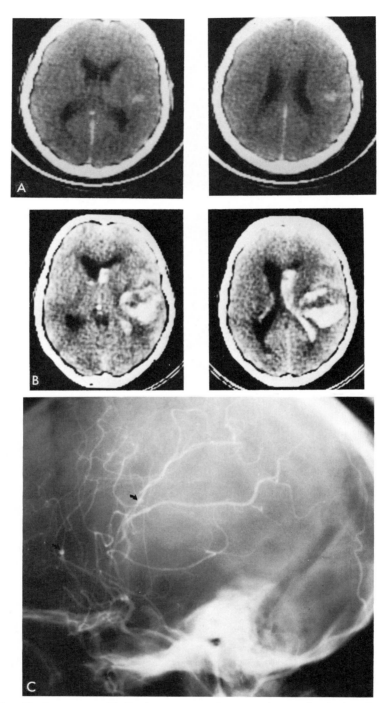

FIGURE 5–36. *Mycotic Aneurysm with Rupture:* Previously, a prosthetic valve had replaced the aortic valve, and the patient developed bacterial endocarditis.

A, The initial CT scans show that the lateral ventricles are mildly enlarged and that there is a small area of enhancement deep in the left hemisphere. This probably represents an area of early abscess formation or cerebritis.

B, CT scans one week later demonstrate a large hematoma in the left temporal lobe region. It has ruptured into the left lateral ventricle and the third ventricle. The scan also reveals a small amount of blood in the dependent portion of the right lateral ventricle.

Illustration continued on the following page

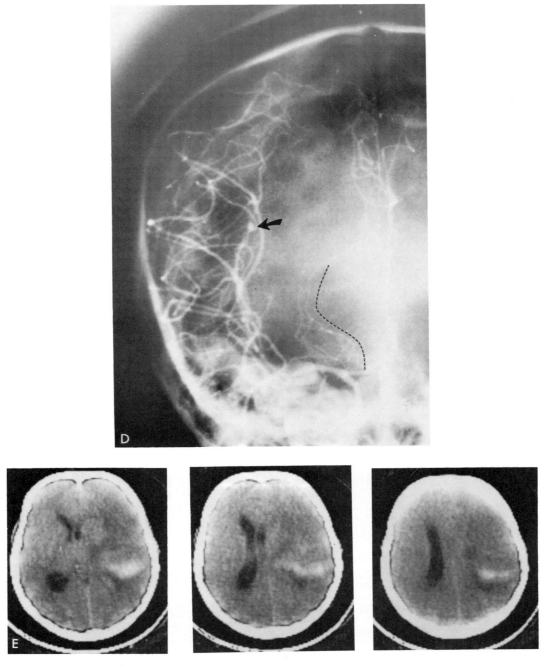

FIGURE 5–36 *Continued.*

C, An angiogram performed at the time of the second CT scan shows a large avascular mass in the temporal lobe. There is elevation of the sylvian triangle and draping of the vessels over the temporal lobe. There is spasm of the supraclinoid portion of the internal carotid artery. Two aneurysms involving the distal portions of the middle cerebral artery vessels also are demonstrated (*arrows*). It is apparently the more superior and posterior aneurysm that has ruptured, leading to the large temporal hematoma.

D, The AP view demonstrates the more posterior aneurysm (*arrow*). There is superior and medial displacement of the sylvian point and medial displacement of the lenticulostriate arteries (*dashed line*).

E, Follow-up scans approximately two weeks later reveal partial resorption of the intracerebral hematoma.

IMP: Mycotic aneurysms (infected) with rupture and hematoma formation.

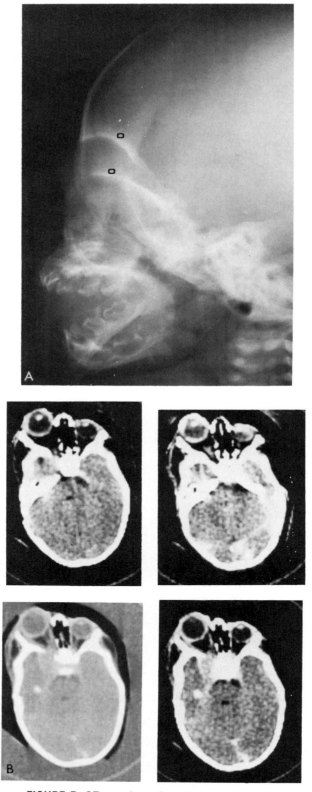

FIGURE 5–37. *See legend on the opposite page.*

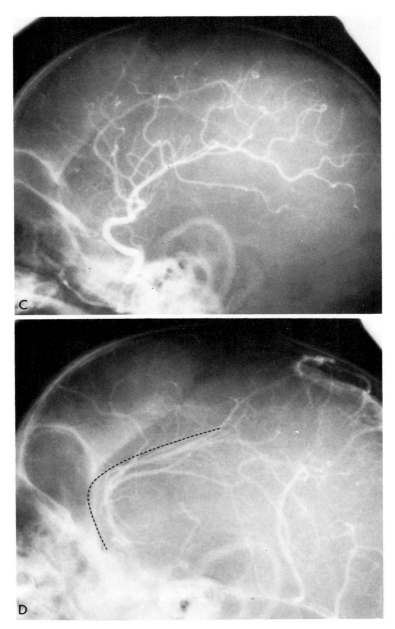

FIGURE 5–37. *Middle Cranial Fossa and Orbital Dysplasia Secondary to Neurofibromatosis:* *A,* On the lateral view of the skull series, the orbital roof on the affected side is much higher than on the opposite side (O), and the greater wing of the sphenoid bone is not seen on the affected side.

B, The CT scans show the expansion of the right middle cranial fossa, the enlargement of the entire orbit on the right and even a globe larger on the right than on the left. There is no evidence of a mass lesion.

C and *D,* The lateral view in the arterial phase of the carotid angiogram reveals opening of the carotid siphon, elevation of sylvian triangle, and elevation and superior displacement of the middle cerebral veins (*dotted line*) secondary to the enlargement of the temporal lobe.

IMP: Neurofibromatosis; temporal fossa dysplasia.

6

ANEURYSMS AND VASCULAR MALFORMATIONS

ANEURYSMS

There are many different types of aneurysms. Determination of the etiology and type of aneurysm directs both the clinical course and subsequent treatment. The aneurysm or aneurysms may be developmental, post-traumatic, dissecting, postoperative, mycotic (septic), secondary to neoplastic emboli, venous, syphilitic, microaneurysm of hypertension, arteriosclerotic, or berry.

Berry Aneurysms

This chapter deals primarily with berry aneurysms—the type most commonly encountered in the day-to-day practice of neuroradiology. Sometimes patients with these aneurysms present with such focal signs as a unilateral third nerve palsy associated with retro-orbital pain caused by a posterior communicating arterial aneurysm that is resting on the third nerve in the wall of the cavernous sinus. More commonly, the patients arrive at the emergency room following the acute onset of severe headache and decreased cerebral function or coma secondary to subarachnoid hemorrhage. An acute ruptured aneurysm may rapidly lead to death.

These aneurysms may be embedded in cerebral tissue, where their rupture causes an intracerebral hematoma as well as subarachnoid hemorrhage. They may thrombose and occlude, or they may result in cerebral emboli and subsequent strokes.

Berry aneurysms may be associated with polycystic kidneys and coarctation of the aorta. A congenital defect in the wall of the blood vessel with interruption of the muscular coat and the internal elastic lamina is present at the site of the aneurysm. Berry aneurysms usually occur at bifurcations of the vessels. Although there may be a congenital tendency to develop these aneurysms, they are rarely seen in children.

Age. The aneurysms usually present in the second to seventh decades, with an incidence of 0.5 to 5.0 per cent of the population as judged by autopsy studies.

Location. Ninety to 95 per cent of berry aneurysms occur in the carotid circulation. The remainder are in the vertebrobasilar system. The most common site for an unruptured berry aneurysm is reported to be the middle cerebral artery bifurcation. The most common locations for ruptured aneurysms, in decreasing order of incidence, are (1) anterior communicating artery, (2) internal carotid artery, (3) posterior communicating artery, (4) middle cerebral artery bifurcation.

Size of Ruptured Aneurysms. Aneurysms 5 to 15 mm in size are most likely to bleed and may demonstrate a small outpouching at the actual site of bleeding, which usually is at the dome of the aneurysm.

Multiple Aneurysms

When multiple aneurysms are present, as is true in approximately 20 per cent of cases, it may be difficult to determine the actual size of rupture or which aneurysm has bled. The CT scan may provide a clue to the bleeding site if a small localized hematoma is seen. Localized vascular spasm demonstrated on arteriography may be helpful in localizing the site of bleeding, although vascular spasm may be remote from the actual bleeding site. Evidence of an intracerebral hematoma also may be present, providing further evidence of the bleeding site. In general, if no secondary signs of hemorrhage are present it is assumed that it is the largest aneurysm that has bled. An increase in size of an aneurysm on serial studies is also suggestive of a bleeding aneurysm.

Giant aneurysms are those measuring 2.5 cm or larger; they rarely bleed.

CT Scanning with Acute Subarachnoid Hemorrhage

The CT scan in a patient with acute subarachnoid hemorrhage (SAH) may be within normal limits. More commonly (in approximately 85 to 90 per cent of cases), the scan demonstrates a diffuse increase in density seen in the basilar cisterns and over the cerebral convexities—a change secondary to blood in the subarachnoid space.

The diffuse increase in density may be very subtle and easily overlooked. Close inspection will show that the usually radiolucent sulci are not seen because they have filled with blood. The blood may even flow retrograde up into the ventricular system, where a "blood–CSF fluid level" will be seen in the dependent portions of the lateral ventricles, or a blood clot cast of the ventricular system may form. The aneurysm may rupture directly into the ventricular system. Occasionally—and I have found this to be of limited help—there will be a focal accumulation of blood in the subarachnoid space associated with a ruptured aneurysm. If present, this sign is helpful in defining a bleeding site in a patient without focal findings. On the other hand, an aneurysm may rupture into the brain substance and produce a large intracerebral hematoma. However, this may simulate the appearance of a primary intracerebral hematoma, and only an unusual anatomic location will point to an aneurysm as the true source of bleeding.

In a small percentage of cases the aneurysm may rupture through the arachnoid layer into the subdural space, causing a subdural hematoma. Again, the true source of bleeding may remain obscure—particularly if an angiogram is not performed.

The use of CT for the diagnosis of aneurysm through direct demonstration is, at this point in our technology, inadequate. The *vast* majority of aneurysms are not visualized by CT scan, even after infusion of contrast material. Those aneurysms that are identified on the CT scan usually are quite sizeable and are commonly partially or even completely clotted. They therefore appear as a well-defined, rounded area of high density, frequently containing flecks of peripheral calcification. If the aneurysm is not clotted, the enhancement has a homogeneous pattern; if the aneurysm is partially clotted, the areas of enhancement are irregular and correspond to the unclotted portion of the aneurysms. If the aneurysm is completely filled with clotted blood there may be no enhancement or only peripheral enhancement secondary to the vasa vasorum that supply the walls of the vessels.

Acutely, there may be ventricular dilatation secondary to clotted blood in the ventricles—especially the third and fourth ventricles—which acts as a mechanical obstruction to ventricular function. Later in the clinical course there may be dilatation of the ventricles because of a communicationg hydrocephalus that develops when blood in the subarachnoid space interferes with the absorption of CSF by the arachnoid villi.

Magnetic Resonance of Aneurysms

Magnetic resonance of an unclotted aneurysm reveals a negative flow defect in the lumen of the vessel because of the flowing blood. If the aneurysm is partially thrombosed, the remaining unthrombosed lumen continues to demonstrate a negative flow defect while the thrombosed portion of the lumen appears as an area of increased signal intensity—a typical appearance seen on both the SE TR530/TE30 and the SE TR3120/TE120 images (T-1 and T-2).

On T-1 weighted MR scans, with a 0.5 Tesla magnet, the acute hematoma has decreased signal intensity and thus mimics a tumor or acute infarct with mass effect. After 48 hours, the hematoma becomes increased in signal intensity. Thus, only on a delayed MR scan does the true nature of the abnormality become apparent.

In the future, thin sections, excellent localization techniques by MR, and perhaps the injection of paramagnetic intravascular contrast agents may allow us to evaluate accurately the presence of aneurysms.

Magnetic Resonance of Subarachnoid Hemorrhage

Magnetic resonance scans obtained shortly after a subarachnoid hemorrhage has occurred reveal that the blood in the subarachnoid space is of low signal intensity. After approximately 48 hours the blood in the subarachnoid space becomes increased in signal intensity on the SE TR530/TE30 images. These initial and later appearances are similar to those reported with intracerebral hematoma. It is thought that the increases in signal intensity with time is related to the chemical alteration in blood, with the hemoglobin molecule changing to methemoglobin. The methemoglobin acts as a paramagnetic agent and causes shortening of the T-1 and a resulting bright or increased signal on the T-1 images. Because acute subarachnoid hemorrhage appears as low signal intensity blood in the subarachnoid space and may not be appreciated, CT is the examination of choice for the diagnosis and evaluation of acute subarachnoid hemorrhage.

Angiography

At one time all patients with subarachnoid hemorrhage and suspected aneurysm underwent emergency angiography to define their anatomic abnormality. However, at the present time there appears to be a general reevaluation and revision of the methodology for work-up of these patients. At our institution the examination begins with an emergency CT scan in an attempt to determine the site of origin of the hemorrhage, to rule out a large intracerebral hematoma, and to determine whether the abnormality may actually be a hypertensive basal ganglionic hemorrhage that has ruptured into the ventricular system, resulting in the clinical appearance of a subarachnoid hemorrhage. A lumbar puncture usually is not performed for diagnosis if a CT scan is available.

Standard grading system:

Grade I (minimal bleed): alert; no neurologic deficit.

Grade II (mild bleed): alert; minimal neurologic deficit or third nerve palsy; stiff neck.

Grade III (moderate bleed): drowsy or confused; stiff neck, with or without neurologic deficit.

Grade IV (moderate or severe bleed): semicoma, with or without neurologic deficit.

Grade V (severe bleed): coma and decerebrate movements.

One higher grade is always assigned to patients over the age of 50, or if another major medical problem exists.

When the patient's clinical condition has improved to a Grade II or less, elective cerebral angiography is performed via the femoral approach using the Seldinger technique. The study is begun with examination of the clinically implicated vascular system. If marked spasm is demonstrated, no further injections are made. If there is no spasm or a mild one, a thorough study of each blood vessel's supply is performed. This includes appropriate oblique views or submentovertex views as necessary. Sufficient views are obtained to demonstrate the neck of the aneurysm so that an appropriate surgical approach can be planned. Following this, the remaining vascular supply to the brain is studied sequentially until all the possible sites of aneurysm have been demonstrated. If other aneurysms are found, appropriate views are obtained to demonstrate the neck of the aneurysm.

If an individual vessel cannot be catheterized for technical reasons, the appropriate percutaneous angiogram should be performed while the patient is in the radiology department so that all four vessels are well demonstrated. Failure to do this may result in failure to diagnose an existing aneurysm. In other words, if a vessel has not been adequately demonstrated it cannot be considered as not involved by an aneurysm.

Bilateral carotid angiography will demonstrate approximately 90 per cent of aneurysms present. In double aneurysm cases, if one aneurysm is demonstrated in the supratentorial circulation, there is a 3 to 5 per cent chance of the second aneurysm arising in the posterior fossa.

Arterial spasm following a subarachnoid hemorrhage is maximal between six and 12 days. Rebleeding after the initial insult is most likely to occur at five to seven days after the initial bleed.

Anterior Communicating Artery Aneurysm

AP, lateral, oblique, and submentovertex views are performed as needed. The submentovertex view is often the most helpful in demonstrating the neck of the aneurysm and its relationship to the anterior cerebral arteries.

Posterior Communicating Artery Aneurysm

AP, lateral oblique views in both oblique projections are performed as needed.

Middle Cerebral Artery Aneurysm

AP, lateral, and "through-the-orbit" view—with the middle cerebral artery bifurcation centered in the mid-portion of the orbit—are performed as needed. The "through-the-orbit" view is often most helpful in demonstrating the neck of the aneurysm and its relationship to the middle cerebral artery. This view frequently separates the multiple overlapping vessels around the genu of the middle cerebral artery. On other views they tend to overlap.

Posterior Fossa Aneurysms

AP, lateral, oblique, and submentovertex views are performed as needed. The author has found the submentovertex view to be especially helpful in the diagnosis of posterior circulation aneurysms.

On the oblique projections, both AP and lateral or single plane studies are performed as needed. In patients with meningismus secondary to blood in the subarachnoid space, it may be difficult to obtain a submentovertex view.

Sedation

I have found it helpful to supplement any premedication with intravenous Valium as needed for adequate sedation and would recommend that the premedication be adjusted for each patient. Valium is then given in 2- to 3-mg doses IV as needed. Often this supplementary medication is given just before an injection of contrast material so that the patient remains immobile for the filming run.

Approximately three quarters of patients with subarachnoid hemorrhage demonstrate an aneurysm as the site of bleeding. Arteriovenous malformations account for another 10 per cent; another 10 per cent are secondary to intracerebral hemorrhage. The remainder are undiagnosed.

Re-Examination

If no aneurysm is demonstrated after thorough examination of both carotid and both vertebral arteries, the patient is treated medically and they restudied with four-vessel arteriography after approximately one week of medical management. This is necessary because focal spasm may have occluded the neck of the aneurysm on the initial study. A vascular lesion of the spinal cord may present as a subarachnoid hemorrhage, and so a myelogram may be necessary for further evaluation.

Figures 6–1 through 6–19 (pp. 273 to 289) represent a variety of aneurysms seen in practice. A somewhat greater than usual emphasis is put on the use of CT scanning in the diagnosis of aneurysm. Although I have not found CT scanning to be of great help in the diagnosis of aneurysm, CT scanning is the procedure of choice in the diagnosis of subarachnoid hemorrage (SAH). CT scanning is also very helpful in evaluating and following any changes in ventricular size that may occur following SAH.

VASCULAR MALFORMATIONS OF THE BRAIN

Pathology

Arteriovenous malformations of the brain are fairly common; other types of vascular malformations of the brain are rare. Consideration of their various angiographic and pathologic features suggests a method of classification (after Russell and Rubinstein) that divides the vascular malformations into the following:

1. Cavernous Angioma. Well-circumscribed mass with large sinusoidal vascular spaces; vessels resemble capillaries without muscle or elastic tissue and no intervening brain parenchyma. Thromboses, calcification, and hemorrhage are common in these 1-mm to several-centimeter lesions.

2. Capillary Telangiectasis. Dilated capillaries without smooth muscle or elastic tissue form these small, solitary, and usually asymptomatic lesions.

3. Arteriovenous Malformations. The most common vascular malformation. The enlarged feeding arteries are thickened and tortuous, as are the veins. The intervening brain degenerates with time owing to hemorrhage and/or vascular insufficiency. The size varies from a few millimeters to many centimeters.

4. Venous Angioma. The rarest of the vascular malformations. There is no arterial component to this lesion, although the large, irregularly dilated venous channels resemble the arteriovenous malformations. The intervening neural tissue is normal.

Arteriovenous malformations (AVMs)—blood vessel abnormalities in which there is an abnormal communication between the arterial and venous circulations—are formed by a tangle of abnormal vessels. These vessels have thickened, malformed walls that make it difficult to identify them angiographically as either arteries or veins. These malformations may be supplied by one or more enlarged feeding arteries and drained by one or more (commonly multiple) large venous channels. The venous channels may drain either superficially or into the deep venous system. Arteriovenous malformations are the type most commonly seen in daily practice.

The vast majority of these lesions will be found in the supratentorial circulation—approximately 6 per cent are in the infratentorial circulation; another 8 per cent occur in the extracranial circulation. Arteriovenous malformations are less common than aneurysms. There is an increased incidence of aneurysms in patients with AVM's.

Clinical Symptoms

The presenting complaints of these patients are quite varied. Symptoms include grand mal seizures, syncopal attacks, transient ischemic attacks, and finally the catastrophic events associated with hemorrhage of the malformations, such as dense hemiplegias and/or coma. When hemorrhage occurs, these lesions may present in a fashion similar to that seen with subarachnoid hemorrhage or intracerebral hematoma secondary to other causes.

Plain Skull

The plain skull films may reveal areas of either curvilinear or punctate calcification that outline a portion or all of the malformation. The areas of curvilinear calcification may resemble those seen with an aneurysm. Frequently, areas of calcification can be identified on the CT scan that cannot be seen on radiographs of the skull. There may be enlargement of the vascular grooves of the skull, particularly if the malformation involves the meningeal coverings of the brain.

If the malformation is associated with obstructive hydrocephalus, as seen with vein of Galen aneurysms, changes may be noted in the sella turcica secondary to the hydrocephalus and to continued pressure on the sella from the dilated third ventricle, with enlargement of the sella and truncation of the dorsum sella and the posterior clinoids.

Computed Tomography of AVMs

The routine preinfusion CT scan appears to be normal in approximately 25 per cent of cases. In the remainder there may be areas of increased density secondary to the deposition of calcium in the walls of the vessels of the malformation. Focal areas of radiolucency secondary to local atrophy may be seen; there may be evidence of hemiatrophy of the hemispheres either ipsilateral or contralateral to the malformation. A mild mass effect secondary to the malformation may be noted, with shift to the contralateral side.

Postinfusion, there is marked enhancement of the malformation, which may have a wedge-shaped appearance that is broad-based superficially. More commonly, there is a "bag of worms" appearance of the malformation, with enhancement of the individual tortuous vessels. In other cases, both the individual feeding arteries and the draining veins can be identified.

The position of the malformation relative to areas of atrophy can be readily identified on the scan.

When the malformation is accompanied by hemorrhage, an area of increased density corresponding to the area of hemorrhage is superimposed on any other findings on the CT scan. If recent hemorrhage has occurred, the infusion of contrast material usually causes no change. With a resorbing hematoma, a ring of enhancement may be seen.

Aneurysms of the great vein of Galen often will be seen as a well-defined area of increased density. This type of malformation may cause obstructive hydrocephalus of varying degree. Vein of Galen aneurysms produce marked enhancement of the vein. The rest of the malformation may or may not be identified.

CT scan may be diagnostic in some cases, but arteriography is necessary for final diagnosis and evaluation. It should be mentioned that when an AVM is suspected the computed tomogram should be performed both without and with infusion of contrast material.

Venous Angioma

The entity of venous angioma has been considered in the literature for some time. However, until the development of CT, a relatively noninvasive test, there has not been a great deal of interest in this abnormality. Venous angiomas are found in both supra- and infratentorial distributions. The preinfusion CT scan may be normal or may reveal an area of amorphous calcification of varying but generally small size. The postinfusion scan demonstrates either a straight or a curvilinear enhancing structure that represents a draining vein. There may or may not be enhancement of the area of calcification. These venous angiomas may hemorrhage, but hemorrhage is more common in the posterior fossa than in the supratentorial region.

Angiography reveals a normal arterial and capillary phase. There is *no* evidence of an early draining vein. The malformation is identified in the venous phase as a tree-like structure of multiple small veins that coalesce into one large vein. This large vein is the structure identified on the CT scan. This rather typical-looking large, straight or slightly curvilinear vein drains directly to the surface of the brain into the cortical veins.

These venous angiomas are often seen as an incidental finding in patients who are examined for other reasons. Because of the possibility of hemorrhage in the posterior fossa, surgery may be considered. Surgery is generally not recommended for supratentorial venous angiomas.

Incidence and Location by CT Scanning

The exact incidence of these malformations is unknown because patients may be asymptomatic. In a review of over 10,000 computed tomograms performed over a three-year period, 23 AVMs were identified (Tables 6–1 and 6–2).

Table 6–1. 23 Arteriovenous Malformations—Presenting Symptoms

Seizures	
Generalized	6
Focal	2
"CVA" (3 hemorrhages)	6
Transient ischemic attack	1
Syncope	1
Visual hallucinations	1
Miscellaneous	5
Asymptomatic (calcifications on skull film)	1

Table 6–2. Findings Preinfusion

Shift or mass effect	Definite	4
	Equivocal	3
Calcification		5
Hemorrhage		3
Focal atrophy		1
Increased density		6
Decreased density		12
Hydrocephalus		2
Normal preinfusion		7

Table 6–3. Clinical Symptoms of the Seven Patients with Normal Preinfusion Scans

Seizures	2
"CVA"	2
Visual hallucination	1
Transient ischemic attack	1
Asymptomatic (calcifications seen on skull film)	1

Table 6–4. 23 Arteriovenous Malformations

	RIGHT	LEFT
Parietal	5	6
Basal ganglia	4	2
Frontal	1	3
Occipital	2	0
Tentorial	0	1

All were subsequently proved by arteriography. Of these 23 patients with arteriovenous malformations, only six presented with a catastrophic event; three patients had intracerebral hematomas and three had cerebrovascular accidents. The remainder had presenting complaints similar to those mentioned above, i.e., syncopal attacks, dizziness, or adult onset of grand mal seizures (see Table 6–3). The low incidence of hemorrhage in this series probably can be attributed to the fact that the computed tomogram represents a noninvasive diagnostic procedure that can be performed in minimally symptomatic patients without the dangers inherent in invasive procedures. With CT, more of the relatively asymptomatic or minimally symptomatic patients with previously unsuspected AVMs are diagnosed. In our series, seven patients had normal preinfusion CT scans (Table 6–3). In this group of seven patients, the symptoms were similar to those of any other group of patients sent for study.

Table 6–4 shows the anatomic positions of the 23 malformations. It is interesting to note that, in spite of the fact tht the parietal lobe is the smallest lobe anatomically, most of the malformations were located predominantly in the parietal lobe.

Radionuclide Studies

Although the subject is beyond the scope of this text, it should be mentioned that radionuclide scanning is very helpful in the diagnosis of arteriovenous malformations. The radionuclide scan is positive in a large percentage of these cases and classically reveals a pattern of early blush on the arteriogram phase of the radionuclide scan followed by rapid wash-out of the radionuclide on subsequent films.

The computed tomogram has proved to be very helpful in the diagnosis of these abnormalities and is positive in a high percentage of cases. It is, however, entirely possible that a small, superficially placed cortical AVM could be missed by the CT scan because of the partial volume phenomenon with the adjacent inner table of the bony calvaria. Therefore, a normal CT scan does not absolutely rule out the presence of AVM. It would appear, however, that if both the radionuclide scan and the CT scan are normal the patient is very unlikely to have an arteriovenous malformation.

Magnetic Resonance of Arteriovenous Malformations

Because of the "negative flow defect" of flowing blood, the appearance of arteriovenous malformations on MR is similar to that on CT, except that instead of serpiginous areas of enhancement on the postinfusion portion of the examination there are serpiginous areas of negative signal secondary to the enlarged feeding arteries and early draining veins. While standard angiography will demonstrate the feeding arteries and draining veins, CT and MR sometimes differentiate between the arterial and venous structures (see Figure 6–21, pp. 292–293). Similarly, the negative flow of a vein of Galen aneurysm can be identified, but neither CT nor MR provides adequate evaluation for surgery. If hemorrhage has occurrred there is an associated area of increased signal intensity because of the hemorrhage. Any intraventricular accumulation of blood can also be identified by the MR scan. Complete evaluation requires standard angiography.

Arteriography

Because of an increased incidence of aneurysms in patients with AVMs, it is advantageous to study these abnormalities by the femoral approach, using selective catheterization of all the great vessels arising from the arch. At the time of fluoroscopy for catheter placement, the carotid and/or vertebral vessels may be noted to be far larger than normal.

The amount of blood flow through the malformation usually far exceeds normal; therefore, an increase in the amount of contrast material injected may be necessary for adequate evaluation. In addition, the arteriovenous circulation time is frequently very rapid, necessitating a more rapid filming technique than ordinarily is used. Instead of the routine two films per second for the first three seconds, it may be necessary to increase this to four or even six films per second for the first three seconds in order to evaluate arterial feeding and venous drainage. This, of course, must be varied for each case. The timing becomes most important when one is attempting to outline the arterial supply and the venous drainage in order to facilitate surgical intervention. In many cases it is also necessary to perform multiple vessel studies to evaluate all the feeding vessels. This serves the additional purpose of ruling out the presence of an aneurysm. It should be noted that malformations in the parietal lobe may feed from the middle cerebral artery on the ipsilateral side while stealing blood from the contralateral side. In these cases, the cross-over from the other side results in a "steal phenomenon" from the contralateral hemisphere; indeed, these patients may become symptomatic from the relatively anemic hemisphere contralateral to the malformation.. We have seen one case where the CT scan revealed apparent atrophy with enlargement of the cortical sulci on the side contralateral to the malformation, but angiography revealed that there was evidence of a "steal" from the atrophic hemisphere.

The diagnostic and frequently pathognomonic arteriographic criteria include enlarged feeding arteries, the malformation itself—which appears as a tangle of blood vessels ("bag of worms")—and early draining veins (see Fig. 6–21, pp. 292–293). The mass is typically non–space-occupying, except in those cases in which hemorrhage has occurred. The malformation may be relatively small, and often is obscured by overlying large feeding arteries and draining veins.

Arteriovenous malformations often first become symptomatic at the time of hemorrhage. The hemorrhage is readily diagnosed by CT scanning, which reveals an area of increased density of variable size that measures between 45 and 90 Hounsfield units. If the hemorrhage is acute there will be no change in the density following infusion of contrast material. An unusual position of the hemorrhage should raise the index of suspicion that the hemorrhage is not hypertensive but may be related to another bleeding source, such as aneurysm or arteriovenous malformation. In those cases, arteriography will be necessary to evaluate the presence of an AVM. Blood in the cerebral tissue or the subarachnoid space is very irritating to the blood vessels; besides the associated intracerebral hematoma, one may also see marked vascular spasm (Fig. 6–24, pp. 298–299) at arteriography.

In addition, there are occasions of "occult" malformations that hemorrhage resulting in total obliteration of the precipitating blood vessel abnormality. These appear as areas of hemorrhage on the CT scan and as an avascular mass lesion at arteriography. The true nature of the lesion is discovered only at surgery, when the typical histologic appearance of the malformation is discovered.

Rarely, a very malignant glioblastoma multiforme may simulate the appearance of an arteriovenous malformation. In occasional rare cases of glioblastoma there is enlargement of the feeding arteries and early draining veins, making differentiation from an AVM difficult. It should be remembered, however, that glioblastomas are space-occupying lesions, whereas AVMs, in the absence of hemorrhage, are non–space-occupying.

Treatment

Surgical correction of these blood vessel abnormalities can be attempted, but has met with only limited success. Follow-up arteriography often reveals that new feeding channels have opened following closure of the original vessels.

In addition to the surgical treatment, instillation of plastic pellets, Gelfoam, sponge, or glue into the feeding arteries has been performed in an attempt to obliterate the malformation or to make it more amenable to a surgical approach. When attempting this method, an arteriogram is first performed for baseline evaluation; then repeat arteriography is performed after each successive instillation of single or multiple pellets. "Superselective" catheterization of the vessel to be embolized is desirable. It is also necessary to monitor the patient's clinical neurologic status carefully during this type of procedure. Balloon catheters also have been used to occlude the arteries in order to prevent materials from moving retrograde out of the vessel and being embolized incorrectly.

Carotid Cavernous Fistula

An additional malformation sometimes seen is the carotid cavernous fistula. This abnormality implies an abnormal direct communication between the internal carotid artery and the cavernous sinus. Although these carotid cavernous fistulas can develop spontaneously, they are seen most often after severe head trauma—apparently when there is tearing of the internal carotid artery at the level of the cavernous sinus. In most cases, this traumatic development of a fistula results in almost immediate symptoms. Rupture of a berry aneurysm at the level of the cavernous portion of the carotid artery also may result in a carotid cavernous fistula with similar findings. The author has seen one case of a spontaneous carotid cavernous fistula in a 23-year-old woman with fibromuscular hyperplasia of the blood vessels.

The clinical findings with a carotid cavernous fistula are a pulsating exophthalmos and an annoying bruit that the patient can hear. The conjunctivae become injected and chemosis may develop. Extraocular muscle palsies and blindness may occur. These changes may be ipsilateral or bilateral; rarely, they involve only the contralateral eye.

Diagnosis is made and/or confirmed at the time of carotid arteriography. The pattern of venous drainage varies from patient to patient but very commonly involves retrograde filling of the superior ophthalmic vein (Figs. 6–26 and 6–28, pp. 301 and 304–305). This vein may become so greatly distended that it causes erosion and enlargement of the bony margins of the superior orbital fissure (Fig. 6–26, p. 301). The retrograde flow into the venous system can also go up into the middle cerebral venous system and to the cerebral convexity to drain into the superior sagittal sinus.

As with studies of any other rapid flow system, films should be shot in quick sequence—usually at a rate of four or, preferably, six films per second for the first three seconds. An increased volume of contrast material is also recommended in many cases for better delineation. The rapid filling of the cavernous sinus and, subsequently, of the superior ophthalmic vein becomes readily apparent at the time of the study.

These carotid cavernous fistulas frighten and discomfort the patient and are a difficult surgical problem. Ligation of the carotid has met with limited success. Obliteration of the cavernous sinus with a balloon catheter has been successful in some cases.

We have seen one unusual case of a carotid venous fistula that drained primarily into the venous structures of the cerebellopontine angle and posterior fossa. This patient presented with a history of tinnitus in the left ear. The plain films revealed enlargement of the internal auditory canal on the side of the fistula. The carotid venous fistula was discovered during the course of work-up for a cerebellopontine angle tumor.

Vein of Galen Aneurysm

This arteriovenous malformation is seen in children; it often presents at birth or in the very young age group as high output congestive heart failure. These vein of Galen aneurysms are actually deep-seated AVMs that drain into the vein of Galen and produce enlargement of the vein because of excessive blood flow (Fig. 6–29, pp. 306–307). This enlargement of the vein of Galen results in obstruction of the aqueduct of Sylvius and the outlet of the third ventricle and consequently in obstructive hydrocephalus. In these cases, "aneurysm of the vein of Galen" is actually a misnomer, but it has become deeply entrenched in our terminology. These AVMs usually are fed by the posterior cerebral arteries. The surgical approach may be very difficult, and the prognosis for these patients is usually very poor.

Dural Arteriovenus Malformations

Malformations that involve the dural covering of the brain (Fig. 6–27, pp. 302–303) also may be seen. These dural malformations are fed by the meningeal vessels and are similar histologically to other malformations. When dural malformations involve the tentorium, arteriography should include study of the carotid arteries in an attempt to visualize an enlarged tentorial artery where it arises from the internal carotid artery at its entrance into the cavernous sinus and proceeds to the free edge of the tentorium. As noted in Chapter 8, enlargement of this vessel is also seen in tentorial meningiomas. Visualization of these vessels helps the surgeon to plan an operative approach.

Scalp Arteriovenous Malformations

Arteriovenous malformations of the scalp may be congenital or may develop secondary to trauma (Fig. 6–32, p. 311). These malformations also may develop following craniotomy. In acquired lesions, one usually can obtain a history of injury, following which a compressible soft tissue mass developed and large draining vessels became visible over the cranial vault. The arteriographic appearance is quite typical, with feeding vessels from the external carotid and enlarged draining veins. Occasionally these scalp malformations can reach a spectacular size (Fig. 6–32, p. 311). In smaller malformations, bright-lighting the soft tissues over the cranial vault will help to differentiate the supplying and draining vessels from intracranial vessels.

Of course, selective internal and external carotid injections with filming in the AP and lateral projections will serve to outline the vascular pattern most accurately. Direct puncture and injection of the scalp malformation has been suggested, but would seem less desirable than selective internal and external carotid injection.

Spinal Cord Arteriovenous Malformations

Arteriovenous malformations of the spinal cord do occur (see Chapter 15). The malformation itself usually is small and is drained by multiple enlarged veins that are visible on the dorsal aspect of the cord. They most frequently are supplied by the artery of Adamkiewicz, which arises from one of the intercostal vessels of the lower thoracic or upper lumbar aorta, but most frequently at the T_{12} level on the left side. Selective catheterization and injection of this vessel will outline the malformation and the draining veins. Care must be taken that the artery is not occluded by the catheter, as this may lead to paralysis of the lower extremities. Paralysis also may occur secondary to a toxic reaction to the contrast material.

It may be necessary to catheterize each of the intercostal vessels in turn. Magnification and subtraction techniques also should be used. Meticulous care should be taken during injection of the vessels to prevent untoward reactions.

Flush aortography and digital angiography are useful to outline any enlarged vascular supply. Spinal arteriography is a time-consuming procedure and sometimes is difficult for both the patient and the physician.

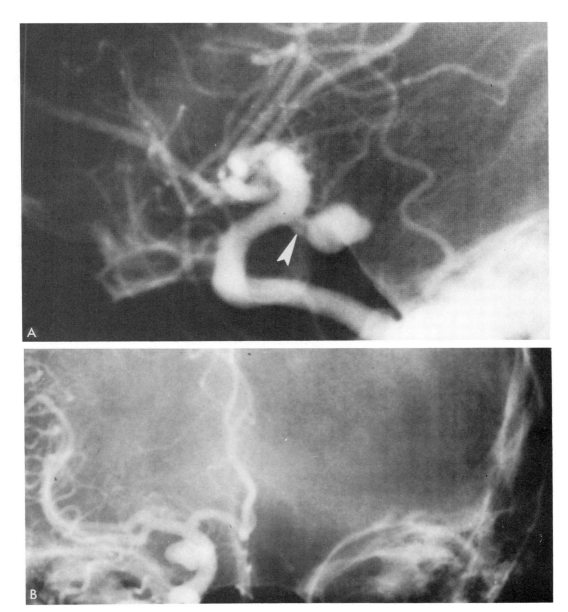

FIGURE 6–1. *Posterior Communicating Artery Aneurysm:* The right common carotid angiogram demonstrates a 1.2-cm aneurysm of the posterior communicating artery. The aneurysm has a well-defined neck (*arrow*) and projects posteriorly on the lateral view (*A*). It is noted to project slightly laterally on the AP view (*B*), just below the bifurcation of the internal carotid artery. The neck of the aneurysm is hidden behind the internal carotid artery on the AP view.

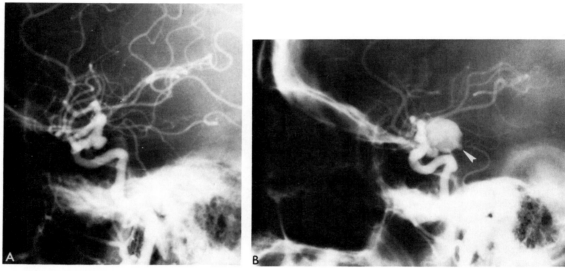

FIGURE 6–2. *Bilateral Posterior Communicating Artery Aneurysms: A*, On this side, a small, broad-necked posterior communicating artery aneurysm projects posteriorly.

B, On the contralateral side, a large, lobulated aneurysm projects posteriorly and superiorly. The patient presented clinically with a subarachnoid hemorrhage and a third nerve palsy on the side of the larger aneurysm. The small localized bulge posteriorly is probably the actual point of hemorrhage *(arrow)*.

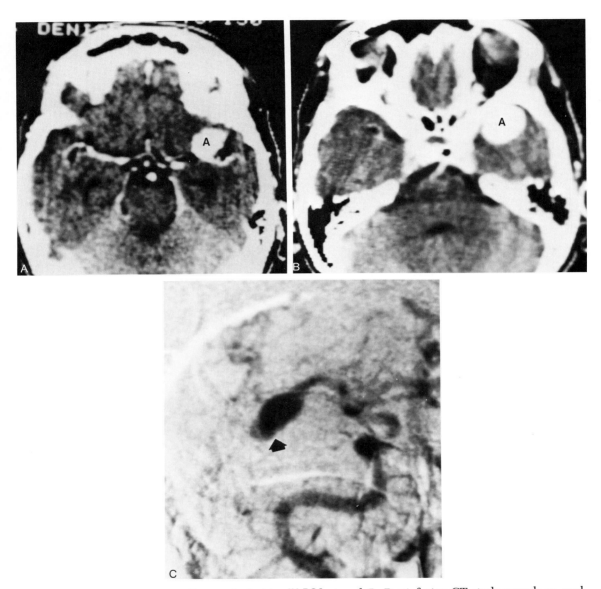

FIGURE 6–3. *Berry Aneurysm Demonstrated by IV-DSA:* *A* and *B*, Postinfusion CT study reveals an oval-shaped area of enhancement in the anterior temporal region. *C*, While an unthrombosed aneurysm or a densely enhancing meningioma may have this appearance, the IV-DSA reveals that this abnormality is actually an unthrombosed middle cerebral artery aneurysm. Although the aneurysm is identified by IV-DSA, it' is better seen with standard angiography (see Figure 6–8).

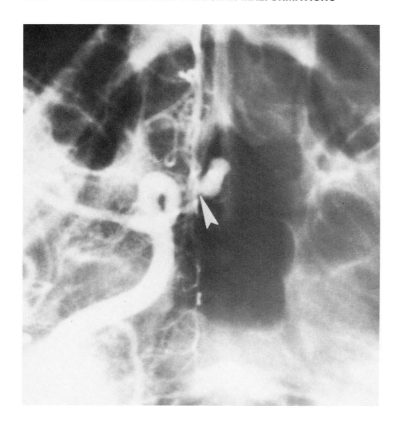

FIGURE 6–4. *Submentovertex View of an Anterior Communicating Artery Aneurysm:* The submentovertex view shows the anterior communicating artery aneurysm as it projects across the midline from its point of origin (*arrow*). The neck is well-demonstrated. In general, the submentovertex view is the best for demonstrating anterior communicating artery aneurysms.

FIGURE 6–5. *Aneurysm Clip on an Anterior Communicating Artery Aneurysm:* The aneurysm clip is well-demonstrated at the level of the anterior communicating artery on the submentovertex view. Patients with aneurysm clips cannot be scanned with magnetic resonance because the magnetic field could torque the clip off the neck of the aneurysm.

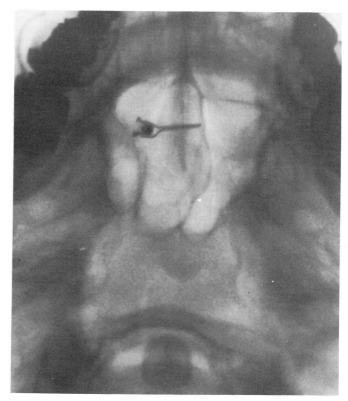

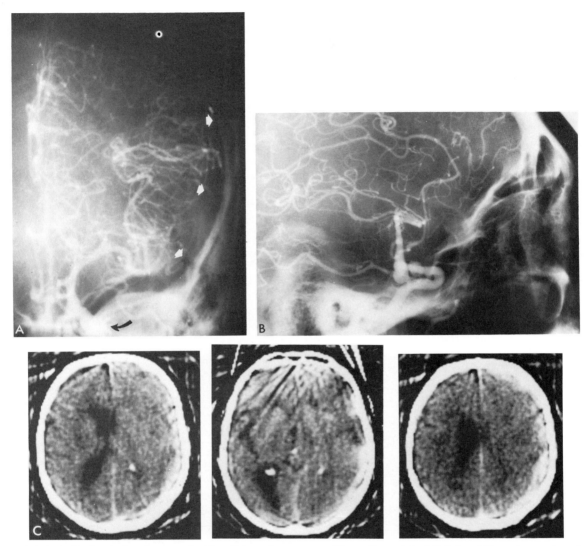

FIGURE 6–6. *Posterior Communicating Artery Aneurysm with an Associated Subdural Hematoma: A* and *B*, A lobulated posterior communicating artery aneurysm is seen on both the AP (*black arrow*) and the lateral view. The supraclinoid portion of the internal carotid artery is straightened and displaced medially, posteriorly, and superiorly. In addition, there is a moderate-sized extracerebral accumulation of blood that displaces the middle cerebral artery vessels away from the inner table of the skull (*white arrowheads*). This subdural hematoma results when the aneurysm ruptures through the arachnoid membrane into the subdural space.

C, CT scans demonstrate an acute subdural hematoma over the right hemisphere. There is shift of the midline to the contralateral side. The straight sinus and the falx cerebri are more dense than normal because they are outlined by blood in the subarachnoid space. The aneurysm is not seen on the CT scan.

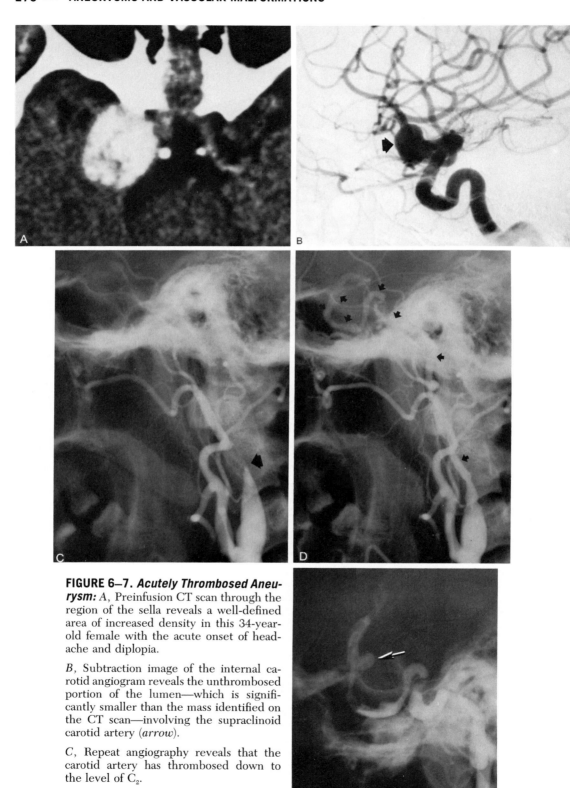

FIGURE 6–7. *Acutely Thrombosed Aneurysm:* A, Preinfusion CT scan through the region of the sella reveals a well-defined area of increased density in this 34-year-old female with the acute onset of headache and diplopia.

B, Subtraction image of the internal carotid angiogram reveals the unthrombosed portion of the lumen—which is significantly smaller than the mass identified on the CT scan—involving the supraclinoid carotid artery (*arrow*).

C, Repeat angiography reveals that the carotid artery has thrombosed down to the level of C₂.

D, Angiography three months later reveals that the vessel has recanalized, and approximately six months later (*E*) a portion of the lumen of the aneurysm (*arrow*) is again demonstrated.

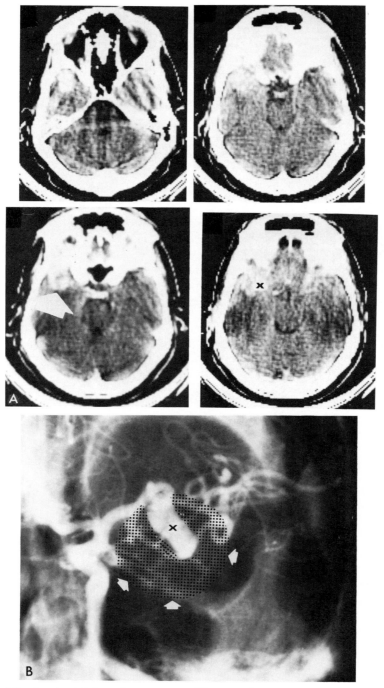

FIGURE 6-8. *Middle Cerebral Artery Aneurysm:* *A,* The preinfusion scan—upper row—reveals a rounded, fairly well-defined area of high density in the anterior margin of the left middle cranial fossa. On the postinfusion scan (lower row), the high density area is again seen (*white arrow*). In addition, there is a small area of enhancement (*x*) more superiorly that was not visible on the preinfusion scan. This is contrast material in the unclotted portion of the aneurysm.

B, The left carotid angiogram demonstrates the unclotted portion of the aneurysm (*x*) that was shown on the postinfusion CT scan. The dotted area (*white arrowheads*) shows the actual size of the aneurysm, which was largely clotted on the scan. The aneurysm acts as a mass and elevates the middle cerebral artery.

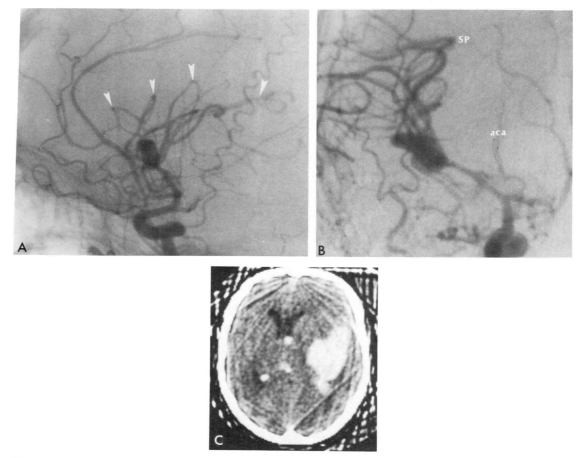

FIGURE 6–9. *Ruptured Trifurcation Aneurysm:* *A,* The lateral view of the carotid arteriogram demonstrates a lobulated aneurysm of the middle cerebral artery. There is spasm of the horizontal portion of the middle cerebral artery and elevation of the sylvian triangle, which is bowed superiorly in its midportion (*arrowheads*).

B, The AP view reveals medial displacement of the genu of the middle cerebral artery, medial displacement of the sylvian point (*SP*), and medial displacement of the anterior choroidal artery (*aca*) as well as contralateral displacement of the anterior cerebral artery. The aneurysm has ruptured, resulting in a large temporal lobe hematoma.

C, The CT scan shows a large area of hemorrhage deep in the hemisphere. Blood has accumulated in the lateral ventricle and in the third ventricle—probably because the aneurysm has ruptured into the temporal horn of the lateral ventricle. There is a moderate shift of the midline structures to the contralateral side.

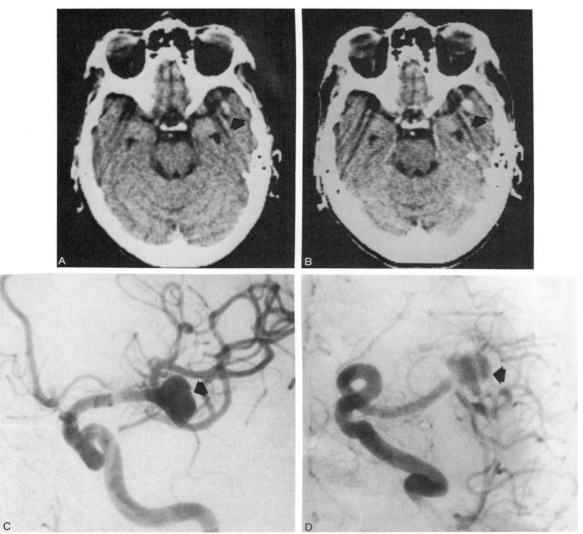

FIGURE 6–10. *Trifurcation Aneurysm:* A, Preinfusion CT scan reveals the aneurysm (*arrow*) in the region of the genu of the left middle cerebral artery. (This is usually an area of rapid bifurcations of the middle cerebral artery but is commonly called "the trifurcation.") The aneurysm contains flowing blood and is similar in density to the basilar artery.

B, The postinfusion CT scan demonstrates dense enhancement of this aneurysm.

C and D, Subtraction angiography in the oblique (C) and submentovertex (D) projections reveals the slightly lobulated aneurysm (*arrows*) and its intimate relationship with the middle cerebral artery vessels.

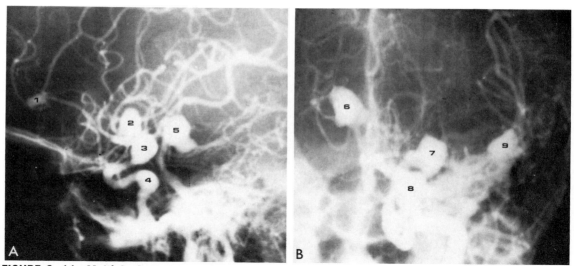

FIGURE 6–11. *Multiple Aneurysms:* This patient has nine aneurysms visible on this right brachial (*A*)–left carotid (*B*) examination. It is difficult or impossible to judge which aneurysm has bled in this case. (Case courtesy of the Radiology Group at the Carle Clinic.)

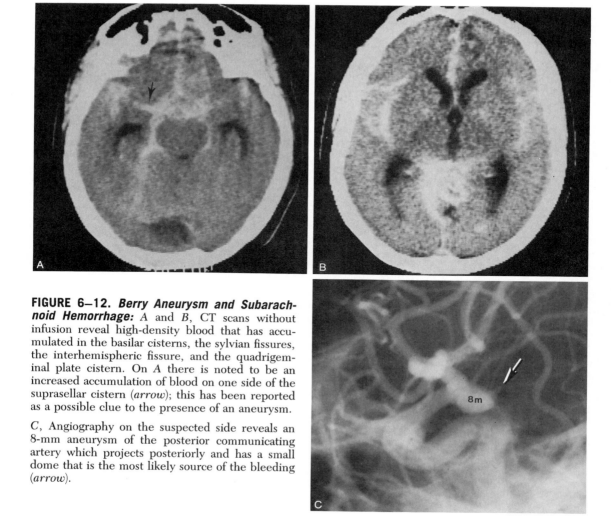

FIGURE 6–12. *Berry Aneurysm and Subarachnoid Hemorrhage:* *A* and *B*, CT scans without infusion reveal high-density blood that has accumulated in the basilar cisterns, the sylvian fissures, the interhemispheric fissure, and the quadrigeminal plate cistern. On *A* there is noted to be an increased accumulation of blood on one side of the suprasellar cistern (*arrow*); this has been reported as a possible clue to the presence of an aneurysm.

C, Angiography on the suspected side reveals an 8-mm aneurysm of the posterior communicating artery which projects posteriorly and has a small dome that is the most likely source of the bleeding (*arrow*).

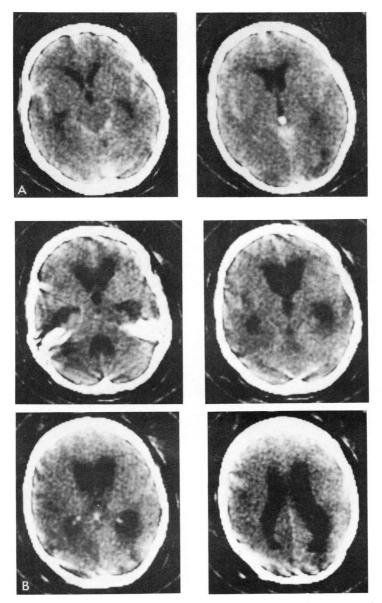

FIGURE 6–13. *CT of Subarachnoid Hemorrhage:* The initial CT scans (A) demonstrate high-density material in the cisterns, in the sylvian fissures, and in the interhemispheric fissure. This finding is secondary to blood in the subarachnoid space.

B, Follow-up CT scans show diffuse enlargement of the lateral, third, and fourth ventricles secondary to a communicating hydrocephalus that developed because of interference with resorption of the CSF by the arachnoid villi. These patients may require a shunting procedure for relief of the communicating hydrocephalus.

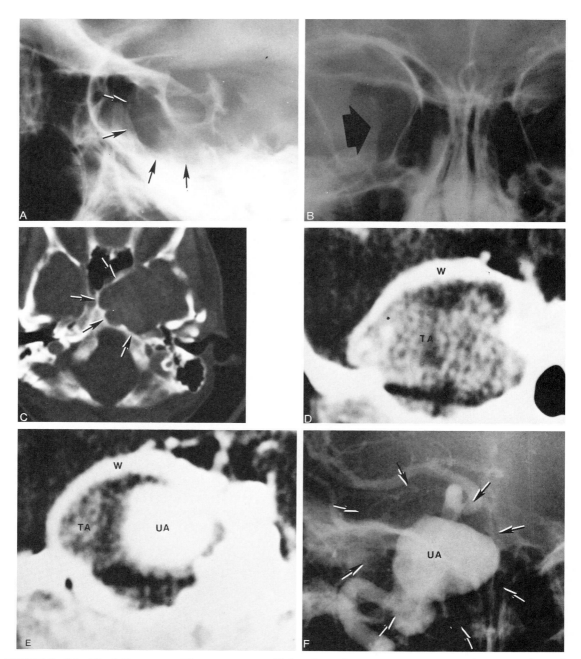

FIGURE 6–14. *Giant Aneurysm:* Thirty-six–year–old female with a cavernous sinus syndrome on the right side. *A,* Lateral view of the sella turcica reveals that one anterior clinoid has been completely eroded, and there is a soft tissue mass that extends into the sphenoid sinus (*arrows*).

B, PA view of the sella reveals enlargement of the superior orbital tissue on the side of the abnormality secondary to pressure erosion of this long-standing lesion (*arrow*).

C, CT scan through skull base reveals a large, smoothly marginated area of bone erosion involving the sphenoid sinus, the lateral margins of the clivus, and the middle cranial fossa (*arrows*).

D and *E,* Coronal CT through the area of interest reveals dense enhancement of the wall (*W*) of the aneurysm, but no central enhancement at this level because the aneurysm is thrombosed (*TA*). Further posteriorly (*E*), the unthrombosed portion of the aneurysm (*UA*) is seen filled with contrast material.

F and *G,* Internal carotid angiography reveals the unthrombosed portion of the aneurysm; the mass effect, however, reveals that the thrombosed portion of the aneurysm is actually much larger (arrows outline aneurysm).

Illustration continued on the following page

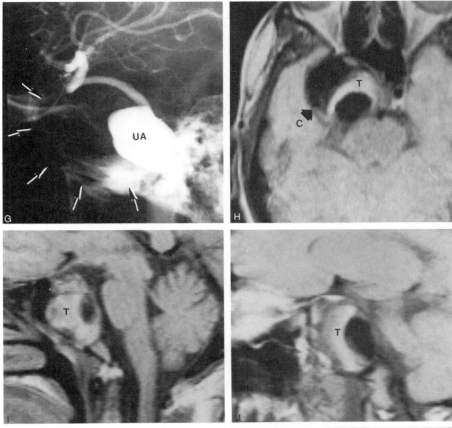

FIGURE 6–14 *Continued.*

H, Axial SE TR530/TE30 image reveals the large parasellar aneurysm. The thrombosed portion of the aneurysm appears as an area of increased signal intensity (*T*), and the unthrombosed portion projects just posteriorly and is a negative flow defect. This area of negative flow defect corresponds to that portion of the aneurysm that fills with contrast material on the CT scan. Far laterally, the patent carotid artery (*arrow-C*) appears as a negative flow defect, and just anterior to it is an area of decreased signal intensity believed to be secondary to an "ancient" thrombosed portion of the aneurysm that, because of iron deposition, behaves as a paramagnetic agent and results in very low signal intensity.

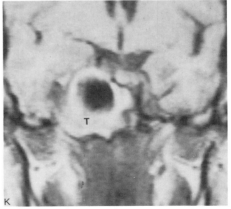

I, Midsagittal SE TR530/TE30 reveals the thrombosed (*T*) portion of the aneurysm with the unthrombosed aneurysm projecting posterior to it. There is erosion of the sphenoid sinus and posterior displacement of the pons.

J, A parasagittal image again demonstrates the thrombosed (*T*) and unthrombosed portions of the lumen.

K, Coronal SE TR530/TE30 again identifies the aneurysm and also demonstrates the mass effect with superior displacement of the ipsilateral temporal lobe and erosion of the base of the skull as illustrated in *C*.

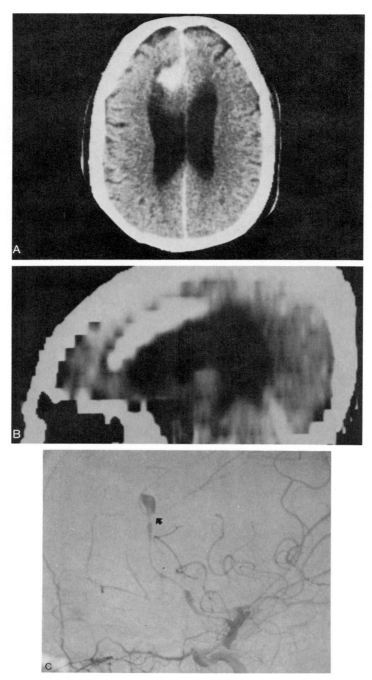

FIGURE 6–15. *Peripheral Berry Aneurysm with Hemorrhage:* *A,* Preinfusion CT scan reveals an area of blood accumulation deep in the frontal lobe just anterior to the body of the lateral ventricle. The increased density of the interhemispheric fissure is secondary to the blood in the subarachnoid space.

B, A parasagittal reconstruction view reveals that the area of hemorrhage follows the upper margin of the lateral ventricle. The ventricles are enlarged secondary to a communicating hydrocephalus that has developed because the blood in the subarachnoid space interferes with the resorption of the CSF.

C, Subtraction image of the internal carotid angiogram reveals diffuse spasm of multiple intracranial branches that alternates with areas of widening of the vessels. There is a large irregular aneurysm at the level of the bifurcation of the anterior cerebral artery into the pericallosal and callosal marginal arteries (*arrow*). This is an uncommon location of a berry aneurysm.

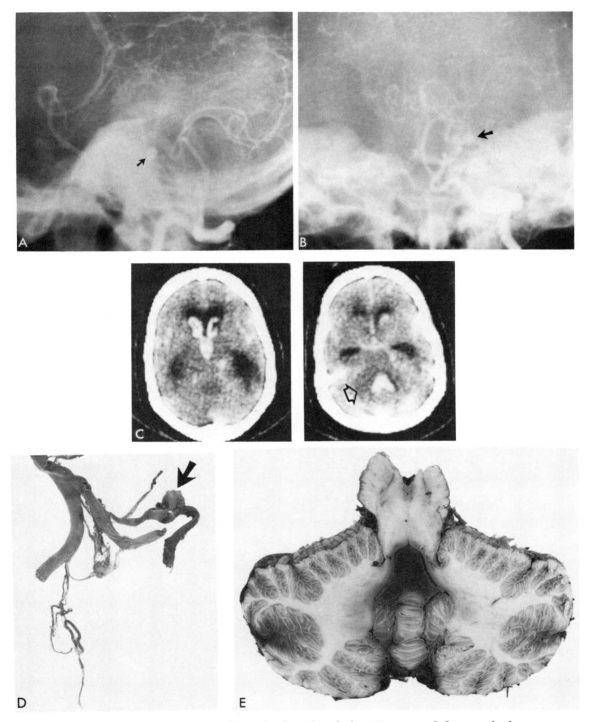

FIGURE 6–16. *PICA Aneurysms:* *A* and *B,* The lateral and the AP views of the vertebral arteriogram demonstrate an aneurysm of the PICA (*arrows*), which lies along the course of the posterior inferior cerebellar artery.

C, The CT scan of this same patient reveals that there is clotted blood in the fourth, third, and lateral ventricles. In addition, there is an area of radiolucency around the right side of the fourth ventricle—an area of infarction (*arrow*).

D, The pathologic specimen reveals the aneurysm (*arrow*) along the course of the PICA.

E, The specimen of the posterior fossa structures shows clotted blood in the fourth ventricle.

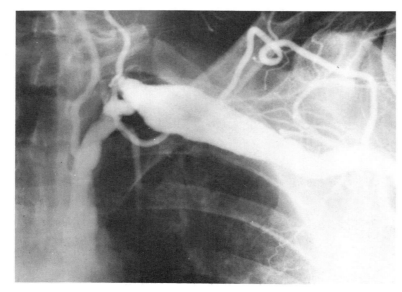

FIGURE 6–17. *Subclavian Artery Aneurysm:* The left brachial arteriogram demonstrates diffuse dilatation of the entire left subclavian artery. The right subclavian artery had a similar appearance. The etiology of this change is unknown.

FIGURE 6–18. *Aneurysmal Change Involving the Entire Brachiocephalic Trunk:* An arch angiogram in the LPO projection demonstrates diffuse dilatation of all the great vessels as they arise from the arch of the aorta. Although all the vessels are patent, there was marked delay in filling of the intracranial circulation.

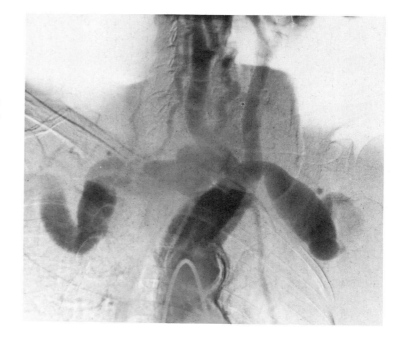

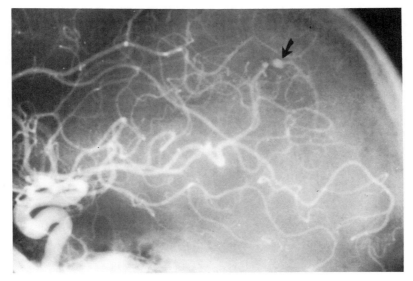

FIGURE 6–19. *Mycotic Aneurysm:* The intracranial circulation demonstrates a small aneurysm (*arrow*) along the distal course of one of the middle cerebral arteries. This is an infected aneurysm that developed because of a septic embolus from the affected heart valve in this patient with subacute bacterial endocarditis.

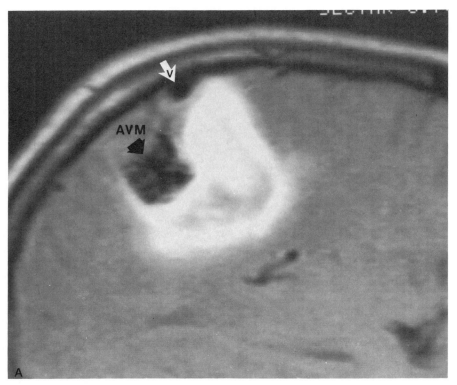

FIGURE 6–20. *Arteriovenous Malformation with Hemorrhage:* A, Parasagittal T-1 weighted image reveals the typical "bag of worms" appearance of a left parietal arteriovenous malformation (AVM). The malformation is decreased in signal intensity because of the negative flow defect of flowing blood in the malformation (AVM). The enlarged draining vein is seen superior to the malformation where it drains into the superior sagittal sinus (V). Anterior to the AVM is a large intracerebral hematoma. The central portion of this hematoma is decreased in signal intensity because of deoxyhemoglobin, and the periphery of this hematoma is increased in signal intensity because of methemoglobin.

B, A more lateral parasagittal section reveals the enlarged distal branch of the anterior cerebral artery (ACA) that supplies the AVM.

C, Axial T-1 weighted image reveals the enlarged middle cerebral artery branches that supply the AVM (MCA). There is slight mass effect with compression of the left lateral ventricle. Angiography confirmed these findings. Surgically proved.

Illustration continued on the following page

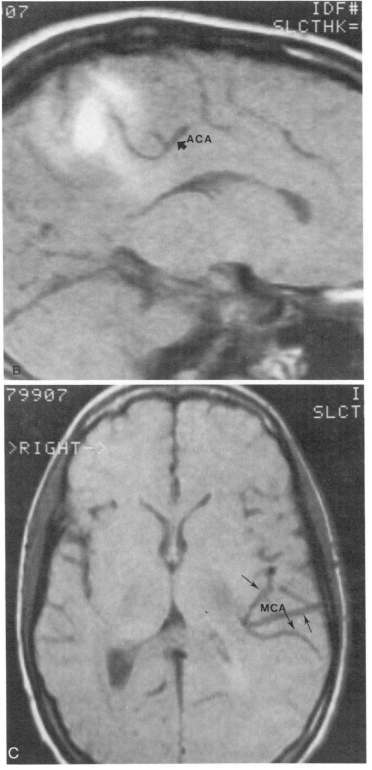

FIGURE 6–20 *Continued.*

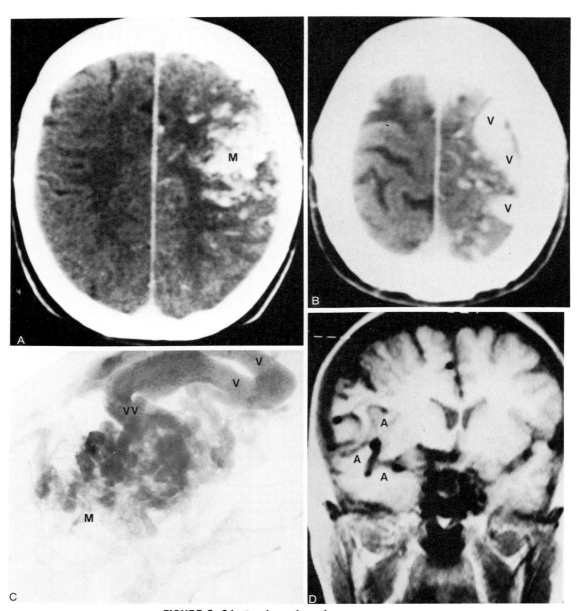

FIGURE 6–21. *See legend on the opposite page.*

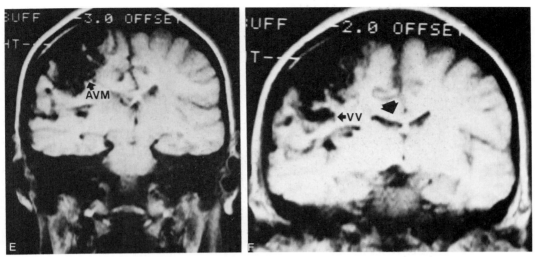

FIGURE 6–21. *Arteriovenous Malformation with CT, Angiography, and MR:* A and B, The postinfusion CT cuts in the high-convexity region demonstrate the malformation (M), and the greatly enlarged single draining vein (V). Note the obliteration of the cortical sulci on the ipsilateral side because the enlarged draining veins act like an extracerebral mass (similar to a subdural hematoma).

C, Angiography demonstrates the malformation (M) and the single enlarged draining vein that is tortuous and drains to the superior sagittal sinus. Point "VV" identifies the origin of the vein and is also identified on the MR scan.

D, The most anterior slice of the coronal MR scan reveals the enlarged feeding arteries that appear as negative flow defects (A) and are branches of the middle cerebral artery.

E, The next slice reveals the malformation as a large negative signal area, and the final slice (F) of this TR530/TE30 MR scan reveals the origin of the vein (VV) and the large extracerebral negative signal area secondary to the enlarged cortical veins. There is a shift of the midline structures because of this mass effect (*arrow*). The appearance is typical of an arteriovenous malformation.

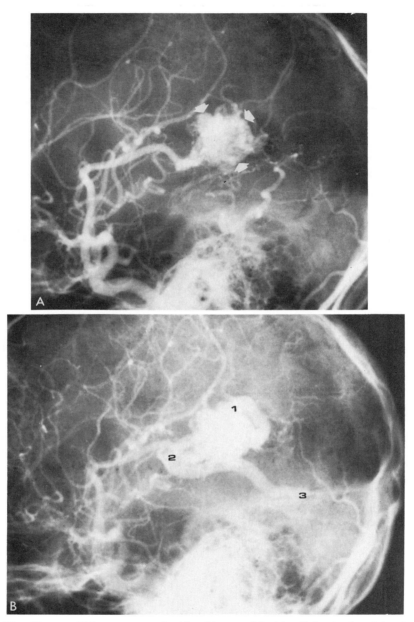

FIGURE 6–22. This 11-year-old boy presented with a history of flashing lights in the right visual field. *A* and *B*, The arteriograms reveal an arteriovenous malformation (*white arrows*) in the posterior temporal parietal region on the left side. It is fed by one enlarged vessel from the middle cerebral artery into the enlarged vein of Labbé.

Illustration continued on the following page

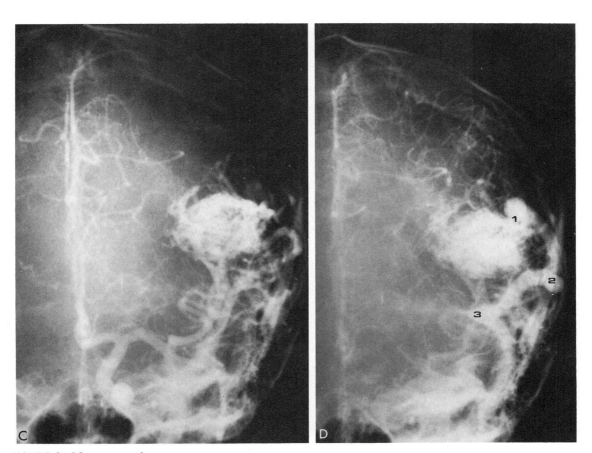

FIGURE 6–22 *Continued.*

C and *D*, The anteroposterior views demonstrate the malformation and the enlarged vein of Labbé. The vein of Labbé is marked (*1*) at its origin in the malformation; this correlates with the lateral view (*B*), which is marked in a corresponding fashion. (*3*) is the point of entrance of the vein of Labbé into the transverse sinus. The transverse sinus then drains into the sigmoid sinus and ultimately into the internal jugular vein.

Illustration continued on the following page

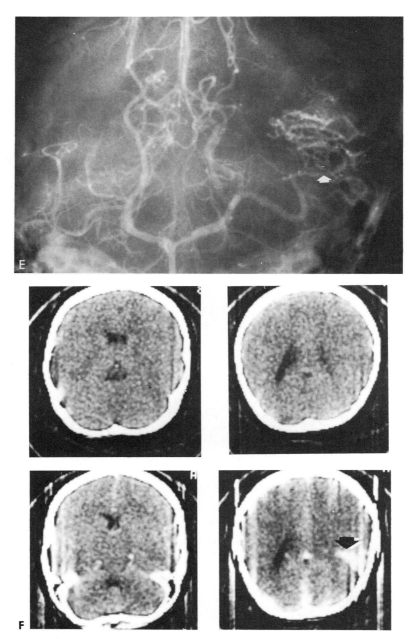

FIGURE 6–22 *Continued.*

E, A small portion of the malformation was seen to fill from the posterior temporal branch of the left posterior cerebral artery (*white arrow*).

F, The preinfusion CT scan is essentially normal; a wedge-shaped area of enhancement is noted on the postinfusion scan (*arrow*). Care must be taken not to confuse the wedge of enhancement with the petrous pyramid on the left side.

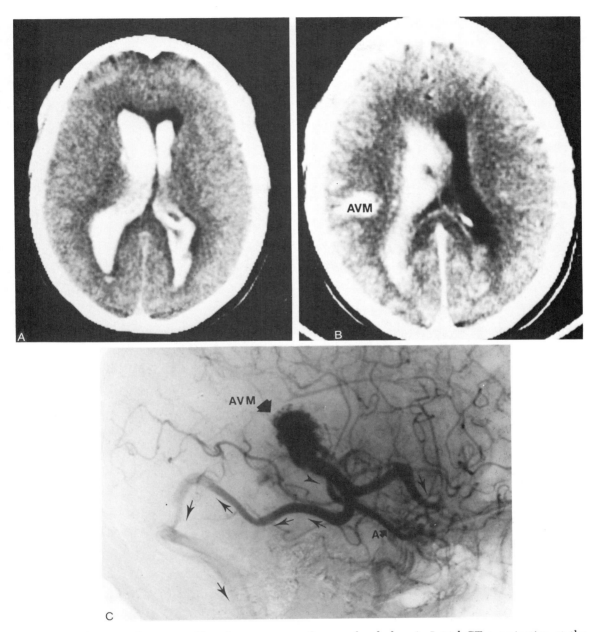

FIGURE 6–23. Forty-five–year–old with acute onset of severe headache. *A,* Initial CT examination at the time of admission reveals that both lateral ventricles are filled with clotted blood (right greater than left).

B, Follow-up CT with contrast infusion reveals that there continues to be a large amount of clotted blood in the right lateral ventricle, and a blood/CSF level in the left lateral ventricle. There is an area of enhancement in the right parietal lobe that subsequently proved to represent an arteriovenous malformation (*AVM*). An enhancing infarct could also have a similar appearance.

C, Right carotid angiogram demonstrates the 2-cm AVM supplied by one enlarged branch of the middle cerebral artery (*A*). The AVM is surrounded by a small avascular area and presumable surrounding edema, and there are two enlarged draining veins (*arrows*). The larger vein drains to the vein of Labbé, sigmoid sinus, and internal jugular vein.

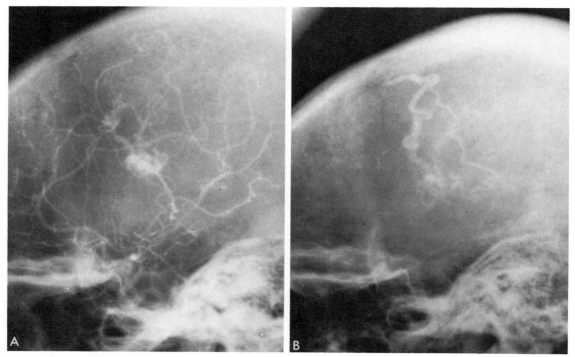

FIGURE 6–24. This 36-year-old woman presented with a sudden onset of unconsciousness and a left hemiparesis. *A* and *B*, The arterial and capillary phases of the arteriogram reveal a small arteriovenous malformation just above the midportion of the sylvian triangle. The malformation is supplied by one moderate-sized middle cerebral artery vessel and drained by several cortical veins. It is surrounded by an avascular area, resulting in stretching of the opercular branches of the middle cerebral artery and downward placement of the sylvian triangle. These findings are consistent with an AVM that is surrounded by an area of hemorrhage. In addition, the vessels exhibit diffuse narrowing secondary to arterial spasm because of irritation by the adjacent blood.

C, The AP view reveals shift of the anterior cerebral artery to the contralateral side and medial displacement of the sylvian point (*arrow*).

D, The postoperative arteriogram shows that the malformation has been obliterated. The branches of the middle cerebral artery have returned to a more normal caliber, and there is less stretching of the opercular branches of the middle cerebral artery because the hematoma has been evacuated. Some downward displacement of the midportion of the sylvian triangle remains (*arrows*).

E, The CT scan reveals a small intracerebral hematoma adjacent to the cortex on the left side. There is shift from left to right. There was no change following the infusion of contrast material.

An arteriogram was performed because the hematoma was not in the anticipated position of a hypertensive hemorrhage. This revealed the arteriovenous malformation.

Illustration continued on the following page

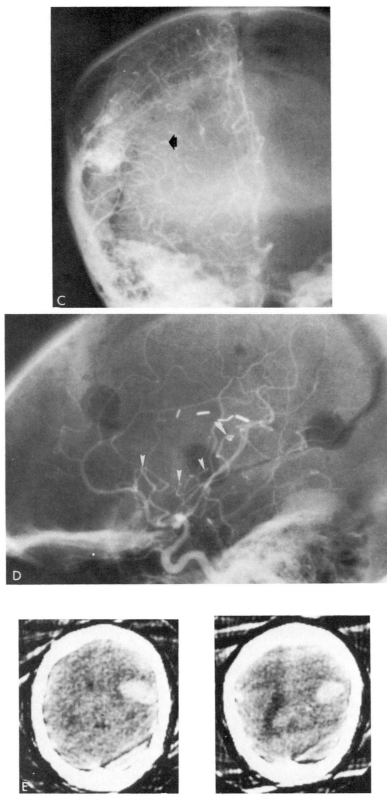

FIGURE 6–24. *See legend on the opposite page.*

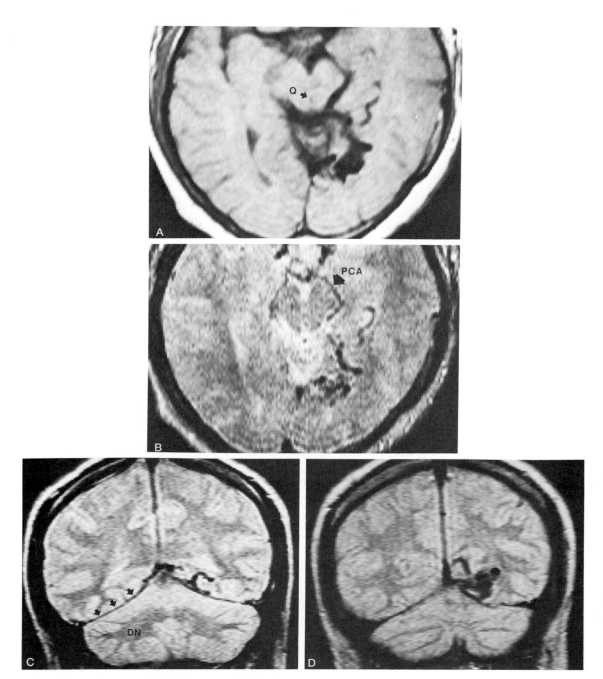

FIGURE 6–25. *MR of Arteriovenous Malformation:* A 42-year-old male with headaches. *A,* Axial SE TR530/ TE30 demonstrates a typical serpiginous area of negative flow defect in the left occipital pole. There is enlargement of the perimesencephalic cistern on the ipsilateral side, probably secondary to focal atrophy. The cerebral aqueduct is well seen (*Q*).

B, SE TR3120/TE120 reveals that the CSF has reached the cross-over point and now has high signal intensity. This allows better visualization of the vessels in the malformation as well as the prominent posterior cerebral artery (*PCA*) on the ipsilateral side as it courses around the midbrain in the perimesencephalic cistern. This vessel is enlarged because it supplies the malformation.

C, Coronal SE TR530/TE30 reveals the malformation as it projects just above the tentorium cerebelli. The tentorium is demonstrated on the contralateral side (*arrows*) as a low signal intensity structure. The tentorium also maintains low signal intensity on the T-2 weighted images. The white matter dentate nucleus is also seen (*DN*).

D, Slightly posteriorly the malformation is better visualized.

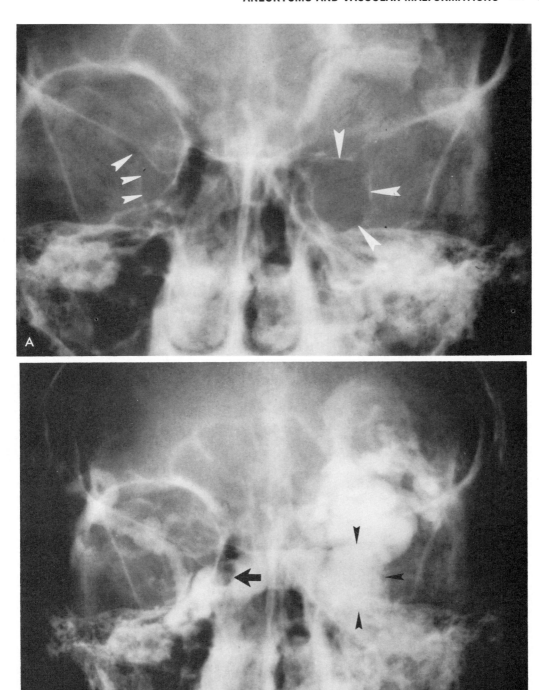

FIGURE 6–26. *Carotid Cavernous Fistula: A*, The plain film reveals marked pressure erosion and enlargement of the superior orbital fissure on the left side. The erosion is secondary to the pressure of the markedly enlarged superior ophthalmic vein (*large white arrows*). The normal superior orbital fissure is demonstrated on the right side (*small arrows*).

B, The left carotid arteriogram reveals the rapid shunting of the blood into the venous system. The markedly enlarged superior ophthalmic vein is marked by the small black arrows. The cavernous sinus is filled and extends in a curvilinear fashion to the opposite side, where the right internal carotid artery is demonstrated (*large black arrow*) as a negative shadow in the contrast-filled cavernous sinus. The right internal carotid artery is visualized because it is filled with unopacified blood.

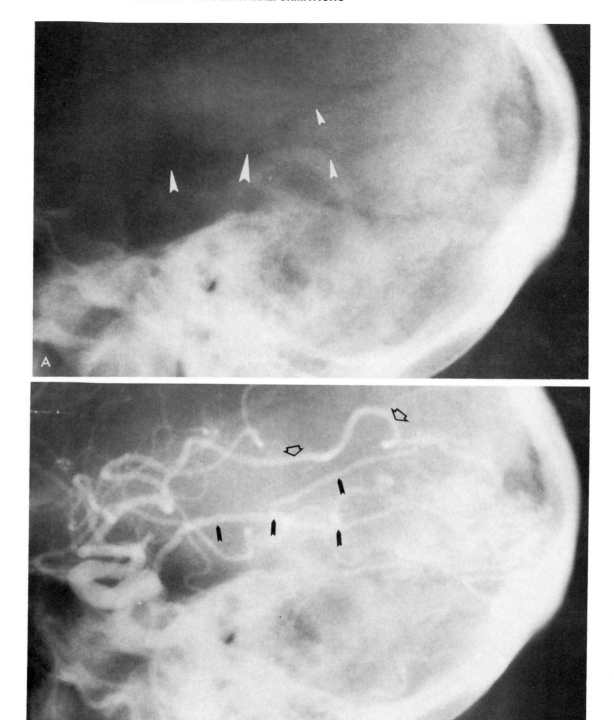

FIGURE 6–27. *Tentorial Arteriovenous Malformation:* *A*, The plain skull films reveal enlarged vascular grooves that carry the enlarged branches of the posterior meningeal artery (*white arrows*) as they course posteriorly to supply the tentorial malformation.

B, The left carotid arteriogram shows the branches of the meningeal artery (*black arrows*) as they lie in the vascular groove noted on the skull film. In addition, an enlarged branch of the left middle cerebral artery (*open arrows*) is also noted to supply the malformation.

Illustration continued on the following page

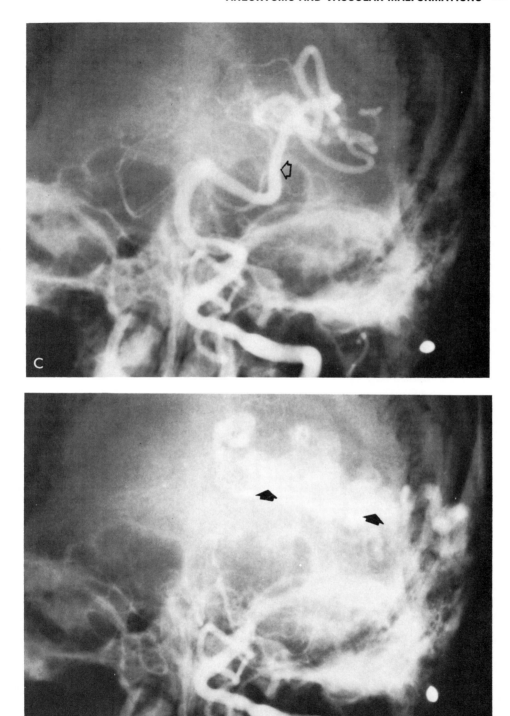

FIGURE 6–27 *Continued.*

C, The left vertebral arteriogram reveals an enlarged left posterior cerebral artery (*open arrow*) that courses posteriorly to supply the malformation.

D, A later arterial film of the left vertebral arteriogram shows a large tangle of vessels resting on top of the tentorium cerebelli and extending from the midline to the region of the sigmoid sinus (*black arrows*).

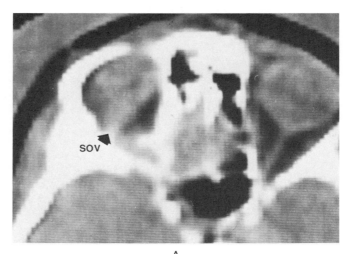

A
Preinfusion

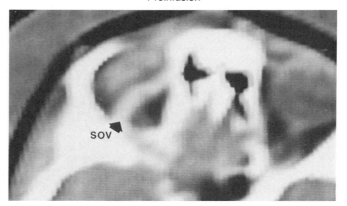

B
Postinfusion

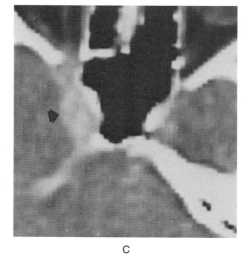

C
Postinfusion

FIGURE 6–28. *See legend on the opposite page.*

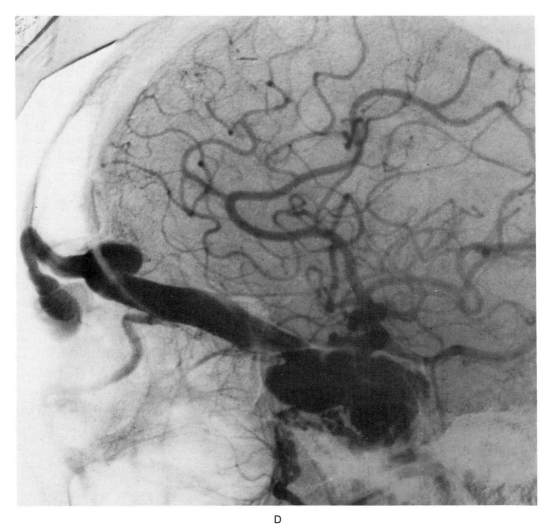

D

FIGURE 6–28. *Carotid Cavernous Fistula:* *A,* Preinfusion CT scan of the orbit reveals dilatation of the superior ophthalmic vein (*SOV*) on the right side.

B, Postinfusion scan shows enhancement of the SOV. There is usually exophthalmos on the side of the fistula, although none was present in this case.

C, The slice through the level of the cavernous sinus reveals that the cavernous sinus is convex laterally (*arrow*). This occurs because the blood flows from the carotid artery to the venous cavernous sinus and results in overfilling of the sinus.

D, The carotid angiogram demonstrates a typical carotid cavernous fistula with retrograde flow into the greatly enlarged superior ophthalmic vein. This is the superior ophthalmic vein that is demonstrated on the CT scan; the cavernous sinus is greatly distended by the direct carotid-venous fistula.

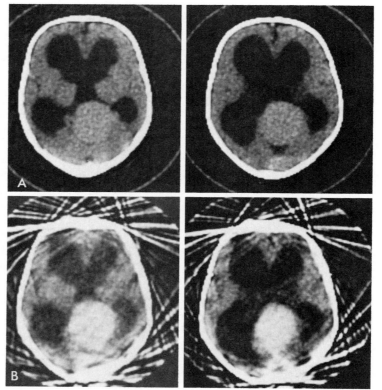

FIGURE 6–29. *Vein of Galen Aneurysm:* *A*, The preinfusion scan reveals a well-defined area of increased density in the midline and extending to the right of the midline. There is moderate obstructive hydrocephalus.

B, The postinfusion scan reveals marked homogeneous enhancement of this area.

C, The right carotid arteriogram demonstrates marked enlargement of the posterior cerebral artery, which communicates directly with the vein of Galen. This is actually an arteriovenous fistula, not a malformation. Note the "jet stream" of contrast material as it enters into the midportion of the vein of Galen. The widened sweep of the pericallosal artery is secondary to the hydrocephalus.

D, The lateral arterial phase reveals better filling of the vein of Galen (*arrow*) and the region of the torcular Herophili, which are densely opacified while the remainder of the vessels are still in the arterial phase.

Illustration continued on the following page

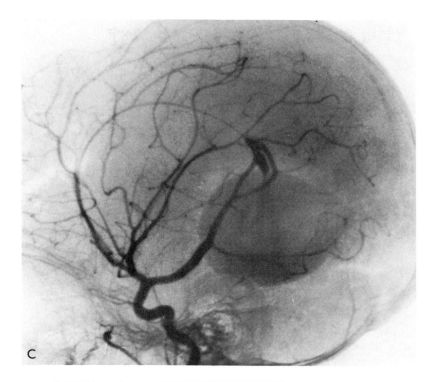

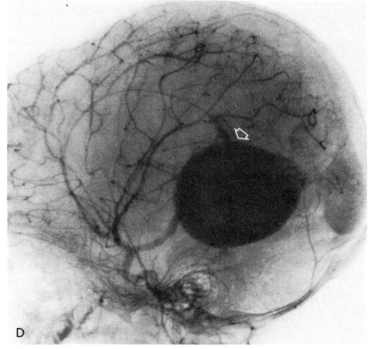

FIGURE 6–29. *See legend on the opposite page.*
Illustration continued on the following page

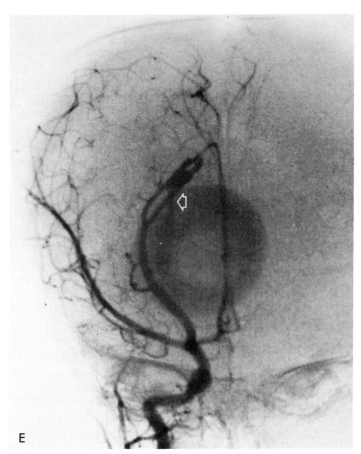

E

FIGURE 6–29 *Continued.*

E, The AP view again demonstrates the fistulous communication between the deformed and enlarged right posterior cerebral artery and the vein of Galen (*arrow*), which is asymmetrically enlarged. The "jet stream" of contrast material is again identified.

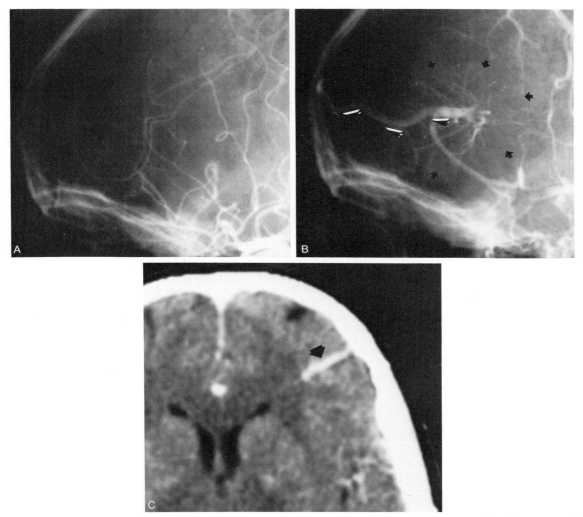

FIGURE 6–30. *Venous Angioma:* A, Postinfusion CT in this patient with headaches reveals a linear area of enhancement extending from deep in the frontal lobe to the cerebral cortex (*arrow*). There is no mass effect. *B* and *C,* Internal carotid angiography reveals that the arterial phase of the study appears normal (*B*) while the venous phase (*C*) reveals a "sunburst" appearance of multiple small veins (*small arrows*) that coalesce into one large vein (*black and white arrows*) that drains superficially. This appearance is very typical of venous angioma.

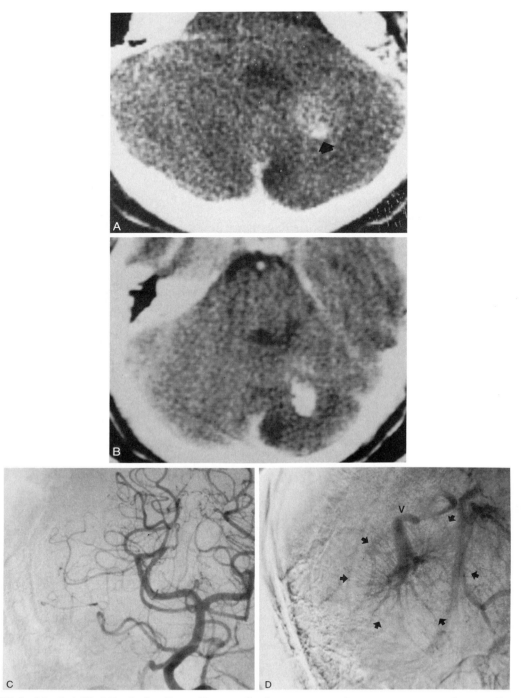

FIGURE 6–31. *Calcified Posterior Fossa Venous Angioma: A,* Preinfusion CT scan reveals a small area of calcification deep in the cerebellar hemisphere (*arrow*) with a larger area of increased density anterior to that. There is no mass effect upon the fourth ventricle.

B, The postinfusion CT scan reveals dense enhancement of the posterior portion of the lesion.

C, Subtraction view of the arterial phase of the vertebral angiogram is normal.

D, The venous phase of the angiogram reveals that multiple tiny veins in a "sunburst" pattern (*arrows*) coalesce to form one large draining vein—the area of enhancement identified by CT. The CT and angiographic appearance are typical of a venous angioma.

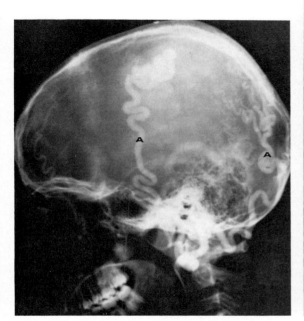 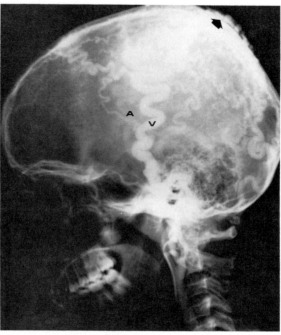

FIGURE 6–32. *Scalp Arteriovenous Malformation:* This patient has a giant scalp arteriovenous malformation that developed following scalp trauma. The selective external carotid arteriogram reveals giant superficial temporal and occipital branches of the external carotid artery (*A*) that supply a large arteriovenous malformation drained by innumerable enlarged draining veins (*V*). The tangential view (*arrow*) reveals that all these vessels lie in the scalp. A similar appearance was seen with arteriography of the opposite external carotid artery.

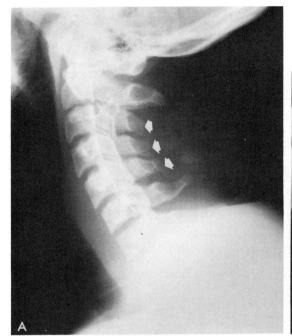
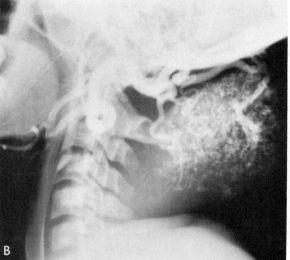
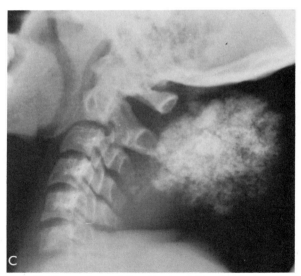

FIGURE 6–33. *Arteriovenous Malformation of the Back of the Neck:* *A,* The lateral view of the cervical spine reveals erosion of the spinous processes of C_3 through C_5 secondary to pressure erosion.

B, Carotid arteriography demonstrates marked enlargement of the common carotid artery and an enlarged occipital branch that supplies the malformation.

C, A later arterial phase shows the large stain of the malformation. Arteriography of the opposite carotid revealed a similar pattern. A portion of the blood supply also arose from the vertebral arteries and from the thyrocervical trunk.

7

DEGENERATIVE, METABOLIC, AND INFLAMMATORY DISEASES

The development of computed tomography provided the neuroradiologist with the opportunity to play a major role in the diagnosis of degenerative and inflammatory disorders of the nervous system. More recently magnetic resonance has been added to our diagnostic armamentarium and has added an even broader dimension to our ability to diagnose degenerative diseases of the brain. The accuracy and noninvasive nature of these tests have greatly aided our work-up of patients with a number of disease processes. It is usually the case that CT or MR will provide the diagnosis in the evaluation of these various diseases. One of the great advantages is not only the ability to make the diagnosis, but also the ability to rule out other diseases or processes, such as a mass lesion, that may mimic the clinical presentation. Because treatment is based upon correct diagnosis, the greater accuracy with which one can now diagnose various diseases has greatly aided our approach to treatment. Following appropriate treatment, CT and MR allow easy and readily reproducible examinations to evaluate the effect of various forms of treatment.

The following is a list of selected disease processes that can be readily evaluated by CT and/or MR:

1. Atrophy

    a. supratentorial   b. infratentorial

2. Subcortical atherosclerotic encephalopathy

3. Multiple sclerosis

4. Metabolic diseases

5. Radiation necrosis

6. Benign postoperative enhancement

7. Carbon monoxide poisoning

8. Cerebral anoxia secondary to respiratory arrest

9. Progressive multifocal leukoencephalopathy

10. Methotrexate leukoencephalopathy

11. Cerebral necrosis secondary to perinatal anoxia

12. Amphetamine toxicity

13. Miscellaneous

Computed tomography and magnetic resonance provide us with more information than was previously available using other diagnostic methods, at the same time causing far less discomfort for the patient. Indeed, a number of abnormalities are easily diagnosed by CT and MR which cannot be evaluated by other methods.

DEGENERATIVE DISEASES ASSOCIATED WITH AN APPEARANCE OF ATROPHY

Alzheimer's Disease. Senile dementia of the Alzheimer type is defined as the gradual onset and progression of intellectual deterioration without a history of cerebrovascular accident or major focal neurologic deficit. Studies have shown that although there is an increase in the amount of atrophy in those patients with dementia, there is sufficient cross-over with the normal population that the diagnosis cannot be made on CT findings alone. Histopathologic studies reveal an excessive number of senile plaques and neurofibrillary tangles.

Parkinson's Disease. The cause is unknown and there are no specific CT findings. The disease itself is considered to be a disorder of the dopaminergic system.

Huntington's Disease. Originally described in 1872 by Dr. George Huntington, it has an autosomal dominant mode of inheritance with uniformity of clinical expression. The disease is usually undetected until the fourth, fifth, or sixth decade. Classically, there is a typical atrophic process involving the head of the caudate nucleus bilaterally. This atrophy can be detected with both CT and MR, but because of cross-over with the normal population an absolute diagnosis cannot be made. Diffuse cerebral atrophy is also present (Fig. 7–1, p. 322).

Olivopontocerebellar Atrophy

There are a large number of degenerative disorders that affect the pons, spinal cord, and cerebellum. This is a complex group of disorders involving various portions of the posterior fossa structures. These atrophic patterns may be focal or diffuse. These diseases include focal cerebellar atrophy that may be seen with familial cerebello-olivary atrophy, cortical cerebellar atrophy, and alcoholic cerebellar atrophy. There may also be diffuse cerebellar atrophy such as is seen with paraneoplastic cerebellar atrophy and congenital atrophy of the granular layer of the cerebellum. The case illustrated in Figure 7–2 (p. 323) demonstrates the appearance of olivopontocerebellar atrophy. This process may be sporadic or familial and is characterized by the involvement of the fibers of pontine and olivary origin. Pathologically there is atrophy of the inferior olives, atrophy of the basis pontis, and cerebellar atrophy. While these changes are characteristic, there is also involvement of the basal ganglia, dentate nuclei, and spinal cord.

CT of olivopontocerebellar atrophy (OPC atrophy) reveals enlargement of the cerebellar folia, cerebellopontine angle cisterns, prepontine cistern, and fourth ventricle. All of these changes reflect the atrophy of the posterior fossa structures and resulting loss of bulk of the various structures in the posterior fossa. It is not unusual for patients with OPC atrophy to carry the clinical diagnosis of Parkinson's disease for many years before the true diagnosis is made. If this diagnosis is entertained then, the CT scan should be performed with thin slices of the posterior fossa, such as 4-mm slices. The entire posterior fossa, including the region of the foramen magnum and the upper spinal cord, should be evaluated. With 4-mm thick slices, reconstruction views can also be obtained in the sagittal view, which facilitates the evaluation of the posterior fossa structures.

Magnetic resonance now provides the ideal tool for evaluation of the posterior fossa. The capability of direct sagittal images provides excellent evaluation of the posterior fossa structures. The exact relationship between the various structures and their surroundings is readily evaluated, and the absence of bone artifact makes MR far superior to CT. The sizes of the pons, medulla, fourth ventricle, superior cerebellar cistern, and vermis are all easily appreciated. The axial and coronal projections image the basilar cisterns to best advantage, and other types of abnormalities such as mass lesions are readily ruled out. Of course, there is no discomfort for the patient, no ionizing radiation, and no need for the injection of contrast material. While Parkinson's disease or some other type of movement disorder cannot be ruled in or out with certainty, the marked atrophic appearance of the posterior fossa structures strongly favors diagnosis of a degenerative disorder of the posterior fossa structure. MR is the procedure of choice for the evaluation of posterior fossa diseases in general and degenerative diseases in particular.

Creutzfeldt-Jakob Disease. Thought to be a familial hereditary disease of as yet undetermined etiology, it is grouped with kuru in humans, and scrapie, an infection of sheep. These diseases appear to have a "slow virus" as an etiologic agent, although dysmetabolic, degenerative, and circulatory causes have not been ruled out. CT scans demonstrate rapid progression of atrophy.

Other Causes of Cerebral Atrophy

The following are additional possible causes of cerebral atrophy:

1. Chronic alcohol abuse
2. Chronic drug abuse
3. Renal failure
4. Heart disease, especially with multiple surgeries
5. AIDS (acquired immunodeficiency syndrome)
6. Anorexia nervosa
7. Late effects of craniocerebral trauma

Chronic Alcohol Abuse. In addition to diffuse atrophy with accentuation of posterior fossa atrophy, alcoholic patients also frequently demonstrate bifrontal, wedge-shaped areas of lucency secondary to post-traumatic encephalomalacia. These post-traumatic areas follow hematoma formation or contusion resulting from repeated falls and head trauma.

AIDS. The acquired immunodeficiency syndrome is a recently recognized disease that is caused by deficiency in cell-mediated immunity, predisposing the individual to opportunistic infectious and unusual malignancies such as Kaposi's sarcoma. The vast majority of cases are in homosexual men. AIDS is caused by the human T-cell lymphotrophic virus type III (HTLV-III), and there is, as yet, no known cure.

In addition to atrophy, patients may develop cerebral infections with such opportunistic organisms as cytomegalovirus or *Toxoplasma*, or may develop microglioma of the brain (Fig. 7–3, p. 324).

Other Degenerative Diseases

Binswanger's Disease. Subcortical arteriosclerotic encephalopathy, or Binswanger's disease, is seen in patients with known hypertension and is thought to be secondary to loss of white matter and gliosis secondary to arteriosclerotic changes involving the small penetrating blood vessels of the brain.

CT demonstrates bilateral areas of lucency in a periventricular distribution that extends into the white matter of the centrum semiovale.

Magnetic resonance is an ideal method of evaluating this entity and demonstrates bilateral increased signal intensity on the T-2 weighted, SE TR3120/TE120 scans. This abnormal area of low density on CT and increased signal intensity on MR is often in a typical bat-wing distribution. MR is more sensitive than CT to these changes. The elderly population may also demonstrate areas of periventricular increased signal intensity that appears to be part of the normal aging process (Fig. 7–4, p. 325).

Multiple Sclerosis

Multiple sclerosis (MS) is the most frequent of the demyelinating diseases. It selectively affects the myelin of the central nervous system but relatively spares the axis cylinders. In this disease the myelin is apparently normally formed but breaks down later in life. The age of onset is between 10 and 50 years, and males and females are about equally affected. The diagnosis is frequently made by the exclusion of other possibilities; in fact, such entities as spinal cord neurofibromas and meningiomas and posterior fossa tumors such as tentorial and foramen magnum meningiomas may mimic the clinical presentation of multiple sclerosis.

This disease is of unknown etiology but is typified by the clinical presentation of neurologic symptoms that are separated by "space and time." In other words, neurologic symptoms arise from varying anatomic locations and occur at different points in time. Permanent neurologic deficit may result. Rather than the typical course of exacerbations and remissions, the disease may follow a steadily progressive course. The cerebrospinal fluid is abnormal in many but not all cases. CSF protein electrophoresis demonstrates an increase in oligoclonal bands; in addition, IgG antibodies directed against myelin basic protein may be found in the CSF of MS patients who have active disease. Sensitivity to basic protein as the etiology of MS remains unproved. Although these theories are attractive, they do not appear to account for the "cause" of MS, and the search for a specific virus or other agent continues.

For a diagnosis of multiple sclerosis, the following six criteria are widely accepted: (1) The results of neurologic examination must be abnormal. (2) There must be evidence that at least two separate parts of the nervous system are involved. (3) Disease of the white matter, i.e., fiber tract damage, must predominate. (4) There must be two or more episodes of worsening separated by one month or more, or else slow or stepwise progression over at least six months. (5) The age at onset is between 10 and 50 years. (6) No other condition can explain the disease process (in other words, rule out other lesions).

Histopathologic examination reveals diffuse dissemination of the plaques throughout the neuroaxis; however, there are a number of preferential locations of involvement and it is common to find the areas of demyelination in a periventricular distribution more prominent in the periatrial region. There is a definite tendency to involve the optic pathways; thus, visual symptoms are a common clinical presentation. The reason for this remains unknown. Both CT and MR evaluation of the optic nerves to identify areas of demyelination have thus far proved unsatisfactory.

Computed Tomography. One of the greatest advantages of the development of CT is that one can so readily rule out the presence of a mass lesion in a patient with MS. On the other hand, the CT scan is often normal in patients with MS. Abnormal CT appearances of MS are:

COMMON

- Enlarged ventricles
- Enlarged cortical sulci
- Combination of enlarged cortical sulci and ventricles
- Areas of periventricular lucency
- Periventricular areas of enhancement

UNCOMMON

- Areas of lucency remote from the periventricular distribution
- Areas of cystic change remote from the ventricles
- Areas of parenchymal as well as periventricular enhancement
- Space-occupying areas of enhancement

There is commonly an appearance of atrophy on the CT scan. It should be noted that this appearance might be considered normal for an older individual, so the degree of atrophy must be correlated with the patient's age. Areas of periventricular lucency correspond to the typical plaques of demyelination and are the next most common abnormality noted. They may be isolated or extensive and extend along the entire periventricular region bilaterally.

Following the infusion of contrast material there may be enhancement of these periventricular plaques, thought to correspond to the acute phase of demyelination. Studies have shown that these plaques may not show enhancement with the standard infusion of 40 grams of iodine but may very occasionally demonstrate enhancement after the intravenous infusion of twice the normal dose of contrast material. These plaques are typically non–space-occupying.

Rarely the areas of lucency may be in a location remote from the typical periventricular distribution. This typical distribution may suggest another diagnosis such as multiple infarcts, areas of cerebritis or abscess formation, or metastases; however, the clinical presentation and laboratory results will confirm the diagnosis. These remote areas of lucency are not uncom-

monly associated with the typical periventricular areas of lucency which make the diagnosis of MS more secure. These scattered remote areas of lucency may or may not enhance with contrast material. Very rarely, there may be cystic-appearing areas of demyelination in a random distribution. These areas usually enhance and are seen in association with fulminant MS. The appearance does mimic multiple abscess. At times, these areas can be minimally space-occupying.

Magnetic Resonance. MR is the procedure of choice for the diagnosis of multiple sclerosis. While even with known, laboratory-proved MS, the MR scan may be normal, at the same time it is not uncommon for the magnetic resonance scan to demonstrate the typical plaques of MS which cannot be identified by any other method. In those cases in which an abnormal area of signal intensity is not identified, the anatomic location of the abnormality is presumably in the brain stem or spinal cord. Plaques can be demonstrated in these areas but are more difficult to demonstrate than in the supratentorial region.

Obviously, the presence of a tumor is ruled out by a normal MR scan. It appears that MR is the procedure of choice as a screening examination in patients with possible or known MS or with any other white matter disease.

Because multiple sclerosis can mimic the presence of a brain tumor, the addition of CT to our diagnostic armamentarium revolutionized our approach to the evaluation of patients with both multiple sclerosis and a suspected brain tumor. In patients with multiple sclerosis it is not uncommon that the CT scan is normal or demonstrates only the presence of cerebral atrophy. This type of "negative" information is very helpful because it does rule out the presence of a brain tumor as the cause of the patient's symptoms. Therefore, one can be more confident that the clinical diagnosis is multiple sclerosis and treatment is begun accordingly. Corroborative laboratory evidence of oligoclonal bands of protein identified with protein electrophoresis of cerebrospinal fluid and neurologic symptoms that are separated in "space and time" also make the diagnosis more secure.

Magnetic resonance demonstrates areas of increased signal intensity in the areas of demyelination, and it is not uncommon that the MR scan is abnormal even when the CT scan is normal. In the author's experience, these abnormal areas of increased signal intensity are best demonstrated using the T-2 weighted images. Some authors have reported that the inversion recovery sequence is the best sequence for demonstration of these abnormal areas; this has not been the author's experience. It appears that the most satisfactory approach to evaluation is to perform the T-2 weighted SE sequence using TR3120/TE60-120. This allows one echo that is to the left (TR3120/TE60) of the cross-over point* of CSF and one echo that is to the right (TR3120/TE120) of the cross-over point. In some patients, the first echo is the more satisfactory, while in others the second echo is the more satisfactory in terms of demonstrating the abnormalities.

If only one echo is possible, then the SE TR3120/TE120 sequence is the better study. In the majority of cases, the examination need be performed only in the axial plane, but if this is normal, additional studies should be performed in the coronal plane. The plaques of MS may be situated just adjacent to the atrium of the lateral ventricles and so be very poorly or not at all demonstrated on the axial scans, but be readily visible on the coronal scans where the periventricular area "stands away" from the lateral ventricle. The partial volume effect also interferes with demonstration of the plaques in the axial plane. The use of multiplanar imaging is also helpful in evaluation of suspected brain tumor because the temporal lobes are best visualized in the coronal images.

The development and availability of MR scanning should aid in the follow-up of patients with multiple sclerosis and similarly allow easy and accurate evaluation of response to treatment (Figs. 7–5 to 7–8, pp. 326 to 330).

Lupus Cerebritis

During the course of examination of patients with lupus, there does appear to be a difference between the appearance of MS and that of lupus cerebritis. In the patients with lupus cerebritis, the areas of increased signal intensity appear to be more laterally placed than the plaques of demyelination seen in multiple sclerosis. The areas of increased signal intensity seen with lupus cerebritis are thought to be secondary to a vasculitis that has resulted in multiple tiny areas of infarction. The positions of the areas of increased signal intensity in lupus cerebritis are only a few millimeters different in location, and it is really premature to predict if MR will be conclusive in differentiating between these two entities. However, since treatment will differ, lupus should be suggested if it is a diagnostic possibility. These abnormal areas of increased

signal intensity in patients with lupus cerebritis may be visualized on the MR scans even when the CT scans are normal.

Schilder's Disease

This might be considered "pediatric multiple sclerosis," as the disease is similar to MS but is characterized by the early age of onset. The disease is usually characterized by a progressive course, although the patients may exhibit the classic intermittent course of multiple sclerosis.

In the rapidly progressive cases, the disease may mimic a mass lesion. There may be headaches, aphasia, cortical blindness, and deafness. Typically this disease affects the posterior part of the cerebral hemispheres. The CT scan demonstrates irregular areas of lucency in the areas of demyelination.

METABOLIC DISEASES

There are a large number of diseases of the brain which may be classified as metabolic. These diseases occur mainly in children and have been divided by Kendall into two groups. One group of diseases is diagnosed by biochemical methods while the second is diagnosed by histologic methods:

BIOCHEMICAL DIAGNOSIS

Mucopolysaccharidoses
Mucolipidoses
GM gangliosidosis
Metachromatic leukodystrophy
Krabbe's leukodystrophy
Adrenoleukodystrophy
Phenylketonuria
Maple syrup urine disease
Homocystinuria
Ornithine transcarbamoylase deficiency
α-Ketoglutaric acidemia
Lowe's syndrome
Methylmalonic acidemia
Propionic acidemia
Menkes' disease
Wilson's disease
Menkes' variant
Glycogen storage disease
Pyridoxine-dependent epilepsy
Transcobalamin II deficiency

HISTOLOGIC DIAGNOSIS

Spongiform degeneration
Alexander's disease
Sjögren-Larsson syndrome
Batten's disease
Niemann-Pick disease

---

*See Figure 3–26.

Leigh's encephalomyelopathy
Congenital muscular dystrophy
Other muscular dystrophies
Mitochondrial cytopathy
Carnitine deficiency
Reye's syndrome
Cornelia de Lange's syndrome
Cockayne's syndrome
Lipoid proteinosis

Wilson's Disease. This is a disease of hepatolenticular degeneration with an autosomal recessive mode of inheritance. In childhood, the disease tends to be rapidly progressive. Onset in adulthood is insidious in the second or third decade. There is deteriorating handwriting, speech difficulty, tremor at rest, difficulty performing purposeful movements, rigidity, and mental deterioration. Serum ceruloplasmin is decreased and total serum copper increased, and physical examination reveals a characteristic Kayser-Fleischer ring in the cornea.

CT demonstrates low-density areas in the putamen, globus pallidus, head of the caudate, and dentate nucleus. MR demonstrates increased signal intensity areas on the T-2 weighted images in the low-density areas seen on CT. There is also diffuse supra- and infratentorial atrophy.

Adrenoleukodystrophy. Adrenoleukodystrophy (ALD) is a hereditary neurologic disorder characterized by rapidly progressing degeneration of the cerebral white matter in association with adrenal insufficiency. There is a sex-linked recessive mode of inheritance, and the disease is seen most commonly in young boys, in whom it is associated with cortical blindness.

ALD is a dysmyelinating disease characterized by widespread dysmyelination of the cerebral white matter. CT demonstrates periventricular low density of the white matter. This has been typically described as affecting the occipital areas and then progressing forward. The author's experiences suggest that these changes are more prominent in the frontal regions. The low-density areas soon resolve, and an appearance of severe atrophy is seen late in the disease.

MR of ALD is probably the diagnostic test of choice. The increased sensitivity of MR to demyelinating disease allows ready detection of abnormal areas. These appear as areas of increased signal intensity on the T-2 weighted images in the areas of low density on the CT scan. MR also has the advantage of not requiring ionizing radiation or the injection of contrast material (Fig. 7–9, p. 331).

Metachromatic Leukodystrophy. This is a metabolic disorder due to a deficiency of the enzyme arylsulfatase A which results in the accumulation of cerebroside sulfate in the neurons, glial cells, and myelin as well as the Schwann cells of peripheral nerves. These granules stain brown rather than blue with acidified cresyl violet, thiozine, or toluidine blue—hence the name metachromatic leukodystrophy. CT demonstrates symmetrical, deep white matter of low density. The end result is diffuse atrophy.

Methylmalonic and Propionic Acidemia. These are inherited disorders of amino acid metabolism, specifically vitamin B_{12} metabolism. The children usually present with unexplained ketoacidosis, failure to thrive, protein intolerance, and early demise. CT demonstrates mild to moderate leukoencephalopathy with low-density areas in the white matter. The end stage has an appearance of diffuse atrophy.

Alexander's Disease. This is macrocephalic leukodystrophy of unknown etiology. There is a paucity of myelin in those areas that myelinate relatively late. CT demonstrates bifrontal, low-density areas that involve the caudate and lentiform nuclei. There is ventricular enlargement that is most marked frontally.

Krabbe's Disease. Also known as globoid cell leukodystrophy, this disease is due to a deficiency of galactocerebroside beta-galactosidase. It is a fatal autosomal recessive disorder of infants. There is widespread demyelination, and the hallmark is the accumulation of large multinuclear globoid cells that contain tubular cytoplasmic inclusions. CT typically reveals bilateral, paratrigonal, low-density areas. The late change is diffuse atrophy. There is no treatment.

Radiation Necrosis

Radiation necrosis of the central nervous system occurs if radiation treatment exceeds approximately 6000 to 7000 rads fractionated at 200 or more rads per treatment. There is usually a delay of nine months or longer following treatment before radiation necrosis occurs. Although possible, it is uncommon for radiation necrosis to occur in the bed of a glioblastoma; rather its occurrence is much more likely following treatment for a tumor such as a pituitary adenoma. In this latter case, there is the opportunity for long survival and the possibility of radiation necrosis in the temporal lobes, which are, of necessity, included in the treatment port.

CT reveals an area or areas of lucency which may or may not be space-occupying and may or may not demonstrate enhancement on the postinfusion portion of the study. There is no specific pattern of enhancement, and differentiation from tumor may be impossible without biopsy.

MR in one pathologically proven case demonstrates an area of increased signal intensity in the area of involvement on the T-2 weighted (TR3120/TE120) SE images. MR will probably prove to be more sensitive than CT; however, the specificity remains to be determined (Figs. 7–10 to 7–12, pp. 332 to 333).

Carbon Monoxide Poisoning

Carbon monoxide poisoning is typically seen in patients who have attempted suicide. Classically, there is necrosis of the globus pallidus, resulting in areas of lucency in the globus pallidus bilaterally on CT examination.

Histopathologically, there are areas of white matter necrosis in addition to involvement of the globus pallidus. Diffuse demyelination may also occur (Fig. 7–13, p. 334).

Methotrexate Leukoencephalopathy

Certain chemotherapeutic agents used intrathecally, especially methotrexate, have been implicated in the development of a leukoencephalopathy. Methotrexate is often combined with cranial irradiation and/or systemic chemotherapy for the treatment of CNS leukemia or as a prophylactic treatment. Toxicity may develop, resulting in encephalopathy with confusion and forgetfulness, progressing to dementia, seizures, spasticity, and ultimately death.

CT demonstrates areas of lucency secondary to white matter necrosis which are typically bifrontal in location. Early there may or may not be enhancement; late in the course of the disease there is an appearance of atrophy (Fig. 7–14, p. 334).

Progressive Multifocal Leukoencephalopathy

PML is a virus-induced, rapidly fatal disease of the white matter which results in multiple areas of demyelination. The virus resembles the papovavirus, which is a variant of the polyoma simian virus 40 subgroup. It is typically seen in patients with chronic lymphoproliferative diseases and in those receiving immunosuppressive therapy. CT demonstrates scattered areas of lucency in the white matter which may enhance. The index of suspicion for this disorder must be high; differentiation from multiple metastases may be difficult (Fig. 7–15, p. 335).

Benign Postoperative Enhancement

Following surgery, there may be areas of enhancement in the bed of the surgical site, even in the absence of tumor, such as that seen with surgery for seizures. Benign postoperative enhancement can also be seen following needle biopsy.

Perinatal Anoxia

In premature infants, intraventricular or subependymal hemorrhages from terminal veins are commonly associated with severe asphyxia. These changes are readily identified on the CT scan.

In addition, with perinatal anoxia there may also be extensive neuronal necrosis, a finding reflected on the CT scan as multiple areas of radiolucency resembling infarcts. Clinically, these patients may have an enlarging head size and bulging fontanelle, while the CT scan demonstrates varying degrees of abnormality. There may be small to massive areas of lucency, with only small amounts of normal-density brain and compressed lateral ventricles remaining. Not uncommonly, on the CT scan the posterior fossa structures appear to have been spared, and pathologic examination confirms the relative sparing of the cerebellum.

If the infant survives, the appearance on the CT scan following intervals of months to years is that of diffuse cerebral atrophy (Fig. 7–16, p. 336).

Respiratory Arrest with Cerebral Anoxia

A variety of changes can occur with circulatory arrest and cerebral anoxia. The late changes demonstrate necrotic foci with cavities or glial scars. These especially affect Ammon's horn and, in the basal ganglia, the globus pallidus. The white matter is better preserved (Fig. 7–17, p. 337).

Amphetamine Toxicity

Drug abuse, particularly the intravenous use of amphetamines, has been shown with angiography to create an appearance of intracerebral vascular spasm. The pathophysiology of this change is not precisely understood (Fig. 7–18, p. 338).

INFLAMMATORY DISEASES

Brain Abscess. The clinical presentation of a patient with a brain abscess is a febrile course followed by neurologic signs. Brain abscesses are commonly associated with other inflammatory processes such as middle ear infections, mastoid infections, and sinus infections, where they develop because of direct spread. Brain abscesses may also be seen in association with pneumonia, in which the hematogenous spread of bacteria results in multiple abscesses identified at the gray/white matter junction. Intravenous drug abuse is a common cause of brain abscess and is also associated with acute or subacute bacterial endocarditis, another cause of brain abscess.

Central nervous system infections are also seen in immunocompromised hosts. This patient population is represented by those on chemotherapy for cancer, organ transplant recipients, those on chronic steroid therapy for other reasons, and more recently those with acquired immunodeficiency syndrome. While in the nonimmunocompromised patient the abscess progresses through the stage of cerebritis followed by capsule formation, in the immunocompromised patient this inflammatory process is less well-localized. It is also common for these immunocompromised patients to develop infections with opportunistic organisms such as cytomegalovirus, *Toxoplasma, Aspergillus, Candida,* and even *Herpesvirus hominis* (herpes zoster).

The CT appearance of an abscess may mimic that of a primary or secondary brain tumor, and so this should also be included in the differential diagnosis. The typical appearance of an abscess is that of an isodense or higher than normal brain density ring on the preinfusion CT scan, with surrounding edema and usually a dense, thick-walled ring of enhancement on the postinfusion portion of the examination. There is usually a low-density central portion of the abscess. Multiple abscesses have a similar appearance, although solid, rounded areas of enhancement may also be seen. Again, the differentiation from multiple metastases may be difficult. Not all brain abscess patients experience a febrile course. It has been this author's experience that patients whose brain abscess is unsuspected until surgery for the tentative diagnosis of brain tumor often have a history of a recent dental visit. This dental work apparently causes a sufficient shower of septic emboli that brain abscess results. This history is usually not volunteered by the patient; therefore if abscess is a diagnostic possibility, the appropriate history should be sought (Figs. 7–19 to 7–21, pp. 339 to 340).

During the early cerebritis stage, and prior to encapsulation, there is central enhancement that becomes less prominent as the capsule forms. In both the cerebritis and abscess stages, there is usually surrounding edema. The author has had the opportunity to use MR to study one patient with multiple abscesses. In this patient the areas of abscess formation appeared as both cystic and solid areas of increased signal intensity on the T-2 weighted images. Areas of edema appear as areas of increased signal intensity surrounding the abscess on the T-2 weighted images (Fig. 7–21, p. 340).

Herpes Simplex Encephalitis. The herpes simplex Type I virus is associated with a rapidly progressive and often fatal encephalitis. Typically, there is involvement of the temporal lobes, although there are commonly additional areas of involvement. Treatment with adenine arabinoside (ARA-A) must be started early in the course of the illness if it is to be effective. Biopsy is usually necessary to confirm the diagnosis and shows intranuclear inclusion bodies with light microscopy and intranuclear viral particles with electron microscopy.

The index of suspicion for this illness must be high so that biopsy can be performed and treatment instituted early in the course of the illness.

CT scan demonstrates areas of lucency in affected regions, usually the temporal lobes. Early in the course of the illness the CT may show only minor changes in density and so careful evaluation is mandatory. There may or may not be mass effect early in the illness, but it is not uncommon that there is a dramatic progression of the CT changes even within a 24-hour period of time. Therefore serial scanning is helpful for diagnosis. There is usually a progressive increase in the size of the low-density area as well as an increase in the mass effect (Fig. 7–22, p. 341).

There may or may not be enhancement of the areas of involvement on the postinfusion portion of the scan. Hemorrhage into the affected area has been reported.

The author has had the opportunity to study (postmortem) with MR one patient with herpes encephalitis (Fig. 7–23, p. 342). The MR scan demonstrated bitemporal involvement with increased signal intensity on the T-2 weighted images in areas of low density demonstrated on the CT scan. Because of its increased sensitivity, and because early diagnosis is essential so that effective treatment can be instituted, MR is probably the procedure of choice. The area of greatest involvement can then be identified and biopsy performed.

Tuberculous Meningitis

Tuberculous meningitis is classically a process that primarily affects the basilar meninges and results in thickening of the meninges with an exudate of lymphocytes and mononuclear cells and tubercles. There are areas of central caseous necrosis, and acid-fast bacilli may be demonstrated in these tubercles. There may be an occlusive endarteritis, and cerebral angiography demonstrates spasm of the blood vessels at the base of the brain (Fig. 7–24, p. 343). The basilar meningitis may cause occlusion of the cisterns and the fourth ventricle and result in ventricular dilation.

If the pachymeningitis extends up over the convexity of the brain, postinfusion CT scan may demonstrate enhancement of the meninges similar to that seen at the base of the brain. However, there is nothing unique about tuberculous meningitis that would differentiate it from a bacterial meningitis. Calcified tuberculomas may also form in the basilar cisterns or in the cerebral parenchyma (Fig. 7–25, p. 344).

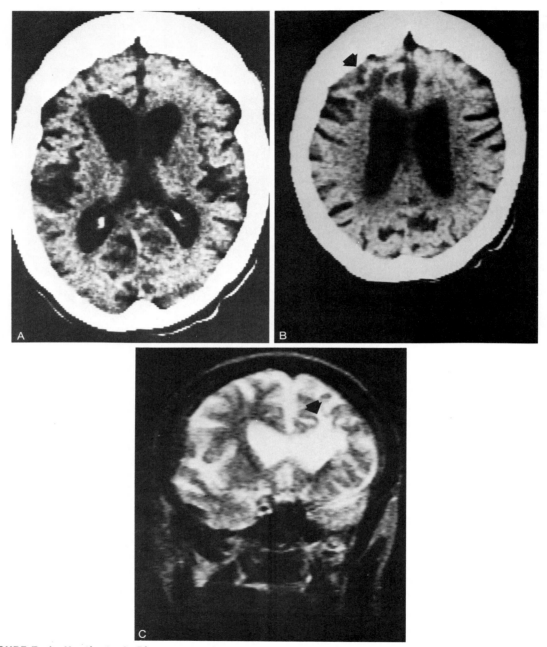

FIGURE 7–1. *Huntington's Disease:* *A* and *B*, CT scans demonstrate diffuse cerebral atrophy in this patient with enlargement of the ventricles and cortical sulci. There is accentuation of the atrophy in the region of the head of the caudate nucleus bilaterally. This caudate atrophy has long been associated with Huntington's disease and has been described as a typical finding; there is, however, cross-over with the normal population so that a diagnosis of Huntington's disease cannot be made with certainty on the basis of the CT scan. Incidentally noted in *B* is an old infarct deep in the frontal lobe (*arrow*).

C, The MR scan using the T-2 weighted SE TR3120/TE120 technique in the coronal plane demonstrates the prominence of the frontal horns of the lateral ventricles secondary to the caudate atrophy. The old frontal infarct is also noted (*arrow*) and is associated with mild focal atrophy of the adjacent frontal horn.

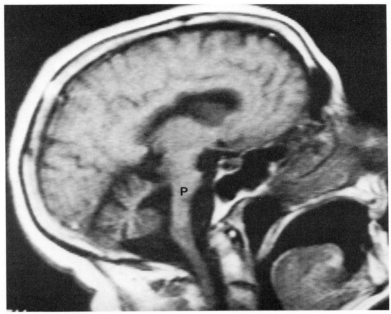

FIGURE 7–2. *Olivopontocerebellar Degeneration:* MR in the midsagittal plane, using the SE TR530/TE30 technique, reveals marked atrophy of the pons (P), medulla, and upper cervical spinal cord. There is also marked cerebellar atrophy with enlargement of the fourth ventricle and shrinkage of the vermis of the cerebellum. Because of the atrophy of the pons there is marked enlargement of the prepontine cistern. Although not well demonstrated, there is also diffuse supratentorial atrophy as well.

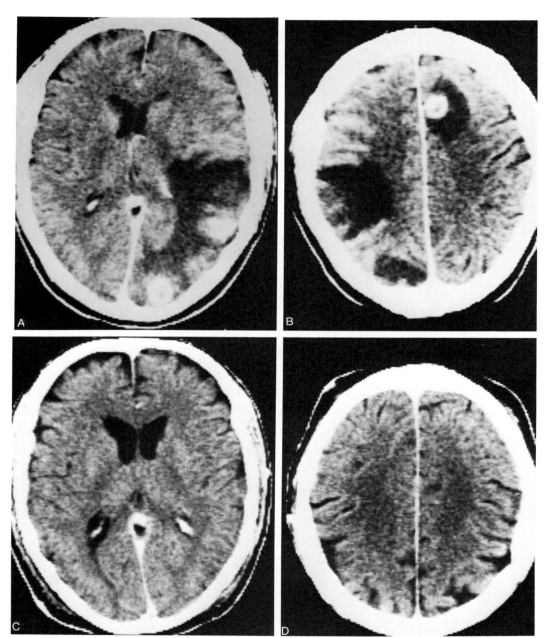

FIGURE 7–3. *Acquired Immunodeficiency Syndrome and Toxoplasmosis:* 35-year-old male with AIDS and toxoplasmosis involvement of the brain. *A* and *B*, Postinfusion CT scan reveals multiple bilateral rounded, both solid and ring-shaped, areas of enhancement with marked surrounding edema. The mass effect was greater on the left side than on the right side, and there is forward displacement of the choroid plexus calcification and shift of the midline structures to the contralateral side. The appearance is not specific for brain abscess, and the diagnosis of toxoplasmosis was proved with brain biopsy. Multiple metastatic deposits could also have this appearance.

C and *D*, After treatment with sulfadiazine and pyrimethamine with folinic acid supplementation, the patient demonstrated marked clinical improvement, and repeat CT scan reveals complete resolution of the multiple enhancing lesions. There is an appearance of diffuse cerebral atrophy, and this appearance has been previously reported in patients with AIDS.

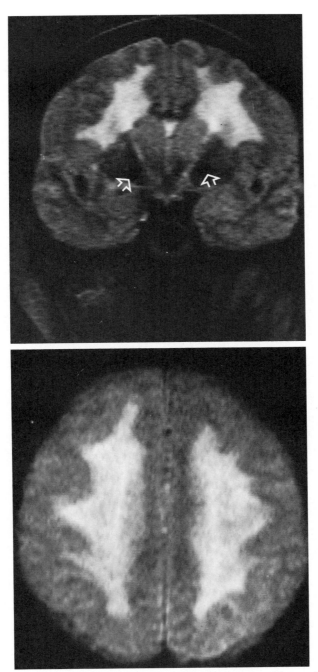

FIGURE 7–4. *Subcortical Arteriosclerotic Encephalopathy (Binswanger Disease):* MR scan using the SE TR3120/TE60 technique demonstrates the typical "bat-wing" appearance of increased signal intensity in a deep, white matter, periventricular appearance. The CT scan reveals this area as a low-density nonenhancing region. The lateral ventricles are mildly enlarged. Bilateral basal ganglia calcification appears as areas of decreased signal intensity (*white arrows*). These changes are thought to be secondary to occlusion of multiple small vessels secondary to arteriosclerotic changes.

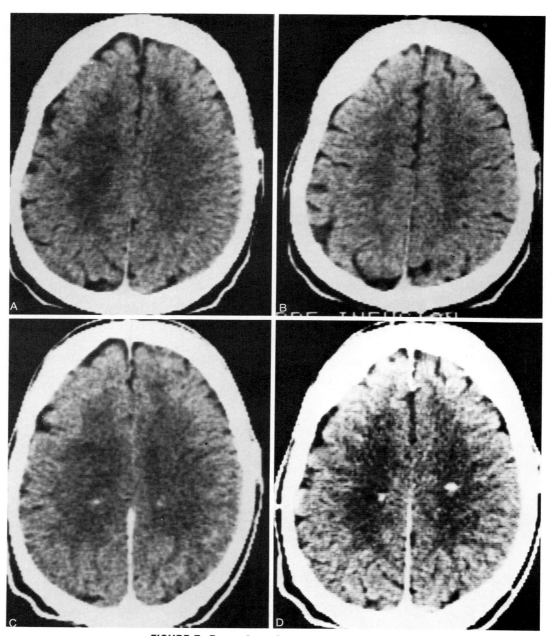

FIGURE 7—5. *See legend on the opposite page.*

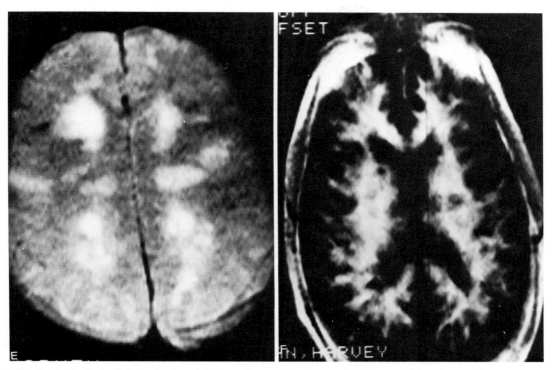

FIGURE 7–5. *Multiple Sclerosis:* A and B, Preinfusion CT scans in this 36-year-old male reveal an appearance of diffuse atrophy.

C and D, The postinfusion CT scan reveals the typical appearance of rounded areas of periventricular enhancement which are present bilaterally.

E, MR using the T-2 weighted SE TR3120/TE120 technique reveals a large number of periventricular areas of increased signal intensity. This appearance is very typical of multiple sclerosis and also reflects the increased sensitivity of MR as compared to CT for the diagnosis of demyelinating disease. There are also parenchymal areas of increased signal intensity. These are also seen with MS but are less common than the periventricular lesions.

F, Inversion recovery (IR) image demonstrates that the areas of demyelination now appear as areas of decreased signal intensity but are less well demonstrated than the SE images. The CT and MR are typical of multiple sclerosis.

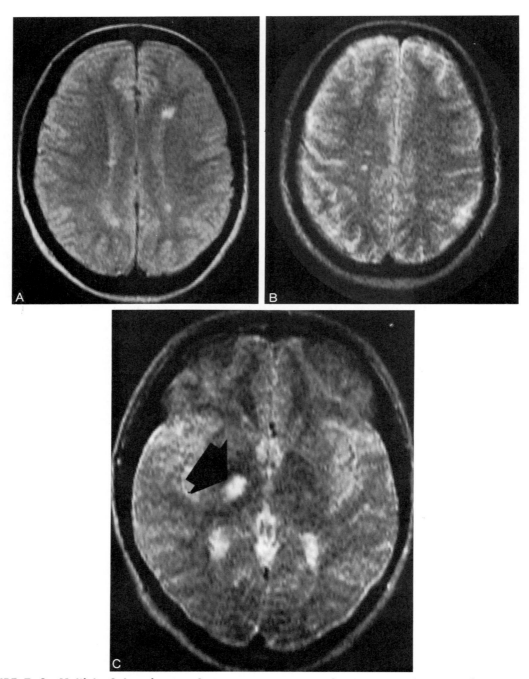

FIGURE 7–6. *Multiple Sclerosis: A* and *B*, MR images using the SE TR3120/TE120 technique reveal multiple, bilateral areas of rounded or oval increased signal intensity in a periventricular distribution.

C, MR SE TR3120/TE120 image at the level of the internal capsule also demonstrates an area of increased signal intensity in the region of the posterior limb of the internal capsule on the right side (*arrow*); this is consistent with an area of demyelination. An infarct could have a similar appearance.

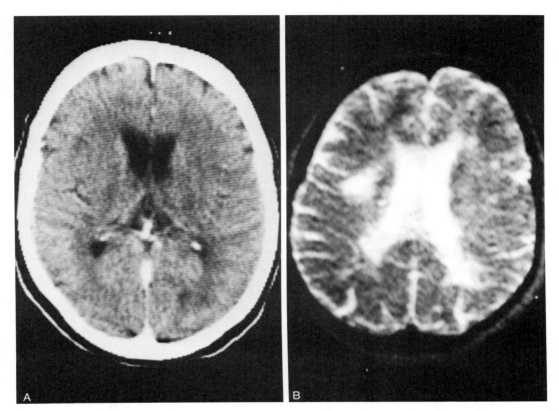

FIGURE 7–7. *Multiple Sclerosis: A*, Postinfusion CT scan demonstrates no evidence of periventricular enhancement. There is mild ventricular enlargement for this 38-year-old female.

B, MR SE TR3120/TE120 image reveals multiple periventricular and parenchymal areas of increased signal intensity. The appearance is typical of MS and reflects the increased sensitivity of MR in the diagnosis of areas of demyelination.

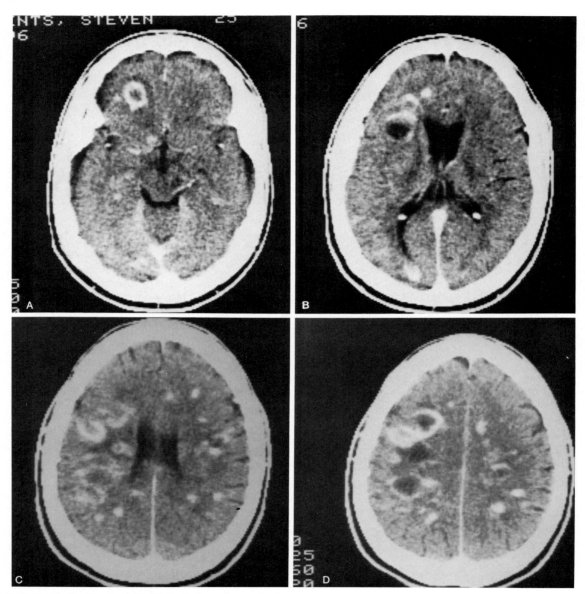

FIGURE 7–8. *Atypical Multiple Sclerosis:* Multiple postinfusion CT scans reveal a large number of cystic areas of enhancement in both a periventricular and parenchymal distribution. In this 25-year-old male there is simultaneously an appearance of atrophy with enlargement of the ventricles and cortical sulci and mass effect with compression of the lateral ventricles toward the midline and elongation of the ventricles. The appearance is typical, although very rare for multiple sclerosis, and represents a fulminant course of active demyelination.

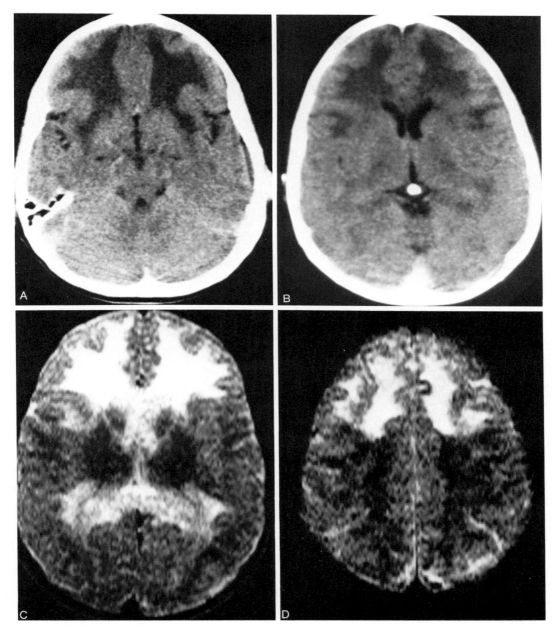

FIGURE 7–9. *Adrenoleukodystrophy:* *A* and *B*, CT scans in this 8-year-old male demonstrate symmetrical, bifrontal lucency involving the white matter distribution. The lucency extends posteriorly into the region of the external capsule.

C and *D*, MR SE TR3120/TE120 images demonstrate that the areas of low density identified on the CT scan appear as areas of increased signal intensity on the T-2 weighted MR images. Patchy areas of increased signal intensity are also visible in a periatrial distribution bilaterally which were not visible on the CT images.

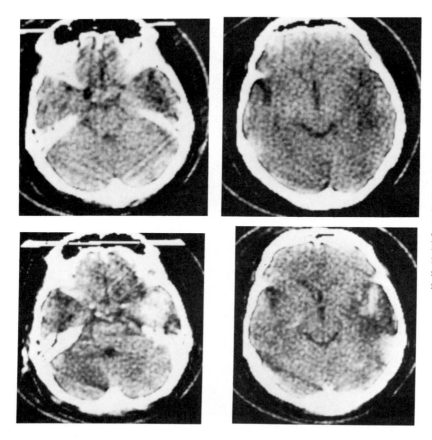

FIGURE 7–10. *Radiation Necrosis:* There is an area of lucency in the right temporal region, with some mass effect and homogeneous enhancement after the infusion of contrast material. The patient had received radiation treatment to the pituitary gland six years previously. Biopsy revealed radiation necrosis.

FIGURE 7–11. *Radiation Necrosis:* Ten-year-old female previously treated with two separate courses of radiation therapy, separated by several years, for neuroesthesioma arising in the frontal region. The patient now presented with progressive paraplegia. MR SE TR3120/TE60 image reveals a streaky area of increased signal intensity involving the medulla (*arrow*) and extending inferiorly to involve the cervical spinal cord. The double arrows illustrate the tumor remaining in the sphenoid sinus. Shortly after this MR scan the patient succumbed secondary to pulmonary metastases. Pathologic examination of the medulla and spinal cord revealed evidence of radiation necrosis. The medulla and cord were of necessity included in the radiation port.

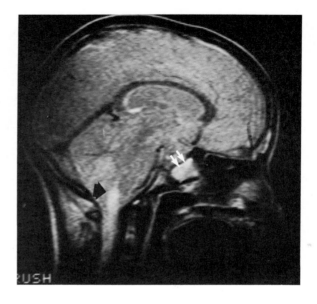

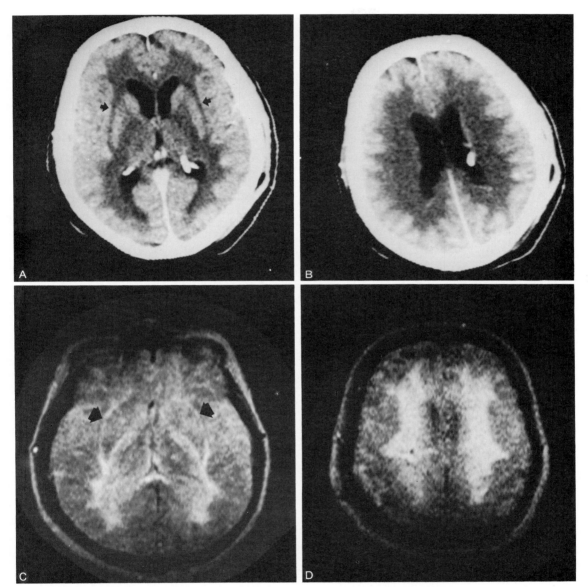

FIGURE 7–12. *Postradiation Change: A* and *B*, CT scans reveal bilateral, diffuse decreased density involving the white matter distribution and extending into the external capsule bilaterally (*arrows*).

C and *D*, T-2 weighted SE MR image reveals that these areas demonstrate increased signal intensity in the same areas that are noted to be abnormal on the CT scan. This change has been identified following whole-brain radiation, although the etiology is unknown.

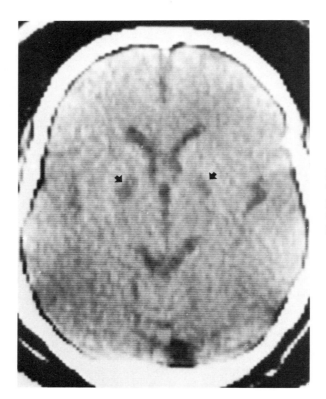

FIGURE 7–13. *Carbon Monoxide Poisoning:* There are areas of low density involving the globus pallidus bilaterally. This appearance is very typical of areas of necrosis following carbon monoxide poisoning.

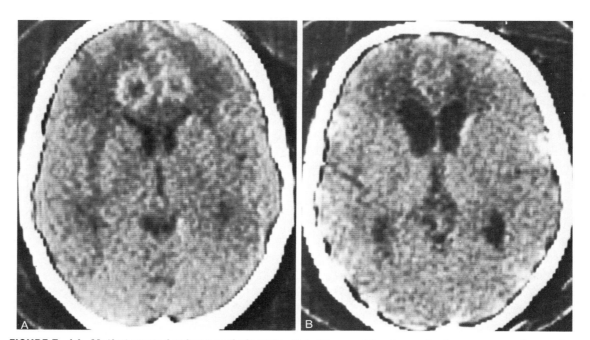

FIGURE 7–14. *Methotrexate Leukoencephalopathy:* This 10-year-old male received treatment with intrathecal methotrexate and also received CNS radiation for leukemia. *A,* Postinfusion CT scan demonstrates bifrontal ring-shaped areas of enhancement with surrounding edema in the deep frontal white matter.

B, Follow-up scan three months later reveals that the areas of enhancement are no longer seen and there is now bifrontal atrophy with dilatation of the frontal horns of the lateral ventricles.

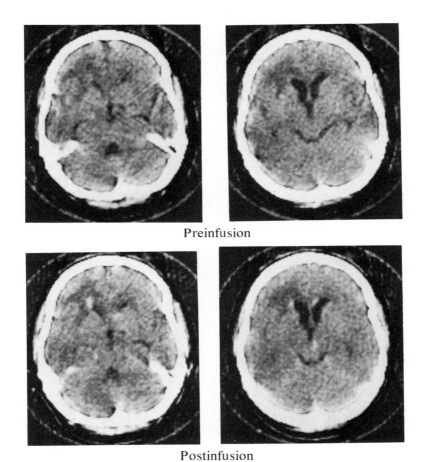

Preinfusion

Postinfusion

FIGURE 7–15. *Progressive Multifocal Leukoencephalopathy:* A and B, The preinfusion CT scans demonstrate patchy areas of lucency and scattered areas of enhancement with surrounding edema on the postinfusion portion of the examination (C and D). Because the clinical presentation may be similar, differentiation from metastases may be difficult without biopsy.

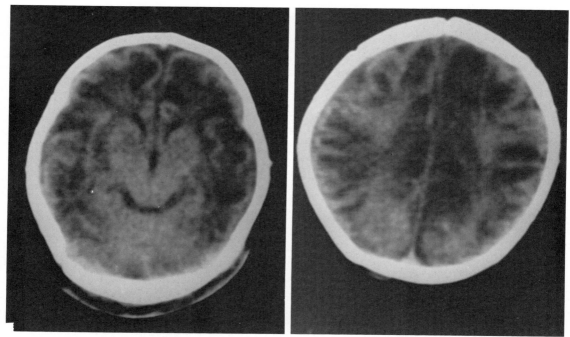

FIGURE 7–16. *Perinatal Anoxia:* CT images obtained within hours of birth in this full-term infant who suffered anoxia at the time of delivery demonstrates bilateral patchy areas of lucency involving both hemispheres. The premature infant may also reveal areas of lucency even in the absence of anoxia, but the distribution then follows a white matter pattern and is secondary to incomplete myelination. In the premature infant, differentiation from anoxic change may be impossible.

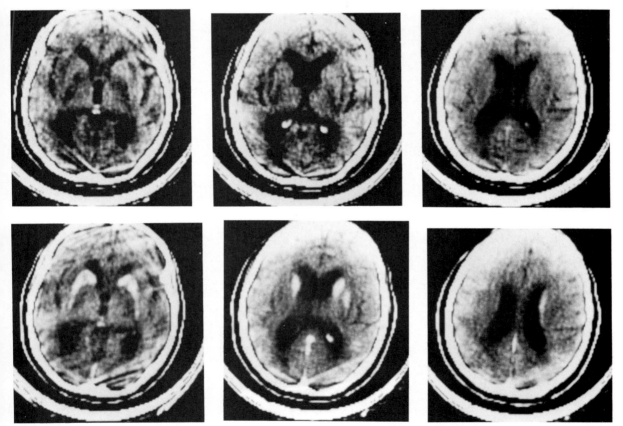

FIGURE 7–17. *Cerebral Anoxia:* The CT scan in this 13-year-old girl following cardiorespiratory arrest reveals moderately severe diffuse cerebral atrophy with areas of radiolucency in the basal ganglia bilaterally. The postinfusion scan (*lower row*) shows marked enhancement of the caudate nucleus.

The general appearance is consistent with cerebral anoxia. The etiology of the caudate nucleus enhancement is unknown, but perhaps it represents an attempt at collateral circulation.

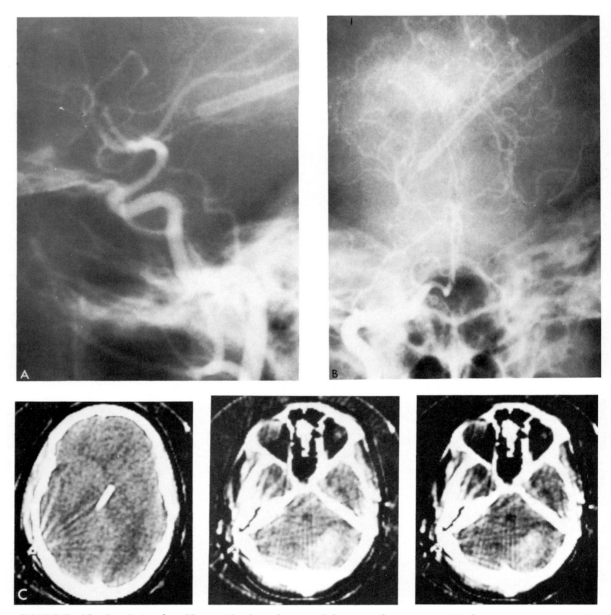

FIGURE 7–18. Amphetamine Abuse: The lateral view of the carotid angiogram (A) demonstrates spasm of the supraclinoid portion of the internal carotid artery. The vertebral angiogram (B) also shows marked spasm of the vertebral and basilar arteries as well as marked attenuation of all the intracranial branches of the vertebrobasilar system. A shunt tubing device is in place.

C, The CT scan shows the shunt tubing device in place in the lateral ventricles. There are scattered areas of radiolucency, which probably are secondary to infarctions caused by vascular spasm. The low cuts also demonstrate a hematoma in the left cerebellar hemisphere. The etiology of the cerebellar hematoma is unknown.

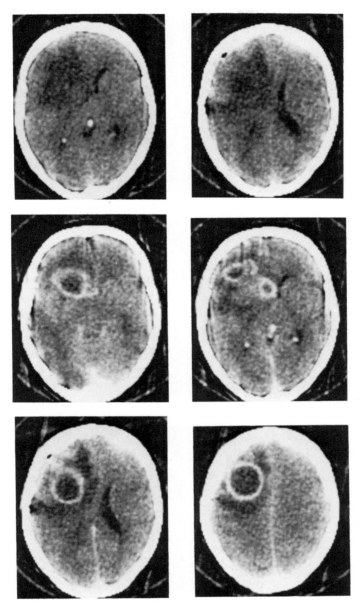

FIGURE 7–19. *Multilobulated Abscess:* The preinfusion scan demonstrates a large lucent lesion in the right frontal and parietal region. Compression of the body of the right lateral ventricle and shift of the midline to the contralateral side are seen. There is posterior displacement of the choroid plexus calcification of the right lateral ventricle as compared to the left. The postinfusion scan shows a multilobulated area of enhancement involving the right frontal and parietal regions with irregular rims of enhancement and surrounding edema. The lesions are multiple abscesses. The differential diagnosis includes multiple metastases.

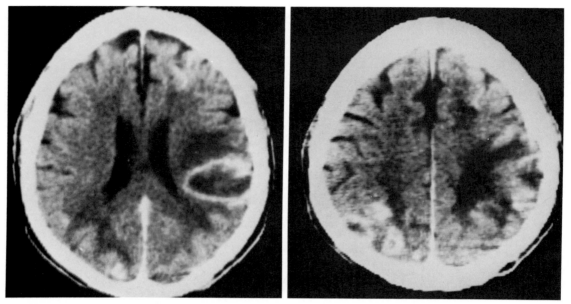

FIGURE 7–20. *Multiple Abscesses:* The patient is a known intravenous drug abuser. Postinfusion CT scans demonstrate multiple bilateral solid and cystic areas of enhancement. The patient had known acute bacterial endocarditis secondary to intravenous drug abuse and has developed multiple brain abscesses following hematogenous spread of bacteria. Surgically proved brain abscesses. Multiple metastases could have a similar appearance.

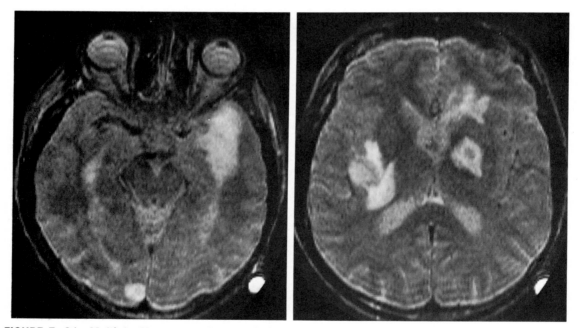

FIGURE 7–21. *Multiple Abscesses, Opportunistic Infection:* Axial MR, SE TR2120/TE120 images reveal multiple abnormal areas of increased signal intensity. The abscesses are lower in signal intensity than the stellate-shaped surrounding edema. More commonly, the abscesses and the surrounding edema are similar in signal intensity, making differentiation between the two impossible. In this regard CT is often more helpful because the enhancing margin of the abscess can be separated from surrounding edema, which is often asymmetric.

Surgically proved multiple abscesses secondary to *Toxoplasmosis* as an opportunistic infection in this patient with AIDS. Multiple metastases would have a similar appearance.

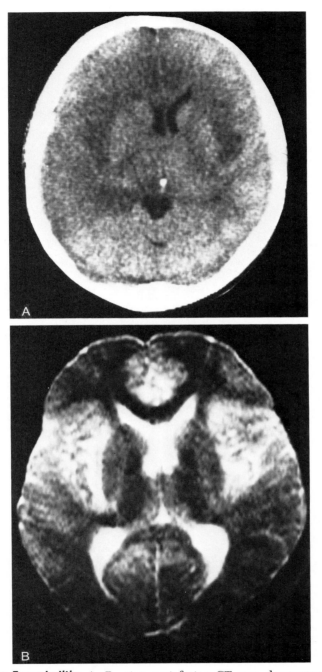

FIGURE 7–22. *Herpes Encephalitis:* *A*, Routine preinfusion CT scan demonstrates bitemporal lucency. There is mass effect that is greater on the right side and displaces the calcified pineal and frontal horn to the contralateral side.

B, Postmortem MR scan demonstrates bitemporal increased signal intensity that reflects the presence of edema typically seen in the temporal lobes in patients with herpes simplex necrotizing encephalitis. Electron microscopic study reveals herpesvirus particles in neuronal and glial nuclei. Time is of the essence in this disease, and if this diagnosis is suspected, brain biopsy should be performed in the temporal lobe region to look for the typical virus particles. Treatment should then be promptly started with cytosine arabinoside (ARA-A) if survival is to be anticipated. Unfortunately, by the time the CT scan is positive the possibilities of successful treatment and survival are remote.

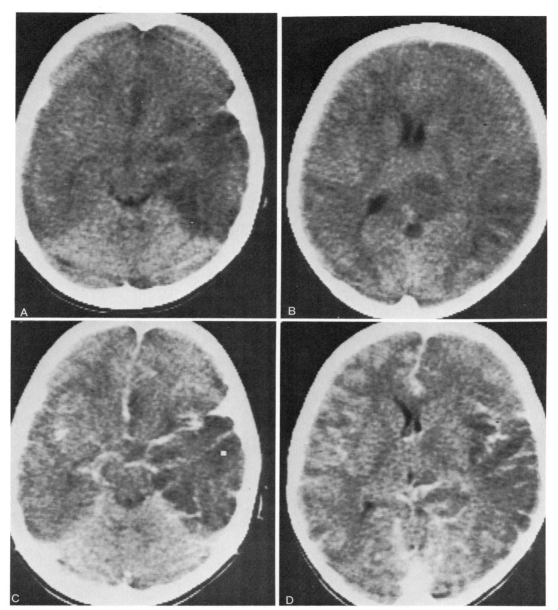

FIGURE 7–23. *Acute Necrotizing Herpes Simplex Encephalitis:* Three-year-old male with fever and progressive obtundation. *A* and *B*, The preinfusion CT scan demonstrates bitemporal lucency greater on the left than on the right. There is also an area of lucency in the left thalamus. *B* demonstrates that the edema extends up into the parietal lobe region on the left. The area of lucency in the thalamus is better demonstrated on this slice. There is greater mass effect on the left side and shift from left to right.

C and *D*, The postinfusion CT scan reveals prominence of the blood vessels of the circle of Willis and middle cerebral arteries but no focal areas of enhancement. The vessels appear more prominent because of the marked lucency of the temporal lobes. Pathologically proved herpes encephalitis.

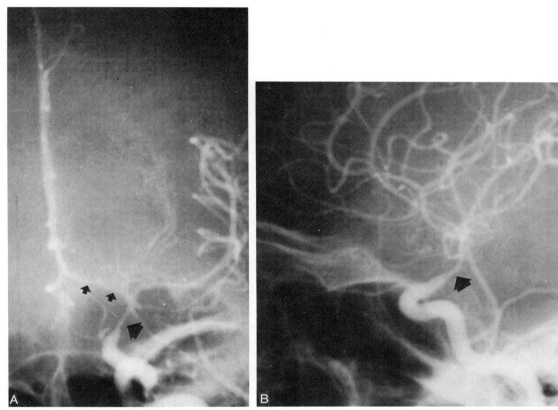

FIGURE 7–24. *Tuberculous Meningitis: A,* AP view of the carotid angiogram reveals spasm of the supraclinoid internal carotid artery *(large arrow)*. The small arrows illustrate the horizontal portions of the anterior cerebral arteries, and the horizontal portions of the middle cerebral arteries are narrowed to the level of the genu of the middle cerebral artery. Note the lack of undulations of the pericallosal artery secondary to enlargement of the lateral ventricles. There is increased filling of the lenticulostriate arteries reminiscent of that seen in "Moya-Moya" disease, probably secondary to an attempt at collateral flow.

B, The spasm of the supraclinoid carotid artery is better seen. On both *A* and *B* there are loss of the normal undulations of the pericallosal artery and widening of the sweep of the pericallosal artery secondary to hydrocephalus. The spasm of the vessels at the base of the brain is typical of basilar meningitis or tuberculous meningitis. The hydrocephalus is secondary to the pachymeningitis over the convexity of the brain and interference with the absorption of the CSF by the pacchionian granulations. (Case courtesy of George Talge, Cook County Hospital.)

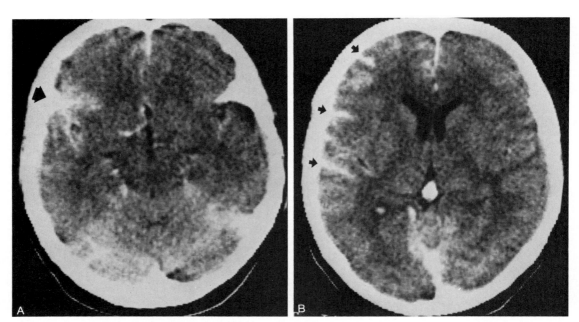

FIGURE 7–25. *CT of Tuberculous Meningitis:* *A,* Postinfusion CT scan demonstrates enhancement of the meninges in the region of the right sylvian fissure (*arrow*).

B, The slightly higher CT slice reveals enhancement of the meninges in the sulci over the right cerebral convexity (*arrows*). The enhancement is secondary to the thickening of the meninges over the convexity. Lumbar puncture confirmed the presence of tuberculous meningitis.

8

MENINGIOMAS

Meningiomas are rather unique tumors that arise from the coverings of the brain, the meninges. They are unique in that they may be considered benign. Meningiomas arise from arachnoid cells embedded in the dura; consequently, almost all meningiomas have a dural attachment.

Meningiomas can be classified as benign because their *total* removal will result in cure. However, while cure is possible, if the tumor arises in an inaccessible location or if it involves critical structures, total excision often is impossible, resulting in tumor regrowth in its original bed after a varying period of time.

Meningiomas are very rare in the first decade of life. They are seen most commonly in the third to sixth decades. The most common presenting complaint is adult onset of a seizure disorder. Anosmia is a common presenting complaint in patients with a subfrontal meningioma. Older patients may have a history of increasing dementia—particularly those who have frontal meningiomas. With posterior fossa meningiomas, the presenting complaints may be secondary to the patient's obstructive hydrocephalus; there may be nausea and vomiting and ataxia as well as headache. Visual disturbances may develop secondary to medial sphenoid wing, parasellar, diaphragma sellae, or orbital meningiomas. Exophthalmos also may accompany these orbital meningiomas.

HISTOLOGY

There are three histologic types of meningiomas: (1) endotheliomatous; (2) fibroblastic; (3) angiomatous. Histologic examination of these tumors always reveals arachnoid cells with tonofilament and desmosomes together with a greater or lesser number of collagen fibers. Meningiomas often show whorls of well-defined cells and a hyalinized and calcified center; these are termed "psammoma bodies."

PLAIN SKULL CHANGES

Findings very suggestive of meningioma are (1) "typical" calcification, (2) "typical" vascularity, (3) reactive hyperostosis.

1. "Typical" calcification implies a well-defined area of speckled calcification or even dense calcification in a typical location for a meningioma. This calcification is psammomatous in nature and may be readily demonstrated by CT scanning even when not visible on the plain skull film.

2. The vascularity seen with meningiomas may be considered "typical" when it reveals enlargement and frequently tortuosity of the grooves of the meningeal arteries as they provide the blood supply to these tumors (Fig. 8–4, pp. 356–357). The venous grooves may also be enlarged to carry the enlarged veins that drain the tumors.

3. Reactive hyperostosis is typical of meningioma. The amount of reactive bone does not necessarily correspond to the size of the soft tissue mass. The tumor may extend through the diploë and project into the scalp, creating a palpable mass.

Meningiomas usually are well-defined tu-

345

mors. However, they also may spread along the deeper surface of the dura and tend to invade the overlying bone, resulting in a diffuse homogeneous hyperostosis. These are meningiomas "en plaque."

Meningiomas of the tuberculum sellae and planum sphenoidal result in a reactive hyperostosis, causing an appearance of a "blister" of the bone. This blistering is quite typical of meningioma. Rarely, meningiomas cause only bony destruction.

In today's practice meningiomas rarely reach a very large size. With the use of such newer noninvasive techniques as radionuclide scanning and, more recently, computed tomography, meningiomas—and brain tumors in general—are being diagnosed earlier. These bony changes may be apparent only on close inspection of the plain skull films and CT scans of the calvaria. If these changes are mild, their significance may only be appreciated in retrospect after the diagnosis has been established.

In addition, other changes secondary to the meningioma may occur, such as shift of the pineal gland or enlargement or erosions of the sella turcica secondary to long-standing increased intracranial pressure.

There have been reports of extracranial metastases of meningiomas, usually in patients who have had an operative procedure upon the primary brain tumor.

ANATOMIC LOCATION

There are certain locations where meningiomas are more commonly seen. Although the list of locations is quite substantial, these tumors exhibit a definite preference for some locations over others. Particular areas and their incidence of occurrence are listed below:

LOCATION	INCIDENCE (%)
Convexity	50
Sphenoid wing (either medial or lateral position)	
Parasellar	40
Olfactory groove	
Posterior fossa	10
a. From the tentorium (origin may be from either the upper or lower surface)	
b. Cerebellopontine angle	
c. Clivus	

Uncommonly, intraventricular meningiomas occur in and arise from the choroid plexus. These meningiomas do not have a dural attachment.

COMPUTED TOMOGRAPHY

Computed tomography of the brain using contrast enhancement is very helpful and is diagnostic in over 95 per cent of cases of meningiomas.

Preinfusion

Because meningiomas contain psammomatous calcification, they frequently are visible on the preinfusion scan as an area of increased density. This increased density may be faint, involving the entire bulk of the meningioma, or there may be some increase in density but also multiple scattered areas of punctate or amorphous calcification. In other cases we have seen small areas of calcification within the bulk of the tumor that do not outline the extent of the lesion. In many cases the meningioma is isodense with normal brain substance, and its presence is identified only by mass effect and/or surrounding edema. Meningiomas may be of lower density than normal brain tissue. Rarely, they may be cystic.

Of particular note is the high parasagittal meningioma, which is not seen unless very high cuts are obtained tangentially through the cerebral convexities. In these cases the edema "below" the meningiomas will be visible before the tumor itself is apparent on the tangential cuts through the convexities.

Edema. The amount of accompanying edema is variable. In some cases there is marked surrounding edema; in others, there is little or none. When edema is present it may be asymmetric in distribution.

Mass. Some cases reveal evidence of the meningioma with surrounding edema and a marked shift to the contralateral side. In other cases, and not uncommonly, the mass is readily visualized but there is little (and in some cases no) shift of the midline structures. It appears in these cases that the tumor grows so slowly that local pressure atrophy of the brain takes place at a rate similar to that of tumor growth—thus, there is no mass effect. In most cases the mass effect is seen to be secondary to a combination of both the tumor mass and the surrounding edema.

Postinfusion

Marked homogeneous enhancement of the tumor is usually seen after the infusion of contrast material. If the lesion is incompletely calcified, the true extent of the tumor will become apparent on the postinfusion scan. Meningiomas that are isodense with brain tissue are readily demonstrated on the postinfusion examination, and full appreciation of both the tumor and the surrounding edema is possible. Rarely, meningiomas may show a "ring" of enhancement. This ring is much more common with gliomas.

Findings of increased density of the tumor combined with a typical location, surrounding edema, and homogeneous enhancement are pathognomonic of many cases of meningioma.

MAGNETIC RESONANCE

Meningiomas frequently contain psammomatous calcification and therefore are often very difficult to demonstrate on the MR scan. Even very large meningiomas may not be appreciated because the calcification results in a low or isodense signal intensity with both the T-1 and T-2 weighted images. In the absence of surrounding edema, a meningioma may not be appreciated on the MR scan. On the other hand, meningiomas are often associated with a large amount of surrounding edema and can, therefore, be demonstrated on the MR scans by virtue of this surrounding edema even if the tumor itself is not visualized. This edema is thought to be secondary to occlusion by the tumor of multiple cortical veins. The surrounding edema is readily demonstrated as an area of increased signal intensity on the T-2 weighted images. It is not understood why with some very large tumors there is no surrounding edema.

The typical location in the frontal or parietal parasagittal or lower convexity region, arising from the falx, as well as in the cerebellopontine angle, aids in arriving at the correct diagnosis. Because meningiomas arise from arachnoid cells embedded in the dura, any broad-based mass apparently arising from the dura suggests a meningioma. The typical location and clinical presentation should confirm the diagnosis.

It is not uncommon that a meningioma, probably because of slow growth, causes pressure atrophy of the adjacent brain tissue. This pressure atrophy causes no apparent distortion of the normal anatomy but rather a combination of invagination of the brain at the level of the tumor and an element of loss of brain substance. This appearance can create a great deal of difficulty in demonstration of the actual presence of a tumor mass. This is particularly true with MR, in which the meningiomas are often isointense with the normal brain. Areas of reactive bone formation are also difficult to appreciate on the MR scan.

Meningiomas frequently occur at the skull base, where they tend to be calcified and so are easily overlooked or missed by MR examination. This is especially true because these tumors cannot be differentiated from the low signal intensity of the bone of the normal skull base. On the other hand, their presence may be appreciated because of the distortion of the normal anatomy at the skull base—a change that is readily demonstrated on the MR scan. Relatively common locations for posterior fossa meningiomas are the region of the cerebellopontine angle, arising from the clivus and/or in the region of the foramen magnum, where they cause distortion at the brain stem and other posterior fossa structures. The ready availability of multiplanar images of the posterior fossa and foramen magnum region makes the evaluation of any mass in this region relatively easy.

One might argue that these small skull base tumors are not life-threatening, but conversely they are most easily "cured" when still small in size. Because of the nearly 100 per cent accuracy of CT in the evaluation of the presence of a meningioma, and because gadolinium-DTPA is not yet available as an MR contrast agent, CT scanning without and with the infusion of contrast material is the method of choice for evaluation of the presence of a meningioma.

Technique for Screening

SE TR530/TE30: axial and coronal or sagittal plane

SE TR3120/TE60-120: axial and coronal or sagittal plane

A single slice, multiecho scan may be helpful for identification of the tumor margin.

It is important to perform the examinations in two planes for complete evaluation. In addition, multiple sclerosis may masquerade as a brain tumor, and the areas of demyelination that are typically seen in the periventricular and periatrial regions may converge with the atrium of the lateral ventricle on the axial view because of the partial volume effect and therefore only be demonstrable in the coronal projection.

Skull Changes with CT

When a meningioma has invaded the bony calvaria at its point of origin or when there is reactive hyperostosis, it is necessary to examine the bony calvaria closely. In fact, it is recommended that in every case of suspected meningioma a thorough inspection of the calvaria be done. Review of the areas of bony density should be performed at standard window width and window level. Following this, the examination should be continued with the unit on the lowest window width, and the window level should be varied to allow accurate examination of the bone. Examination should also be performed when the window width is very high—400—and at varying window levels. Bony change may become apparent only after this type of inspection of the CT scan with varying window widths and window levels. The CT findings will correlate with the plain skull films, but subtle changes may be more apparent on the CT scan.

VASCULAR SUPPLY

Most commonly, meningiomas take their blood supply from the meninges. This vascular supply may derive from any of the blood vessels that normally serve the coverings of the brain. The internal maxillary artery, one of the branches of the external carotid artery, in turn gives rise to the middle meningeal artery. From its origin from the internal maxillary artery, the middle meningeal artery courses laterally and slightly anteriorly below the base of the skull until it enters and passes through the foramen spinosum. The vessel then turns laterally to lie in a groove in the inner table of the skull—the middle meningeal artery groove (see Fig. 8–1, p. 351). This groove is not seen in children; it develops with age and normally is apparent only in adults. The middle meningeal artery bifurcates most commonly into two main divisions—the anterior and posterior branches. The anterior branch ascends in a groove at or near the coronal suture. The posterior branch runs posterosuperiorly in the squamosal portion of the temporal bone; because of its very straight course, it may simulate a fracture.

Although most meningiomas receive their blood supply from the external carotid circulation, falx meningiomas and parasagittal meningiomas may be supplied by the terminal portion of the pericallosal artery or terminal branches of the middle cerebral artery. Because the blood supply is usually from the external carotid artery, it is often quite helpful to perform a selective external carotid arteriogram to achieve better definition of the area of tumor involvement. It also may be desirable to perform a selective internal carotid arteriogram or a common carotid arteriogram so that the relationship between the two circulations can be evaluated independently. With common carotid arteriography the overlap between the internal and external carotid circulations may make it difficult to evaluate the area of tumor involvement as accurately as with the selective external carotid injection. When using the femoral approach and the catheter technique, the external carotid artery can be selectively catheterized in a large majority of cases. Under fluoroscopic control, the catheter is placed in the common carotid artery and then slowly advanced until its tip reaches the external carotid. In most cases, the external carotid artery courses anteriorly and medially relative to the internal carotid at the level of the bifurcation. Because of this, the curved tip of the catheter should be directed anteriorly and medially to facilitate correct placement. The use of a guidewire can help in selective catheterization. The wire may be introduced into the external carotid and the catheter then advanced over the wire until it rests in the vessel. At this time, a test dose of contrast material should be instilled under fluoroscopic control to confirm the positioning in the external carotid artery. During visualization of the branches of the external carotid artery, the patient will experience a good deal of discomfort from the injection because the contrast flows to the mucosal surface of the oral cavity. To achieve patient cooperation, a preliminary warning of this discomfort should be given before the examination.

This manipulation of the external carotid artery and contrast injection may result in localized spasm of the artery at the time of arteriography. If spasm should occur, there will be poor filling of the external carotid circulation and "wash-out" of the contrast material down into the internal and common carotid systems. When this problem does not occur, the examination can be facilitated by the fact that the external carotid system often is enlarged if a meningioma is present. Similarly, an enlarged foramen spinosum should be looked for in any patient with a suspected meningioma. This foramen is readily visualized on the submentovertex view of the skull. It should also be noted that normal variations in the size of the foramen spinosum occur; therefore, the presence of an enlarged foramen or a variation in its size is not absolute proof of meningioma—only further confirmatory evidence.

In patients with arteriosclerotic changes involving the carotid bifurcation with narrowing of the vessel lumen, particular care must be taken that the narrowed lumen is not occluded by the needle or catheter.

Because these tumors originate from the meninges, arteriography will reveal changes secondary to an extracerebral mass lesion. In the case of a supratentorial meningioma, the routine common carotid arteriogram reveals that the cerebral convexity blood vessels fail to reach the inner table of the skull because of the presence of the tumor over the convexity of the brain. Instead, the vessels will be seen to course around the mass lesion and to be "draped" over the mass rather than separated by it. This change is readily apparent in the presence of a sphenoid wing meningioma, where the tumor is visible in the AP projection as a mass with medial displacement of the vessels of the middle cerebral artery away from the inner table of the skull (see Fig. 8–9, pp. 366–367).

Often one can also see the enlarged middle meningeal vessel as it feeds the tumor. The lateral view is also quite characteristic in this case, frequently demonstrating the typical blush of the meningioma.

Commonly, the stain of the meningioma has a "sunburst" pattern. With this appearance it will be seen that the meningeal vessel feeding the tumor is enlarged and tortuous; upon reaching the tumor itself it branches into myriad very tiny vessels that appear to begin at a central point and to branch out in a sunburst pattern.

The blush seen with meningioma often is described as "cloudlike" because of its dense appearance, which persists into the venous phase. This cloudlike blush is to be distinguished from that of glioblastoma multiforme, in which the tumor blush appears quite early but then fades quickly as it is washed out by unopacified blood. Multiple early draining veins can be seen with meningioma, but this finding is not common.

PARIETAL CONVEXITY MENINGIOMA

The classic parasagittal meningioma presents a typical arteriographic picture. In these cases, however, it is unlikely that the radionuclide scan and the computed tomogram will not have strongly suggested the diagnosis before arteriography. The carotid arteriogram reveals downward displacement of the sylvian triangle by the suprasylvian mass and displacement of the branches of the anterior cerebral and middle cerebral artery away from the inner table of the skull. The middle meningeal artery will be seen to be enlarged and to become even larger and more tortuous in its distal segment. In many cases the distal meningeal vessels will develop a "corkscrew" appearance. The tumor itself demonstrates the typical sunburst pattern of vascularity, with vessels radiating out from the center of the tumor. The typical cloudlike blush remains throughout the venous phase of the arteriogram. When this very typical pattern is seen, it is safe to make a diagnosis of meningioma.

Parasagittal convexity meningiomas frequently invade the superior sagittal sinus. If this is the case, the venous phase of the arteriogram will demonstrate absence of filling of the sinus at the level of the meningioma. This may be better demonstrated by using subtraction techniques. This invasion of the superior sagittal sinus makes surgical removal more difficult. DSA also evaluates the presence of sagittal sinus invasion to excellent advantage.

MENINGIOMAS OF THE ANTERIOR CRANIAL FOSSA

Olfactory groove and other subfrontal meningiomas and meningiomas of the anterior cranial fossa are common. When an anterior cranial fossa meningioma is present, one can frequently identify an enlarged anterior falx artery or an enlarged anterior meningeal artery. This vessel enters the cranial vault through the cribriform plate. Like other abnormal meningeal vessels, this one will be seen to become enlarged and tortuous and to demonstrate a "corkscrew" appearance. This anterior falx or anterior meningeal artery may be noted in many normal arteriograms, but it is seen more frequently when there is enlargement secondary to a meningioma. The enlargement of the anterior meningeal artery as it arises from the ophthalmic artery is not always readily appreciated and should be specifically looked for when a meningioma of the anterior cranial fossa is suspected.

On occasion myriad small meningeal vessels may be seen to arise from an enlarged ophthalmic artery and to supply the tumor in the subfrontal area. These small vessels enter the cranial vault through the cribriform plate.

In addition to the standard arteriogram, magnification views and subtraction techniques will make possible a better evaluation of the vascular supply to the tumor and the extent of the tumor mass. The typical "cloudlike" blush seen with meningiomas in other locations is also seen with these tumors.

Olfactory groove meningiomas and other subfrontal meningiomas produce backward displacement of the pericallosal artery and the vessels that supply the frontal lobes. The pattern of vessel displacement is that of an extracerebral mass lesion. The anterior cerebral artery vessels will be seen to be displaced up and away from the orbital roofs, frequently outlining the tumor location.

The typical "cloudlike" blush will be seen in the subfrontal area. Subfrontal and olfactory groove meningiomas often rest close to the midline of the cranial vault; consequently, there may be little if any shift of the anterior cerebral and pericallosal arteries across the midline. This finding is also consistent with any extracerebral mass lesion, where mass lesions within the frontal lobe shift the anterior cerebral artery and its branches across the midline.

Meningiomas of the planum sphenoidale typically promote hyperostosis of the bone, causing a "blistered" appearance.

Tumors of the "clinically silent" areas—such as the frontal region—may be quite sizable when first examined.

PARASELLAR AND SUPRASELLAR MENINGIOMAS

Parasellar meningiomas are not uncommon and are frequently supplied by myriad small meningeal vessels that arise from the cavernous portion of the carotid. There may also be hypertrophy of the meningohypophyseal trunk as it arises from the internal carotid at the entrance of the cavernous sinus. Depending upon the location of the tumor, there may be opening or closing of the carotid siphon; there may be medial or lateral displacement of the cavernous and supraclinoid portions of the internal carotid artery.

Magnification and use of subtraction techniques allow better demonstration of the vascular supply and the typical blush of the meningioma.

Meningiomas also may originate from the diaphragma sellae. Their blood supply is similar to that noted above.

TENTORIAL AND POSTERIOR FOSSA MENINGIOMAS

When meningiomas of the posterior fossa are present, there will frequently be an enlarged posterior meningeal artery arising from the vertebral artery at the level of the entrance of the vertebral artery into the cranial vault through the foramen magnum. In addition, with tentorial meningiomas and some other posterior fossa meningiomas—particularly those that originate from the clivus or cerebellopontine angle—one may see an enlarged tentorial artery. The tentorial artery, also known as the artery of Bernasconi and Cassonari, originates from the internal carotid artery at the level of its entrance into the cavernous sinus. It should be noted that the vessel is present normally, but that it becomes enlarged in the presence of a tumor or arteriovenous malformation that arises from the meninges. As the name implies, this small blood vessel is one of the sources of supply to the meninges and can be seen normally—particularly when lateral magnification technique is used. The meningohypophyseal trunk arises from the internal carotid artery just at the level of its entrance into the cavernous sinus; it may also supply a posterior fossa meningioma or give rise to the tentorial artery.

In the presence of a posterior fossa meningioma, the tentorial artery becomes enlarged and tortuous to supply the tumor, producing the typical sunburst and/or cloudlike blush seen with meningiomas in the supratentorial compartment. The presence of such a vessel strongly suggests the possibility of a meningioma (see Fig. 8–13, pp. 374–375).

Note: The persistent trigeminal artery also has its origin from the internal carotid artery at this point, and a small trigeminal artery may resemble the tentorial artery.

Posterior fossa meningiomas may cause obstructive hydrocephalus. Cerebellopontine angle meningiomas present clinically with a cerebellopontine angle syndrome, but usually with little or no hearing loss.

ORBITAL MENINGIOMAS

Intraorbital meningiomas are occasionally seen. They may arise intracranially or from within the orbit from the dural extension of the meninges that follows the optic nerve into the orbit. They may or may not cause exophthalmos, and usually there is interference with vision. Plain film examination may reveal reactive hyperostosis around the optic canal. Orbital meningiomas are well demonstrated by computed tomography but do not present pathognomonic findings.

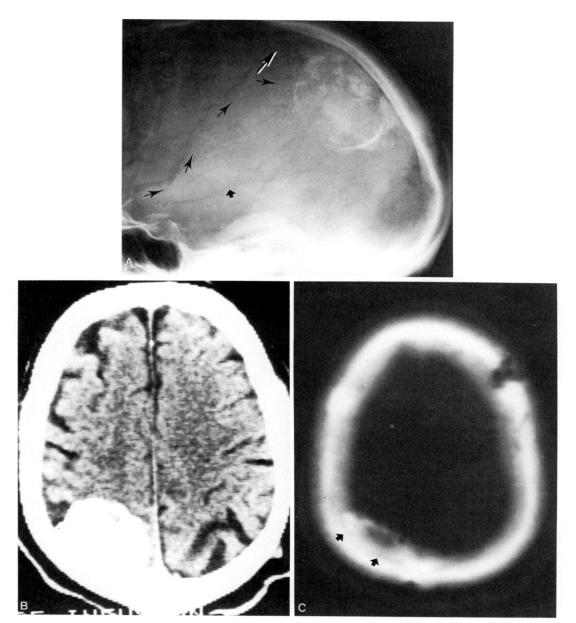

FIGURE 8–1. *Parasagittal Meningioma:* Sixty-five–year–old male with long history of headaches. *A,* Lateral skull radiograph reveals a calcified meningioma in the parietal region. The middle meningeal artery groove is enlarged and courses superoposteriorly to supply the meningioma (*long arrows and black and white arrow*). The posterior branch of the middle meningeal artery is also enlarged (*small arrow*) and can also be identified coursing posterior to the tumor.

B, CT scan at standard viewing level reveals the densely calcified mass in the parietal parasagittal region. There is no surrounding edema and no mass effect. The long-standing, slow-growing nature of this tumor has resulted in focal atrophy of the brain.

C, At "bone" window widths the calcified mass and reactive bone formation, typical of meningioma, are readily identified (*arrows*). (A defect in the contralateral bone is a venous lake.)

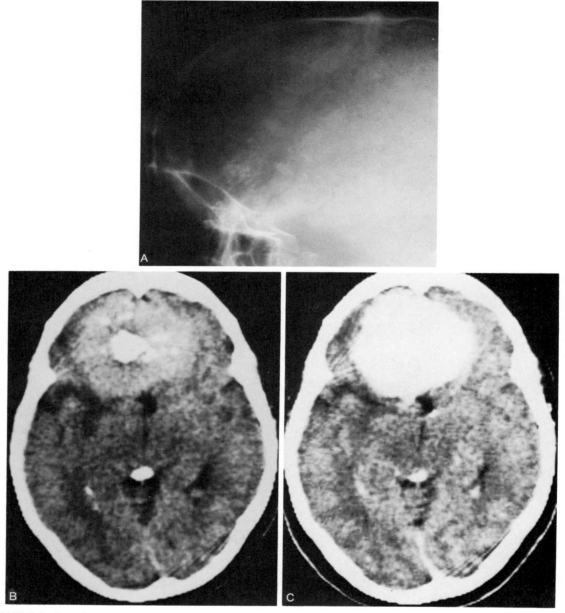

FIGURE 8–2. Fifty-six–year–old female with progressive dementia. *A,* Lateral view of the skull demonstrates multiple amorphous areas of calcification that project just above the planum sphenoidale. Note the reactive hyperostosis of the planum sphenoidale.

B, Preinfusion CT scan reveals the large areas of calcification demonstrated on the skull film. Faint psammomatous calcifications outline the actual tumor location and cause the mass to appear diffusely increased in density.

C, Postinfusion CT scan demonstrates dense homogeneous enhancement of the slightly lobulated tumor.

Illustration continued on the following page

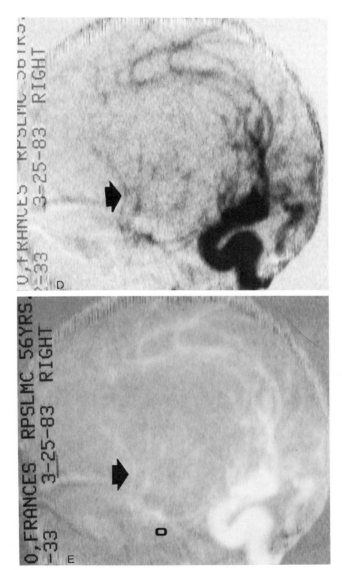

FIGURE 8–2 *Continued.*

D and *E*, IV-DSA photographed in the positive and negative modes reveals the posterior and superior displacement of the anterior cerebral arteries around the large subfrontal mass. The ophthalmic arteries are easily demonstrated bilaterally ("O" in *E*) and give rise to multiple small meningeal feeders (*arrow* in *D* and *E*) that supply the subfrontal meningioma. These multiple small feeders enter the skull base via the cribriform plate (surgically proved).

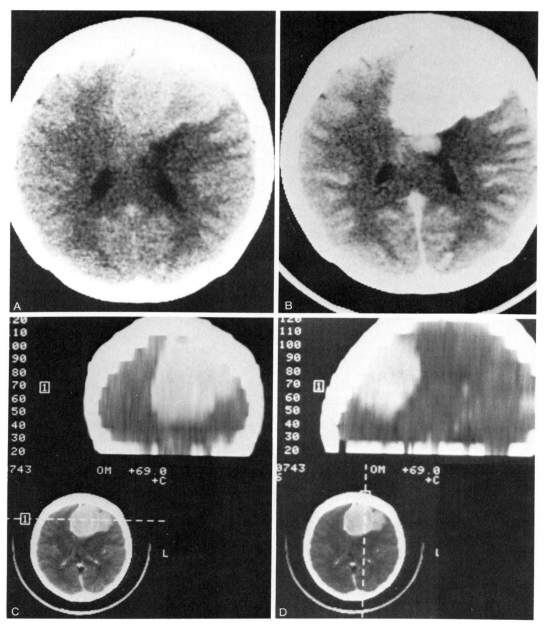

FIGURE 8–3. *See legend on the opposite page.*

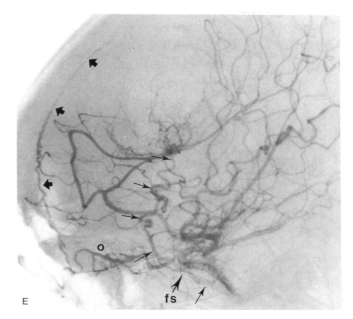

FIGURE 8–3. *Frontal Meningioma:* Sixty-seven–year–old female with progressive dementia. *A,* Preinfusion scan demonstrates a higher than normal brain density mass in the frontal region.

B, The postinfusion CT scan demonstrates homogeneous enhancement of the mass that shows lobulated borders—a somewhat unusual appearance for a meningioma, shift of the falx, and minimal surrounding edema.

C and *D,* Coronal and sagittal reconstruction views further define the location of the mass, which probably arose from the frontal convexity region, although an origin from the falx cannot be ruled out. The meningioma invades the superior sagittal sinus, which does not preclude surgical removal in this case because only the anterior one third of the sinus can be safely removed surgically, and the tumor appears to be limited to this portion of the sinus.

E, Lateral subtraction view of the common carotid angiogram reveals blood supply to the tumor arising from the middle meningeal artery (*small arrows*), which enters the calvarium via the foramen spinosum (*fs*). The anterior falcine artery (*large arrowheads*), which arises from the ophthalmic artery (*o*) and is enlarged and becomes more tortuous distally, also supplies the tumor. This latter vessel enters the base of the skull via the foramen cecum or the cribriform plate, is a midline structure, and courses along the inner table of the skull. The pericallosal artery is depressed, and its branches are displaced around the mass in curvilinear fashion.

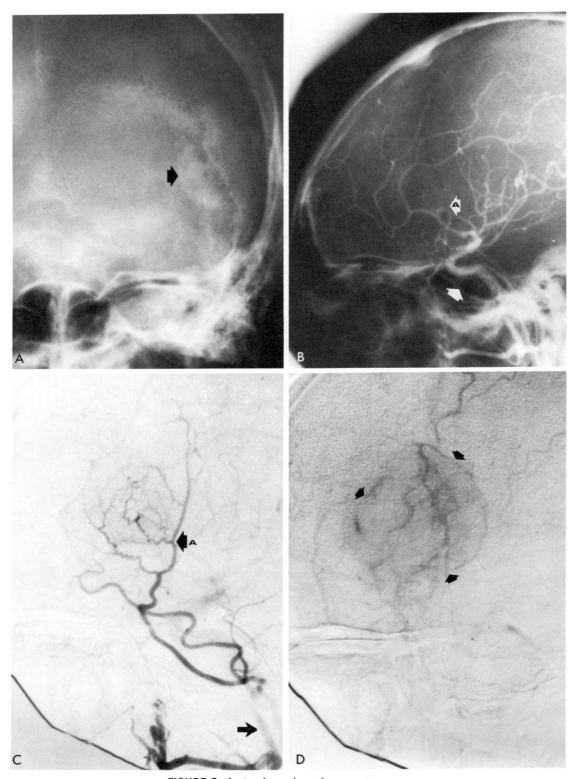

FIGURE 8–4. *See legend on the opposite page.*

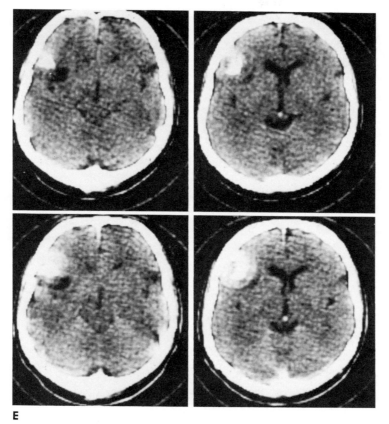

E

FIGURE 8–4. *Posterior Frontal Meningioma:* A, The AP skull radiograph reveals a calcified tumor that projects deep in the cerebral substance (*black arrow*). The tumor actually lies adjacent to the inner table of the calvaria; however, because of the narrow width of the frontal region relative to the biparietal diameter, it appears to lie deep in the brain.

B, The lateral view of the common carotid arteriogram demonstrates stretching of the branches of the middle cerebral artery in the region of the anterior aspect of the sylvian triangle. An enlarged meningeal vessel (*white arrows* and Point "A") courses toward the area of calcification. The unlettered arrow indicates the more proximal point of the vessel.

C and D, The selective external carotid arteriogram with subtraction technique better demonstrates this meningeal vessel (*large black arrow*). The smaller arrowhead (Point "A") shows the meningeal vessel at a point similar to that shown in B. There are multiple small corkscrew vessels that supply the tumor. The venous phase (D) demonstrates the "cloudlike blush" (*black arrows*) so typical of meningioma.

E, The preinfusion scan (*upper*) shows a densely calcified mass adjacent to the inner table of the skull in the posterior frontal region on the right side. On the postinfusion scan (*lower*), this is surrounded by an area of enhancement, which reveals that the extent of the tumor is actually larger than the calcified portion of the mass.

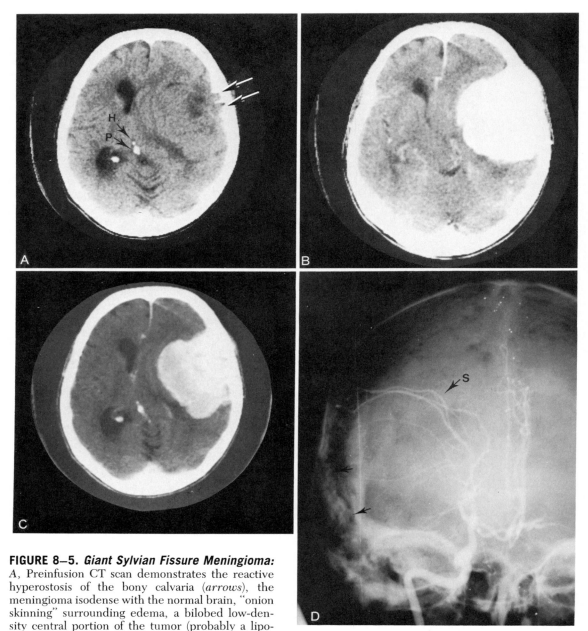

FIGURE 8–5. *Giant Sylvian Fissure Meningioma:*
A, Preinfusion CT scan demonstrates the reactive hyperostosis of the bony calvaria (*arrows*), the meningioma isodense with the normal brain, "onion skinning" surrounding edema, a bilobed low-density central portion of the tumor (probably a lipomatous portion), shift of the pineal body (*P*) and habenular commissure (*H*), and compression of the ipsilateral lateral ventricle.

B, Postinfusion scan demonstrates the typical homogeneous enhancement of the tumor.

C, The image at high window widths and window levels reveals that there are actually internal variations in the amount of enhancement.

D, AP internal carotid angiogram reveals the thickening of the bone secondary to reactive hyperostosis (*arrows*), marked elevation of the sylvian point (*S*), stretching of the branch of the middle cerebral artery, and displacement of these vessels away from the inner table of the skull—findings typical of an extra-axial mass. There is approximately equal shift of the anterior cerebral artery in its proximal and distal portions.

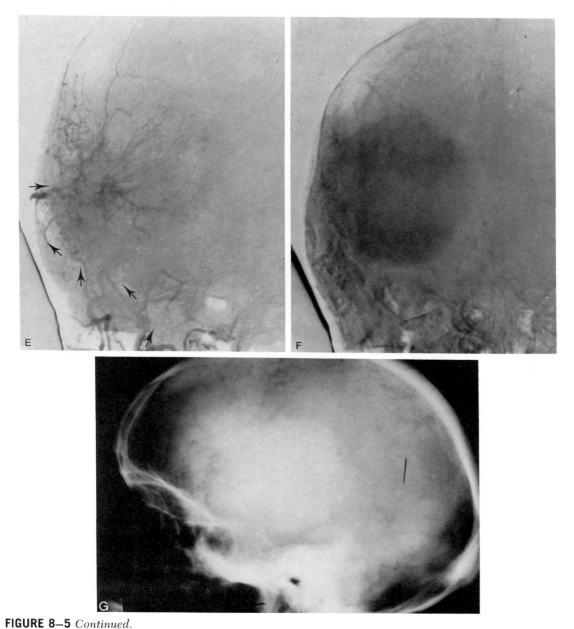

FIGURE 8–5 *Continued.*

E to *G*, APP and early and late serial images from the external carotid angiogram reveal the enlarged, tortuous middle meningeal artery (*arrows*), with the typical "sunburst" pattern of vascularity and pathognomonic delayed cloudlike blush persisting into or even beyond the venous phase of the angiogram.

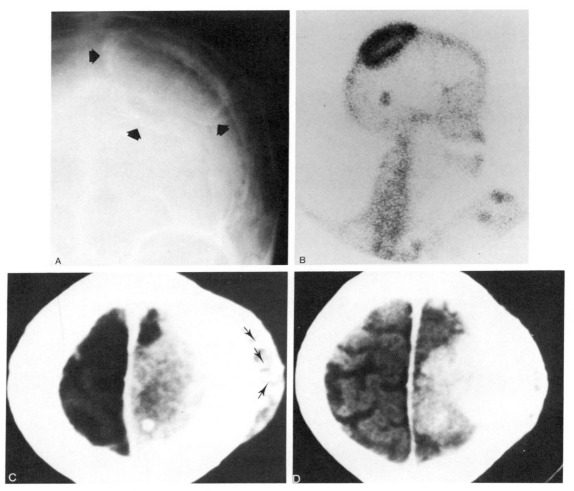

FIGURE 8–6. *Parasagittal Meningioma:* Seventy-three–year–old female with palpable mass of the skull. *A,* AP skull radiograph reveals the mass, which contains prominent peripheral calcification (*arrows*).

B, The radionuclide bone scan reveals the dense uptake in a doughnut-shaped configuration.

C and *D,* The postinfusion CT scan demonstrates dense enhancement of the tumor as well as through-and-through involvement of the bony calvaria with spicules of bone that project outside of the calvaria (*arrows*).

Illustration continued on the following page

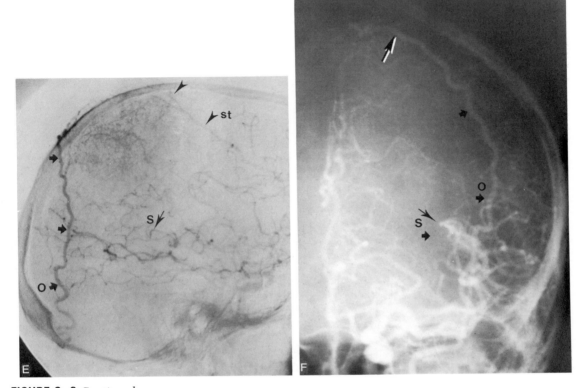

FIGURE 8–6 *Continued.*
E and *F*, Lateral subtraction and AP views of the common carotid angiogram reveal marked downward displacement of the sylvian point (S) and a blood supply that arises from the occipital branch of the external carotid (O) as well as the superficial temporal branch of the external carotid (*st*). The unusual blood supply has probably resulted from the fact that the tumor has grown through the calvaria and into the soft tissue of the scalp. (Case courtesy of the Palos Community Hospital Radiology Group.)

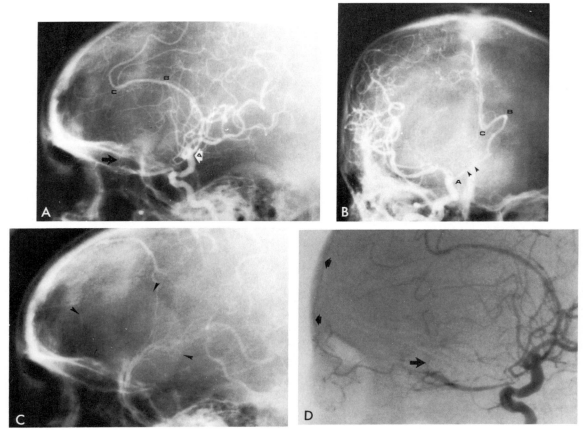

FIGURE 8–7. Subfrontal Meningioma: *A* and *B*, The lateral and AP views of the selective internal carotid arteriogram reveal marked posterior displacement of the anterior cerebral artery, which is also bowed upward and around a large mass positioned below the frontal lobes bilaterally. The corresponding points of the anterior cerebral artery are marked on both the AP and lateral views. The small arrowheads in *B* identify the irregularly narrowed horizontal portion of the anterior cerebral artery—perhaps secondary to encasement by tumor. The AP view also reveals a shift toward the left side, demonstrating that the tumor is larger on the right side.

C, There is a homogeneous stain that remains well into the venous phase (*arrows*).

D, The subtraction view demonstrates the enlarged ophthalmic artery and the treelike branch that courses directly upward through the cribriform plate to provide blood supply to the tumor (*large arrow*). A large anterior meningeal artery also arises from the terminal portion of the ophthalmic artery and courses along the inner table of the skull (*small arrows*).

Illustration continued on the following page

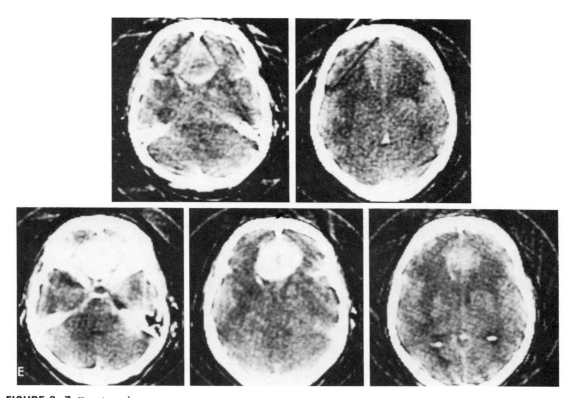

FIGURE 8–7 *Continued.*

E, The preinfusion scan reveals a large dense tumor mass in the midline arising from the floor of the middle cranial fossa. The mass is surrounded by large scalloped areas of cerebral edema. Postinfusion there is marked homogeneous enhancement of the tumor. The frontal horns of the lateral ventricles are displaced posteriorly and splayed apart.

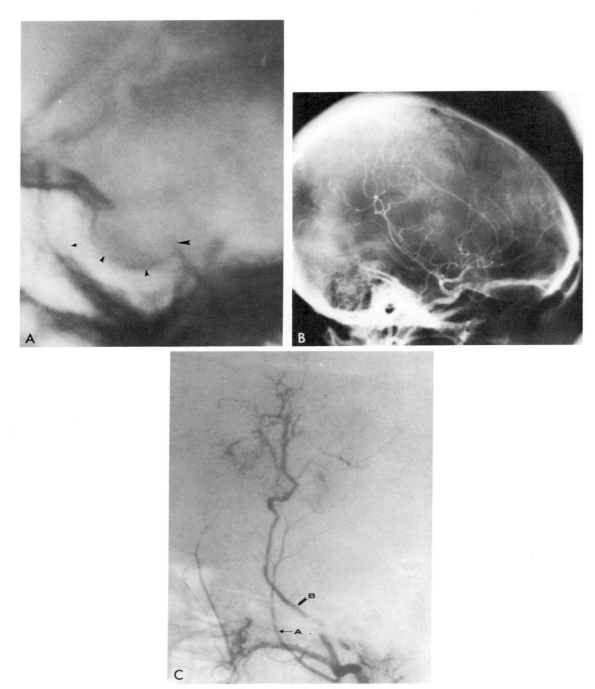

FIGURE 8–8. *See legend on the opposite page.*

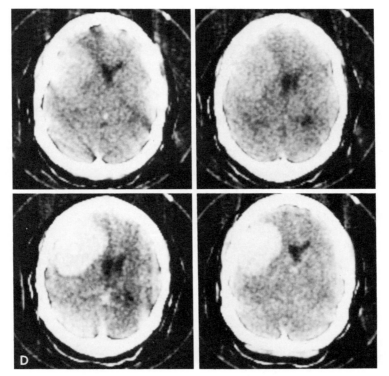

FIGURE 8–8. *Convexity Meningioma: A,* The skull radiograph reveals erosion and destruction of the posterior clinoids and the dorsum sellae as well as demineralization and thinning of the floor of the sella (*arrows*). These changes are secondary to chronic increased intracranial pressure.

B, The common carotid arteriogram reveals downward displacement of the sylvian triangle and stretching of the opercular branches of the middle cerebral artery. A large middle meningeal artery is seen to become more tortuous and enlarged distally in order to provide blood supply to the tumor.

C, Selective external carotid arteriography with subtraction technique demonstrates that both the middle meningeal artery (Point "A") and an accessory meningeal artery (Point "B") supply the meningioma. These arteries enlarge distally and demonstrate a tree-branching pattern with multiple, small twiglike vessels seen frequently with meningioma.

D, The preinfusion CT scan shows a large tumor mass of higher density than normal brain substance. There is no surrounding edema, but marked shift from left to right is evident. The tumor appears to rest against the inner table of the skull in the left posterior frontal region. Postinfusion, there is marked homogeneous enhancement of the tumor.

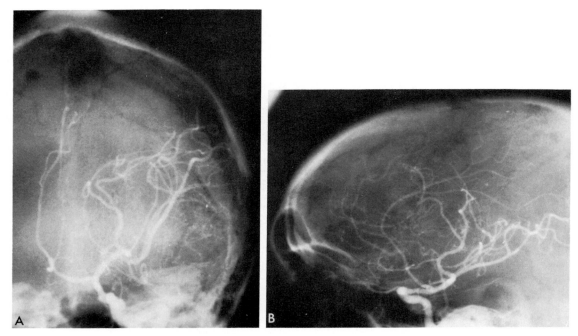

FIGURE 8–9. *Frontal Convexity Meningioma:* A, The common carotid arteriogram shows proximal and distal shift of the anterior cerebral artery with medial posterior displacement of the anterior portion of the middle cerebral arteries.

B, The lateral view reveals total disruption of the anterior portion of the sylvian triangle with posterior telescoping of the posterior branches of the triangle. A large meningeal vessel supplies the tumor, which demonstrates the sunburst pattern of vascular staining seen with meningioma.

Illustration continued on the following page

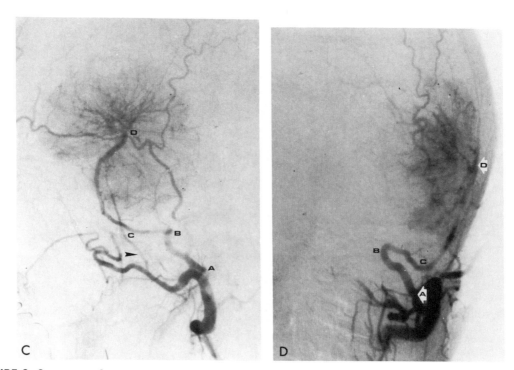

FIGURE 8–9 *Continued.*

C and D are subtraction views of the selective external carotid arteriogram. Corresponding points are marked on the AP and lateral views. "A" is the point of origin of the vessel from the internal maxillary artery. "B" is the point where the vessel enters the cranial vault via the foramen spinosum—which would be expected to be enlarged in this case. "C" demonstrates the vessel as it grooves into the bony calvaria along the inner table of the skull. The vessel enlarges distally and demonstrates a symmetric sunburst pattern of vascularity that appears to originate from point "D." The small black arrowhead in C marks a smaller meningeal vessel that appears to enter the base of the skull via the foramen ovale.

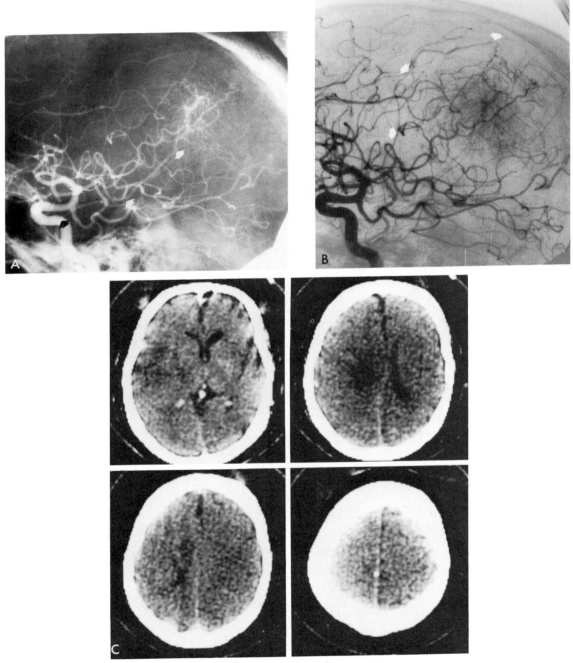

FIGURE 8–10. *See legend on the opposite page.*

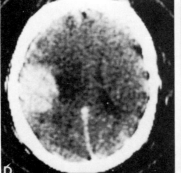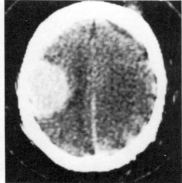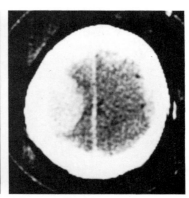

FIGURE 8–10. *Parietal Convexity Meningioma:* A, The common carotid arteriogram reveals downward displacement of the sylvian triangle and a large posterior branch of the middle meningeal artery, which becomes enlarged and more tortuous in its distal portion (*arrows*). The artery supplies a large tumor in the midparietal convexity region.

B, A later arterial phase shows the anterior branch of the middle meningeal artery as it courses posteriorly to provide additional blood supply to the tumor (*arrows*). This subtraction view better demonstrates the sunburst pattern of vascularity.

C, The preinfusion scan shows a tumor that is isodense with brain tissue and surrounded by a thin rim of edema. There is only minimal shift of the midline structures. The slow growth of the tumor probably has resulted in pressure atrophy of a portion of the brain, since only a modest shift to the left is seen.

D, Postinfusion, the tumor enhances in a homogeneous fashion.

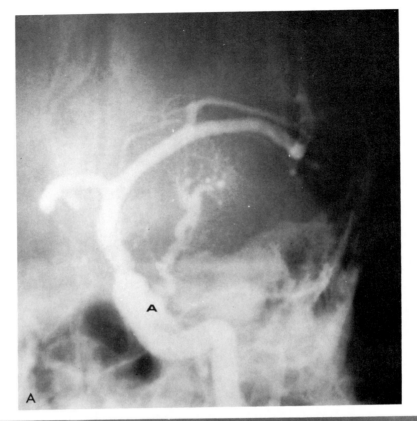

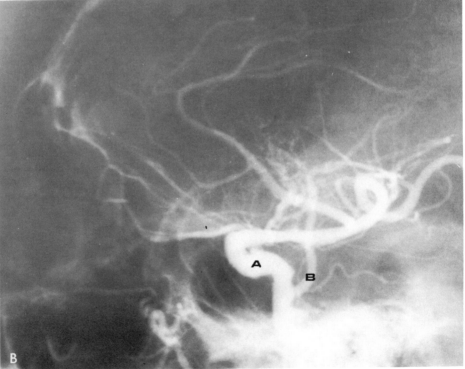

FIGURE 8–11. *See legend on the opposite page.*

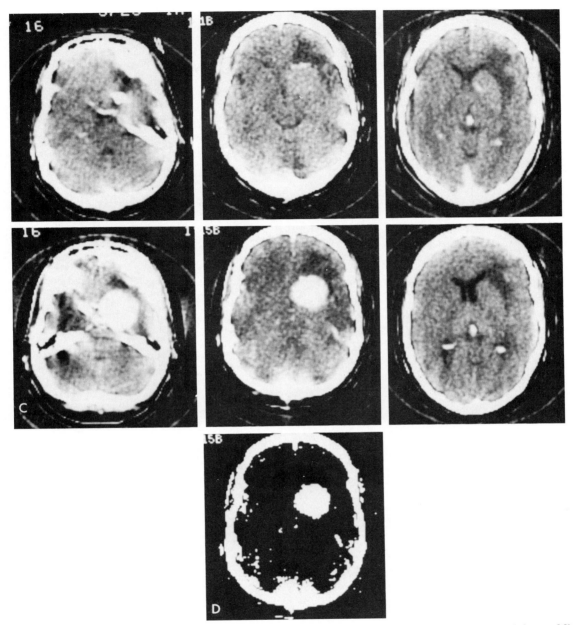

FIGURE 8–11. *Parasellar Meningioma: A* and *B,* Marked elevation of the horizontal portion of the middle cerebral artery and medial displacement of the internal carotid artery are seen as they follow a curvilinear course around the tumor. This meningioma arises from the medial aspect of the sphenoid wing and may be accompanied by hyperostosis of the greater wing of the sphenoid around the superior orbital fissure. If hyperostosis is present, this may strongly resemble fibrous dysplasia. Point "A" on the AP and lateral views marks the origin of an unnamed meningeal vessel at its point of origin from the internal carotid artery. This large vessel becomes even larger and more tortuous as it projects superiorly and posteriorly to supply the tumor. Point "B" is a large superficial temporal artery that could be seen in the soft tissues on the AP view.

C, The preinfusion scan reveals that the tumor is isodense with brain tissue and is surrounded by a rim of edema. There are a few scattered areas of calcification around the periphery of the tumor. Postinfusion there is homogeneous enhancement. Differentiation from an aneurysm may be difficult.

D, On the measure mode the meningioma is readily identified as a high-density area of enhancement.

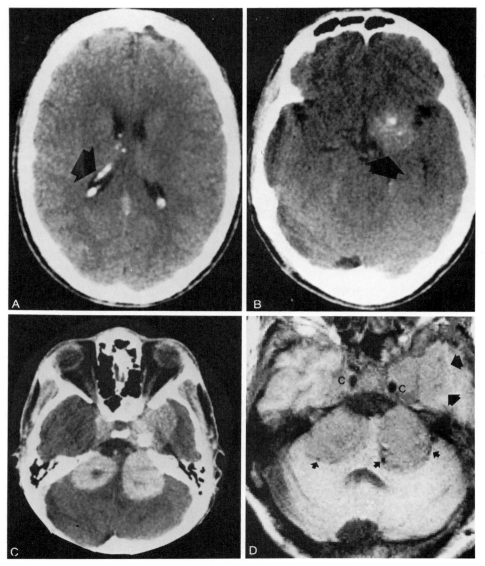

FIGURE 8–12. *Meningioma and Bilateral Acoustic Neuromas:* Seventeen-year-old male with known neurofibromatosis. *A,* Preinfusion CT scan demonstrates increased calcification in the choroid plexus of the lateral ventricle *(arrow).* This increased calcification is typical of patients with neurofibromatosis. Patients with neurofibromatosis have an increased incidence of all types of brain tumors, but particularly meningiomas and acoustic neuromas, as illustrated by this case.

B, There is homogeneous as well as dense amorphous calcification in a large parasellar meningioma *(arrow).*

C, Postinfusion scan shows homogeneous enhancement of the parasellar meningioma. There are also bilateral, homogeneously enhancing acoustic neuromas that demonstrate cystic areas, a common finding with acoustic neuromas.

D, Axial SE TR530/TE30 MR scan demonstrates that because of the calcification the parasellar meningioma is only poorly visualized *(large arrows).* The cavernous internal carotid arteries are seen as negative flow defects bilaterally *(C).* There are also bilateral low signal intensity acoustic neuromas, and the fourth ventricle is compressed along its anterior margin and displaced posteriorly. Small, rounded, negative signal areas are probably negative flow defects from blood vessels supplying or draining the tumors *(small arrows).* Note the greatly enlarged prepontine cistern (also visible in *C*) because of posterior displacement of the pons by the large extra-axial acoustic neuromas.

Illustration continued on the following page

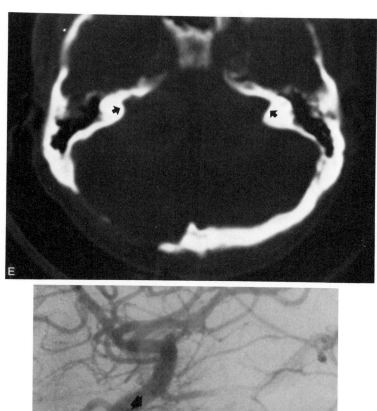

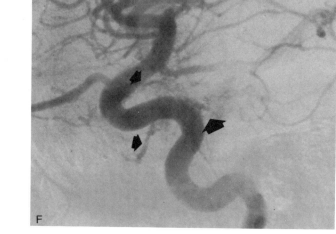

FIGURE 8–12 *Continued.*

E, The "bone window" CT image reveals flaring of the internal auditory canals bilaterally (*arrows*) and a postoperative defect in the occipital bone.

F, Subtraction view of the internal carotid angiogram reveals multiple enlarged meningeal vessels supplying the parasellar meningioma (*arrows*).

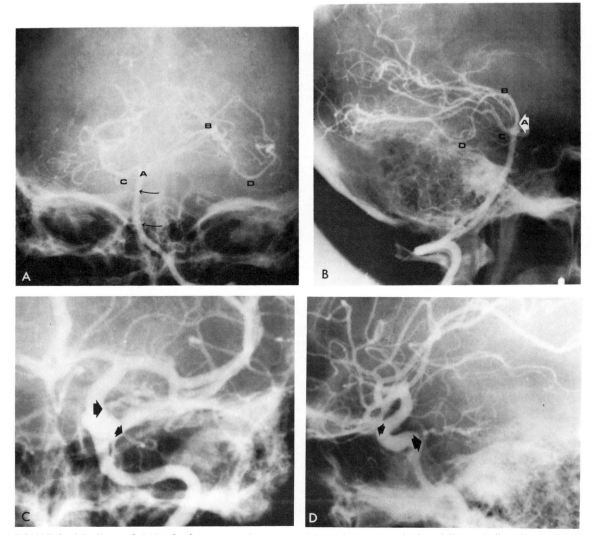

FIGURE 8–13. *Tentorial Meningioma: A* and *B,* AP and lateral views marked as follows: "A" is the origin of the left posterior cerebral artery; "B" is the uppermost point of the left posterior cerebral artery as it is displaced over the tentorial meningioma just below it; "C" is the lowest point of the normally positioned right posterior cerebral artery; "D" is the lowest point of the abnormal left posterior cerebral artery as it is displaced laterally and posteriorly. There is such gross distortion of the left posterior cerebral artery that both the normal and abnormal positions can be readily demonstrated. The basilar artery is displaced to the right (*arrows*).

C and *D,* The left internal carotid arteriogram reveals a large tentorial artery—the artery of Bernasconi and Cassonari—which provides the main blood supply to the tumor (*large arrowhead*). The ophthalmic artery is also visualized on both the AP and lateral views (*small arrowhead*).

E, A subtraction view reveals the ophthalmic artery (*small arrowhead*), the tentorial artery of Bernasconi and Cassonari (*large arrowhead*), and the blush of the meningioma in the posterior fossa and along the free edge of the tentorium as it is supplied by myriad small vessels (*open arrowheads*).

F, The preinfusion CT scan (viewed from above) shows the tumor along the edge of the petrous bone on the left side, extending medially just across the midline and superiorly to the left of the third ventricle. The posterior portion of the third ventricle is thinned and displaced to the right. The tumor is of higher than normal brain density and contains small areas of calcification. There is moderate obstructive hydrocephalus. Postinfusion there is homogeneous enhancement of the tumor, providing a beautiful illustration of the exact location of the mass.

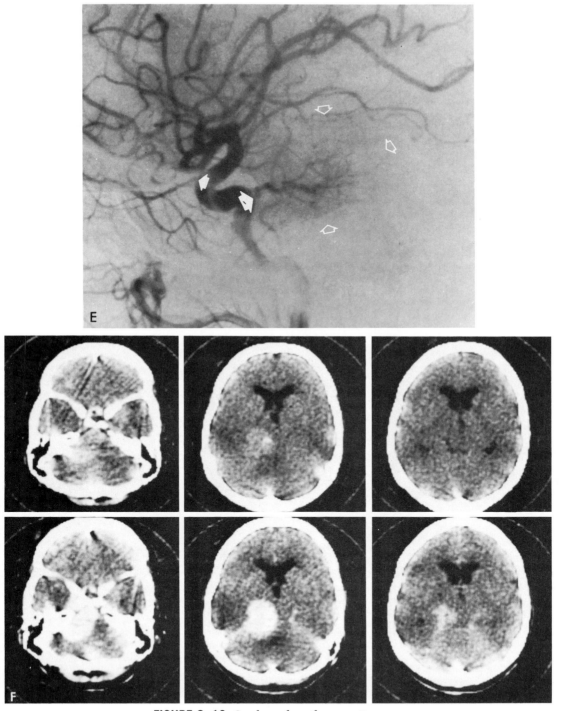

FIGURE 8–13. *See legend on the opposite page.*

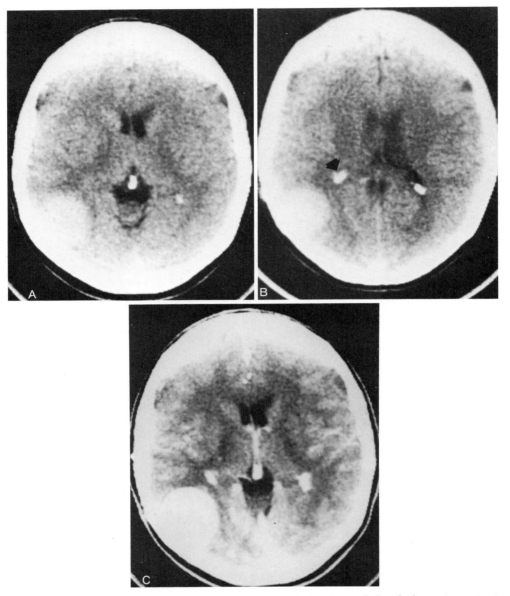

FIGURE 8–14. *Tentorial Meningioma:* Thirty-five–year–old female with headaches. *A* to *C*, Pre- and postinfusion scans demonstrate a high-density, well-defined mass with minimal surrounding edema that enhances homogeneously. There is very slight mass effect with compression of the ipsilateral lateral ventricle and forward displacement of the calcified glomus of the choroid plexus of the lateral ventricle (*arrow*).

D, Subtraction view of the common carotid angiogram reveals that the blood supply to the tumor is from the posterior branch of the middle meningeal artery as well as the occipital branch of the external carotid artery (*o*).

E, The venous phase reveals the typical delayed "cloudlike" blush of the meningioma. There is also invasion of the transverse sinus (*TS*) by a portion of the tumor (*arrows*).

F and *G*, Direct coronal postinfusion CT (*F*) and the AP angiogram (*G*) reveal the tumor as it rests on top of the tentorium cerebelli just where the tentorium attaches to the transverse sinus.

H, The pathologic specimen was removed in contiguity with the invaded portion of the transverse sinus.

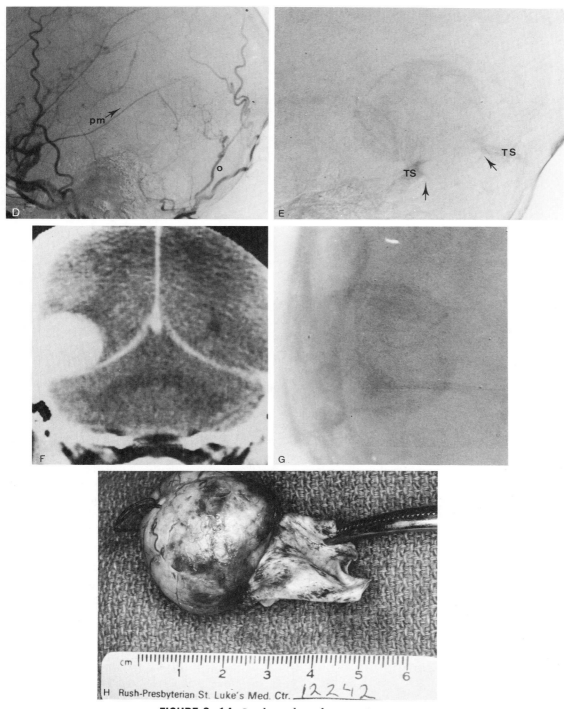

FIGURE 8–14. *See legend on the opposite page.*

9

DEEP HEMISPHERE AND MIDLINE LESIONS

Masses that arise in the midline in the supratentorial compartment are difficult to demonstrate by angiography. In fact, even in the presence of relatively large lesions, the angiogram may demonstrate hydrocephalus but may otherwise be uninformative. Angiography usually does not characterize the lesion or identify its exact position. Abnormal vascularity, if demonstrated, can of course reveal the extent of the mass; however, it is not uncommon to find that the mass is avascular.

Pneumoencephalography, necessary for evaluation before the availability of CT, is no longer required. CT easily demonstrates the nature and position of most abnormalities. In the absence of magnetic resonance, metrizamide cisternography may be necessary for evaluation of a mass in the region of the sella turcica. Magnetic resonance is also an excellent method for evaluation of these midline lesions and is particularly helpful for evaluation of pituitary adenomas. The unique usefulness of MR in the region of the sella is discussed extensively below. Magnetic resonance will probably replace other diagnostic methods for evaluation of sella turcica abnormalities.

Midline lesions outside the sella include:

1. Pinealoma
2. Teratoma
3. Hypothalamic glioma
4. Vein of Galen aneurysm
5. Colloid cyst of the third ventricle

Lesions within and immediately adjacent to the sella include:

1. Ectopic pinealoma
2. Pituitary adenoma
3. Aneurysm of internal carotid artery
4. Craniopharyngioma
5. Empty sella
6. Meningioma of diaphragma sellae or medial sphenoid wing
7. Optic glioma
8. Basal ganglionic hematoma

BASAL GANGLIONIC HEMATOMA

Hemorrhages that occur in the region of the basal ganglia are secondary to the rupture of small aneurysms arising from the lenticulostriate arteries. These basal ganglia hemorrhages most commonly are seen in hypertensive patients and are especially prevalent among the black population. The clinical presentation is dramatic, with the sudden onset of severe headaches, a dense contralateral hemiplegia, and decreased sensorium and/or coma. Complete recovery from a large hemorrhage is rare, and many patients die following a basal ganglia hemorrhage.

Because these hemorrhages can rupture into the ventricular system, their clinical appearance may mimic a subarachnoid hemorrhage. With rupture into the ventricular system, a lumbar puncture will reveal bloody cerebrospinal fluid. In the past, angiography was necessary to rule out an aneurysm as the cause of the bloody CSF. With basal ganglionic hemorrhage, angiography may also be helpful and diagnostic.

On the other hand, the angiogram may be normal or may demonstrate only a shift of the internal cerebral vein to the contralateral side. Other abnormalities that may be seen are displacement of the lenticulostriate arteries (either medially or laterally, depending on the position of the hemorrhage), a widened distance between the anterior cerebral artery and the laterally displaced middle cerebral artery group and, in some instances, a shift of the anterior cerebral artery to the contralateral side.

Since the availability of CT scanning, the diagnosis of basal ganglionic hemorrhage can be made with nearly 100 per cent accuracy. In most instances no other diagnostic tests are necessary.

PITUITARY ADENOMA

Pituitary tumors are usually seen from the third through the fifth or sixth decade. Because pituitary tumors are rare in the first two decades, craniopharyngioma is a more likely possibility in those under 20 years of age. In the past, pituitary tumors were traditionally classified as eosinophilic, basophilic, or chromophobe adenomas. At this time, however, all pituitary adenomas are considered as one type. Microadenomas are less than 1 cm in size and are usually associated with a clinical presentation of amenorrhea and galactorrhea. With the macroadenomas, the usual clinical presentation is that of headaches and a bitemporal hemianopia secondary to suprasellar extension of the tumor. In addition, the patient may complain of decreasing libido and secondary sex characteristics and a change in voice.

Skull. With macroadenomas, there is enlargement of the sella turcica greater than the 14 × 17 mm size that is the upper limit of normal. There may be destruction of the floor of the sella with invasion of the sphenoid sinus. There may be undercutting of the anterior clinoid processes. There is commonly posterior displacement or even destruction of the dorsum sellae and the posterior clinoid processes. Rarely, pituitary adenomas may calcify. With the "basophilic" adenoma associated with Cushing's disease, there is usually no change in the size of the sella, although there may be diffuse demineralization of the skull and sella secondary to the disease itself.

Microadenomas usually show no change in the configuration of the sella, although at times there is focal erosion of the floor of the sella.

Computed Tomography of Macroadenomas

Computed tomography should be performed in the axial projection using 4-mm slices parallel to the optic nerve. The scan is performed pre- and postinfusion. The author does not recommend postinfusion only scans for initial evaluation. The study may also be performed in the direct coronal projection if the patient is able to assume this position. With newer scanners, 4-mm slices overlapping by 2 mm through the area of abnormality and extending both above and below allow ready evaluation in the sagittal and coronal projections by the use of reformatting techniques. Microadenomas will be considered separately.

For solid tumors, the mass is usually isodense with the brain on the preinfusion scan. The extension into the sphenoid sinus is easily evaluated and is best appreciated on CT slices done at wide window widths. With suprasellar extension these masses obliterate the five-pointed, CSF density, suprasellar cistern. Following the infusion of contrast material, there is dense homogeneous enhancement in all cases. Usually these tumors are smoothly marginated but may uncommonly be multilobulated. At times they may rarely become very large in size, even extending forward into the subfrontal region. Meningioma and aneurysm should be considered in the differential diagnosis. If the adenoma is sufficiently large in size, it will extend up to the level of the foramen of Monro and cause obstructive hydrocephalus.

Occasionally these tumors are cystic or multicystic, apparently secondary to areas of hemorrhage or infarction of varying size which ultimately become areas of cystic necrosis. There may be one large cyst or multiple small cysts. The cysts do not demonstrate enhancement, although the periphery of the cyst and the remainder of the gland do enhance.

Rarely pituitary apoplexy (a sudden hemorrhage into the gland) occurs. If this is the case, the patient may present acutely ill, with cranial nerve palsies and the sudden onset of blindness—an emergency situation if vision is to be preserved. The CT scan usually demonstrates a cystic pituitary adenoma with a fluid/fluid level within the cyst, although hemorrhage may also occur into a solid tumor. The fluid in the dependent portion of the cyst is of high density because it contains blood. Areas of hemorrhage are easily identifiable on MR scans and appear as areas of increased signal intensity on the T-1 weighted images.

Microadenomas of the Pituitary

Microadenomas are best examined using the coronal only, postinfusion only technique. A rapid injection of contrast material should be performed and the scan should be begin immediately following injection. The normal height should not exceed 8 mm in women and 7 mm in men. Using this method, most microadenomas will appear as low-density areas in the lateral portion of the gland. There is usually upward convexity of the gland, with the upward convexity, often focal, above the adenoma. High-resolution scans should be performed using thin, 2-mm or preferably 4-mm cuts overlapping by 2 mm. Occasionally microadenomas will appear increased in density early in the study, but more commonly the low density originally identified will become increased density later in the study or isodense with the gland, thus making visualization impossible. For this reason early postinfusion scanning is mandatory.

In addition to routine window widths, close examination of the floor of the sella with wide window widths may demonstrate areas of erosion at the level of the microadenoma.

A Word of Caution

It is not uncommon that patients with large pituitary tumors experience panhypopituitarism. This is reflected in their clinical history of decreased, abnormal, or absent menstruation in women, decrease in axillary and pubic hair in both sexes, and decreased beard growth in men. There may also be a change in voice. Less commonly appreciated, there is also a decrease in the adrenal-stimulating hormones, resulting in clinical or subclinical hypoadrenalism. Because of this decrease in adrenal function, these patients respond poorly to stressful situations and may become hypotensive at the time of examination with such tests as angiography. Obviously, an episode of hypotension in an older individual could lead to a stroke, but in any case, treatment with steroids prior to examination will obviate this possibility. If not administered in anticipation of the study, then 100 mg of Solu-Medrol can be given intravenously immediately prior to beginning the procedure.

Magnetic Resonance of the Pituitary

Magnetic resonance imaging of the pituitary region has added a new dimension to the clinical evaluation of this region. Even with the 1-cm slices available with the early scanner, and now with the development of thinner slices and, in some cases, overlapping slices, this area of the base of the skull can be exquisitely evaluated. In addition, the ability to scan in a variety of different planes makes the study of the pituitary fossa convenient, especially in the patient who is unable to remain in the sometimes awkward positions necessary for CT evaluation. The carotid arteries can be demonstrated because of the negative flow defect visualized on the MR scans. In addition, the exact relationship of the carotid arteries to the surrounding tumor is readily distinguished.

The normal pituitary fossa is easily demonstrated on all MR scans, and its relationship to surrounding structures is easily seen. The pituitary gland is seen in the floor of the pituitary fossa, and in some cases the anterior lobe (adenohypophysis) can be differentiated from the posterior lobe (neurohypophysis), and the pars intermedia is seen as an area of low signal intensity between the two. In addition, and best demonstrated on the lateral view, there is a small area of high signal intensity in the posterior aspect of the sella turcica which represents a small collection of fat and is a normal finding in MR of the sella. Just above the sella the optic chiasm is demonstrated on the T-1 weighted images as an area of relatively increased signal intensity bathed by the low signal intensity of the CSF in the suprasellar cistern. Below the pituitary gland the sphenoid sinus is demonstrated as an area of very low signal intensity because it is air-filled. The cortical margin of the sella is poorly visualized because it is so thin and because of its very low signal intensity. The clivus is very high in signal intensity because of the fatty bone marrow that is present in the clivus. The low signal intensity of the aerated sinus and the high signal intensity of the clivus nicely outline the pituitary fossa. It should be mentioned here that sinusitis is readily demonstrated by MR scanning and appears as areas of increased signal intensity either with areas of mucosal thickening or with retention cysts, both of which are easily demonstrated (see Fig. 9–29, p. 427).

As with CT scanning, the MR scan is abnormal in similar ways: (1) upward convexity of the gland as opposed to the normal upward concavity, (2) a height greater than 8 mm in the female and 7 mm in the male, (3) destruction of the sphenoid sinus, (4) a mass that extends from within the sella up into the suprasellar cistern. In addition to these changes, MR has the capability to demonstrate areas of hemorrhage within the tumor which appear as areas of increased signal intensity on the T-1 weighted images. This increased signal intensity is easy to appreciate on the MR scans and should be helpful in diagnosing pituitary apoplexy in those patients who present with acute onset of loss of vision. In addition, it is not uncommon for there to be areas of cyst formation within the gland which probably are caused by small areas of hemorrhage or infarction and result in areas of cystic necrosis within the gland. These appear as areas of decreased signal intensity on the T-1 weighted images but are especially easy to demonstrate on the T-2 weighted images, where the cystic areas appear as rounded increased signal intensity areas. These areas are different and higher in signal intensity than the remainder of the gland, which also increases in signal intensity on the T-2 weighted images. The identification of cystic areas allows one to alert the surgeon that these areas are present and can be aspirated at the time of surgery; this is helpful if only subtotal removal is possible. We use the SE TR3120/TE60-120 to excellent advantage when evaluating the pituitary fossa; the first echo TR3120/TE60 usually best demonstrates the cystic portions of the tumor as separate from the remainder of the enlarged gland. Again, the ready availability of multiplanar imaging allows excellent evaluation of the gland.

The exact location of the tumor and its relationship to surrounding structures are easily seen. This obviously allows for evaluation without the need for other invasive types of examinations such as metrizamide cisternography. While in the majority of cases surgery can be performed on the basis of CT and MR, occasionally angiography is necessary for evaluation. The ready demonstration with MR of the relationship to the optic chiasm, optic tracts, brain stem, and basilar artery, encroachment upon the suprasellar cistern, and subfrontal extension greatly facilitates the decision regarding the surgical approach and whether a transphenoidal or frontal craniotomy will be necessary.

One of the real benefits of MR imaging in the region of the pituitary is the fact that the carotid arteries appear as negative flow defects. Therefore, the exact relationship of the vessels to the tumor, the cavernous sinus, and other surrounding structures can be easily evaluated. The Technicare scanner generates the multiple slices in a predetermined fashion, i.e., from left to right; therefore, the amount of superior displacement of the carotid siphon can be readily

estimated from the sagittal slices. Also the lateral displacement as well as any superior displacement of the carotid arteries can be easily evaluated in coronal projection. As mentioned previously, the tumor appears as increased signal intensity on the T-2 weighted images and therefore can be easily demonstrated if it surrounds the negative flow defect of the carotid artery. This obviously makes preoperative evaluation of the feasibility of surgical tumor removal much easier and more accurate. In this regard MR is superior to CT because with the postinfusion portion of the CT scan, the tumor, the cavernous sinus, and the carotid artery all enhance homogeneously, making differentiation between these structures impossible.

Differential Diagnosis

Craniopharyngioma. These tumors are usually cystic. The cystic portion of the tumor may have either low or increased signal intensity on the T-1 weighted SE TR530/TE30 sequences. On the T-2 weighted SE TR3120/TE60-120 sequences the cyst demonstrates increased signal intensity in most cases. These tumors are not uncommonly calcified, and this area of calcification may or may not be demonstrated on the MR scan. They are often slightly lobulated in appearance.

Medial Sphenoid Wing or Diaphragma Sellae Meningioma. Meningiomas contain psammomatous calcifications and so are difficult to demonstrate on the MR scan. On the other hand, there is often surrounding edema that is readily demonstrated on the MR scan as areas of increased signal intensity. Therefore, the meningioma can be localized although it may not be directly demonstrated.

Carotid Artery Aneurysm. If the aneurysm is not clotted it is readily demonstrated as a negative flow defect on the MR scan. If the aneurysm is partially thrombosed, it will appear as an area of increased signal intensity, with the unthrombosed lumen appearing as an area of low signal intensity secondary to the negative flow defect.

Empty Sella Syndrome. This syndrome is more common in females than in males and clinically is associated with headaches and, rarely, decreased vision. There is commonly a minimal enlarged sella turcica, without marked erosion or areas of calcification. CT scanning reveals CSF density material within the enlarged sella turcica and a pituitary gland that is flattened and positioned in the very floor of the sella. The pituitary stalk is displaced posteriorly adjacent to the dorsum sellae. Magnetic resonance reveals CSF density material within the sella turcica. With older scanners that lack the ability to do thin, high-resolution sections, it may be difficult to evaluate these changes. If there is a question of a cystic mass in the sella that mimics an empty sella syndrome, then metrizamide cisternography may be necessary for complete evaluation.

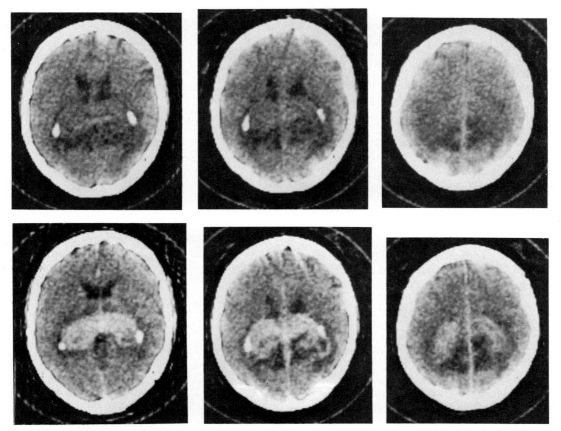

FIGURE 9–1. *Butterfly Glioblastoma:* The pre- and postinfusion scans demonstrate a large enhancing mass deep in the cerebral hemispheres. It exhibits a mixed pattern of high and low density on the preinfusion scan. The tumor extends from one hemisphere to the other via the corpus callosum in a classic "butterfly" distribution.

These tumors may be very difficult to demonstrate by angiography unless they exhibit neovascularity; however, they are beautifully outlined by the CT scan.

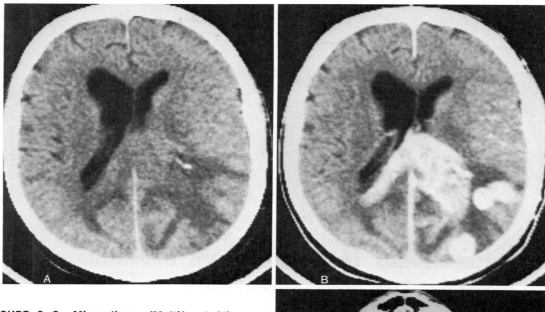

FIGURE 9–2. *Microglioma (Multifocal Glioma, Reticulum Cell Sarcoma, Lymphoma) of the Brain:* Sixty-five–year–old male with progressive confusion and headaches. *A,* Preinfusion CT scan demonstrates a mass that is isodense with the normal brain, has obliterated the posterior body of the left lateral ventricle, extends across the midline, and has irregular surrounding edema extending away from the mass along white matter pathways.

B, The postinfusion CT scan demonstrates dense enhancement of the mass and multiple parenchymal areas of enhancement peripheral to the main mass. The tumor extends across the midline via the splenium of the corpus callosum.

C, A slightly lower section reveals the periventricular distribution of the enhancement in a subependymal distribution as well as the side-to-side appearance in a "butterfly" distribution. The appearance is typical of microglioma of the brain, although metastatic disease may have a similar appearance. Treatment with steroids leads to marked clinical improvement in patients with microglioma, and a follow-up CT scan may reveal complete disappearance of the enhancing lesions, only to have the area of tumor recur several months later, often with an entirely different appearance and distribution.

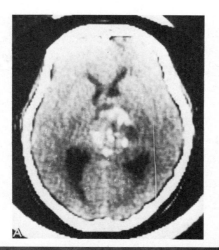

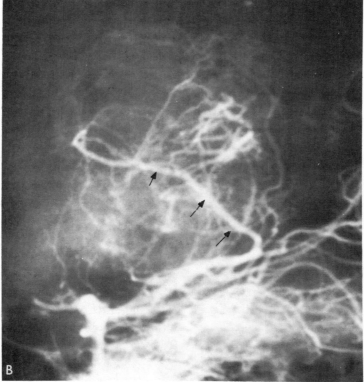

FIGURE 9–3. *Ependymoma:* *A*, The CT scan demonstrates an irregularly calcified mass arising in the region of the third ventricle and off to either side—slightly more on the right than the left. There are areas of both peripheral and central calcification. The third ventricle is compressed, and a curvilinear portion of the third ventricle projects just anterior to the mass. The frontal horns of the lateral ventricles are distorted by the mass, and there is mild obstructive hydrocephalus.

B, The lateral view of the vertebral angiogram reveals marked enlargement of the medial posterior choroidal vessels (*arrows*) and multiple small abnormal vessels that extend from this vessel to supply a large area of abnormal vascularity. There was no blood supply to the tumor from the carotid artery system.

Surgically proved ependymoma arising from the third ventricle. Differential diagnosis includes pinealoma, teratoma, astrocytoma, and oligodendroglioma. (Case courtesy of Dr. Gregory I. Shenk.)

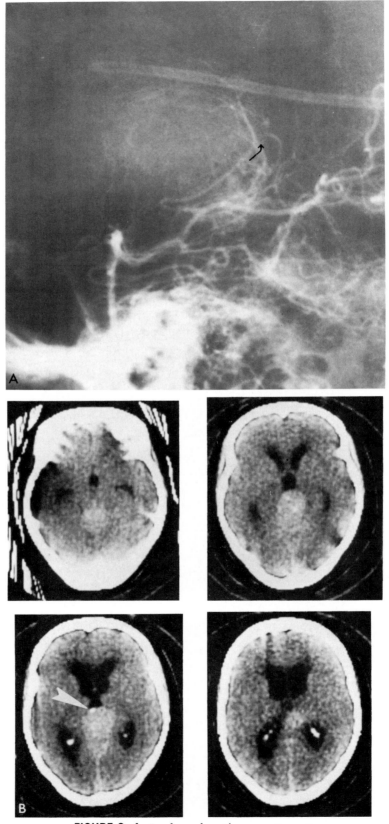

FIGURE 9–4. *See legend on the opposite page.*

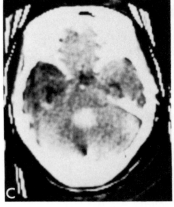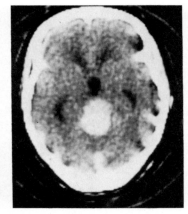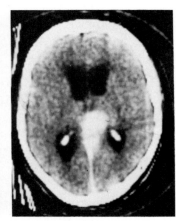

FIGURE 9–4. *Pinealoma: A,* The lateral view of the vertebral angiogram reveals enlargement of the medial posterior choroidal artery, which courses in a curvilinear fashion around the tumor mass (*arrow*). A very faint tumor blush is seen anterior to this vessel. The carotid angiogram revealed hydrocephalus but was otherwise unremarkable. A shunt tubing device is seen in place.

B, The preinfusion CT scan reveals a fairly well-defined mass in the region of the pineal gland which appears to displace the calcified pineal anteriorly (*arrow*). The mass appears to extend into the posterior fossa at the level of the tentorial notch.

C, There is marked homogeneous enhancement of the tumor on the postinfusion scans. There is moderate obstructive hydrocephalus.

Differential diagnosis includes pinealoma, aneurysm of the vein of Galen (unlikely), and metastasis.

Surgically proved pinealoma.

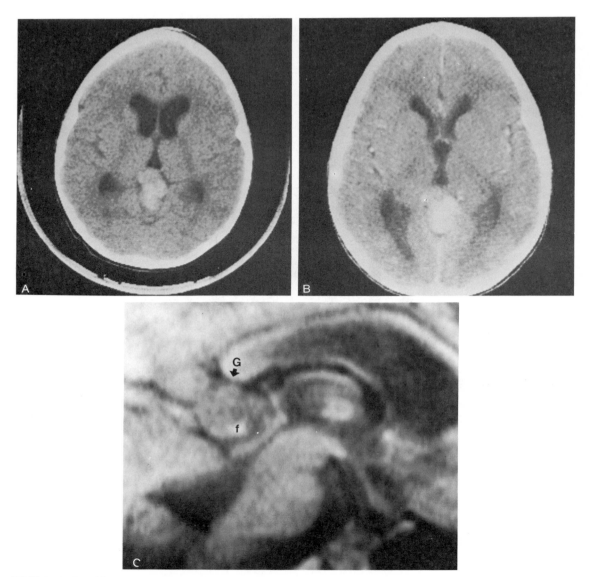

FIGURE 9–5. *Pinealoma:* Ten-year-old female with headache and vomiting. *A,* Preinfusion CT scan demonstrates a higher than normal brain density mass in the region of the pineal gland. The third ventricle is displaced anteriorly and effaced by the mass. There is moderate obstructive hydrocephalus secondary to obstruction of the outlet of the third ventricle and the sylvian aqueduct.

B, Postinfusion CT scan demonstrates dense enhancement of the mass.

C, Midsagittal SE TR530/TE30 image reveals an inhomogeneous signal intensity mass in the region of the pineal gland. The quadrigeminal plate is compressed and displaced anteriorly. The area of increased signal intensity within the mass is presumably an area of fat within the tumor mass. On the basis of CT and MR the patient was treated with radiation therapy to the region of the pineal gland and became symptom free. Approximately eight months later the patient presented with inability to walk, and repeat CT revealed moderately severe hydrocephalus and bilateral to extracerebral low-density collections. CSF obtained at the time of shunt placement revealed tumor cells. The vein of Galen is seen as a negative flow defect (*G*). The fourth ventricle is also seen (*f*).

Illustration continued on the following page

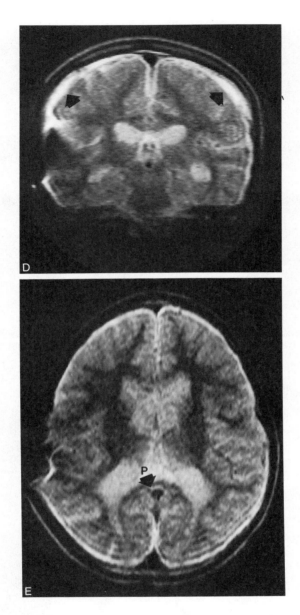

FIGURE 9–5 *Continued.*

D and *E*, MR in the coronal and axial planes with SE TR3120/TE120 reveals the enlarged lateral ventricles, the bilateral increased signal intensity, extracerebral collections (*arrows*), and prominence of the white matter secondary to the radiation treatment. Artifacts along the periphery of the scan in both views are secondary to distortion of the field by the metal in the shunt tubing device. The patient now has carcinomatous meningitis. It is not uncommon to see suprasellar or spinal metastases with pineal type tumors. Meningeal carcinomatosis is less common. The pineal (*P*) is normal in size.

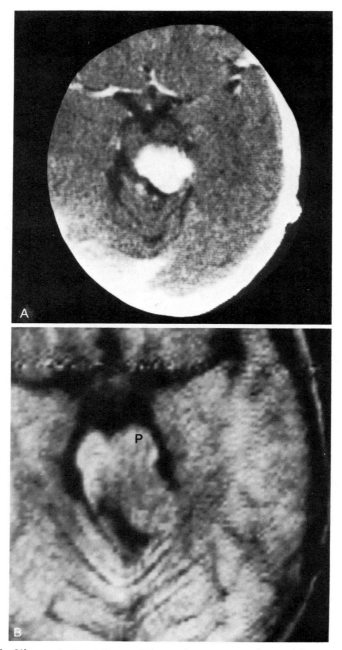

FIGURE 9–6. *Midbrain Glioma:* *A,* Postinfusion CT scan demonstrates dense enhancement of the tumor mass arising from the left side of the midbrain in the region of the quadrigeminal plate. The mass compromises the ambient and superior cerebellar cisterns.

B, SE TR530/TE30 images exquisitely demonstrate the exophytic nature of this midbrain glioma. The mass arises from the left side of the midbrain, enlarges the left cerebral peduncle (*P*), and extends into the ambient (perimesencephalic) cistern.

Illustration continued on the following page

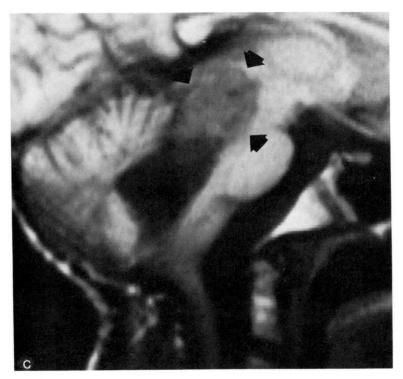

FIGURE 9–6 *Continued.*
C, Midsagittal SE TR530/TE30 image demonstrates the mass as a lower than normal signal intensity mass arising from the dorsal aspect of the midbrain (*arrows*), distorting the quadrigeminal plate beyond recognition and extending into the quadrigeminal plate cistern. Surgically proved glioma.

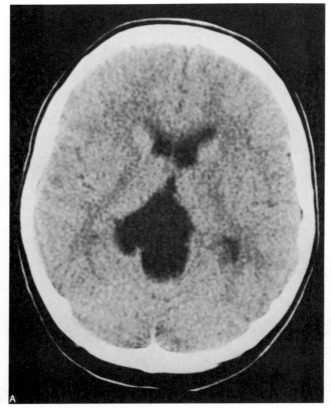

FIGURE 9–7. *Quadrigeminal Plate Cyst:* Twelve-year-old male with headaches. A, Preinfusion CT scan demonstrates a slightly lobulated CSF density mass in the region of the quadrigeminal plate cistern. There was no enhancement on the postinfusion portion of the examination.

Illustration continued on the following page

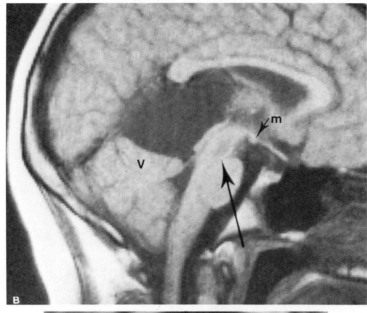

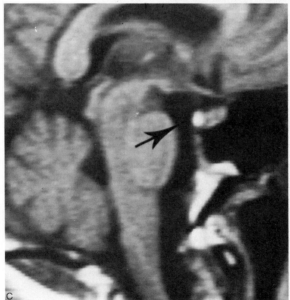

FIGURE 9–7 *Continued.*

B, Midsagittal SE TR530/TE30 image demonstrates the cystic structure in the region of the quadrigeminal plate cistern. The anterior vermis (*V*) is effaced and compressed inferiorly. The quadrigeminal plate is compressed and elongated, and the sylvian aqueduct is narrowed. The large arrow indicates the red nucleus in the midbrain. The mammillary bodies are also well seen (*m*).

C, The normal SE TR530/TE30 image is shown for comparison. The arrow illustrates the high signal intensity from a small amount of fat that can be seen in the posterior portion of the sella turcica. The pituitary stalk can be faintly seen extending directly superiorly from the small area of fat. The appearance is typical of a quadrigeminal plate cyst.

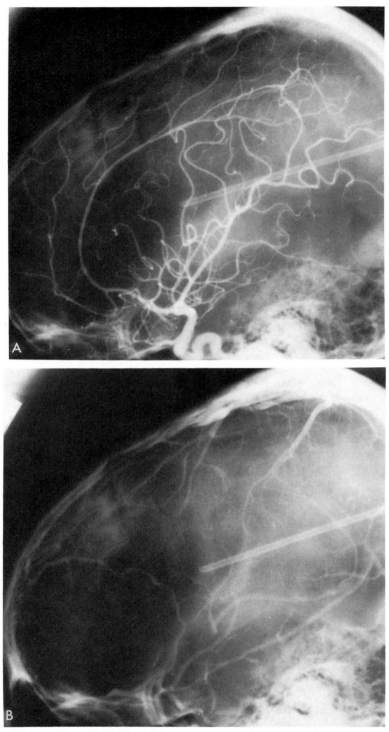

FIGURE 9–8. *Colloid Cyst of the Third Ventricle:* Colloid cysts that arise in the anterior third ventricle have been shown to develop from residual epithelial cells of the paraphysis in the anterior portion of the third ventricle. The arterial (*A*) and venous (*B*) phases of the carotid angiogram reveal marked hydrocephalus but are otherwise unremarkable. The venous phase AP (not shown) demonstrated that the internal cerebral veins are displaced apart by the large mass lesion growing between them.

Illustration continued on the following page

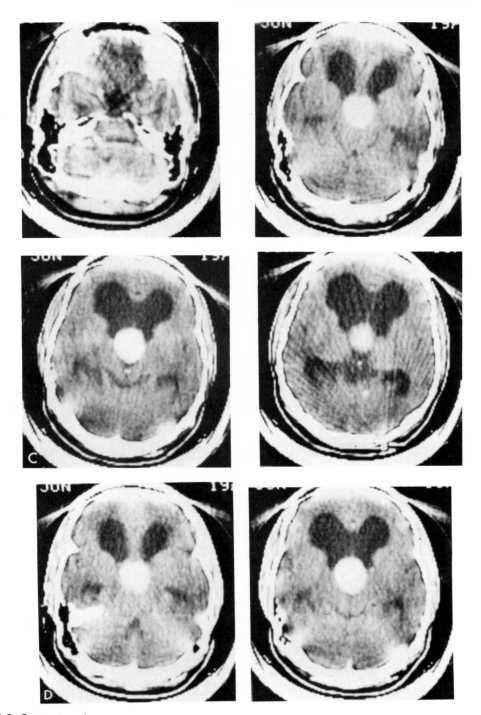

FIGURE 9–8 *Continued.*

C, The preinfusion CT scans reveal a large, high-density mass in the midline occupying the position of the third ventricle and leading to obstructive hydrocephalus secondary to bilateral blockage of the foramen of Monro. There is marked obstructive hydrocephalus.

Choroid plexus papillomas also may develop in the third ventricle and may at times cause unilateral occlusion of the foramen of Monro as it leads into the lateral ventricles. Patients with choroid plexus papillomas may have positional headache because of an intermittent obstruction of the foramen of Monro that leads to ipsilateral hydrocephalus when the patient assumes a certain position.

D, No change is seen following the infusion of contrast material.

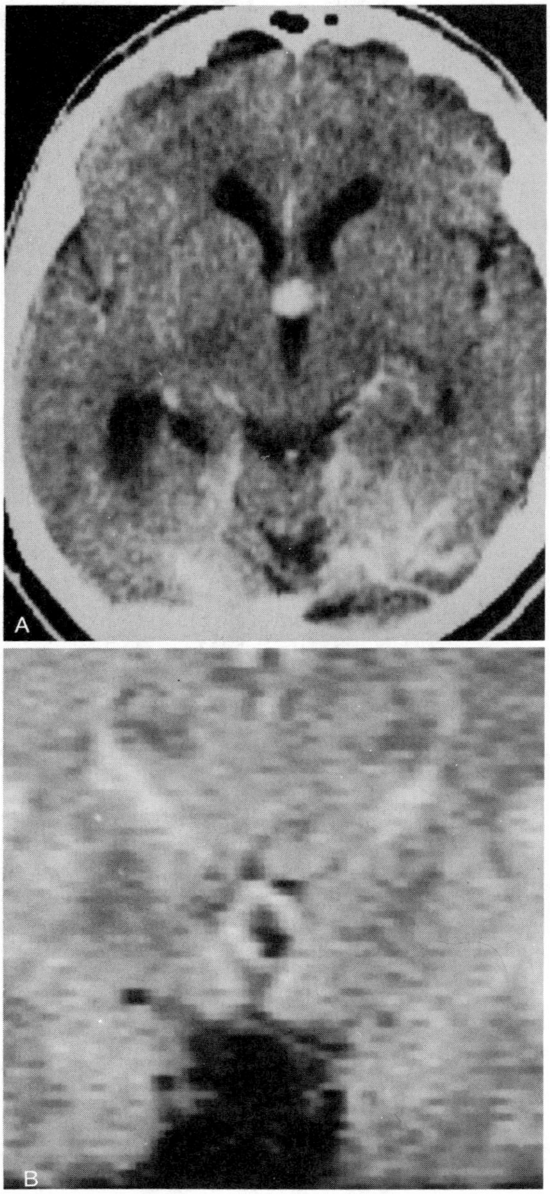

FIGURE 9–9. ***Colloid Cyst of the Third Ventricle:*** Thirty-six–year–old female with increasing headaches. *A*, Postinfusion CT scan at the level of the foramen of Monro demonstrates a densely enhancing 1-cm mass that arises from within the third ventricle along its anterior margin.

B, SE TR3120/TE60 image in the coronal plane reveals that the colloid cyst appears as an increased signal intensity mass with a low signal intensity central nidus. The enlarged lateral ventricles are isodense with this SE sequence.

Illustration continued on the following page

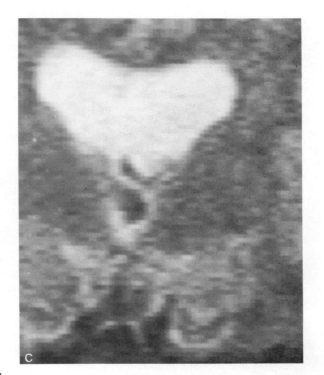

FIGURE 9–9 *Continued.*

C, The SE TR3120/TE120 image in the coronal plane continues to demonstrate the "target" lesion of the colloid cyst. The enlarged lateral ventricles now appear of increased signal intensity because the TR is long and the TE is now greater than 90 milliseconds. The author has had the opportunity to study one additional case of colloid cyst of the third ventricle that had a similar MR appearance. Surgically proved.

Examination of colloid cysts by CT reveals that these masses, which arise in the anterior portion of the third ventricle, may be isodense or of higher than normal brain density on the preinfusion scan. Colloid cysts usually, but not always, enhance on the postinfusion portion of the examination.

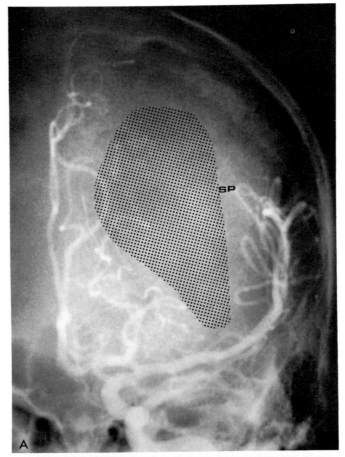

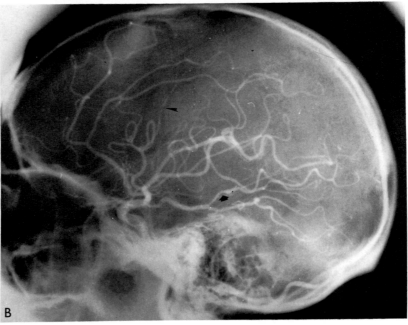

FIGURE 9–10. *See legend on the opposite page.*

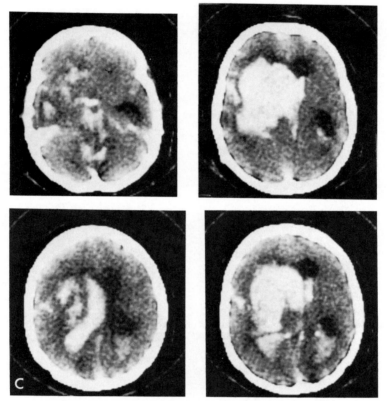

FIGURE 9–10. *Basal Ganglionic Hemorrhage:* A, The AP view of the carotid angiogram reveals shift of the anterior cerebral artery to the contralateral side, more marked in the mid- and distal portions than in the proximal. The sylvian point and the middle cerebral artery branches are displaced laterally (*SP*); the shaded area outlines the approximate position of the bulk of the basal ganglionic hemorrhage.

B, The lateral view demonstrates widening of the sweep of the pericallosal artery. The sylvian triangle appears to be in a relatively normal position. Branches of the middle cerebral artery and the posterior cerebral artery show areas of focal spasm secondary to blood in the subarachnoid space (*arrows*).

C, The CT scans demonstrate a large basal ganglionic hematoma. In addition, there is rupture into the ventricular system, with blood in the lateral, third, and fourth ventricles. There is blood in the dependent portions of the lateral ventricles, giving the appearance of blood/CSF fluid levels. The hemorrhage has also ruptured into the subarachnoid space and can be seen outlining multiple cortical sulci.

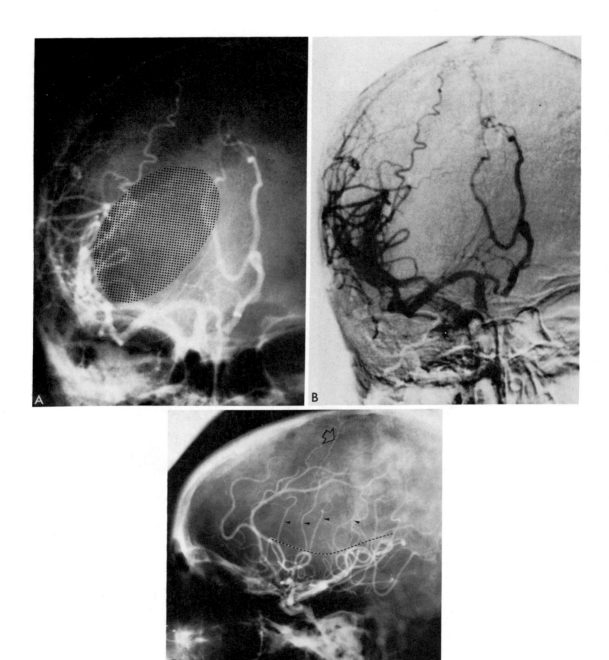

FIGURE 9–11. *See legend on the opposite page.*

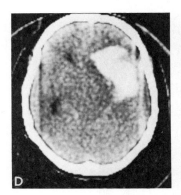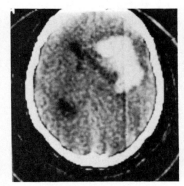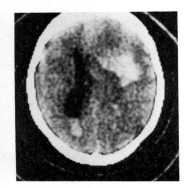

FIGURE 9–11. *Basal Ganglionic Hemorrhage:* A, The AP view of the carotid angiogram reveals both proximal and distal shift of the pericallosal artery. There is lateral displacement of the sylvian point and the remaining branches of the middle cerebral artery as they run in the isle of Reil. The shaded area outlines the approximate position of a large avascular mass in the region of a putamen of the basal ganglia. The lenticulostriate arteries are displaced medially by the mass.

B, The subtraction view of the angiogram better demonstrates the lenticulostriate arteries and the large avascular area in the region of the putamen. There is spasm of the distal horizontal portion of the middle cerebral artery.

C, The lateral view demonstrates downward displacement of the midportion of the sylvian triangle (*dashed line*) and stretching of all the opercular branches of the middle cerebral artery in the posterior frontal and anterior parietal regions (*arrows*). The mass extends high up to affect these vessels. The meningeal artery is quite prominent, probably because of excessive filling of the external carotid artery system secondary to increased intracranial pressure.

D, The CT scans demonstrate a large intracerebral hematoma in the region of the putamen of the basal ganglia. The isle of Reil is poorly visualized but is displaced laterally. The hematoma has ruptured into the ventricular system and demonstrates a blood/CSF level in the dependent portion of the right lateral ventricle. There is shift to the opposite side and dilatation of the left lateral ventricle.

IMP: Classic hypertensive basal ganglionic hemorrhage.

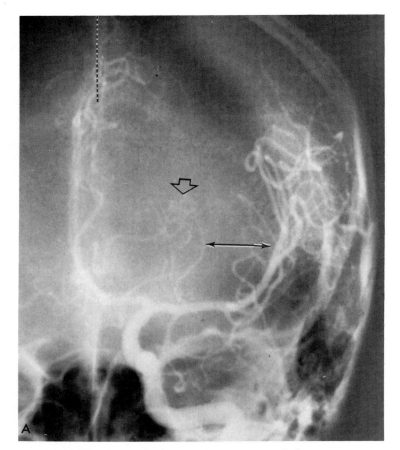

FIGURE 9–12. *Basal Ganglionic Hemorrhage:* A, The AP view of the angiogram reveals an increased distance between the anterior cerebral and middle cerebral arteries as well as medial displacement of the lenticulostriate arteries (*double-headed arrow*). There is a proximal and distal shift of the anterior cerebral artery and its branches. The distal portions of the lenticulostriate arteries appear to be dilated and tortuous (*open arrow*), perhaps reflecting small aneurysm formation thought to be responsible for these hypertensive basal ganglionic hemorrhages. Dotted line marks the normal falx.

B, The CT scans show a large basal ganglionic hemorrhage that has ruptured into the ventricular system. Clotted blood is also present in the fourth ventricle.

C, The pathologic specimen demonstrates a classic basal ganglionic hemorrhage.

Illustration continued on the following page

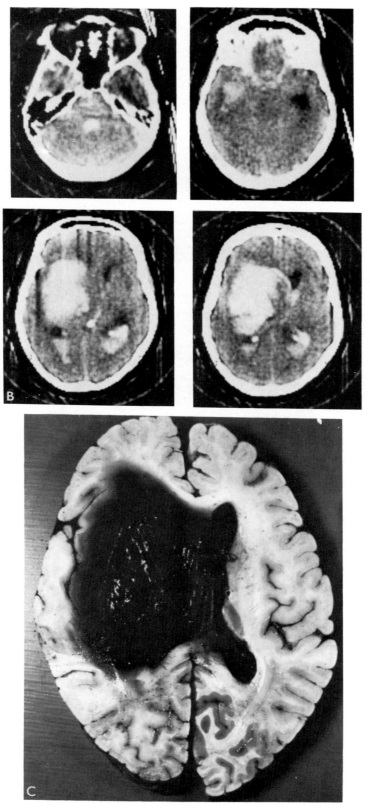

FIGURE 9–12 *Continued.*

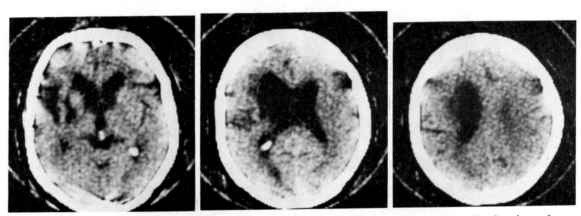

FIGURE 9–13. *Old Basal Ganglionic Hemorrhage:* With time, the hemorrhage ultimately absorbs and may lead to the development of a closed porencephalic cyst in the bed of the hematoma. In this example there is also enlargement of the right lateral ventricle and cortical sulci on the side of the hematoma, secondary to atrophy.

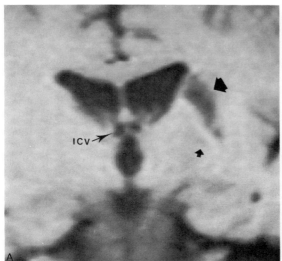

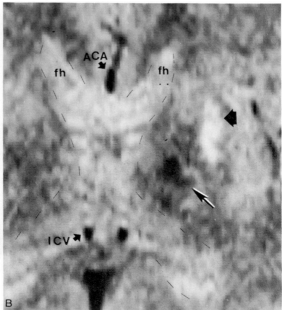

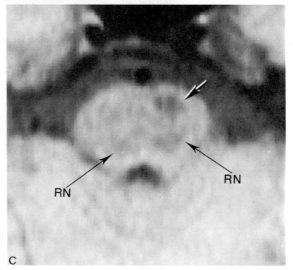

FIGURE 9–14. *MR of Old Basal Ganglia Hematoma:*
A, Coronal SE TR530/TE30 image reveals the wedge-shaped area of decreased signal intensity in the putamen of the basal ganglia on the left side (*large arrow*). This represents a postinfarction area of encephalomalacia and/or porencephaly. There is also a second faint area of decreased signal intensity (*small arrow*) that is believed to be iron from an ancient area of hemorrhage. The internal cerebral veins (*ICV*) appear as two small negative flow defects adjacent to the midline.

B, Axial SE TR3120/TE120 image demonstrates that the area of encephalomalacia is not increased in signal intensity (*large arrow*), while the area of residual iron deposition secondary to hemorrhage appears as low signal intensity (*black and white arrow*) because of its paramagnetic effect. The dashed lines outline the lateral ventricles. The frontal horns (*fh*), anterior cerebral arteries (*ACA*), and internal cerebral veins (*ICV*) are all visible.

C, The axial SE TR530/TE30 image at the level of the pons also demonstrates the residue of the previous hemorrhage with a small area of iron deposition in the anterior portion of the pons (*black and white arrow*). The red nucleus appears as an area of low signal intensity (*RN*) which is rounded in contour. The substantia nigra is located just anterior to the red nucleus and is linear in configuration. The fourth ventricle appears as an area of low signal intensity dorsal to the pons and triangular in shape.

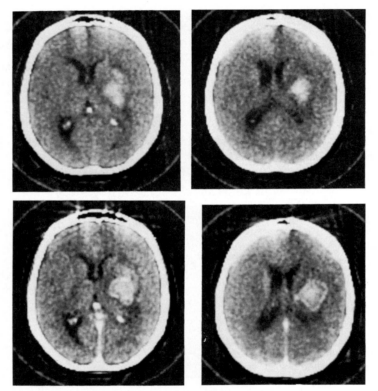

FIGURE 9–15. *Resolving Basal Ganglionic Hematoma:* The CT scans reveal a partially resorbed basal ganglionic hematoma on the left side. There is a small amount of surrounding edema and slight compression of the body of the left lateral ventricle. The postinfusion scan demonstrates a ring of enhancement around the hematoma—a finding not uncommonly seen with resorbing hematoma.

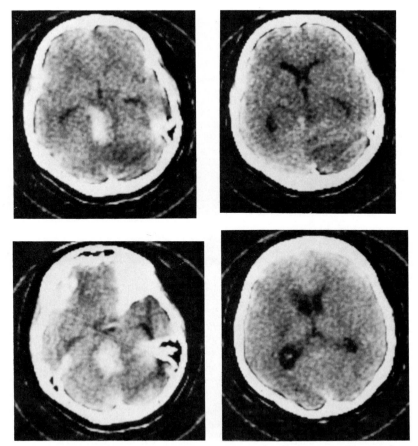

FIGURE 9–16. *Pontine Hemorrhage:* The CT scans demonstrate a large area of hemorrhage in the pons that extends superiorly to involve the right cerebral peduncle. There is a small amount of blood in the dependent portions of the lateral ventricles, creating blood/CSF levels. There is moderate obstructive hydrocephalus.

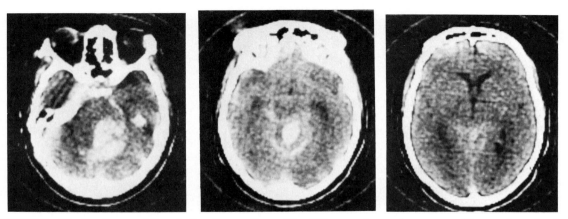

FIGURE 9–17. *Pontine and Cerebellar Hemorrhage:* The CT scans show a large area of hemorrhage in the left cerebellum and the left side of the pons. The blood also has entered the subarachnoid space; it outlines the basilar cistern in the posterior fossa and fills the cerebellar folia.

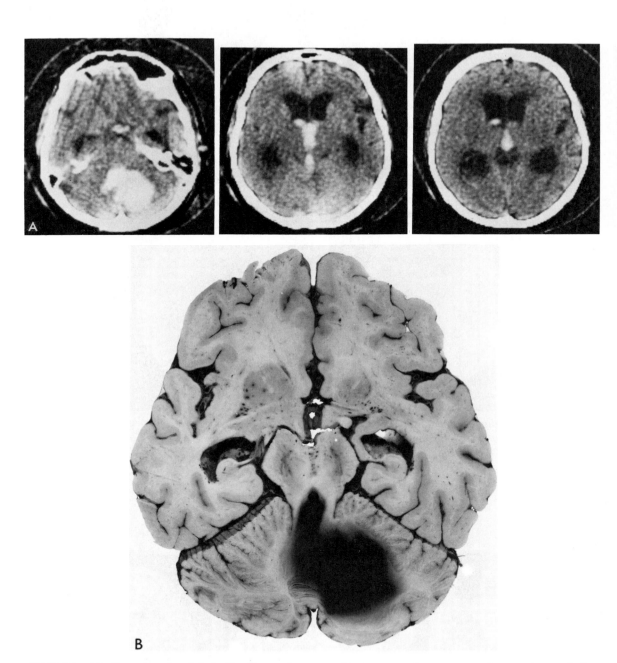

FIGURE 9–18. *Hypertensive Cerebellar Hemorrhage:* A, The CT scans demonstrate a large right cerebellar hematoma. The hemorrhage has ruptured into the fourth ventricle, and clotted blood is also present in the third and lateral ventricles. There is moderately severe obstructive hydrocephalus. The pathologic specimen (B) shows the precise correlation between the CT scan and the pathologic anatomy (viewed from above to match pathologic specimen).

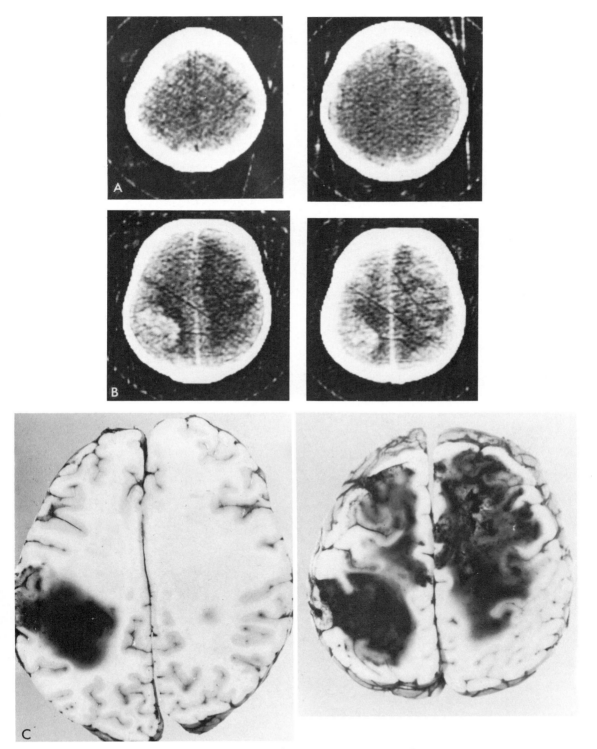

FIGURE 9–19. *Superior Sagittal Sinus Thrombosis:* A, The initial CT study appears within normal limits. One week later (B), a second CT scan demonstrates an irregular area of hemorrhage in the left posterior parietal region and large areas of radiolucency throughout both hemispheres—slightly more marked on the right side than on the left. The falx is displaced in a curvilinear fashion toward the left side.

C, The pathologic specimen reveals large areas of hemorrhage in the high parietal regions bilaterally as well as marked edema of both cerebral hemispheres. There was also evidence of superior sagittal sinus thrombosis and bilateral cortical vein thrombosis. The areas of hemorrhage occur in the distribution of the occluded cortical veins, resembling a hemorrhagic infarct (viewed from above).

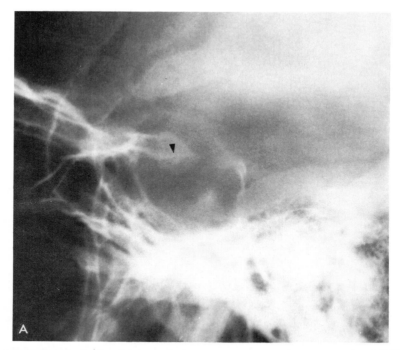

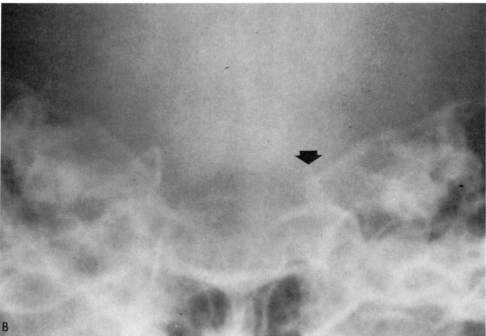

FIGURE 9–20. *Pituitary Adenoma:* The lateral and AP views (*A* and *B*) of the sella reveal that the sella turcica is enlarged and that the posterior clinoids and the dorsum sellae are thinned and displaced posteriorly. Undercutting of one of the anterior clinoids is seen on both views (*arrows*). Both anterior clinoids are also thinned along their medial margins secondary to the enlarging intrasellar tumor.

Illustration continued on the following page

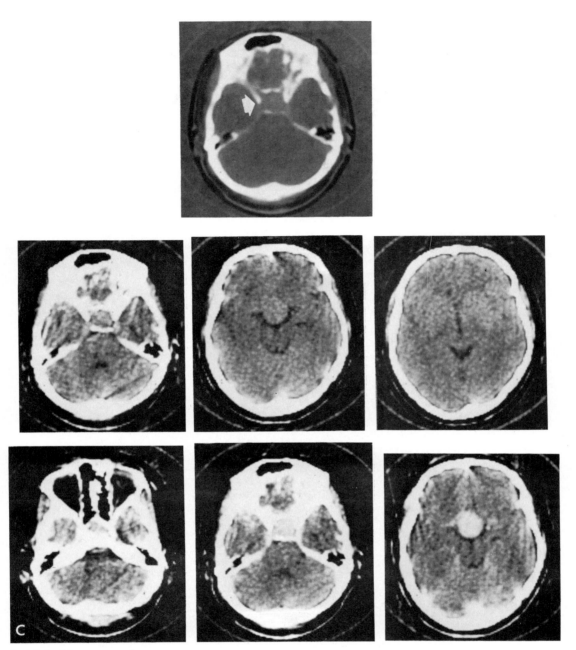

FIGURE 9–20 *Continued.*

C, CT scans of the region of the bony sella show the enlargement of the sella; they also confirm the presence of erosion of the medial side of the anterior clinoid process (*arrow*). A mass is visible in the region of the sella; it extends up into the suprasellar cistern, which is obliterated. The postinfusion scan demonstrates marked enhancement of the tumor in a homogeneous fashion.

Surgically proved adenoma of the pituitary.

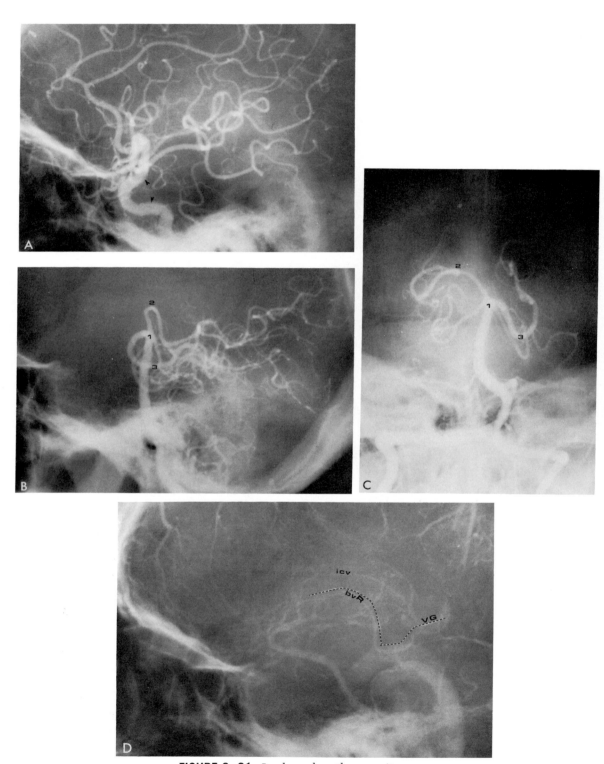

FIGURE 9–21. *See legend on the opposite page.*

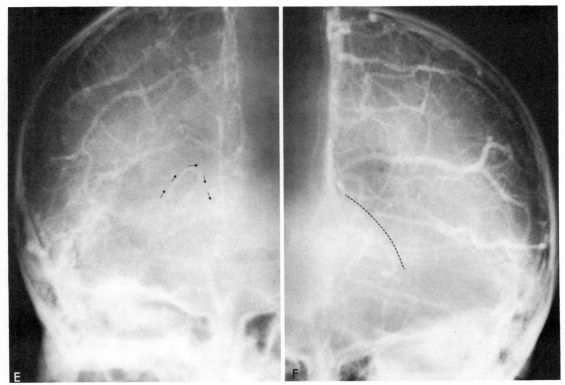

FIGURE 9–21. *Pituitary Adenoma:* *A,* The carotid angiogram demonstrates opening of the carotid siphon (*arrows*). No abnormal vessels are seen.

B and *C,* AP and lateral views of the vertebral angiogram show the enlarged sella and (*1*) tip of basilar artery; (*2*) highest portion of the superiorly displaced posterior cerebral artery on the right side; (*3*) the normal course of the posterior cerebral artery on the left side.

On the right side, the pituitary tumor has grown into the suprasellar cistern and posteriorly to such an extent that it affects the posterior cerebral artery, which passes in curvilinear fashion up, over, and around the adenoma.

D, The lateral view of the venous phase demonstrates the marked superior displacement of the anterior and midportions of the basal vein of Rosenthal (*bvR*) as it courses over the lateral extent of the tumor on the right side. The internal cerebral vein is also superiorly displaced (*icv*). Both veins join to form the vein of Galen (*VG*).

E and *F,* The AP views also demonstrate the superior displacement of the basal vein of Rosenthal on the right side (*small arrows*) and the normal course of the basal vein on the left side (*dashed line*).

Illustration continued on the following page

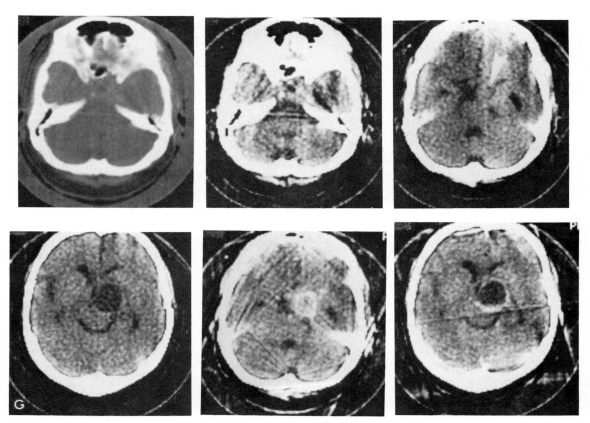

FIGURE 9–21 *Continued.*

G, CT scans of the region of the sella confirm the presence of a large sella and show evidence of a tumor mass in the region of the sella that is both solid (*white arrow*) and cystic in its superior portion and larger on the right side than on the left. The third ventricle is displaced to the left. The postinfusion scan demonstrates homogeneous enhancement of the solid portion of the tumor and a ring of enhancement around the cystic mass on the right side (viewed from above).

Surgically proved partially cystic chromophobe adenoma.

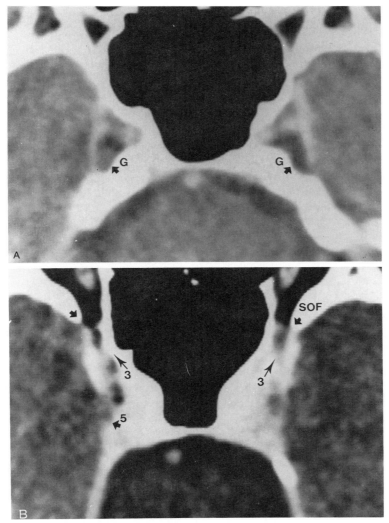

FIGURE 9–22. *Normal Anatomy Around the Sella Turcica:* A, CT slice at the level of the well-aerated sphenoid sinus reveals that the cavernous sinus is opacified by contrast material bilaterally, and the gasserian ganglion is identified (G) as it projects into the cavernous sinus posteriorly. The gasserian ganglion is not seen on all CT scans but can usually be identified on thin-section, high-resolution slices. The ganglion can also be identified on coronal sections and should not be mistaken for a tumor mass. The basilar artery is seen as a dotlike area of enhancement in the midline just anterior to the pons.

B, CT slice through the cavernous sinus demonstrates the oculomotor nerve (cranial nerve III, labeled "3") as it is embedded in the superolateral wall of the cavernous sinus. The oculomotor nerve courses anteriorly, from its point of origin between the midbrain and pons, between the posterior cerebral artery and the superior cerebellar artery in the wall of the cavernous sinus, and enters the orbit via the superior orbital fissure (SOF). A small portion of the gasserian ganglion is also seen (5).

Illustration continued on the following page

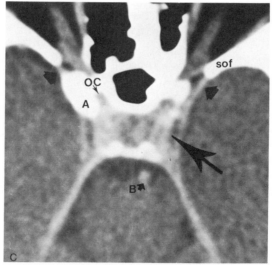

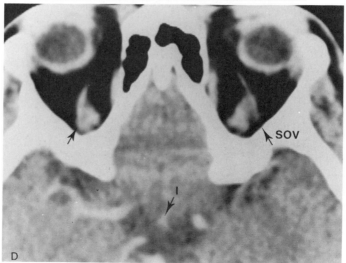

FIGURE 9–22 *Continued.*

C, The patient is positioned slightly asymmetrically in the scanner and therefore demonstrates the optic canal on only one side (*OC*) and the superior orbital fissure on the opposite side (*sof*), as well as on the ipsilateral side (*large arrowheads*). The anterior clinoid can be seen (*A*) on the same side as the optic canal, and the optic nerve can be seen coursing through the optic canal to enter the orbit. The oculomotor (III) nerve is again identified in the wall of the cavernous sinus (*large arrow*). Within the sella there is CSF density material as well as enhancement of the pituitary gland in the floor of the sella. The basilar artery is also enhancing (*B*). Note that the cavernous sinus is *concave* laterally, the normal configuration.

D, The infundibulum enhances (*I*), and the superior ophthalmic veins (*SOV*) can also be seen as they course obliquely across the orbit to exit via the superior orbital fissure and enter into the cavernous sinus.

Illustration continued on the following page

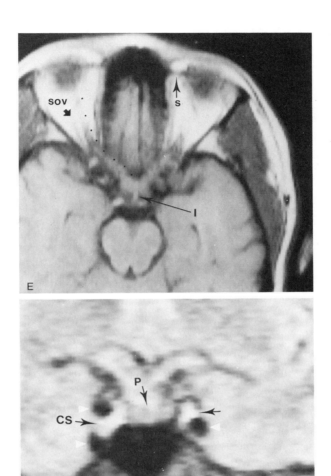

FIGURE 9–22 *Continued.*

E, Magnetic resonance of the orbit using the SE TR530/TE30 technique demonstrates that the retro-orbital fat has increased signal intensity. The superior ophthalmic vein can be faintly visualized as it crosses the optic nerve (*SOV*). The course of the optic nerve can be identified by the dotted line along the medial side of the nerve. The infundibulum appears as an area of relatively high signal intensity because of slow blood flow in the venous plexus and projects just posterior to the optic chiasm. Both optic nerves are enlarged, as is the optic chiasm, but are illustrated here for demonstration purposes. Incidentally, the orbital septum (*S*) can also be seen (see Chapter 12, The Orbit).

F, Coronal MR, SE TR530/TE30 image through the region of the sella demonstrates the pituitary gland in the floor of the sella (*P*), with its normally concave upward superior margin. The carotid arteries in the region of the carotid siphon appear as negative flow defects (*white triangles*), and the cavernous sinus (*CS*) appears of high signal intensity, probably because of slow blood flow. The supraclinoid carotid arteries as well as the horizontal portions of the anterior and middle cerebral arteries are visualized as negative flow defects. The exact relationship between the pituitary, the sella, and the surrounding vascular structures is readily appreciated. The advantage of MR, which does not require the injection of contrast material, is obvious.

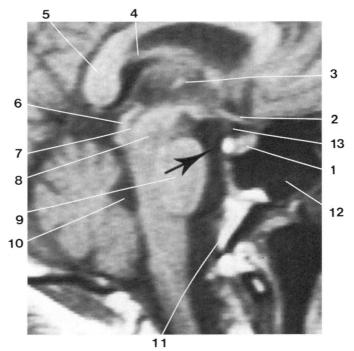

FIGURE 9–23. The normal SE TR530/TE30 midsagittal image delineates the normal anatomy to excellent advantage. Structures that can be identified are:

1 Pituitary gland.	8 Midbrain.
2 Optic chiasm and tract.	9 Pons.
3 Massa intermedia.	10 Fourth ventricle.
4 Fornix.	11 Fat in clivus.
5 Splenium of corpus callosum.	12 Air in sphenoid sinus.
6 Quadrigeminal plate.	13 Pituitary stalk (infundibulum).
7 Aqueduct.	

The arrow illustrates the small collection of fat in the posterior portion of the pituitary fossa—a normal finding.

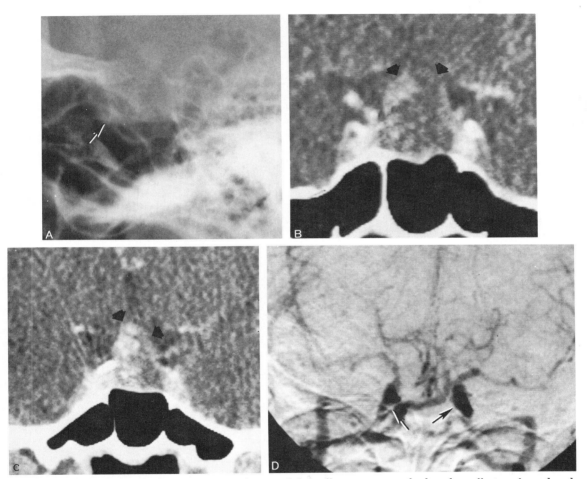

FIGURE 9–24. *Pituitary Adenoma:* *A,* Lateral view of the sella turcica reveals that the sella is enlarged and the floor, the posterior clinoids, and the dorsum sellae are eroded and no longer visible. A soft tissue mass extends into the sphenoid sinus (*arrow*).

B and *C,* The coronal CT scan performed with high-resolution, thin-section cuts (obtained post-DISA) demonstrates the intrasellar mass that extends up into the suprasellar cistern. The tumor is both cystic and solid and therefore enhances inhomogeneously. Arrowheads mark the superior extent of the tumor.

D, DISA (digital intravenous subtraction angiography) reveals no aneurysm and demonstrates that the cavernous portions of the carotid arteries are displaced laterally bilaterally (*arrows*). Surgically proved partially cystic pituitary adenoma.

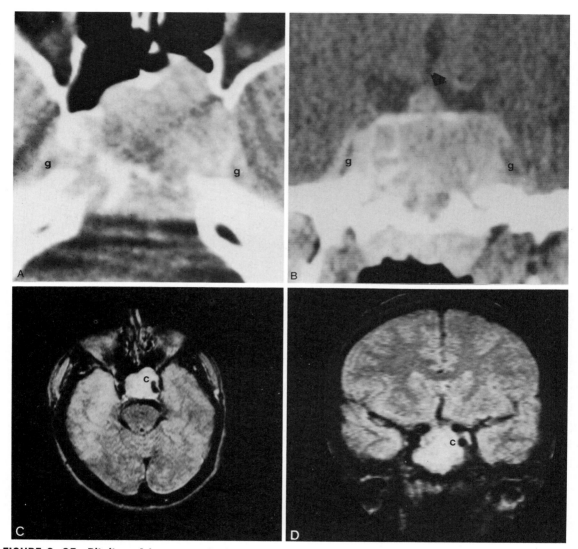

FIGURE 9–25. *Pituitary Adenoma:* Fifty-five–year–old male with panhypopituitarism. *A,* Postinfusion axial CT scan reveals a large intrasellar mass that has eroded the floor of the sella, the dorsum sellae, and posterior clinoids and extends into the sphenoid sinus.

B, The coronal CT scan demonstrates the intrasellar mass that projects in the midline into the suprasellar cistern (*arrow*). The gasserian ganglion (*g*) is seen as a low-density filling defect within the cavernous sinus on both the axial and the coronal images.

C and *D,* The SE TR2120/TE60 images in the axial and coronal planes reveal the pituitary tumor as an area of increased signal intensity. The tumor is larger on one side and encases the carotid artery. The cavernous carotid artery is identified as a negative flow defect in both the axial and the coronal planes (*C*). One of the advantages of MR is this ability of easy differentiation between the tumor and the carotid artery, both of which enhance on the postinfusion CT scan.

Illustration continued on the following page

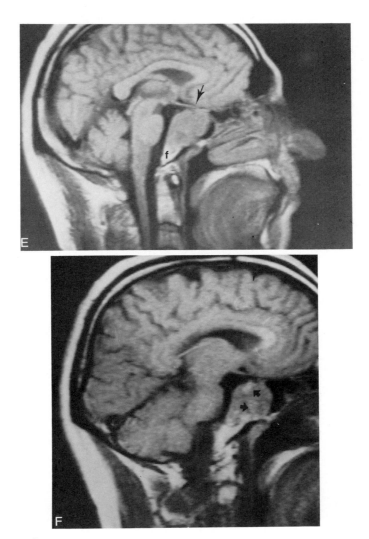

FIGURE 9–25 *Continued.*

E, SE TR530/TE30 image reveals the large mass, which has destroyed the floor of the sella, the posterior clinoids, and the dorsum sellae. The mass extends inferiorly into the clivus and has replaced most of the fatty marrow of the clivus (*f*) with tumor tissue. The optic chiasm and optic tracts are stretched and displaced superiorly (*arrow*).

F, SE TR120/TE60 image reveals mottled signal intensity of the tumor. The areas of increased signal intensity (*arrows*) are secondary to areas of cyst formation, probably related to old hemorrhage. Surgically proved pituitary adenoma.

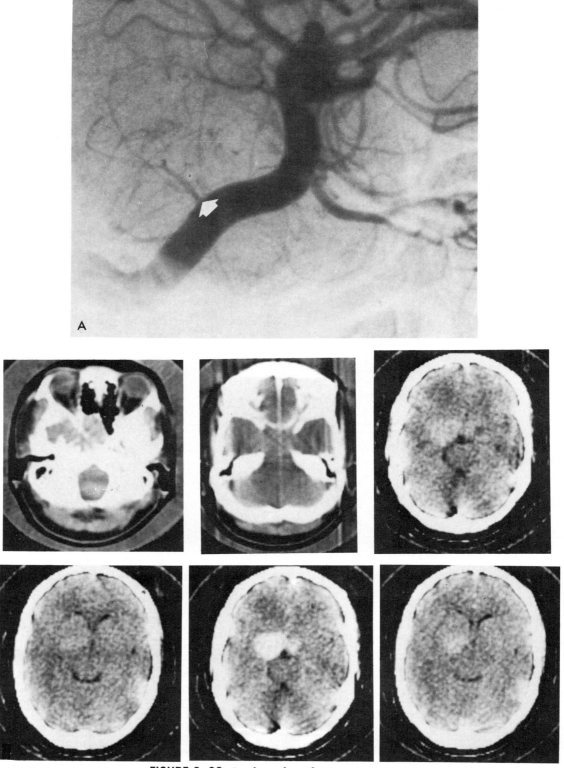

FIGURE 9–26. *See legend on the opposite page.*

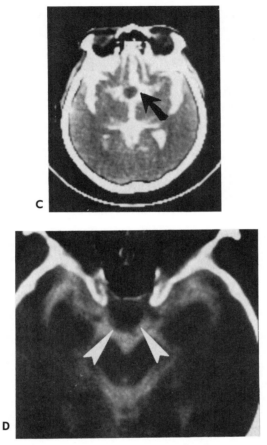

FIGURE 9–26. *Pituitary Adenoma:* *A*, Using magnification and subtraction techniques, the lateral view of the carotid angiogram demonstrates opening of the carotid siphon and an enlarged meningohypophyseal trunk that has multiple small vessels distributed in a curvilinear fashion around the pituitary tumor (*white arrow*).

B, The CT scans show the enlarged sella turcica, which is larger on the right side than on the left; there is a well-defined, bilobed rounded mass in the region of the sella that extends to the right of the sella. The mass is of higher than normal brain density on the preinfusion scan. Postinfusion, there is marked homogeneous enhancement of the bilobed tumor, which extends up into the suprasellar cisterns.

C, This CT scan from another patient was obtained after the instillation of 5 cc of 180 mg of I/cc solution of Amipaque. The CT scan demonstrates a mass lesion (*arrow*) extending up into the suprasellar cistern.

D, The adenoma appears as a lucent lesion bathed by the higher density Amipaque in the suprasellar cistern (*arrowheads*).

Differential diagnosis includes meningioma as well as pituitary adenoma. Surgically proved pituitary adenoma.

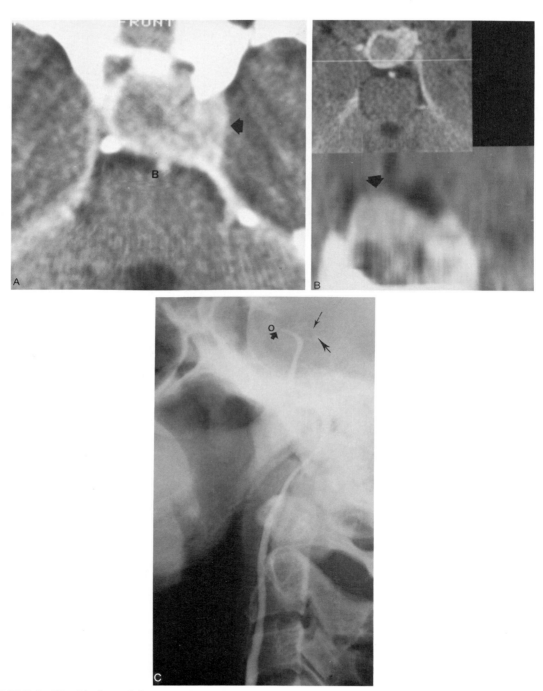

FIGURE 9–27. *Pituitary Adenoma:* Twenty-four–year–old female with amenorrhea and bitemporal hemianopsia and diplopia. *A,* Axial postinfusion CT scan reveals an intrasellar mass, larger on the left side, with lateral convexity of the cavernous sinus on the ipsilateral side secondary to involvement with tumor (*arrow*). The dorsum sellae and posterior clinoids are destroyed. The basilar artery is displaced posteriorly (*B*).

B, Coronal reconstruction image demonstrates the suprasellar extension of the tumor (*arrow*).

C, Right internal carotid angiography reveals that the IAC on the right side is small in size, demonstrates very slow flow, and tapers to occlusion (*o*) at the level of the cavernous sinus with only a few twiglike branches that supply the tumor (*arrows*).

Illustration continued on the following page

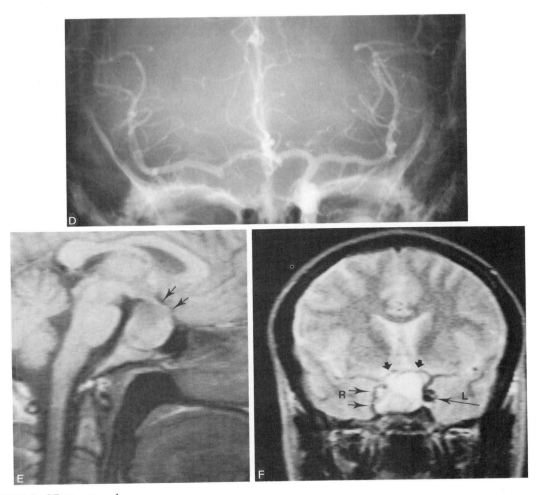

FIGURE 9–27 *Continued.*

D, AP left carotid angiogram reveals cross-over to fill the right internal carotid distribution.

E, SE TR530/TE30 image reveals the mottled signal intensity mass within the sella and extending into the suprasellar cistern. The optic chiasm and optic tracts are displaced superiorly (*arrows*). The tumor extends into the sphenoid sinus and clivus.

F, The coronal SE TR3120/TE120 image reveals that the relatively lower signal intensity seen in the upper portion of the tumor on the T-1 weighted midsagittal image (*E*) now appears as an area of increased signal intensity and is higher in signal intensity than the CSF in the lateral ventricles. This was a cystic portion of the pituitary adenoma at surgery. The left carotid artery is seen as a negative flow defect and is laterally displaced by the cystic and solid portions of the adenoma (*long arrow*). The right cavernous carotid artery is displaced far laterally, the floor of the sella is depressed more on the right than the left side, and the artery demonstrates less negative flow than the contralateral side; these findings correlate with the right carotid angiogram, which reveals markedly decreased flow and terminal occlusion. The horizontal portions of the anterior cerebral arteries are displaced superiorly and appear as negative flow defects on the T-2 weighted image (*arrowheads*). Surgery via frontal craniotomy revealed multiple cystic areas within the tumor and demonstrated that the right internal carotid artery was encased by tumor. The nerves within the cavernous sinus were also encased by tumor, and this had resulted in inability to move the extraocular muscles and therefore the clinical presentation of diplopia.

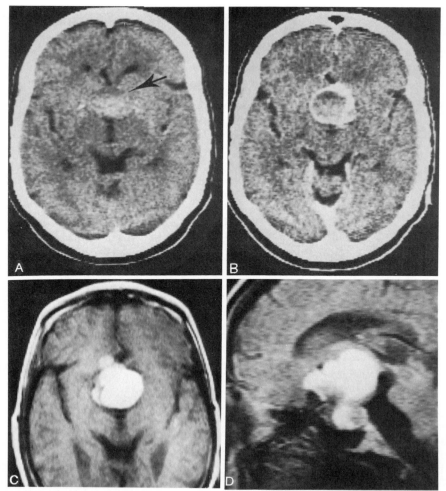

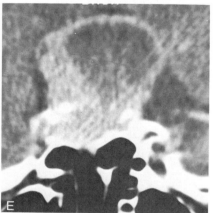

FIGURE 9–28. *Pituitary Apoplexy:* *A,* The preinfusion CT scan demonstrates a fluid/fluid level (*arrow*) in this patient who presented with sudden onset of headache and blindness. The fluid/fluid level is secondary to hemorrhage into the cystic pituitary tumor. The heavier blood accumulates in the dependent portion of the cystic tumor.

B, The postinfusion CT scan demonstrates peripheral enhancement around the tumor. The level between the fluid within the cyst and the blood is still faintly visible.

C, Axial SE TR530/TE30 image on the same patient obtained shortly after the CT scan demonstrates that the mass is lobulated and exhibits increased signal intensity.

D, Midsagittal SE TR530/TE30 readily confirms the multilobulated intra- and suprasellar nature of this adenoma. The third ventricle is obliterated, and the midbrain and the pons are displaced posteriorly. The areas of varying signal intensity represent both cysts and hemorrhage within the adenoma.

E, Coronal only/post-only CT scan approximately two months later demonstrates both peripheral and solid areas of enhancement within the mass. (A fluid level should also be visible with the patient in position for a direct coronal scan, and therefore the hemorrhage has presumably resolved.) The patient refused surgery. The appearance is typical of a pituitary tumor with hemorrhage or apoplexy.

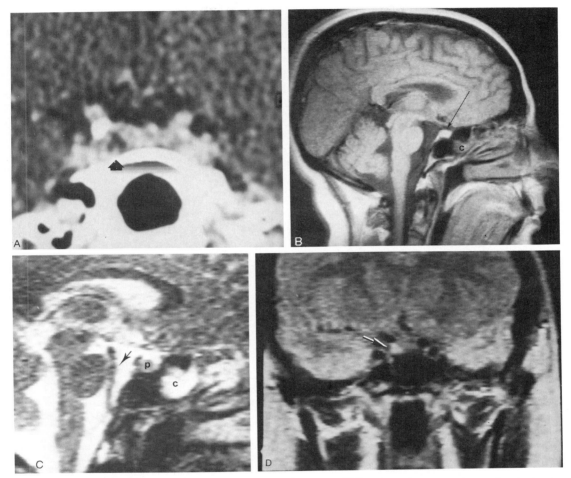

FIGURE 9–29. *Microadenoma of Pituitary:* Twenty-eight–year–old female with amenorrhea and galactorrhea. *A*, Postinfusion coronal cuts through the sella reveal a low-density area within the gland (arrow), upward convexity of the gland above the tumor, and focal erosion of the floor of the sella on bone window widths (not shown).

B, Midsagittal MR slice with SE TR530/TE30 image reveals upward convexity (*arrow*) of the normally upwardly concave pituitary. Note the incidental finding of a retention cyst (*C*) in the sphenoid sinus that becomes increased in signal intensity on the SE TR3120/TE120 image (*C*).

C, The SE TR3120/TE120 image reveals that the CSF has reached the "cross over" point and is now of high rather than low signal intensity. The pituitary gland (*P*) remains of low signal intensity. The retention cyst becomes increased in signal intensity, and the basilar artery appears as a negative flow defect (*arrow*) in the prepontine cistern just anterior to the pons.

D, The coronal SE TR3120/TE60 image reveals the microadenoma as an increased signal intensity area (*arrow*). The negative flow defect of the carotid arteries in the region of the carotid siphon is seen bilaterally. This is typical appearance of a microadenoma of the pituitary with both CT and MR. It appears that MR will replace CT for the evaluation of pituitary abnormalities.

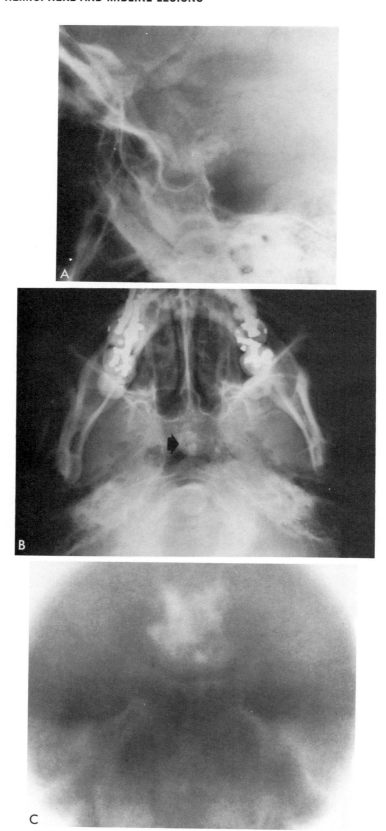

FIGURE 9–30. *See legend on the opposite page.*

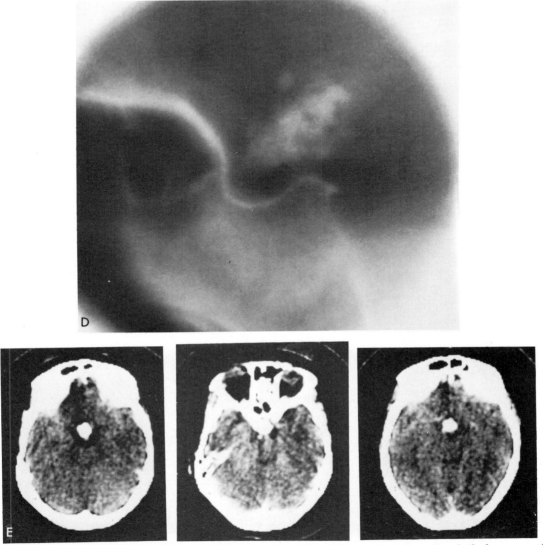

FIGURE 9–30. *Craniopharyngioma: A,* The lateral view of the skull reveals a densely calcified mass in the sella that extends into the suprasellar cisterns.

B, The calcification is also seen on the submentovertex view of the skull (*arrow*).

C, The AP tomographic view demonstrates the area of calcification just superior to the dorsum sellae in the midline.

D, The lateral view also shows the calcified mass, which is in the suprasellar cistern but extends into the sella.

E, The CT scans confirm the presence of a densely calcified mass in the suprasellar cistern and extending into the sella.

The appearance is that of a calcified craniopharyngioma. These tumors are usually cystic.

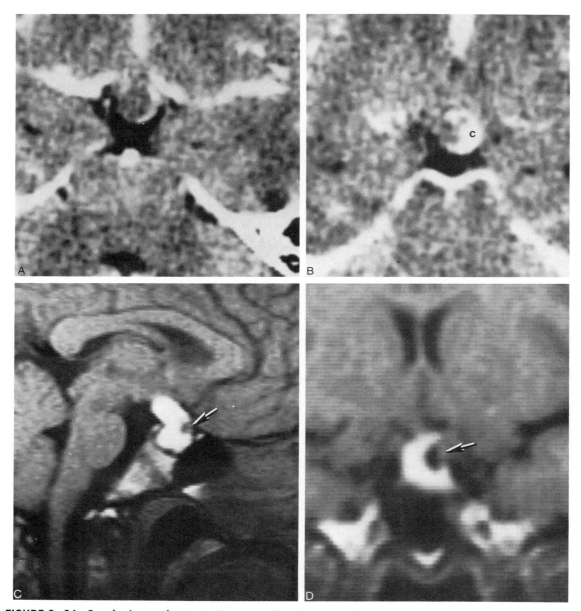

FIGURE 9–31. *Craniopharyngioma:* Twelve-year-old male with diabetes insipidus. *A* and *B,* Two postinfusion axial images reveal a low-density, peripherally enhancing mass in the suprasellar cistern which extends into the sella turcica. A small area of calcification (*c*) was identified on the preinfusion CT scan.

C, Midsagittal SE TR530/TE30 image reveals an increased signal intensity mass that is lobulated and is both intrasellar and suprasellar. There is slight enlargement of the sella, and a small area of calcification appears as a low signal defect within the high signal portion of the tumor (*arrow*).

D, Coronal T-1 weighted image again demonstrates the increased signal intensity of the cystic portion of the tumor as well as the low signal intensity of the area of calcification (*arrow*). This combination of CT and MR appearance is very typical of craniopharyngioma, although the cystic portion of some craniopharyngiomas are of low signal intensity on the T-1 weighted images and only become increased in signal intensity on the T-2 weighted images.

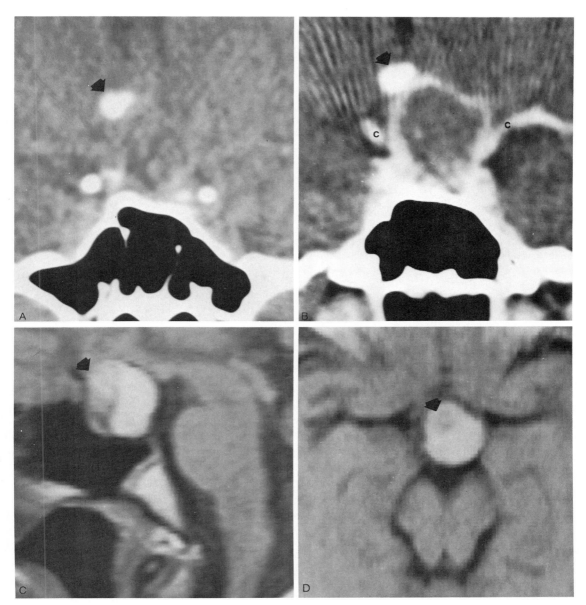

FIGURE 9–32. *Craniopharyngioma:* Twenty-year-old female with primary amenorrhea. *A,* Preinfusion coronal CT scan demonstrates an area of amorphous calcification (*arrow*) in the suprasellar cistern. The suprasellar cistern is obliterated by an isodense mass.

B, The postinfusion CT scan reveals a low-density mass with peripheral enhancement and the area of calcification embedded in the enhancing wall of the tumor. The contrast-filled carotid arteries (*c*) are displaced slightly laterally by the tumor. Surgically proved craniopharyngioma. Note that while calcification can occur within a pituitary adenoma, it is rare. Calcification is present in approximately 80 per cent of younger patients with craniopharyngioma.

C, Sagittal SE TR530/TE30 reveals that the craniopharyngioma is increased in signal intensity and is both intrasellar and suprasellar. There is a fluid/fluid level, apparently secondary to settling of the inhomogeneous fluid within the cyst.

D, The axial SE TR530/TE30 again reveals inhomogeneous increased signal within the cystic tumor.

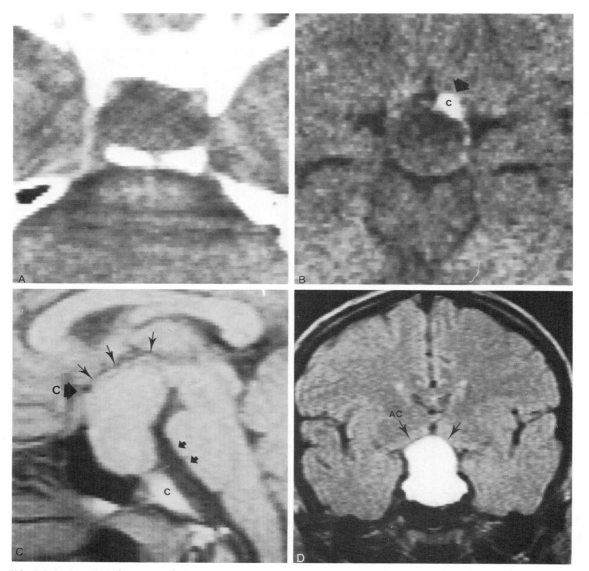

FIGURE 9–33. *Craniopharyngioma:* Thirty-seven–year–old male with decreasing beard growth and change in voice. *A,* The preinfusion CT scan through the region of the sella turcica reveals that the sella is enlarged and filled with homogeneously low-density material.

B, The slightly higher slice demonstrates obliteration of the suprasellar cistern by a cystic mass. There is a small area of calcification along the anterior margin of the cyst (*C-arrow*) and very faint calcification along the lateral margin of the cystic mass just posterior to the larger area of calcification.

C, Midsagittal SE TR530/TE30 reveals the bean-shaped, isodense mass in the sella and extending into the suprasellar cistern. The sella is enlarged. The area of calcification appears as a small area of decreased signal intensity (*C-arrow*), and the optic chiasm and optic tracts are displaced markedly superiorly (*long arrows*). The optic chiasm and optic tracts are separated from the tumor by a thin low signal intensity area of CSF. The pons is effaced (*short arrows*) and displaced posteriorly away from the clivus (*C*).

D, The coronal SE TR2120/TE60 reveals that the cystic tumor has increased signal intensity, obliterates the inferior portion of the third ventricle, displaces the cavernous and supraclinoid portions of the carotid arteries laterally, and elevates the horizontal portions of the anterior cerebral arteries (*AC-arrows*).

Surgically proved craniopharyngioma.

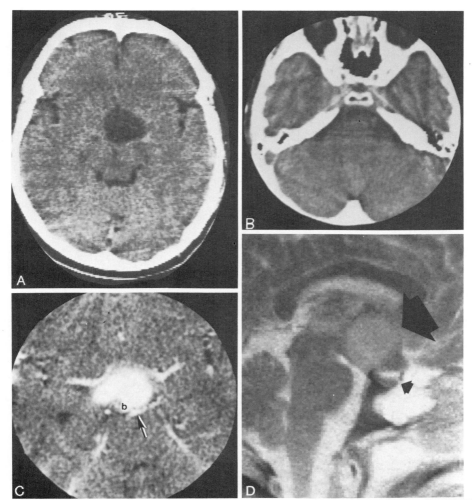

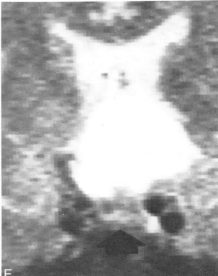

FIGURE 9–34. *Hypothalamic Glioma:* Fifty-year-old male with headaches. *A*, Preinfusion CT scan demonstrates low-density mass in the supraseller cistern which obliterates the third ventricle.

B, The postinfusion CT scan through the sella turcica reveals that the sella is normal in size and configuration and that there is *no* evidence of an enhancing mass within the sella.

C, A higher slice reveals dense homogeneous enhancement of the slightly lobulated suprasellar mass. The mass abuts the basilar artery and effaces the proximal portion of the posterior cerebral artery (*arrow*).

D, SE TR3120/TE60 sagittal image reveals that the tumor mass remains of relatively low signal intensity (*large arrow*). The sella turcica and its contents are normal (*small arrow*).

E, The coronal SE TR3120/TE120 image reveals that the mass has increased signal intensity, and its suprasellar location is easily appreciated. The negative flow defects of the cavernous and supraclinoid carotid arteries flank the normal-appearing sella turcica (*arrow*). Surgically proved hypothalamic glioma. Care should be taken to evaluate the *lack* of involvement of the sella in cases, such as this hypothalamic tumor, that might be mistaken for a pituitary tumor with suprasellar extension.

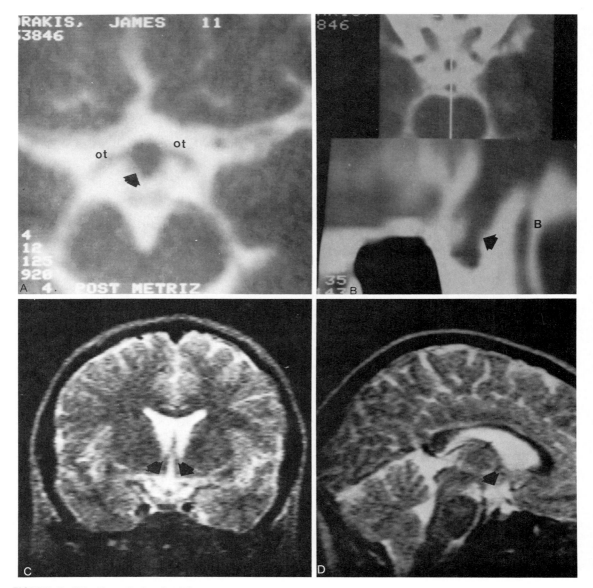

FIGURE 9–35. Hypothalamic Glioma: The patient is an 11-year-old male with diabetes insipidus and rage attacks. *A,* The axial image of the metrizamide cisternogram reveals marked enlargement of the pituitary stalk (*arrow*) in the region of the hypothalamus. The optic tracts are also outlined by contrast material (*ot*) in the suprasellar cistern.

B, The midsagittal reconstruction image again demonstrates the enlarged pituitary stalk (*arrow*) as it projects just above the bilobed pituitary gland and just below the anterior recesses of the third ventricle. The basilar artery (*B*) is seen as a filling defect in the prepontine cistern because it is surrounded by the metrizamide in the basilar cisterns.

C, MR SE TR3120/TE120 image demonstrates that the hypothalamus, which is located on either side of the anterior, inferior portion of the third ventricle, is visible as an area of increased signal intensity (*arrows*). The carotid arteries appear as areas of negative flow in the parasellar region.

D, The midsagittal SE TR3120/TE120 demonstrates the increased signal intensity area in the region of the hypothalamus (*arrow*). Probable hypothalamic glioma (not surgically proved).

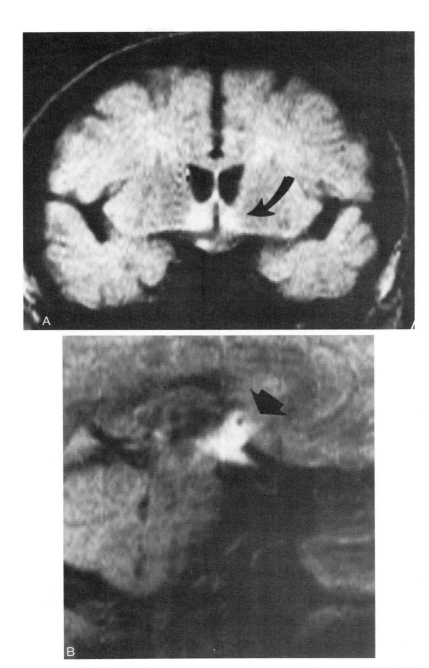

FIGURE 9–36. *Hypothalamic Glioma:* The magnetic resonance scans in the coronal (*A*) and sagittal (*B*) planes demonstrate an area of increased signal intensity in the region of the hypothalamus (*arrows*). This is the SE TR530/TE30 sequence. The area of increased signal intensity extends down to the region of the optic chiasm on both views, where it also appears as an area of increased signal intensity.

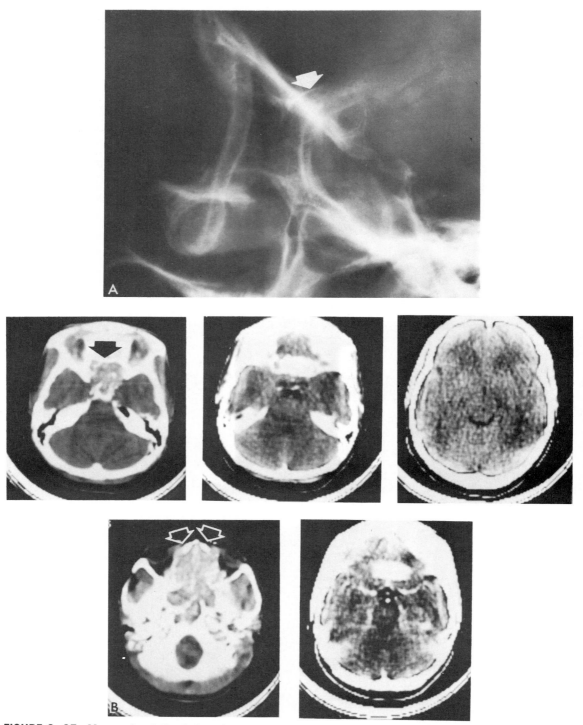

FIGURE 9–37. *Mucocele of the Sphenoid Sinus:* *A,* The lateral view of the skull demonstrates destructive changes and irregular opacification of the sella. The planum sphenoidale is displaced superiorly and is markedly thinned (*arrowhead*). There is obviously an expanding lesion in the region of the sphenoid sinus.

B, CT scans demonstrate an area of increased density in the region of the expanded sphenoid sinus (*black arrow*) and the superiorly displaced planum sphenoidale. The third ventricle appears to be normal in size and position.

The lower cuts through the nasal cavity reveal an extensive soft tissue mass throughout the nasal cavity (*open arrows*); physical examination disclosed multiple nasal polyps. There is no change on the postinfusion scan.

Surgically proved mucocele of the sphenoid sinus.

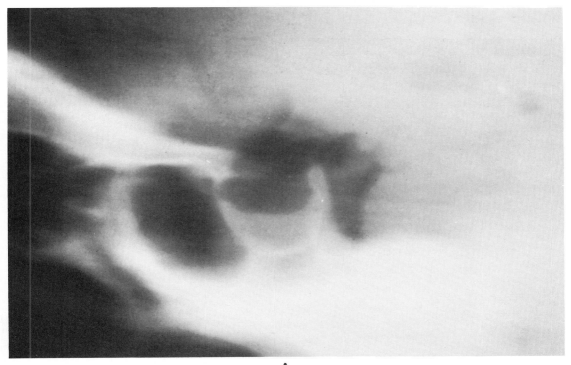

A

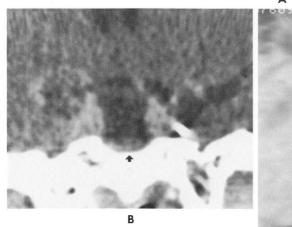

B

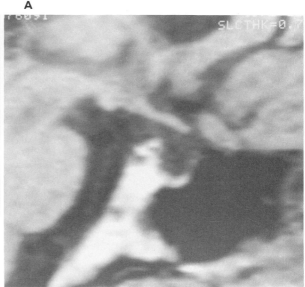

C

FIGURE 9–38. *Empty Sella Syndrome:* This syndrome is usually seen in women. The clinical symptoms are headache and, occasionally, visual difficulties. The sella is usually enlarged. Air will enter the sella during pneumoencephalography.

A, The size of the sella is slightly enlarged in this patient. A midline tomogram with the patient in the inverted position demonstrates that the sella turcica fills with air, although a small amount of pituitary tissue remains in the floor of the sella.

B, CT in the coronal AP projection of the postinfusion scan demonstrates only a small amount of visible tissue in the floor of the sella (*arrow*). The remainder of the sella is filled with CSF density material. The enhancement of the cavernous sinus and carotid arteries is visible on either side of the "empty sella."

C, MR, SE TR530/TE30 image in the sagittal plane reveals material of CSF signal intensity within the sella turcica and no visible pituitary tissue. The infundibulum is displaced posteriorly in the sella, a finding typical of the empty sella syndrome.

CT and MR have replaced pneumoencephalography for diagnosis of empty sella syndrome.

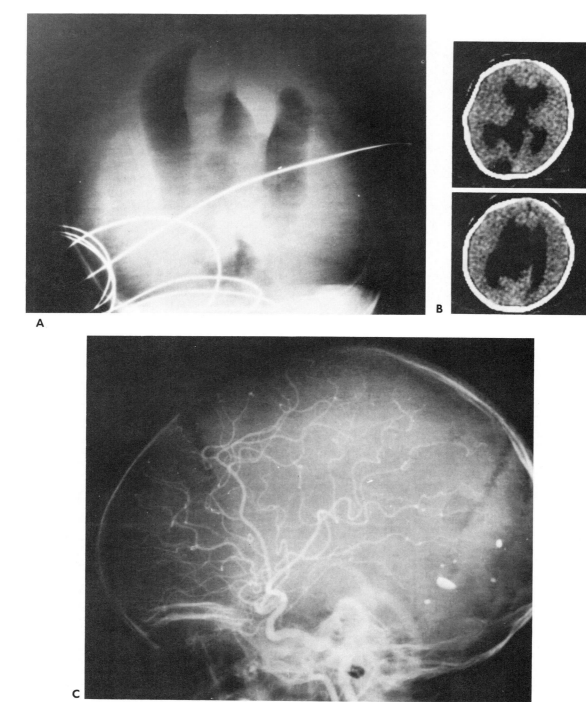

FIGURE 9–39. _Agenesis of the Corpus Callosum:_ The pneumoencephalogram (_A_) demonstrates that the lateral ventricles are wide-spread and that the third ventricle pushes superiorly between the lateral ventricles. The CT scans (_B_) confirm those findings, and the appearance is quite typical for an agenesis of the corpus callosum.

_C_, The angiogram reveals a straightened and meandering course of the pericallosal artery—another finding typical of agenesis of the corpus callosum.

10

HYDROCEPHALUS, PORENCEPHALY, AND METASTASES

HYDROCEPHALUS

Computed tomography revolutionized the approach to the evaluation of hydrocephalus. CT allows readily available, accurate, and easily reproducible evaluation of the ventricular size as well as the presence or absence of a mass lesion obstructing the ventricular system. The more recent addition of MR has further aided the work-up of hydrocephalus. The convenient availability of multiplanar imaging makes magnetic resonance the procedure of choice for evaluation. The midsagittal images allow direct visualization of the cerebral aqueduct and the fourth ventricle as well as the third ventricle. Because hydrocephalus is frequently seen in association with the Chiari malformation (see below) and the accompanying aqueduct stenosis or occlusion, MR has specific advantages in that it allows visualization of these structures as well as the position of the cerebellar tonsils and the configuration of the brain stem.

With hydrocephalus, there may be transependymal resorption of CSF with an appearance of periventricular low density on the CT scan and a similar distribution of increased signal intensity on the T-2 weighted MR images.

The obvious advantage of MR is the absence of ionizing radiation and the ability to directly visualize the midbrain and posterior fossa structures without the artifact secondary to the surrounding bone. The ability to visualize the position of the cerebellar tonsils without the use of contrast material is obviously a great advantage in pediatric patients. In addition, there is an associated syrinx in a large number of patients with the Chiari malformation, and this can also be directly visualized without the use of contrast material. Magnetic resonance scanning of the spine also provides accurate evaluation of the remainder of the spinal cord and vertebral column. The presence or absence of a lipoma of the lower spine can also be determined, again, in multiplanar fashion without the use of contrast material and obviously without the need for needle placement, a significant advantage in the pediatric patient (see Chapter 15).

The term "hydrocephalus" implies the presence of large ventricles, but these may or may not be associated with increased head size. An obstructive hydrocephalus usually is secondary to a mass lesion that obstructs the ventricular system. This obstruction can be at any level—e.g., at the foramen of Monro because of a colloid cyst of the third ventricle; at the cerebral aqueduct because of a pinealoma or aqueduct stenosis; or at the fourth ventricle because of an ependymoma. The obstruction causes enlargement of the ventricle and an enlarging head size in children; in adults, there is changed or increased intracranial pressure.

In a "communicating" hydrocephalus there is

439

no mass lesion. Rather, one finds interference with the absorption of CSF by the arachnoid granulations secondary to a subarachnoid hemorrhage or interference with the normal flow of CSF through the tentorial notch because of adhesions following meningitis.

With an atrophic process such as that seen with toxoplasmosis or cytomegalic inclusion disease, there will be large lateral ventricles but a small head size.

Several examples of hydrocephalus associated with the Chiari malformation and aqueduct stenosis are illustrated in this chapter. Examples of many other types of hydrocephalus are presented elsewhere in this book.

Aqueduct Stenosis and Insufficiency

Aqueduct occlusion may be a congenital finding in some cases. At birth or shortly thereafter the child's head begins to enlarge. It is not clear why the head does not grow large in utero—although in some cases it may be large even at birth. The aqueduct may be forked, having two blind ends along its more cephalad portion. The distal end of the aqueduct will be closed and will not communicate with either limb of the proximal aqueduct.

In addition to forking of the aqueduct, there may be a gliosis about the aqueduct that ultimately leads to its occlusion.

If there is narrowing of the aqueduct without distal occlusion, the subsequent development of a meningitis may cause enough reactive fibrosis to occlude the small opening totally.

In some patients with aqueduct insufficiency, the fluid pathway may be sufficiently patent so that enlargement of the head does not develop during the pediatric period. Indeed, some of these patients may live into adulthood and even to old age before their abnormality is discovered. In these cases it seems that the lateral ventricles enlarge very slowly over a long period of time because their borderline aqueduct sufficiency allows only minimal flow of CSF out of the ventricular system. However, an episode of meningitis or subarachnoid hemorrhage may be all that is needed to create occlusion or critical insufficiency of the pathway, and the patient develops the signs and symptoms of hydrocephalus. In these older patients it is of the utmost importance to be certain that it is not a tumor that is creating the problem. Care must be taken to rule out tumor because adult aqueduct insufficiency is only possible, not common.

A CT scan with contrast enhancement or MR is sufficient in most cases to rule out the presence of a mass lesion as the cause of obstructive hydrocephalus.

Plain Skull. Because increased intracranial pressure is so insidious in its onset and often long-standing, its secondary changes often are reflected in the sella turcica. There is enlargement of the sella turcica and erosion of the dorsum sellae and posterior clinoids associated with demineralization and destruction of the sella. These changes occur because of the marked dilatation of the third ventricle, which continues to pound down on the dorsum sellae with each transmitted pulsation secondary to heartbeat and respiration. There may also be an increase in the digital markings of the calvaria because of the increased intracranial pressure.

If the aqueduct stenosis is associated with the Chiari malformation, there may be an associated small posterior fossa because of the inferior displacement of the posterior fossa structures into the cervical region.

Arnold-Chiari Malformation

The Arnold-Chiari malformation is a developmental abnormality of the hindbrain. With this congenital abnormality, alterations in the growth of the brain stem, midbrain, and cerebrum lead to characteristic alterations in the posterior fossa structures. The main feature of this abnormality is the displacement of the cerebellar tonsils into the region of the cervical canal. This appears to be related in part to the failure of the pons to flex during its course of development. In addition to low-lying cerebellar tonsils, the Arnold-Chiari malformation also may be associated with abnormal development of the spinal cord, resulting in meningoceles or myelomeningoceles and spinal dysraphia. One theory of the development of the malformation is that the meningomyelocele holds the spinal cord in the lumbar region, resulting in the downward displacement of the tonsils. This traction theory does not, however, explain all cases of this abnormality because the hindbrain malformation may occur without a meningomyelocele.

Arnold described the displacement of the cerebellar tonsils into the upper cervical canal; Chiari described the downward protrusion of the medulla and fourth ventricle into the cervical spinal canal, which causes the primitive cervical flexure of the embryo to be retained and the medulla to lie dorsal to the cervical spinal cord in the region of the cervical spinal canal.

This anomaly is now called the Chiari malformation. There are four types:

Type I. This is a variable downward displacement of the tonsils and inferior cerebellum into the cervical canal. This type of Chiari malformation is not associated with a meningomyelocele. There may be an associated basilar impression and platybasia. Although an aqueduct stenosis may be present, it appears that these patients—who may live into adulthood without difficulty—suffer from a "foramen magnum syndrome" with resulting failure of CSF to circulate out of the fourth ventricle and over the cerebral hemispheres, where resorption recurs, leading to hydrocephalus.

Type II. There is downward displacement of the cerebellar tonsils into the cervical canal, but these patients also exhibit caudad displacement of the lower pons and medulla. The fourth ventricle is also displaced inferiorly and can be identified on the pneumoencephalogram as an elongated and distorted air shadow in the cervical region. In addition to the hindbrain malformation, a myelomeningocele is also present in Type II Chiari malformation. Harwood-Nash and Fitz consider the Type II malformation to be the classic abnormality seen in neuroradiologic practice. This malformation becomes apparent at birth or shortly thereafter. Hydrocephalus develops early in the clinical course and is secondary to the aqueduct stenosis or occlusion present in every case. This stenosis is secondary to forking, compression, or inflammatory gliosis, and occlusion may occur by intracerebral hemorrhage or infection.

Although a simple meningocele may be present in the absence of the Chiari malformation, a meningomyelocele is always associated with the malformation. However, the malformation may have either a meningocele or meningomyelocele. The CT and MR findings include a large massa intermedia and a pointed floor of the lateral ventricles. An accessory commissure may be present in the region of the lamina terminalis, and, of course, the elongated aqueduct and the inferiorly positioned fourth ventricle will be seen in the region of the cervical canal.

Type III. This is a displacement of the medulla and fourth ventricle and all of the cerebellum into an occipital and high cervical encephalomeningocele. Type III Chiari malformation may come to the radiologist's attention if CT or MR is performed to determine how much of the cranial contents are contained in the encephalocele; ventricular connections with the encephalocele may be demonstrated.

Type IV. Aplasia of the cerebellar hemispheres, the vermis, and the pons is associated with a small, funnel-shaped posterior fossa. Usually the third and lateral ventricles are not enlarged. There is marked dilatation of the fourth ventricle and the cisternae magnae. The pons has a "pigeon-breast" shape. This is an uncommon malformation, and some believe that it does not fall in the category of Chiari malformation.

CT Scan. The CT scan reveals a varying degree of obstructive hydrocephalus. The lateral and third ventricles will be noted to be enlarged, while the fourth ventricle is very small. Frequently there is differential enlargement of the occipital horns of the lateral ventricles as compared to the frontal horns. This appears to be secondary to a dysplastic development of the ventricular system. In some cases the fourth ventricle is not seen in the posterior fossa. This is because of the inferior displacement of the aqueduct and fourth ventricle into the cervical canal.

MR Scan. MR is the diagnostic procedure of choice. Shunt placement can then be performed and follow-up MR or CT can be used for the evaluation of shunt efficacy.

Dandy-Walker Syndrome

The underlying abnormality in the Dandy-Walker syndrome is congenital occlusion of the foramina of Magendie and Luschka. This results in cystic dilatation of the fourth ventricle. There is also dysgenesis of the cerebellar roof. In some cases, the foramina are patent, and so the anomaly is more complex than simple cystic dilatation of the fourth ventricle. Classically, the torcular is displaced superior to the lambdoid suture—torcular-lambdoid inversion. There is variable obstructive hydrocephalus, and associated anomalies such as agenesis of the corpus callosum may also be seen.

Communicating Hydrocephalus

A "communicating hydrocephalus" implies that there is *no* evidence of a mass blocking the ventricular system. One cause is meningitis. It appears that a communicating hydrocephalus develops from meningitis because of apparent interference with the absorption of CSF by the arachnoid villi. Not all patients with meningitis develop a communicating hydrocephalus.

Another cause is subarachnoid hemorrhage. This communicating hydrocephalus is thought to develop because the blood in the subarachnoid space over the cerebral convexities interferes with the absorption of CSF by the arachnoid villi. It should be remembered that an acute obstructive hydrocephalus may develop following a subarachnoid hemorrhage from the accumulation of clotted blood in the aqueduct and fourth ventricle.

A communicating hydrocephalus also may develop in the presence of excess CSF production, as seen with choroid plexus papilloma.

Chronic subdural hematomas also have been associated with ventricular enlargement and the picture of a communicating hydrocephalus. In the case of patients with chronic extracerebral accumulations of fluid, it is felt that the local pressure over the cerebral convexities interferes with the reabsorption of CSF and results in ventricular enlargement.

Low-pressure hydrocephalus has a CT and MR appearance similar to communicating hydrocephalus but is associated with the clinical triad of (1) dementia, (2) ataxia, and (3) urinary incontinence.

Hydrocephalus ex vacuo refers to fluid accumulations following brain atrophy. This term is now obsolete and should not be used.

All the varied causes of communicating hydrocephalus produce enlargement of the lateral ventricles without significant enlargement of the cortical sulci. With cerebral atrophy the cortical sulci also are enlarged. This diagnosis can be readily suggested by computed tomography or MR.

Subarachnoid Hemorrhage

The blood vessels that feed the cerebral tissues are carried by the pia mater of the leptomeninges. Following a ruptured aneurysm, the blood accumulates in the subarachnoid space. In addition, the aneurysm may rupture into the cerebral tissue, producing an associated intracerebral hematoma. The hemorrhage usually is associated with severe headache, nausea and vomiting, and frequently with a syncopal episode. Localizing physical findings may or may not be observed following the episode of hemorrhage. The patient develops a stiff neck secondary to the irritation of the meninges by the blood in the subarachnoid space. The CT scan of a subarachnoid hemorrhage without an intracerebral hematoma reveals areas of increased density in the basilar cisterns, sylvian fissures, and interhemispheric fissure and over the cortical sulci. The blood in the subarachnoid space appears white on the CT scan, whereas the normal scan reveals areas of radiolucency in these distributions.

In addition, subarachnoid hemorrhage may even result in the appearance of blood in the ventricular system. It seems that the blood in these cases enters the fourth, third, and lateral ventricles via the foramina of Luschka and Magendie and then through the aqueduct and foramen of Monro into the lateral ventricles. It is this free circulation of blood in the subarachnoid space that results in the accumulation of blood in the lumbar subarachnoid space that is found at the time of lumbar tap.

Acutely there may be an obstructive hydrocephalus because of clotted blood in the fourth ventricle and cerebral aqueduct that acts as a mechanical obstruction to the flow of CSF. This hydrocephalus may resolve after the dissolution of the clot. On the other hand, the ventricles may never return to normal size.

Following the acute hemorrhage, a communicating hydrocephalus may develop as soon as the first week after the initial insult. A simple and probably incomplete explanation of the development of this communicating hydrocephalus after a subarachnoid hemorrhage is that the blood in the subarachnoid space over the cerebral cortex interferes with the normal function of the arachnoid villi to reabsorb the circulating CSF. Although the progression of hydrocephalus from initial obstruction to communicating hydrocephalus may be a continuum, there may be no evidence of acute obstructive hydrocephalus but a later development of a communicating or low-pressure hydrocephalus.

A communicating hydrocephalus develops over a highly variable period of time. In addition, not all patients who develop large ventricles and apparent communicating hydrocephalus become symptomatic. Patients who do become symptomatic will be improved by the placement of a shunt tubing device.

The presence and development of hydrocephalus can be readily followed by CT scans or, if a scanner is not available, by angiography.

Magnetic Resonance of Subarachnoid Hemorrhage

Patients with acute subarachnoid hemorrhage are probably not candidates for magnetic resonance imaging. These patients are frequently clinically unstable and because of various life-support systems cannot be placed into the scanning room. In addition the varying level of consciousness interferes with the patient's ability to cooperate and remain immobile for the duration of the scan. Most importantly, the acute hemorrhage is not visible on the MR scan because it is of low, rather than high, signal intensity. CT is accurate in greater than 95 per cent of acute subarachnoid hemorrhage and so is the procedure of choice (see Chapter 6).

PORENCEPHALY

Areas of porencephaly are readily identified on CT scans. They have a well-defined border, contain fluid the same density as cerebrospinal fluid, and do not change in density following the use of contrast material. Before the advent of CT scanning, the diagnosis of porencephaly depended on a combination of plain radiographic findings, angiography, pneumoencephalography, and ventriculography. However, even with all these techniques, the radiographic appearance was that of any space-occupying lesion, and surgery was required for definite diagnosis. Since the development CT, it usually is possible to diagnose the abnormality and treat the patient without additional diagnostic work-up.

The term "porencephaly" was coined by Heschl in 1859, who defined it as a "pore" in the brain. The term "porencephalic cyst" implies a lesion that has an ependymal lining and communicates with the lateral ventricles or subarachnoid cyst. A broader definition of porencephalic cyst also includes "closed" porencephaly, which does not communicate with either the ventricular system or the subarachnoid space. By any diagnostic examination other than CT, these areas of closed porencephaly would appear as a mass lesion. The examples illustrated here include some porencephalic cysts and a variety of other CSF-containing lesions.

Areas of porencephaly may have a variety of etiologies:

1. Germ plasm defects
2. Intrauterine cerebrovascular accidents
3. Birth trauma
4. Vascular thrombosis or embolism
5. Postinflammatory changes
6. Focal atrophy
7. Hemorrhage
8. Postsurgical changes

Care must be taken not to mistake a cystic neoplasm for a porencephalic cyst. However, when a tumor is present, the fluid within the cyst is of higher density than CSF, and usually a ring or solid area of enhancement is noted after the infusion of contrast material.

Post-traumatic hematomas, spontaneous hematomas, and infarcts have all been observed to progress to areas of porencephaly on serial CT scans. The areas of postsurgical porencephaly are readily correlated with the surgical procedure. Usually no further diagnostic tests are necessary to determine the correct diagnosis.

These patients may be neurologically intact, or they may demonstrate seizure disorders, mental retardation, or hemi- or monoparesis.

METASTASES

Now that CT scanning is available, it can be stated that the CT scan with infusion of contrast material is the diagnostic procedure of choice for cerebral metastases. It is recommended that at the time of initial work-up each patient should first have a preinfusion scan, followed by infusion of contrast material and another scan. For follow-up examination, only a postinfusion scan may be performed if there is no suspicion of intracerebral hemorrhage.

There is no doubt that, of all the tests available, the CT scan provides the most accurate evaluation of the presence or absence of metastases. The CT scan will detect lesions as small as 1 cm in diameter. Because the scan can have a normal appearance before infusion of contrast material, a postinfusion scan is essential. Most metastatic lesions are space-occupying; however, even sizable metastases may be present without significant mass effect, or there may be symmetrical bilateral metastases that result in no shift of the midline. Most metastases demonstrate contrast enhancement on the postinfusion study.

Multiple metastatic lesions occur frequently; however, a certain number of patients have only one intracranial metastasis. The patient's symptoms reflect the position of the lesion, although it is not uncommon to have a patient present with a clinical history consistent with transient ischemic attacks. CT with infusion is much more sensitive than the radionuclide scan for diagnosing metastatic lesions—especially those located in the midbrain and posterior fossa.

Both routine and postinfusion studies are useful for treatment planning for radiation therapy and for estimating response to treatment with radiotherapy or chemotherapy.

Magnetic Resonance of Cerebral Metastases

Magnetic resonance is useful for the diagnosis of cerebral metastases. MR is probably the procedure of choice for evaluation of posterior fossa metastases and may eventually replace CT for the evaluation of metastases. The advantages of MR are the lack of ionizing radiation and the ability to perform the study without the use of contrast agents. On the other hand, while there is increased sensitivity of MR for cerebral abnormalities, the lack of specificity remains. As the examples included in this chapter illustrate, metastases may simulate the appearance of multiple abscesses and vice versa; therefore, while a multiplicity of lesions is helpful in confirming the diagnosis of metastatic disease, it is not pathognomonic.

The recommended screening technique for metastatic disease is:
SE TR530/TE30 axial plane
SE TR3120/TE60-120 axial plane
SE TR3120/TE60-120 coronal plane, if necessary.
The above spin-echo sequences should rule out the presence of an abnormality with a high degree of certainty.

The development of contrast agents such as gadolinium DTPA will aid in evaluation in the future.

The multislice technique should be used. The multiplanar imaging capabilities are ideal for lesion localization and treatment planning.

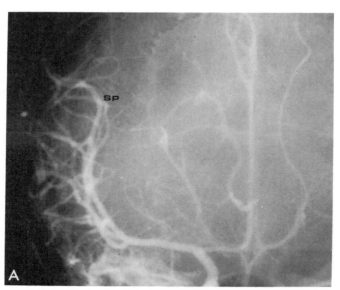

FIGURE 10–1. *Angiographic Appearance of Hydrocephalus:* Carotid angiography: *A,* The AP view of the arterial phase demonstrates that the anterior cerebral artery and its branches are straightened and closely applied to the midline. They show no undulations.

The sylvian point (*SP*) and all the middle cerebral artery branches in the isle of Reil are displaced laterally by the dilated temporal horn. This results in a widened distance between the anterior and middle cerebral artery groups.

Illustration continued on the following page

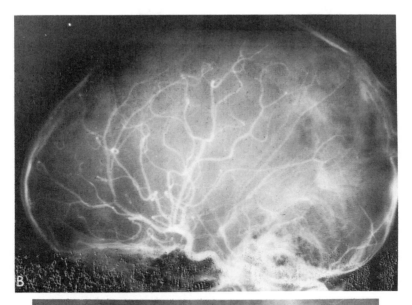

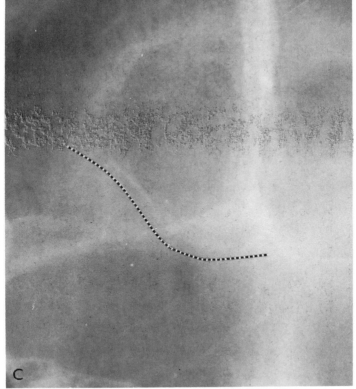

FIGURE 10–1 *Continued.*

B, The lateral view demonstrates a widened sweep of the pericallosal artery. There is elevation of the sylvian triangle secondary to dilatation of the temporal horn.

C, The AP view of the venous phase demonstrates a widened sweep of the thalamostriate vein secondary to dilatation of the lateral ventricle (*dotted line*).

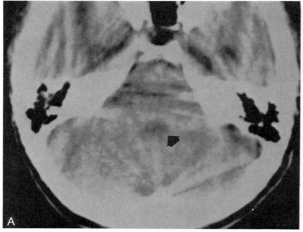

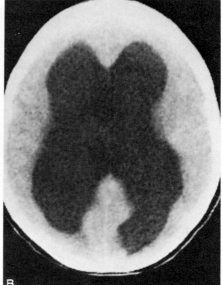

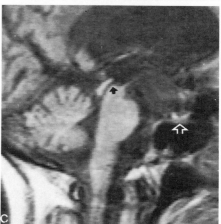

FIGURE 10–2. *Adult Aqueduct Stenosis/Insufficiency:* *A*, CT scan reveals that the fourth ventricle is small or normal in size (*arrow*) for this 34-year-old female with severe headaches.

B, CT scan at the ventricular level reveals moderately severe enlargement of the lateral ventricles without enlargement of the cortical sulci.

C, Midsagittal SE TR530/TE30 image reveals enlargement of the lateral and third ventricles without dilatation of the third ventricle down to the level of the upper aqueduct (*black arrow*). At this point the aqueduct returns to a normal size and configuration. The fourth ventricle is normal in size and position, and no mass is present. Because of the long-standing increased intracranial pressure and dilatation of the third ventricle, there is enlargement of the sella turcica (*white arrow*). This appearance is typical of adult aqueduct insufficiency/stenosis. Following shunt placement, it is not uncommon to find bilateral extracerebral collections of blood which may or may not be symptomatic.

D, Postoperative CT scan reveals a large right-sided and a small left-sided chronic subdural fluid collection (*arrows*), associated with shift from right to left, although the patient improved after shunt placement. The subdural collections apparently occur because there is an element of brain atrophy secondary to the long-standing hydrocephalus, and following shunt placement the brain falls away from the inner table of the skull and is unable to expand.

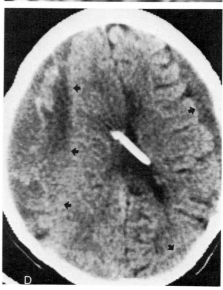

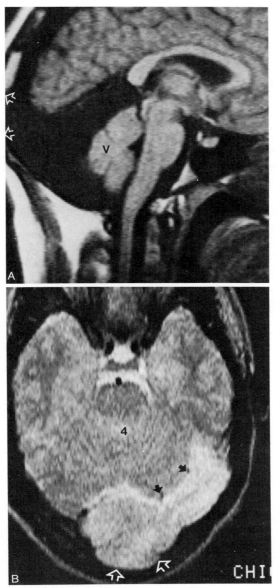

FIGURE 10–3. *Posterior Fossa Arachnoid Cyst:* A, Midsagittal MR, SE TR530/TE30 image reveals a large CSF-containing cyst of the posterior fossa. The vermis is hypoplastic (V), and the fourth ventricle is displaced forward relative to its anticipated normal position. There is pressure erosion of the inner table of the skull (*white arrows*). There was no evidence of ventricular obstruction, although the ventricles were enlarged in size.

B, Axial SE TR3120/TE60 image reveals that the CSF-containing arachnoid cyst projects behind the hypoplastic vermis. The erosion of the inner table of the skull can be seen (*white arrows*), and the vermian veins (*black arrows*) can be seen displaced anteriorly and appear as negative flow defects. The fourth ventricle (*4*) is seen, and the basilar artery appears as a negative flow defect anterior to the pons. The appearance is typical for a posterior fossa arachnoid cyst and should not be mistaken for a Dandy-Walker cyst.

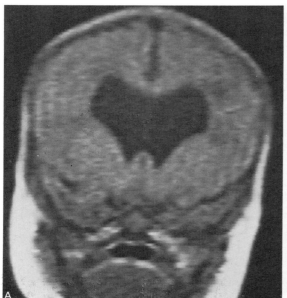

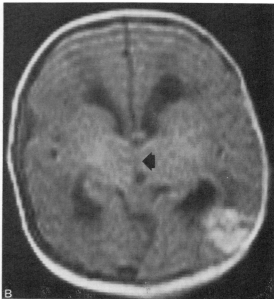

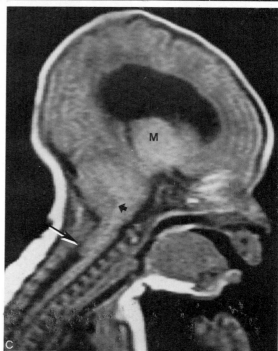

FIGURE 10–4. *Chiari Type II Malformation:* The patient is a newborn with a meningomyelocele. *A,* Coronal SE TR530/TE30 demonstrates the enlarged lateral ventricles secondary to aqueduct stenosis and resulting obstructive hydrocephalus. There is also downward pointing of the floors of the lateral ventricles—typical of the Chiari malformation.

B, Axial SE, TR530/TE30 image reveals large lateral ventricles and an enlarged massa intermedia *(arrow).* There is also an area of increased signal intensity in the left parietal lobe secondary to an intracerebral hematoma following a traumatic delivery because of the large head size.

C, Midsagittal SE TR530/TE30 image again demonstrates the large lateral ventricles. The posterior fossa is small and the fourth ventricle is displaced anteriorly and inferiorly and is elongated *(black arrow).* The "peglike" tonsils project far below the foramen magnum *(black and white arrow).* The upper cervical cord is compressed anteriorly, and the cervical subarachnoid space is consequently narrowed anterior to the cord and widened posterior to the cord just below the level of the herniated tonsils. The appearance is very typical of the Chiari type II malformation. MR is probably the only diagnostic test necessary for evaluation.

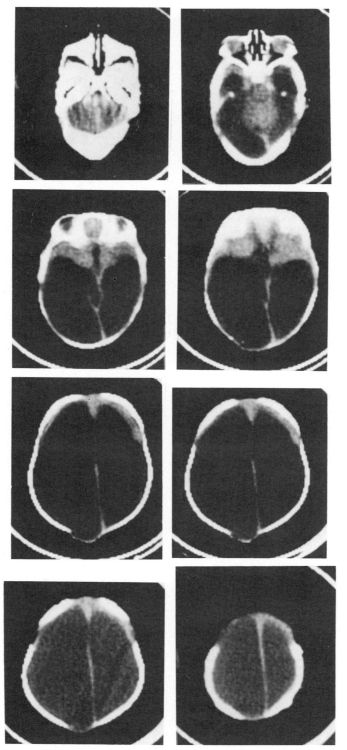

FIGURE 10–5. *Aqueduct Stenosis Associated with the Chiari Malformation:* There is massive ventricular dilatation, with only a thin mantle of remaining cerebral tissue detectable in the frontal regions. Some preservation of the deep midline structures and the posterior fossa structures can be seen. The sutures and fontanelles are widely patent. The fourth ventricle is never seen; it is displaced inferiorly because of the Chiari malformation and lies in the upper cervical region. An associated aqueduct stenosis has resulted in the marked ventricular enlargement.

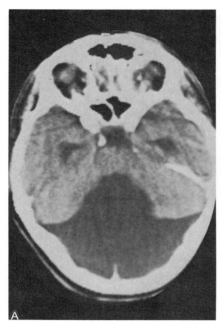

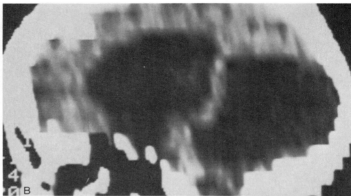

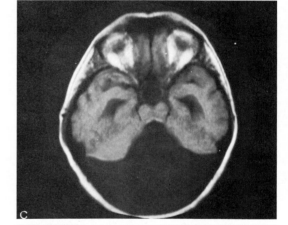

FIGURE 10–6. *Dandy-Walker Cyst:* The patient is an elderly female with a history of gait disturbance for many years. *A*, CT scan demonstrates that the fourth ventricle has been replaced by a large cystic structure that is actually the dilated fourth ventricle. This dilatation is secondary to occlusion of the foramina of Magendie and Luschka. There is usually, but not always, dilatation of the third and lateral ventricles.

B, The midsagittal reformatted image of the CT scan reveals the dilatation of the third and lateral ventricles. The greatly dilated fourth ventricle causes distortion of the occipital bone. The torcular Herophili projects above the level of the lambdoid suture, a change typically seen with the Dandy-Walker cyst.

C, Axial SE, TR530/TE30 image reveals changes similar to those seen on the CT scan. In addition, the dilatation of the anterior recesses of the third ventricle is also seen, and the third ventricle extends into the sella turcica and enlarges it. The pons is compressed and the cerebellar hemispheres are hypoplastic.

D, Midsagittal SE, TR530/TE30 nicely demonstrates the nature of the abnormality. The greatly dilated fourth

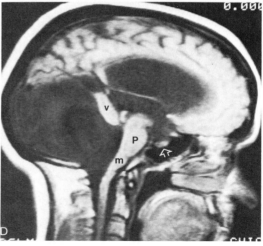

ventricle acts as a mass and compresses the hypoplastic vermis (*V*); the pons (*P*) and medulla (*m*) are compressed and closely applied to the clivus. The quadrigeminal plate is rotated counterclockwise; the reason for this is unknown but may be related to dilatation of the upper aqueduct. The appearance is very typical of the Dandy-Walker syndrome, and MR is the ideal method of evaluation. The pituitary gland is compressed in the floor of the sella turcica (*arrow*).

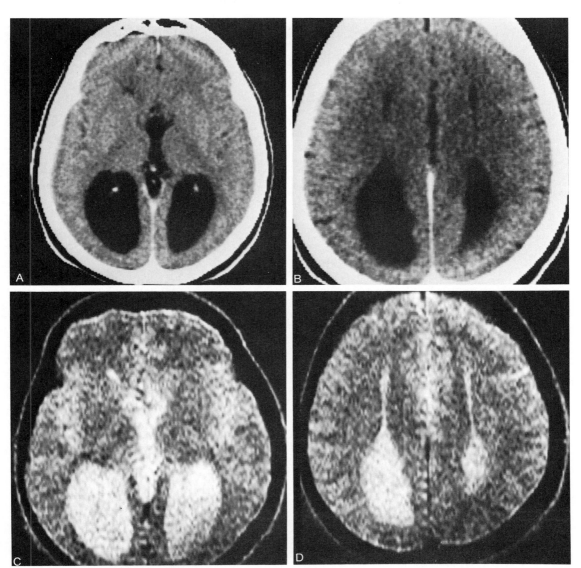

FIGURE 10–7. *Agenesis of the Corpus Callosum:* Both the CT (*A* and *B*) and the MR (*C* and *D*), SE TR3120/TE120 scans demonstrate the typical appearance of agenesis of the corpus callosum. The lateral ventricles are widespread, and the third ventricle extends between the lateral ventricles. The third ventricle extends superiorly above its normal position between the widespread lateral ventricles, as if the absent corpus callosum is no longer present to limit the upward projection of the third ventricle. In the example shown, as in many but not all cases, there is disproportionate enlargement of the occipital horns of the lateral ventricles.

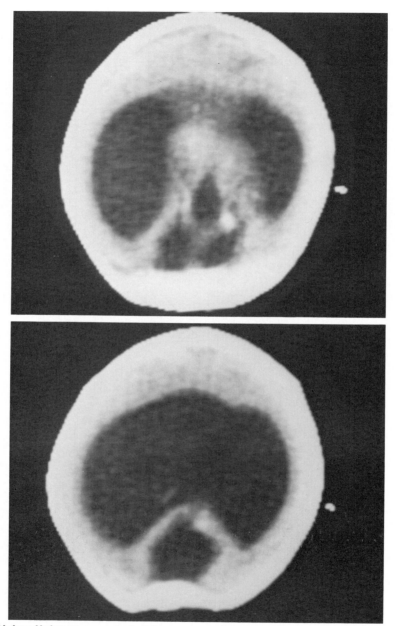

FIGURE 10–8. *Alobar Holoprosencephaly:* This congenital malformation, usually incompatible with life, is characterized by a monoventricle and thin cortical tissue. The third ventricle is incorporated into the lateral ventricles and the thalami become fused. The falx and other midline structures are absent. There are associated anomalies of the facial structures such as cleft lip and palate, microphthalmia, anophthalmia, micrognathia, and trigonocephaly.

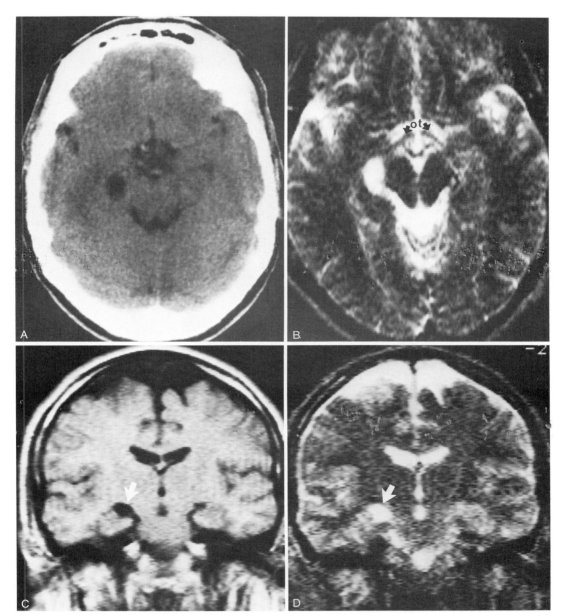

FIGURE 10–9. *Deep Hemispheric Porencephalic Cyst/Lacunar Infarct:* A, CT reveals an oval area of low density deep in the right hemisphere just lateral to the cerebral peduncle.

B, Axial MR using SE TR3120/TE120 image reveals that the area identified on the CT is now an area of increased signal intensity that projects just lateral to the cerebral peduncle. Note that the optic tracts (*ot*) are identified in the suprasellar cistern and that the appearance is that of a metrizamide cisternogram. The posterior cerebral arteries project just posterior to the optic tracts.

C and D, Coronal T-1 and T-2 weighted images reveal that the abnormal area (*white arrow*) responds similar to CSF to the magnetic resonance techniques. There is also diffuse cerebral atrophy.

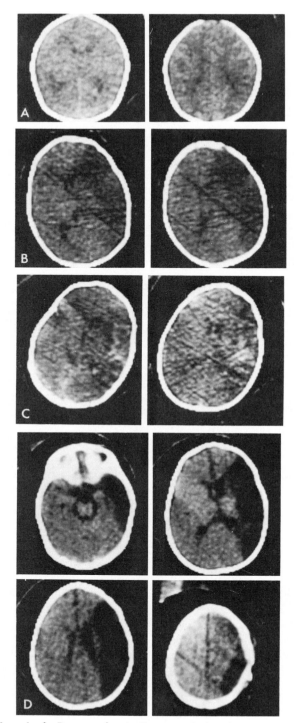

FIGURE 10–10. *Encephalomalacia Progressing to Porencephaly:* The initial CT scan (*A*) reveals scattered areas of radiolucency throughout both hemispheres. A scan one week later (*B*) demonstrates a large area of radiolucency occupying the entire right hemisphere, apparently secondary to infarction (etiology—probably cerebral anoxia).

A follow-up scan (*C*) two weeks later showed an area of irregular enhancement in the region of the right middle cerebral artery. The final scan (*D*) several months later shows that this area of infarction has progressed to a large area of porencephaly occupying almost the entire right hemisphere.

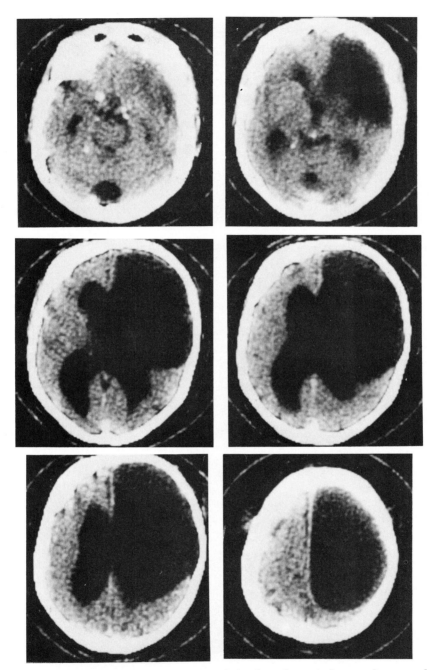

FIGURE 10–11. *Large Porencephalic Cyst:* Both of the lateral ventricles are large, and a large cystic extension of the left lateral ventricle extends to the high convexity region, thinning the overlying bony calvaria. The fluid measures of CSF density and represents porencephalic dilatation of the left lateral ventricle. The patient shown is an adult who has exhibited left hemiatrophy since birth. The changes presumably are secondary to a germ plasm defect or to birth trauma. Although it appears that the left lateral ventricle communicates freely with the cyst, pathologic studies show that there may be a thin ependymal lining between the cyst and the ventricle.

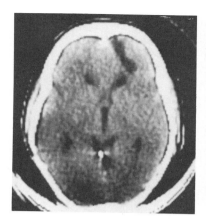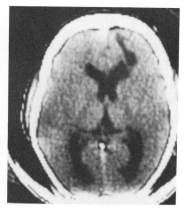

FIGURE 10–12. *Postsurgical Porencephaly:* An area of radiolucency can be seen in the left frontal region; it is well-defined and non–space-occupying and contains fluid of CSF density. The lateral ventricles are mildly dilated. The left frontal lesion is a porencephalic cyst that developed after placement of a catheter for ventriculography.

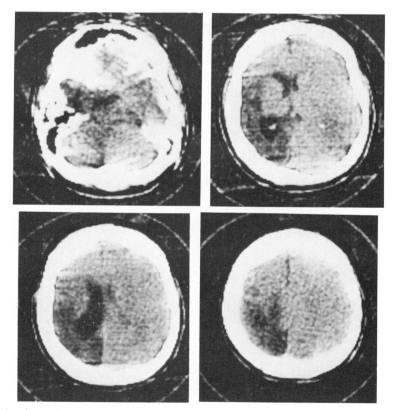

FIGURE 10–13. *Hemiatrophy:* There is dilatation of the right lateral ventricle as compared to the right. Shift toward the atrophic right side and atrophy of the hemisphere on the right side with areas of radiolucency over the right hemisphere also are seen. There is thickening of the bony calvaria of the right hemisphere. The appearance is that of classic right hemiatrophy.

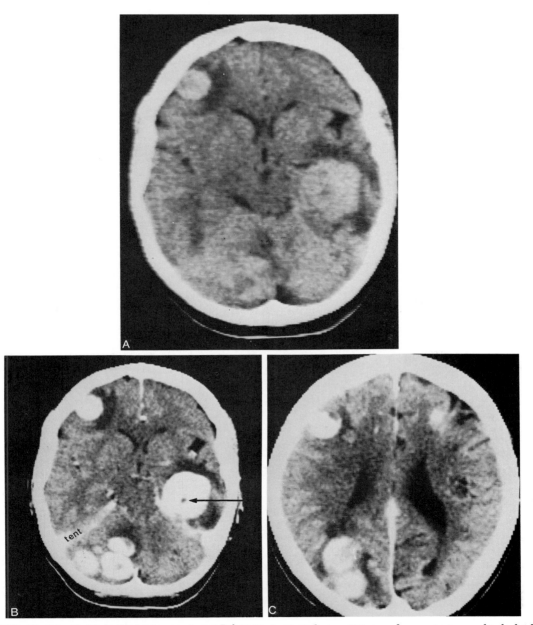

FIGURE 10–14. *Multiple Metastases, Lung Primary:* A, Preinfusion CT scan demonstrates multiple higher than normal brain density and rounded masses with surrounding edema. Because of the "balancing" nature of these multiple metastatic deposits, there is no shift of the midline structures.

B and C, Postinfusion CT reveals homogeneous enhancement of these lesions, with a small area of central necrosis within the large left temporal lesion (*arrow*). Multiple posterior fossa metastases are also seen, as they project medial to the tentorium cerebelli (*tent*). Direct coronal or coronal reconstruction views are helpful if there is a question of whether the mass is supra- or infratentorial.

This appearance is very typical of multiple metastases, which tend to be spread hematogenously and to appear rounded in configuration. The amount of edema is variable with metastatic disease.

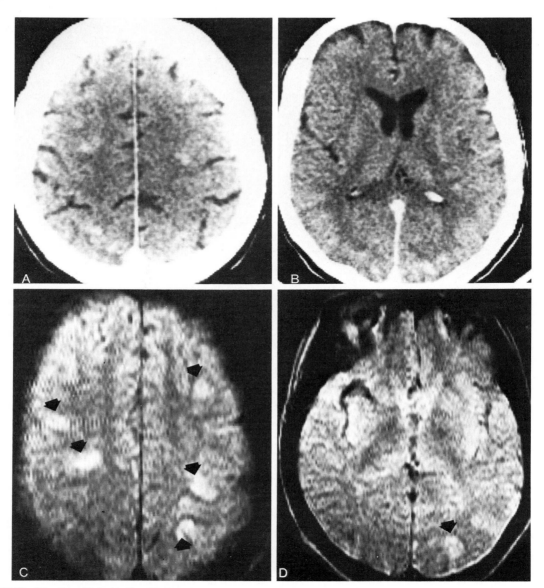

FIGURE 10–15. *Metastatic Melanoma: A* and *B*, Postinfusion CT scans reveal multiple small faintly enhancing lesions throughout both hemispheres. The preinfusion CT scan was normal.

C and *D*, Magnetic resonance scans using the SE TR3120/TE120 reveal multiple scattered areas of increased signal intensity (*arrows*). The findings are consistent with metastatic disease.

FIGURE 10–16. *Multiple Metastases:* Elderly female presented with symptoms of a transient ischemic attack. *A* and *B*, Preinfusion CT scan is within normal limits.

C to *F*, Postinfusion CT scans demonstrate innumerable rounded metastatic deposits, which are visible on every slice of the scan. These deposits are located in both the supra- and infratentorial distribution. This case illustrates the obvious value of the postinfusion CT scan, which should be obtained in all patients being evaluated for metastatic disease. It is not uncommon for patients with multiple metastases to present with signs and symptoms of a transient ischemic attack. These multiple rounded lesions were found to be secondary to primary breast carcinoma.

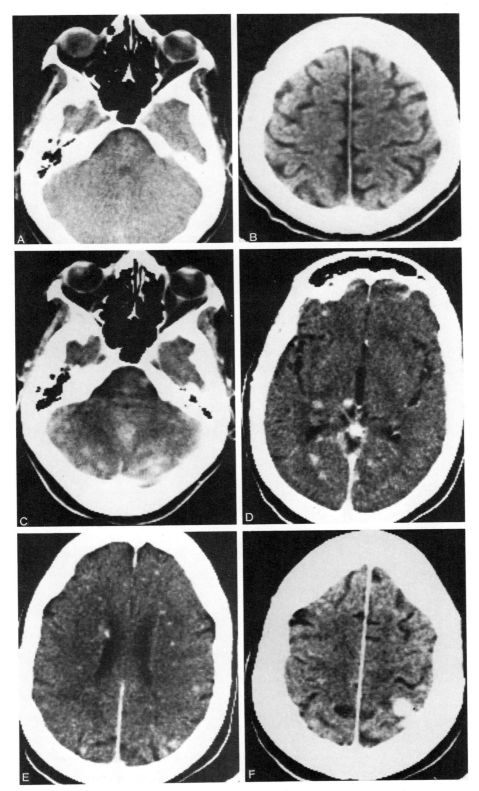

FIGURE 10–16. *See legend on the opposite page.*

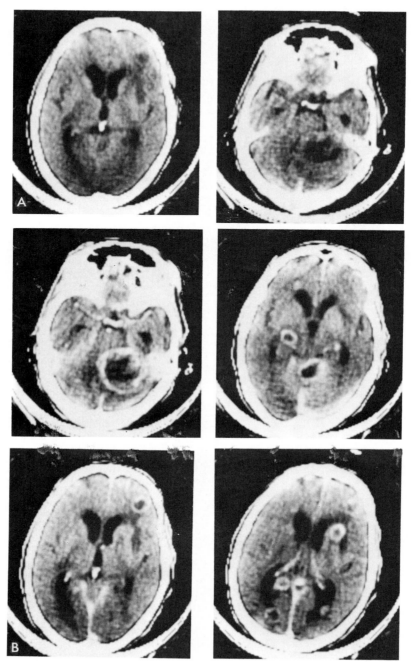

FIGURE 10–17. *Multiple Metastases, Supra- and Infratentorial:* A, The preinfusion scan reveals multiple areas of radiolucency in both hemispheres and in the infratentorial region. There is mild obstructive hydrocephalus. Because the lesions are balancing, there is no shift of the midline.

B, The postinfusion scan reveals that the lesions enhance in a ring-shaped fashion; all are surrounded by varying amounts of cerebral edema.

IMP: Multiple metastases; primary lung cancer. Multiple abscesses could have a similar appearance.

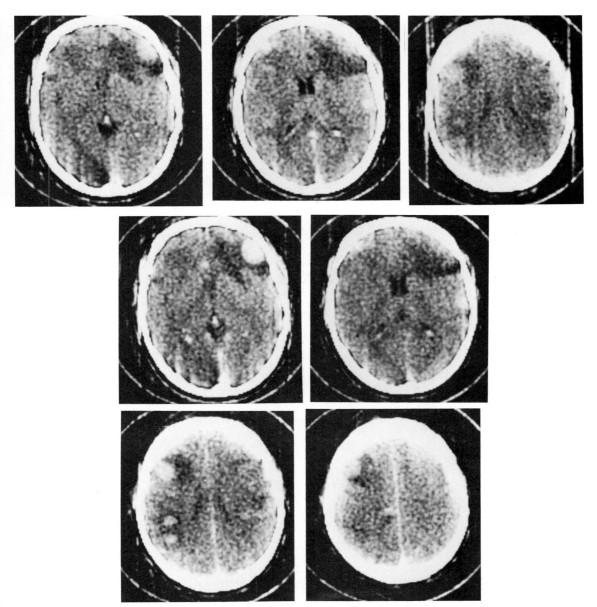

FIGURE 10–18. *Metastatic Melanoma:* The preinfusion scan reveals scattered high-density lesions throughout both hemispheres. The postinfusion scan reveals marked homogeneous enhancement of the lesions. This appearance is quite typical of metastatic melanoma, which often is very vascular and therefore of high density on the preinfusion scan; it enhances greatly on the postinfusion scan. Scans in metastatic melanoma may also demonstrate that the metastatic nodules are hemorrhagic.

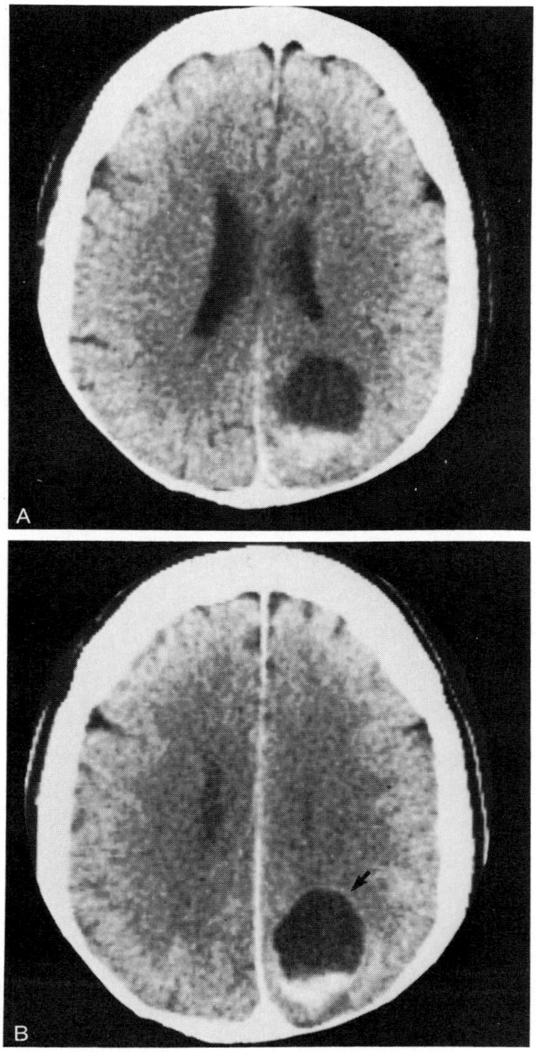

FIGURE 10–19. *Metastatic Lung Cancer:* *A,* The preinfusion CT scan demonstrates a cystic lesion high in the left parietal lobe. There is a fluid/fluid level in the dependent portion of the mass secondary, most likely to hemorrhage into the cyst. There is slight mass effect with compression of the ipsilateral lateral ventricle.

B, Postinfusion CT scan reveals a faint rim of enhancement around the cystic portion of the mass (*arrow*). Close examination for this type of change with peripheral enhancement should be performed, because in the absence of a nodule of enhancement or hemorrhage this could be mistaken for a porencephalic cyst. There is also slight increase in the density of the fluid in the dependent portion of the cyst, probably because some of the contrast material has leaked into the cyst.

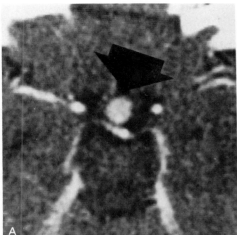

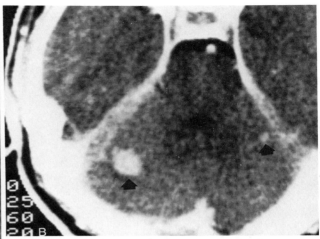

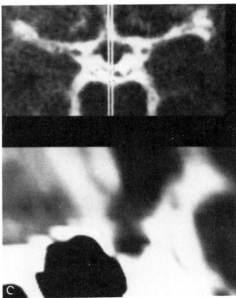

FIGURE 10–20. *Metastases Involving Pituitary Stalk and Cerebellum, Lung Primary:* *A* and *B*, Postinfusion CT scans reveal a round mass in the region of the pituitary stalk that measures 1 cm in diameter (*arrow* in *A*); the normal stalk is 4 mm or less in size. Two small cerebellar metastases are also seen (*arrows* in *B*).

C, Midsagittal reconstruction view of the metrizamide cisternogram reveals the greatly enlarged pituitary stalk and prominent hypothalamus.

D, Midsagittal SE TR3120/TE60 reveals the enlarged infundibulum (*arrow*) extending up to the hypothalamus. There is also an area of increased signal intensity in the region of the hypothalamus (*H*). The patient presented with the clinical signs of diabetes insipidus, and the findings are consistent with multiple metastases with involvement of the pituitary stalk and hypothalamus, which led to diabetes insipidus.

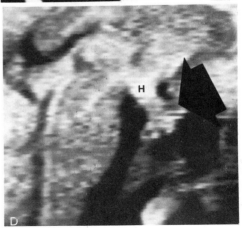

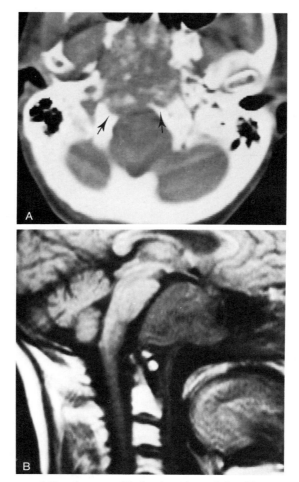

FIGURE 10–21. *Nasopharyngeal Carcinoma with Destruction of the Skull Base:* A, CT scan through the region of the sella turcica reveals marked destructive changes of the sella, the sphenoid sinus, and the medial ends of the petrous bones, and even extends back to the anterior margin of the foramen magnum (*arrows*).

B, Midsagittal SE TR530/TE30 reveals the large isointense mass that has destroyed the clivus, the sphenoid sinus, and the sella turcica. The optic chiasm is displaced superiorly, and the pons is effaced and displaced posteriorly.

Biopsy proved nasopharyngeal carcinoma. Metastases or chordoma could have a similar appearance.

11

TRAUMA

FRACTURES OF THE SKULL

Plain Skull Film Examination

Skull fractures may be classified as linear, comminuted, depressed, or compound.

Linear fractures may occur in any area of the calvaria. Fractures involving the base of the skull are particularly difficult to detect. The routine skull series should be inspected closely, with emphasis on the area of interest. It may be necessary for the radiologist to perform a physical examination of the patient to determine the point of injury. If the patient is not present in the department, the films should be "bright lighted" to determine whether there are any areas of soft tissue swelling that might aid in identifying the point of injury.

Linear fractures of the calvaria are radiolucent, with a very well-defined border (see Fig. 11–1, p. 476). A thorough knowledge of the normal anatomy of the skull will help the radiologist avoid mistaking a normal suture line or vascular groove for a linear fracture. This is particularly true in pediatric patients, in whom sutures and areas of synchondrosis may simulate the appearance of a fracture line. Fractures may be visible on only one view of the skull; therefore, multiple views are obtained for complete evaluation. Simple linear skull fractures extend through both tables of the skull and therefore are more lucent than normal vascular grooves. They do not have the sclerotic border seen with a vascular groove, and they rarely bifurcate—another finding seen with vascular grooves.

The suture line on the outer table of the skull has a serrated appearance, whereas the suture on the inner table of the skull is a straight line. This straight line of the inner table may be mistaken for a fracture.

The posterior branch of the middle meningeal artery courses posterosuperiorly in the squamosal portion of the temporal bone and not uncommonly is mistaken for a fracture—particularly when the history relates to an injury in that region. If the vascular groove is visualized bilaterally, its true nature is more easily established; however, in some cases it may be impossible to differentiate this groove from a fracture.

On the Towne's view of the skull, the occipitomastoid suture frequently is viewed "on-end," and because of its rather straight appearance may easily be mistaken for a fracture. Comparison with the opposite side is helpful for complete evaluation but may not provide absolute proof of the presence or absence of a fracture. The pediatric skull presents unique problems because of the persistence of normal suture lines and synchondroses in the early years of life (Fig. 11–9, p. 483). In particular, the mendosal suture of the occipital bone may have the appearance of a fracture. Usually the mendosal suture is bilateral (Fig. 11–9).

Depressed Fractures. The amount of depression of the fracture fragments varies greatly depending on the injury. A depression of 0.5 cm or more is likely to cause damage to the underlying brain and therefore is usually surgically elevated. A tangential view is helpful in determining the amount of depression (see

465

Chapter 2 and Figs. 11–3, p. 478, and 11–10, p. 483).

Compound Fractures. External compound fractures result from a communication with the scalp. Internal compound fractures communicate with the paranasal sinuses. Osteomyelitis may occur as a result of compound fractures, and safeguards should be taken to prevent its occurrence.

Base-of-Skull Fractures. Not all fractures of the base of the skull will be identified on the plain films. There may, however, be secondary signs of fractures involving the base of the skull. Clinically, these patients may present with CSF rhinorrhea or CSF otorrhea; if the fracture involves the facial canal, there may be facial nerve palsy. The skull films may reveal an air-fluid level in the sphenoid sinus because CSF has leaked into the sinus or because of the accumulation of blood in the sinus. These air-fluid levels also may be seen in the frontal sinus or in the ethmoid sinus. For these reasons it is strongly recommended that skull films be obtained with the patient in the upright position if at all possible. On the other hand, the air-fluid level can also be demonstrated in cross-table lateral films with the patient in the supine position (see Fig. 11–11, p. 484).

With high-resolution CT scanning, a high percentage of base-of-skull fractures can be identified. To prove the presence of a CSF leak, cotton pledgets are placed in the nose or the ear, and radioactive material is then instilled in the lumbar-subarachoid space. Later, the pledgets are removed from the nose or ear and scanned. The presence of radioactivity in the plegets confirms leakage of CSF.

CT scanning of the sinuses after the instillation of Amipaque also may be used to demonstrate a CSF leak. The Amipaque that leaks from the subarachnoid space will be seen to accumulate in a small puddle in the nose.

Medicolegal Aspects of Skull Fractures

In one study of adult patients with head trauma who were examined with skull radiographs, less than 10 per cent exhibited skull fractures. Most of these were linear and were seen in the cranial vault. No correlation was demonstrated between the physical findings, the patient's symptoms, and the radiographic findings. In only two of the 49 patients studied radiologically was the proposed treatment altered.

In one study of a large number of pediatric patients with head trauma, approximately 25 per cent had radiographic evidence of a skull fracture. The skull fracture did not correlate with the clinical seriousness of the patient's symptoms and did not alter the decision for medical care, except in children with depressed or compound fractures. The incidence of serious intracranial sequelae in head injuries, regardless of the presence or absence of a skull fracture, is 9 per cent; the incidence of these sequelae in children without a fracture is 8 per cent. However, because of the need for as thorough an evaluation as possible in patients who have a history of head trauma and possible skull fracture, a routine skull series probably should be obtained in these patients. This is particularly true if there is external evidence of severe head trauma. On the other hand, if one considers cost effectiveness as well as the potential hazards of radiation, one might argue that more stringent criteria be applied to patients selected for skull radiography.

Such criteria might include a history of unconsciousness, gunshot wound or skull penetration, or previous craniotomy with shunt tube in place. During the physical examination, one should look for:

1. Palpable skull depression or skull fracture
2. CSF discharge from nose
3. Battle's sign
4. CSF discharge from ear
5. Raccoon's eyes
6. Blood in the middle ear cavity
7. Coma or stupor
8. Focal neurologic signs

Fracture Healing

Linear fractures may remain apparent for many years after the initial injury. In some cases they may never be completely obliterated. Healing does not occur with callus formation as it does in the long bones; instead, there is gradual bony overgrowth of the fracture site (Fig. 11–6, p. 480).

TRAUMA—AN OVERVIEW

Specific entities will be discussed later in this chapter. The changes following head trauma are related to the type and severity of the injury and also to the point of injury. Because these changes may or may not be visible on the plain film examination of the skull, a thorough knowledge of normal anatomy is needed in order to evaluate the plain skull examination and any areas of suspicion.

Soft tissue injury will appear radiographically as an area of soft tissue prominence that becomes visible when the skull films are examined under a bright light. This examination for swelling of soft tissues is of particular importance when the history does not indicate the area or point of interest. Skull fractures may appear as small, thin linear areas of radiolucency to the shattered skull seen with severe head injury (Figs. 11–1, p. 476, and 11–10, p. 483).

It is important to remember that most patients who have suffered life-threatening head trauma also have severe injuries to other parts of the body. This will, of necessity, limit the patient's ability to cooperate fully during radiographic examination. It may be necessary to re-examine the patient after the other critical injuries have become stabilized to the point where more particular attention can be given to the bony calvaria. In cases of multiple injury, AP and lateral films may be all that can be obtained at the initial examination. An attempt should be made to evaluate these films as completely as possible, noting any abnormalities that could be associated with intracranial problems and any areas of suspicion that need re-examination (Figs. 11–2, p. 477, and 11–3, p. 478).

If possible, when there are no other life-threatening problems, a routine skull series should be obtained. The series should include right and left lateral views, PA view, Towne's view, and the submentovertex, if possible. As noted earlier, a skull fracture may be visible on only one view; therefore, multiple views are necessary for complete evaluation. Particular attention should be paid to the point of soft tissue injury. Linear skull fractures appear as thin, well-defined areas of radiolucency. If visible on the lateral view, they will appear finer and more distinct on the film closest to the side of the injury.

Fractures in the frontal and occipital areas may be visible on only one view. Particular care should be taken to visualize the occipital region on the Towne's view. Likewise, a fracture placed far laterally in the frontal bone or an occipital area may be difficult to visualize on both the PA and the lateral views of the skull. If any such area of suspicion cannot be evaluated by the films available, additional studies, such as oblique views, should be made to rule out a fracture.

The presence of a skull fracture does not imply that there is severe or even *any* intra-cranial injury. However, it does mean that there has been a certain degree of injury beyond soft tissue damage. On the other hand, the absence of a skull fracture does not rule out the presence of severe and even life-threatening intracranial damage. Trauma may result in extracerebral collections of blood in the subdural or epidural space. Contusion of the brain with edema or clot formation also may be seen. An individual patient may have any combination of these processes. It should be mentioned that the plain film examination remains the best method for evaluation of the presence of a linear skull fracture. The CT scan *may* reveal the fracture line—but if the plane of the fracture is in the same plane as the scan slice, the fracture will not visualize. The bony calvaria should be evaluated by examination of each slice of the CT scan on the viewing screen with manipulation of the window widths and window levels.

Late Effects

Leptomeningeal Cyst. If the skull fracture has resulted in a tear in the dural layer of the meninges, the arachnoid membrane may be tethered in the fracture line after protruding through the dural tear. Over a long period— months or years—the continued transmitted pulsations of the heart beat and respirations to the arachnoid caught in the linear fracture result in a smoothing and widening of the margin of the fracture and a palpable cystic mass outside the bony calvaria—a leptomeningeal cyst (see Chapter 2).

Porencephalic Cysts. Head trauma that has resulted in significant intracranial damage destroys a portion of the cerebral tissue. This damage may present initially as an area of edema, areas of infarction, hemorrhage, or a combination of these processes. Eventually the acute cerebral damage resolves, sometimes leaving an area of porencephaly in the bed of the previous abnormality. The development of such post-traumatic porencephalic cysts can be observed on serial CT scans. The cysts contain cerebrospinal fluid and consequently are of similar density to the ventricular fluid on the CT scan.

Extracerebral Hematomas

If a fracture extends across the meningeal artery grooves, there is a possibility of shearing the vessel lying in the groove. Damage to the middle meningeal artery may result in an epidural hematoma; therefore, any fracture with this appearance should alert one to the real possibility of intracranial hemorrhage (see Fig. 11–36, p. 509). Typically, an epidural hematoma is of arterial origin from the middle meningeal artery, but venous bleeding into the epidural space also may occur. Without proper care, this injury may lead rapidly to death.

Head injuries also may result in a subdural hematoma. The amount of trauma necessary to create a subdural or epidural hematoma varies from individual to individual and in different age groups. Very young and very old persons develop subdural hematomas more readily than individuals in other age groups.

Intracerebral Hematomas

In addition to extracerebral accumulations of blood, there may be evidence of intracerebral hematoma formation. The intracerebral hematoma may be remote from the point of skull trauma and may be secondary to "contra-coup" injury to the brain—brain injury opposite the point of skull trauma. This results when there is rapid deceleration of the brain—as from a high-speed motor vehicle accident—and the brain opposite the initial point of injury is stopped suddenly by hitting the cranial vault. This occurs because there is a certain amount of mobility of the brain within the bony calvaria.

The development of intracerebral hematoma may, of course, be at the site of direct trauma. There may be an associated subdural hematoma, an epidural hematoma, or a combination of these. The contra-coup damage may occur in any portion of the brain. Commonly affected areas are the anterior temporal lobes, as they are limited by the greater wings of the sphenoid bone, which is a firm bony margin; the frontal lobes; and the occipital lobes of the brain. In addition to hematoma formation or in its absence, there may be contusion of the cerebrum, which results in small petechial hemorrhages or edema. Any of these cerebral changes may produce a similar clinical picture, and, in many cases, arteriography will assist in defining the problem but not the true pathologic nature of the intracranial lesion. Only since the development of CT scanning has it become possible to differentiate with certainty between cerebral edema and hemorrhage.

Computed Tomography

The development of computed tomography has brought an entirely new approach to the evaluation of patients with head trauma. When these facilities are available, the CT scan should be the first diagnostic procedure performed on a patient with signficant head trauma. *The CT scan provides a more accurate picture of intracranial injury than any other type of diagnostic procedure.* A CT scan of adequate diagnostic quality offers a highly accurate evaluation of intracranial anatomy, and comparison with anatomic sections shows excellent correlation between the scans and the pathologic anatomy.

CT scanning provides a totally new approach to the problems of head injury. Although plain radiography may reveal a skull fracture, the *absence* of a skull fracture does not rule out any of the complications of head trauma discussed earlier. Therefore, any patient who has sustained significant head trauma and in whom there are clinical signs or suspicion of intracranial damage should have an emergency CT scan. It may be necessary to sedate these patients in order to obtain a good quality study. If sedation is used, careful monitoring is necessary. In some cases general anesthesia is needed—especially in the combative or intoxicated patient when immobilization by any other method proves impossible. Indeed, it is these patients who not uncommonly are sent from the emergency room to the scanning room and then directly to the operating room.

In any patient who has suffered severe central nervous system damage, consultation with the neurosurgical service should be obtained as quickly as possible. This is essential because occasional emergency room patients will require bur holes before a diagnosis is made if there is such rapid deterioration that further delay will lead to certain death.

Specific CT Scan Appearance in Trauma

With diffuse *cerebral edema* the lateral ventricles will be very small or even invisible, although the CT scan may not reveal a detectable alteration in the density of the brain. Accumulation of blood in the subarachnoid space may make the falx cerebri more readily visible than would be expected because it is outlined by blood on either side. With intraventricular hemorrhage the blood may accumulate in the dependent portions of the lateral ventricles when the patient lies in the supine position. Localized areas of edema may be revealed as areas of radiolucency, with shift of the midline structures; high-resolution CT scanning often demonstrates disruption of the normal gray-white relationship. Even small areas of intracerebral hemorrhage are readily demonstrated by the CT scan.

If the scan reveals a subdural hematoma, epidural hematoma, or a large intracerebral hematoma, the patient can be taken directly to the operating room for surgical correction. Further diagnostic procedures might only delay appropriate treatment. In *selected* cases it may be appropriate to obtain only one midsection cut through the brain. If a large epidural or subdural hematoma is demonstrated, appropriate therapeutic measures may be taken without further delay.

Following acute head trauma there may be dilatation of the lateral ventricles without any other abnormalities. This ventricular dilatation may be caused by a communicating hydrocephalus secondary to subarachnoid hemorrhage, although the etiology in some cases is unknown. The lateral ventricles may then remain unchanged in size, return to normal size, or continue to increase in size. Ventricular enlargement not present acutely may later be seen on a follow-up scan. It is believed that this communicating hydrocephalus develops because blood in the subarachnoid space interferes with the absorption of cerebrospinal fluid by the arachnoid villi. CT scans are the ideal method to follow this alteration in ventricular size.

SUBDURAL HEMATOMAS

Subdural hematomas develop between the inner layer of the dura and the arachnoid membrane—hence, the name "subdural hematoma." An acute subdural hematoma is a life-threatening event that results in death in many individuals and in significant morbidity in others.

Plain Film Examination

Plain film radiography may or may not reveal a skull fracture. A shift of the pineal gland contralateral to the side of the subdural hematoma may be noted. However, the absence of shift does not rule out a subdural hematoma because the subdural accumulations may be bilateral. Also, there may be significant edema on the contralateral side secondary to a contra-coup lesion, preventing a shift of the midline structures even when there is significant intracranial damage. In addition, the pineal gland may be uncalcified—and thus of no help in diagnosis. Subdural hematomas also may develop in the posterior fossa. Indeed, posterior fossa subdural hematomas can cause compression of vital structures and the very rapid demise of the patient.

Computed Tomography

In acute subdural hematoma a crescentic extracerebral collection of clotted blood is seen over the affected hemisphere. There will be shift of the midline structures to the contralateral side (see Fig. 11–16, p. 488). These accumulations vary from small to very large amounts of blood. Sometimes the extracerebral accumulation of blood may be so small that it is barely appreciable (Fig. 11–22, p. 494). In these cases there is a varying amount of shift of the midline structures to the contralateral side. It is important and often necessary to manipulate the density control system on varying window widths and window levels to better outline the abnormality. Clotted blood measures from 50 to 90 Hounsfield units.

Density manipulation of the CT scanning unit should also be performed so that the bony calvaria also can be viewed and examined for evidence of skull fracture. Both linear and depressed skull fractures can be identified by CT scan. Linear fractures may not be identified if they are not in a plane visualized by the cuts. Failure to visualize a skull fracture on the CT scan therefore does not rule out its presence.

Large acute subdural hematomas may develop the appearance of a hematocrit level (Figs. 11–16, 11–18, and 11–19, pp. 488, 489, and 490–491). This occurs because the blood components settle when the patient remains in the supine position for a prolonged period. The settling of the relatively heavy hemoglobin molecule produces this appearance; at the time of surgery, there is no difference in the appearance of the clotted blood—unlike a hematocrit determination.

Acute subdural hematomas are readily identified by CT scanning, whether uni- or bilateral. In addition, the scan may show edema surrounding these extracerebral accumulations and/or evidence of contusion of the brain.

Subacute Subdural Hematomas

A gradual decrease in density of the extracerebral accumulations of blood takes place post-injury. This results in a mottled appearance of the subdural blood, rather than the white density seen in acute hematomas. It is not known how much time is required before this change in density occurs, because it is often impossible to determine when the patients initially sustained their head trauma. However, early density changes probably occur in the first week post-injury. These patients are frequently alcoholic or demented and may even give a history of multiple instances of head trauma. Not uncommonly these unfortunate individuals are brought to the emergency room without any useful history.

An associated shift of the midline to the contralateral side is seen in the subacute stage. The subdural accumulation will be less crescentic and more lentiform.

Chronic Subdural Hematomas

CT Scan. During the progression of a subdural hematoma from the acute to the chronic stages, the density of the blood accumulation may be similar (isodense) to the normal brain substance. If this is the case, there may be a shift of the midline but no evidence of a mass lesion or extracerebral accumulation. There may even be an appearance of hemiatrophy on the contralateral side, the shift of the midline appearing to be toward the atrophic side. The greatest danger in these fortunately uncommon cases is that isodense subdural accumulations may be bilateral (Fig. 11–21, p. 494), thus producing no shift of the midline. It is helpful for diagnosis if the index of suspicion for a subdural hematoma is high in these cases. In patients with isodense bilateral subdural hematomas, the lateral ventricles appear to be elongated and compressed toward the midline.

The lateral ventricles may appear to be smaller than one would normally anticipate for a patient in the older age group because of compression by bilateral subdural hematomas. As these lesions occur frequently in older patients, the absence of cortical sulci provides further evidence of an abnormal scan. The sulci may be obliterated unilaterally or bilaterally, depending on the nature of the lesions.

If bilateral isodense subdural hematomas are a consideration, arteriography may be necessary for more definitive evaluation. A membrane develops around a subdural hematoma 10 to 14 days post-injury. Chronic subdural hematomas may cause enhancement of this membrane on the postinfusion study. This enhancement may be quite subtle (Fig. 11–27, p. 498) and should be looked for by using varying window widths and window levels; all the cuts should be reviewed, with particular attention given to the very highest cuts. Displacement of the cortical veins away from the inner table on the postinfusion study also may be seen.

Following evacuation of bilateral subdural accumulations, the follow-up CT scan reveals that the lateral ventricles have returned to a more normal size for the patient's age group; also, there may be visualization of the cortical sulci that had not been visible prior to evacuation.

In pediatric patients, *chronic* bilateral subdural hematomas may be associated with dilatation of the lateral ventricles. The CT appearance of enlarged ventricles and small cortical sulci is consistent with a communicating hydrocephalus. The lateral ventricles are dilated and there is evidence of bilateral low-density extracerebral accumulations of fluid. The enlargement of the lateral ventricles is thought to be a result of interference with absorption of CSF by the arachnoid villi because of the presence of the bilateral subdural hematomas; however, the exact pathophysiology is not understood.

The author has seen cases in which evacuation of subdural accumulations has resulted in collapse of the cerebrum and accumulation of air in the cranial cavity. It appears that in these cases there is a pre-existing decrease in the normal amount of brain substance. Following removal of the subdural accumulation, the brain is unable to expand and refill the intracranial space.

Magnetic Resonance of Trauma

The patient with acute craniocerebral trauma is probably not a candidate for magnetic resonance scanning. This is because the acutely injured patient often has sustained multisystem injury and is likely to be on life-support systems that will not function properly in a magnetized environment or, because of their magnetic properties, cannot be brought into the scanning arena. In addition to these basic mechanical and technical problems, acute hemorrhage— less than 48 hours old—may appear as low signal intensity and therefore be difficult to appreciate by MR scanning (see below). Another problem that militates against the use of MR for the acutely injured patient is the fact that the MR scans may require 5- to 15-minute scanning times. These long scanning times require that a patient remain immobile throughout the scanning period, and thus the patient must be able to cooperate or the scan will not be successful. Although the ready availability of multiplanar imaging makes MR attractive for the evaluation of the exact anatomic location of a blood collection, it is immediately obvious that the scan slices of less than five seconds which are possible with CT make CT the procedure of choice for the patient with acute craniocerebral trauma.

The experience with MR to date suggests that acute hemorrhage less than 48 hours old will be of low signal intensity on the T-1 weighted SE sequences. Therefore, an acute extra- or intracerebral collection of blood, such as that seen following trauma or with a hemorrhagic contusion, may not be appreciated on the MR scan obtained early in the course of the illness. Therefore CT is the procedure of choice under these circumstances because it is exquisitely sensitive to the presence of blood—either intracerebral or extracerebral. On the other hand, blood that is greater than 48 hours old is readily appreciated on the MR scans and appears as an area of markedly increased signal intensity on the T-1 weighted images. The exact location of this blood is easily identified, and whether it is intracerebral or extracerebral is easily appreciated. The multiplanar capability of MR is extraordinarily useful for localization.

Changing Signal Intensity with Time

The signal intensity of blood appears to change with time because the hemoglobin molecule in the blood changes to methemoglobin in the course of its metabolism. This alteration in the chemical structure from deoxyhemoglobin to methemoglobin makes the blood more paramagnetic and results in shortening of the T-1 and therefore a higher signal intensity on the T-1 weighted images. This change in appearance over time can be used to advantage. In the patient with an isodense subdural hematoma, as identified by CT—a condition that is often very difficult, but simultaneously very important, to diagnose—the obvious advantage of MR is easily appreciated. These older blood collections are exquisitely identified by MR, and the surgical approach can be easily planned, particularly because the multiplanar capability of the MR scan allows for accurate localization of the extracerebral collections. In particular, coronal images are helpful for evaluation and differentiation of infra- vs a supratentorial extracerebral collection.

The metabolism of intracerebral hematomas presents a unique appearance with MR. With very old blood collections, probably greater than three months (the exact time has not yet been determined), the MR signal again becomes decreased in intensity, probably because of the deposition of hemosiderin. Hemosiderin is a paramagnetic contrast agent that shortens the T-1, but also shortens the T-2, resulting in a decreased signal intensity on the T-1 weighted images. The areas of hemosiderin deposition also remain decreased in signal intensity on the T-2 weighted images.

Older extracerebral hematomas, such as chronic subdural hematomas, may present as isointense extracerebral collections on the T-1 weighted images. Their presence may be appreciated because the cortical veins appear as areas of negative flow defects that are displaced away from the inner table of the bony calvaria. In some cases the blood flow in the cortical veins is sufficiently slowed that the displaced veins appear as dotlike areas of high signal intensity. These chronic extracerebral collections are easily identified on the T-2 weighted images, where they appear as increased signal intensity. Chronic subdural collections can be diagnosed by the typical lentiform or biconvex configuration similar to those identified by CT scanning.

Epidural Hematoma

MR demonstrates the typical lentiform configuration that is pathognomonic of the epidural hematoma. The blood appears of increased signal intensity on the T-1 weighted images, and the dura appears as low signal intensity outlining the periphery of the blood collection. The dura remains of low signal intensity on both T-1 and T-2 weighted images. Associated abnormalities such as intracerebral hematomas and contralateral lesions are easily identified.

Shearing Injuries

Shearing injuries were originally described several decades ago in the neurosurgical literature. At that time, it was thought that all individuals who sustained this type of injury died. We now know that many individuals with shearing injuries may live, but return to a normal level of functioning is unlikely.

Shearing injuries result from rapid deceleration such as occurs when an individual is propelled through the windshield of a car or hits the steering wheel in a motor vehicle accident. The name is descriptive. The white matter and gray matter of the brain have two different densities; when rapid deceleration occurs, the white matter stops at one rate of speed while the gray matter stops at a different rate of speed. This results in a "shearing" off of the nerves at the gray-white junction.

CT of Shearing Injury

In the acutely severely injured, even the comatose patient, the CT scan may be entirely within normal limits or may demonstrate small ventricles secondary to diffuse cerebral swelling. Acutely, rapid changes in the clinical condition of the patient may necessitate several CT scans within the first 24 hours and additional CT scans within the first week following injury to rule out a potentially surgically treatable problem. Subtle changes that may be present acutely are (1) blood in the subarachnoid space, (2) blood in the lateral ventricles, (3) rounded or oval areas of hemorrhage at the gray-white junction, and (4) small lateral ventricles. The hemorrhages at the gray-white junction also may be delayed and may occur hours or days after injury. The appearance of small lateral ventricles may be secondary to diffuse cerebral edema. Care must be taken in interpreting small lateral ventricles, depending upon the patient's age. Small ventricles in a very old individual are more suggestive of diffuse cerebral edema than are small lateral ventricles seen in a younger patient, in whom they are a normal finding.

Very late changes, seen in surviving patients, are an appearance of either a communicating hydrocephalus or diffuse cerebral atrophy with enlargement of the ventricles and cortical sulci. There may also be areas of lucency at the gray-white junction secondary to encephalomalacia or porencephaly following resorption of the hematomas. These severely injured patients rarely return to a normal life and frequently survive in a vegetative state.

Magnetic Resonance of Shearing Injury

ACUTE CHANGES. Magnetic resonance is more sensitive to the changes seen following a shearing injury than is any other diagnostic method. The MR scan demonstrates typical areas of increased signal intensity on the T-1 weighted images if bleeding has occurred at the gray-white junction. If no bleeding has occurred, the MR scan demonstrates areas of increased signal intensity at the gray-white junction on the T-2 weighted images. Because of the increased sensitivity of MR as compared to CT, the MR scan may be abnormal even if the CT scan is normal. Shearing injuries may also affect the midbrain region, and this area is best demonstrated by MR. Similarly, changes may also occur in the corpus callosum. For the comatose patient with abnormal CT scan following head injury, MR may be helpful not only as a diagnostic test, but also as a predictive test for possible late effects and/or permanent damage.

CHRONIC CHANGES. MR is also sensitive to the very late changes of craniocerebral trauma. In those patients with persistent mental deterioration or progressive mental changes, MR may be grossly abnormal, even if other tests are normal. MR demonstrates areas of increased signal intensity on the T-2 weighted images at the gray-white junction and enlarged lateral ventricles with or without enlarged cortical sulci, secondary to diffuse atrophy or a communicating hydrocephalus. These changes may be apparent by MR even though the CT scan does not reveal any areas of abnormal density. The identification of these late changes is helpful for future life-style planning for both the patient and the family.

Spinal Trauma

Because MR allows direct visualization of the spinal cord, it is an ideal method to evaluate any change in cord size secondary to hematoma formation or edema. MR also demonstrates fracture deformity of the vertebral column and associated hematoma formation. MR may well become the procedure of choice for evaluation of spinal or vertebral injury (see Chapter 15).

Arteriography of Subdural Hematomas

The AP view is usually most helpful. With a subdural hematoma in the parietal convexity area, the AP view will demonstrate that the branches of the middle cerebral artery group will not reach the inner table of the skull; instead, they are displaced away from the inner table, revealing an avascular crescentic mass outside the cerebral substance. The midline structures will be shifted to the contralateral side.

In the venous phase the cortical veins also will be displaced away from the inner table of the skull in a fashion similar to that noted for the arteries. Both the arteries and the cortical veins run in the subarachnoid space and therefore will be displaced by a subdural accumulation of blood. In addition, there will be a shift of the internal cerebral vein to the contralateral side. Note that subdural accumulations do not cross the midline because they are limited by the reflection of the dura that forms the falx cerebri. Inspection of the films reveals that the cortical veins at the level of the subdural hematoma curve superiorly as they approach the parasagittal region (Fig. 11–32, p. 504) in order to drain into the superior sagittal sinus in normal anatomic fashion. It is because of the falx and superior sagittal sinus and its attachment to the cortical veins that subdural hematomas do not cross the midline.

Subdural hematomas also may develop in the interhemispheric fissure on either side of the falx. This is more readily demonstrated on the CT scan.

When a subdural hematoma is demonstrated by arteriography and there is no shift of the midline structures, one should strongly suspect the presence of a contralateral subdural hematoma or contusion. A study of the contralateral side should be performed in such patients. This may be done by using the cross-compression technique or, if this is unsuccessful in visualizing the opposite side, by subsequent arteriography of that side. The position of the internal cerebral vein should be determined by linear measurement—not by the use of the "eye-ball" technique.

Pitfalls in Diagnosis. If the subdural accumulation is positioned anteriorly, the branches of the middle cerebral artery—which are at the widest biparietal diameter of the skull—will appear to reach the inner table, whereas in reality there is displacement of the branches *away* from the inner table more anteriorly, where the bony calvaria is narrower. This results in failure to visualize the extracerebral accumulation. Although there will be shift of the pericallosal artery to the contralateral side and a less marked shift of the internal cerebral vein, an oblique view of the AP projection toward the side of the suspected subdural hematoma will be required. This allows a tangential view of the vessels where they fail to reach the inner table of the skull (Fig. 11–33, p. 505).

If the subdural accumulation is positioned posteriorly, a similar arteriographic appearance is noted. Again, the branches of the middle cerebral artery will reach the inner table, while the more posterior branches that are displaced away from the inner table will not be seen because of the narrowing of the skull posteriorly. If this is the case a distal shift of the pericallosal artery under the falx and a more marked shift of the internal cerebral vein will be seen. Again, an oblique view away from the side of the hematoma will allow a tangential view of these vessels posteriorly (Fig. 11–33, p. 505). In fact, when CT scanning is unavailable and an emergency arteriogram is done for a suspected subdural hematoma, a practical and expeditious method of arteriographic study is a standard AP and lateral projection followed immediately by AP runs (arterial phase only),

turning the patient obliquely, first toward the ipsilateral side and then toward the contralateral side. This way, either an anteriorly or posteriorly placed subdural hematoma will not be overlooked. The technique is especially helpful if the hematoma happens to be bilateral and is not associated with a shift of the anterior cerebral artery or internal cerebral vein.

If the supratentorial circulation is normal, the infratentorial circulation may require additional study. This is particularly true if hydrocephalus is demonstrated in the supratentorial circulation.

The Lateral View. The lateral view not uncommonly gives a normal or nearly normal appearance in a large percentage of cases. This occurs because the structures are simply displaced out of the plane of view toward the side opposite the hematoma and are frequently not distorted. In other words, the vessel relationships are not changed, but simply moved from their normal positions. This relatively normal appearance is more likely to be seen when the hematoma is over the low convexity and covers a large area. It must be remembered that this is true only when the subdural hematoma is not complicated with other findings, such as an intracerebral hematoma, a cerebral contusion, or focal areas of cerebral edema.

On the other hand, if the hematoma is situated in the high convexity or parasagittal area there will be downward displacement of the sylvian triangle. If a subdural hematoma is anterior in its location, the sylvian triangle will be displaced posteriorly, and it will be noted that the vessels in the frontal area do not reach the inner table of the skull (Fig. 11–34, p. 506). Although absence of vessels adjacent to the inner table of the skull also may be seen with atrophy of the frontal lobes of the brain, if atrophy is present there will be no shift to the contralateral side. This, of course, is true only in the absence of bilateral subdural accumulations. Because the cortical veins must join with the superior sagittal sinus high in the convexity region, these veins will not *appear* to be displaced from the inner table on the lateral view (Fig. 11–34, p. 506). However, they will be displaced away from the inner table on the AP view obtained in the oblique projection with the patient's head turned toward the side of the hematoma. This is not to say that displacement has not occurred—only that it cannot be appreciated on the lateral view. The sylvian triangle may be displaced posteriorly as well as inferiorly. With a subdural accumulation in the occipital region, the sylvian triangle may be telescoped anteriorly if the mass is retrosylvian—and/or displaced inferiorly if the mass is superior to the sylvian triangle. Obviously, any combination of these changes may be seen, depending on the location of the hematoma.

Other Associated Changes. If there has been *contusion* of the brain, or even an element of subarachnoid hemorrhage, spasm of the vessels may be seen that is similar to that which occurs with a subarachnoid hemorrhage secondary to an aneurysm. If this is the case, the CT scan will demonstrate very small areas of high density secondary to the intracerebral hematoma or petechial hemorrhage, together with some associated edema that appears as areas of radiolucency surrounding the areas of hemorrhage. There may be no evidence of hemorrhage on the CT scan, only areas of lucency secondary to infarction because of spasm or to the edema that follows contusion. This will be associated with shift of the midline structures to the contralateral side. If this is the case, the arteriogram may show a mass effect that is confined to a localized area of edema, or it may reveal diffuse splaying of the vessels if there is massive cerebral edema. With diffuse edema there is no evidence of any specific mass; rather, diffuse changes secondary to the edema are evident.

Most often, trauma results in involvement of the frontal and occipital poles as well as the anterior temporal tips of the brain. In rapid deceleration injuries, primary injury to the brain may occur at the initial point of impact, with secondary edema and contusion at the pole opposite the initial injury—the so-called "contra-coup" lesion. On the other hand, most of the damage may occur at the point of initial injury. Contra-coup lesions develop because the cerebrum is somewhat mobile as it floats in the CSF. Consequently, in rapid deceleration injuries the brain may slide either forward or backward and then be halted by the inner table of the frontal or occipital regions; or, very commonly, the anterior temporal lobes may be injured as they abut the greater wings of the sphenoid that form the anatomic limit of the middle cranial fossa.

Frontal lobe injuries can cause posterior displacement of the anterior cerebral arteries and diffuse splaying of the vascular branches in the frontal poles. If the injury to both frontal poles has been of equal severity, there will be no shift of the midline structures. With an asymmetric injury, the arteriogram will show asymmetric changes that correspond to the extent of damage. Frontal lobe damage will cause posterior displacement of the sylvian triangle. If the damage was severe enough to affect both frontal lobes, frequently there is damage to both anterior temporal lobes as well. The insult to the temporal lobes results in upward displacement of the sylvian triangle secondary to hematoma, contusion, or edema of the lobes.

The author has seen two cases in which severe trauma to the back of the skull resulted in a linear fracture of the occipital bone, apparent forward motion of the cerebrum, and resulting total anosmia—apparently from shearing of all the olfactory nerves where they pass through the cribriform plate—without any other evidence of damage to the cerebral structures.

SUBARACHNOID HEMORRHAGE SECONDARY TO TRAUMA

If an element of subarachnoid hemorrhage is associated with trauma, accumulation of blood in the dependent portions of the lateral ventricles may be evident. A more subtle manifestation is a diffuse increase in density of the falx cerebri that occurs because blood in the subarachnoid space accumulates along the falx and is then apparent on the CT scan. In the older patient, however, the falx may be diffusely calcified even when there is no blood in the subarachnoid space; therefore, this sign must be evaluated on an individual basis. If an old scan is available that did not show this increased density of the falx, or if the increased density resolves on follow-up, the diagnosis of subarachnoid hemorrhage is substantiated.

EPIDURAL HEMATOMAS

An epidural hematoma, as its name implies, is situated outside the dura. It is an extracerebral accumulation of blood in the space between the outer layer of the dura and the inner table of the skull. Generally speaking, epidural hematomas result from arterial bleeding—most frequently from the middle meningeal artery branches. They are frequently, but not always, associated with a fracture that crosses the groove of the meningeal artery branches. Classically, they have a lentiform configuration that is readily demonstrated on both the arteriogram and the CT scan.

Patients with an epidural hematoma may experience a so-called "lucid interval." If this occurs, the patient may have a history of unconsciousness immediately after the injury followed by an interval of total lucidity and a subsequent episode of coma. If the patient is examined during the lucid period, the presence of an epidural hematoma may not be appreciated, and care must be taken not to discharge such a patient from care before a satisfactory period of observation has passed. In our experience this "lucid interval" occurs rarely.

Plain Skull. The plain skull film may be normal. One should look for a fracture that extends across a groove that carries one of the meningeal artery branches. In older patients, the meningeal artery becomes grooved into the inner table of the skull and is more or less fixed in this groove. Therefore, if a fracture extends across the meningeal artery groove, the fixed meningeal artery is very likely to be severed—resulting in hemorrhage into the epidural space.

Epidural hematomas also occur in the posterior fossa; these are frequently associated with a fracture of the occipital bone. Posterior fossa epidural hematomas compress the vital brain stem structures, leading to rapid demise of the patient. They also produce an obstructive hydrocephalus. Thus, if this diagnosis is suspected, appropriate steps should be taken to confirm the diagnosis as rapidly as possible so that appropriate treatment may be undertaken without delay.

Computed Tomography. The CT scan is the diagnostic procedure of choice. The epidural accumulation appears as a lentiform area of blood density in the extracerebral space and is associated with shift of the lateral ventricles to the contralateral side. On occasion, epidural hematomas may resemble a subdural hematoma. Both supratentorial and infratentorial epidural hematomas have a lentiform configuration.

Occasional cases of subfrontal epidural hematoma have a unique and typical configuration in which the classic lentiform configuration is seen in the frontal lobe region but there is only *minimal* shift of the midline structures in spite of the rather large appearing mass (Figs. 11–42 and 11–43, pp. 514–515 and 516). The blood accumulates in the subfrontal region and displaces the brain upward and posteriorly; consequently, the anterior cerebral artery is displaced upward and posteriorly in much the same way as with a subfrontal meningioma. CT scans done in the coronal section are very helpful in confirming the diagnosis of a subfrontal epidural hematoma (Fig. 11–42, pp. 514–515) but are not necessary for diagnosis when the axial CT scan demonstrates the typical appearance of this disorder. The use of high window widths and window levels may help in the identification of small skull fractures.

Arteriography. The arteriographic changes seen with an epidural hematoma are much the same as those seen with subdural hematomas, and the same diagnostic principles apply. In general, it is nearly impossible to make an absolute differential diagnosis between the two types of abnormalities. Only *rarely* will one be able to demonstrate that the middle meningeal artery is displaced away from the inner table of the skull. This finding, in association with an extracerebral accumulation of blood, will enable one to make the diagnosis of epidural hematoma.

Since the epidural hematoma is outside the dura, one may also see separation of the superior sagittal sinus away from the inner table of the skull by an epidural accumulation of blood that extends across the midline. This is in contradistinction to subdural hematomas, which do not cross the midline but are limited by the falx cerebri.

In the posterior fossa, the torcular and lateral sinuses also may be displaced away from the inner table (Fig. 11–45, pp. 518–519). Subtraction films may be helpful and sometimes necessary to evaluate these subtle posterior fossa changes.

BIRTH TRAUMA

Trauma to the head at the time of birth may result in subarachnoid hemorrhage and subsequent enlargement of the lateral ventricles secondary to communicating hydrocephalus. There may be actual post-traumatic intracerebral hematoma formation. In addition, other post-traumatic abnormalities such as subdural hematomas also may be evaluated by the CT scan.

POSTOPERATIVE TRAUMA

It is not uncommon to observe subdural extracerebral accumulations on CT scans performed following shunting procedures in patients with markedly or even moderately dilated ventricles. Generally speaking, these subdural accumulations do not cause clinically significant changes in the patients' condition; indeed, the clinical condition is so improved by the shunt procedure that small changes in condition probably are not appreciated. These subdural accumulations are not uncommon, but their incidence was not appreciated until the development of CT scanning and, with it, the ability to follow these patients without the need for invasive procedures. On rare occasions these extracerebral accumulations have been treated with moderate success with subdural shunt tubes. In other cases, this treatment has resulted in re-expansion of the lateral ventricles.

If a craniotomy has been performed, the CT scan will reflect the type of procedure done. The CT scan will reflect these changes following removal of cerebral tissues for decompression or tumor removal.

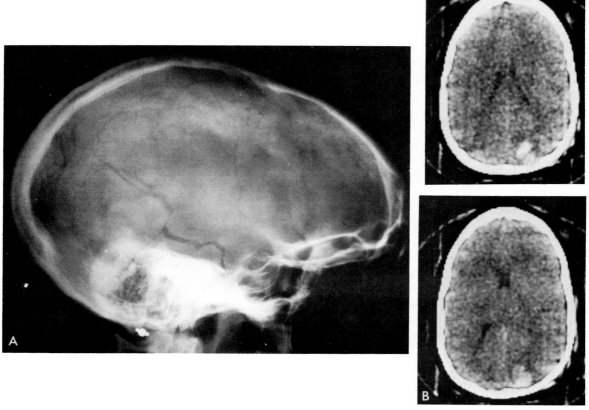

FIGURE 11–1. *Linear Skull Fracture: A,* The linear skull fracture extends from the squamous portion of the temporal bone posteriorly to the posterior parietal bone. There is diastasis of the fracture fragments, and the fracture line has a wavy configuration. There is a second fracture high in the posterior parietal region just above the lambdoid suture.

B, The CT scan reveals a small intracerebral hematoma in the left occipital pole just beneath the inner table of the skull. There is a small amount of surrounding edema and slight compression of the left lateral ventricle.

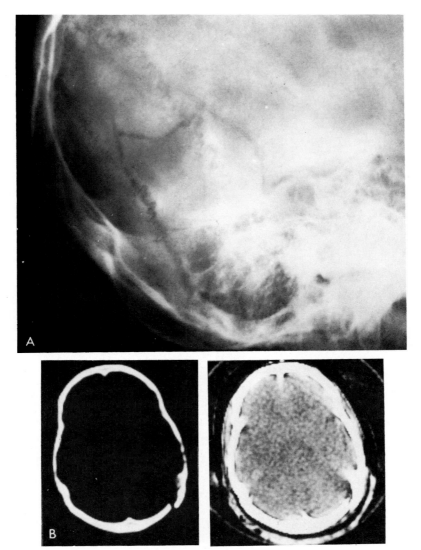

FIGURE 11–2. *Depressed Fracture, Left Occipital:* A, The plain skull film reveals an irregular fracture line extending from above the mastoid air cells posteriorly and then superiorly through the lambdoid suture and into the occipital bone.

B, The CT scan reveals diastasis of the fracture and depression of the occipital bone at the point of the fracture. There is no evidence of intracerebral hematoma.

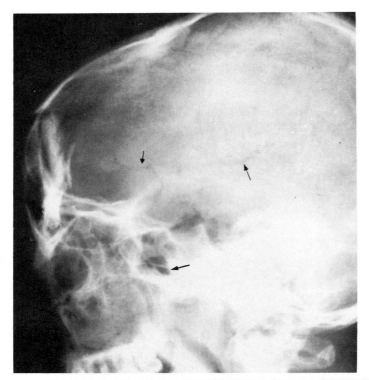

FIGURE 11–3. *Comminuted Depressed Skull Fracture and Traumatic Pneumocephalus:* There is a large comminuted and depressed fracture in the frontal region. Air is noted in the suprasellar cisterns, and a small amount of air outlines the cerebral gyri (*small arrows*). The horizontal beam lateral view reveals an air-fluid level in the sphenoid sinus (*large arrowhead*) secondary to CSF or blood in the sphenoid sinus. Note the complete opacification of the paranasal sinuses secondary to hemorrhage and multiple associated facial bone fractures.

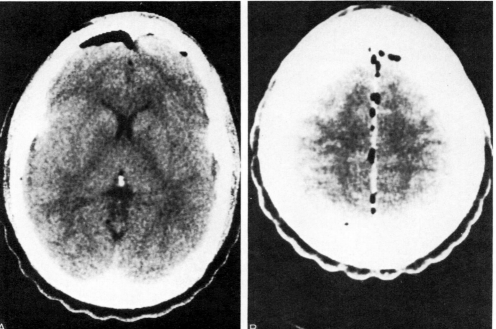

FIGURE 11–4. *Traumatic Pneumocephalus:* *A,* CT scan reveals a small accumulation of air beneath the inner table of the skull in the right frontal region, a tiny bubble of air in the left frontal region, and another tiny bubble in the interhemispheric fissure.

B, In the convexity region there are multiple small bubbles of air in the interhemispheric fissure. This type of accumulation of intracranial air seen following craniocerebral trauma means that there is a fracture into the paranasal sinuses or elsewhere that allows air to enter the cranial vault. While readily demonstrable by CT, this small accumulation of air is very difficult to visualize by plain skull radiographs. (Case courtesy of Justo Rodriguez, M.D., Cook Country Hospital.)

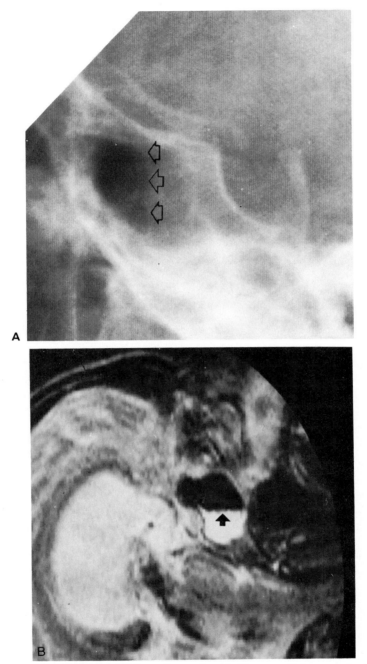

FIGURE 11–5. *Air-Fluid Level Sphenoid Sinus Secondary to Trauma:* Films are obtained with the patients in the supine position; thus, air-fluid levels are demonstrated on the horizontal beam "shoot-through" lateral views. *A*, The arrows outline an air-fluid level in the sphenoid sinus secondary to either CSF or blood in the sinus following a base-of-the-skull fracture.

B, SE MR TR3120/TE120 image reveals an air-fluid level in the sphenoid sinus (*arrow*) in a different patient.

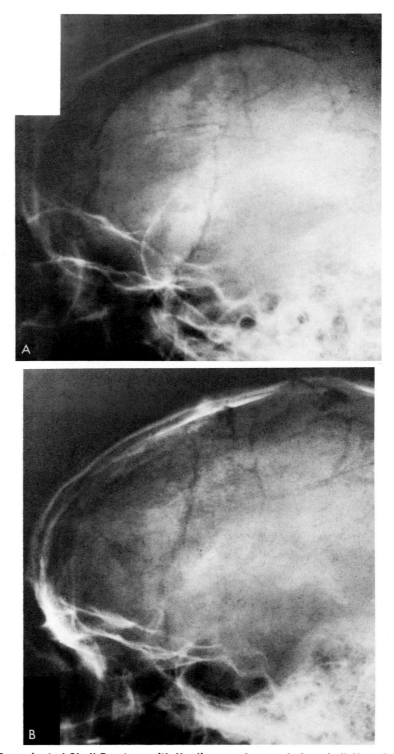

FIGURE 11–6. *Comminuted Skull Fracture with Healing:* *A*, The initial plain skull films show a comminuted skull fracture involving the frontal and anterior parietal regions.

B, Follow-up examination six months later reveals that the fracture lines have become indistinct owing to secondary bony overgrowth at the fracture sites. Bony union does not occur with callus formation.

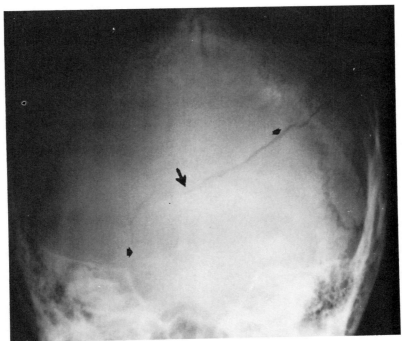

FIGURE 11–7. *Linear Fracture of the Occipital Bone:* The plain film examination reveals a long diastatic fracture that extends from the left posterior parietal region inferiorly and obliquely across the occipital bone, through the torcular (*large arrow*) and into the foramen magnum (*small arrows*). See also Figure 11–45. This fracture was associated with a posterior fossa epidural hematoma and a contra-coup contusion of the right frontal and parietal lobes.

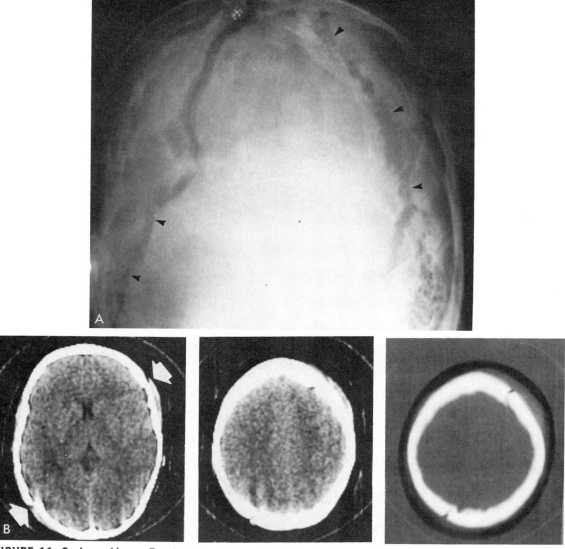

FIGURE 11–8. *Long Linear Fracture:* *A*, A long linear fracture is noted to extend from the right posterior frontal to the left posterior parietal region. There is some diastasis of the fracture line. Extracranial soft tissue swelling is noted, but the cranial contents appear to be within normal limits.

B, The fracture and its true extent are readily demonstrated on the CT scan viewed at high window width.

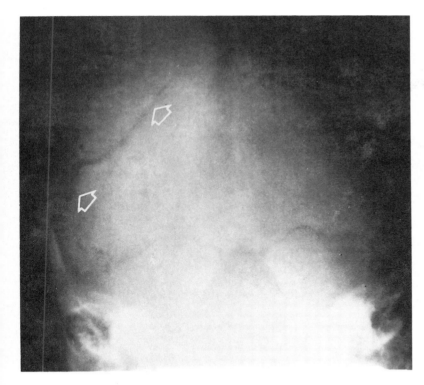

FIGURE 11–9. *Occipital Fracture Simulating Mendosal Suture in a Child:* A linear fracture extends across the occipital bone on one side (*arrows*). The normal mendosal suture is usually bilateral and originates at the posterolateral fontanelle. The mendosal suture is frequently mistaken for a fracture (see Chapter 2).

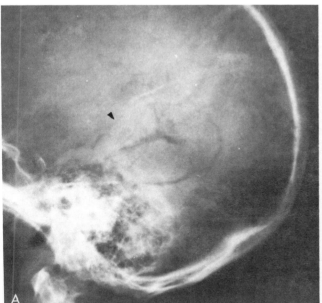

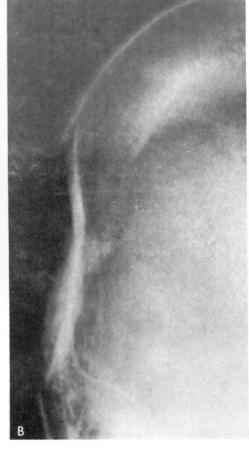

FIGURE 11–10. *Depressed Fracture: A,* The patient has sustained a sharp blow to the calvaria that has resulted in a round and stellate fracture that is depressed in the center portion.

B, The tangential view affords the best method to evaluate the amount of depression of the bony fragments. If the depression of the fracture is greater than 5 mm, it is elevated surgically.

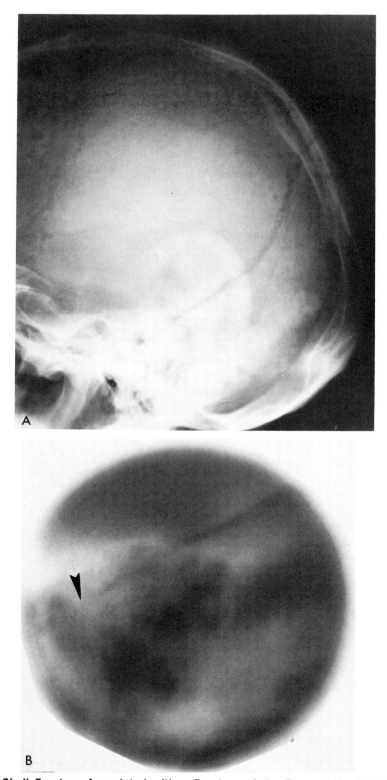

FIGURE 11–11. *Skull Fracture Associated with a Fracture of the Base of the Skull:* A, This patient presented with CSF otorrhea following severe head trauma. A long linear fracture extends into the petrous bone.

B, The tomogram of the petrous bone best demonstrates the fracture extending into the base of the skull.

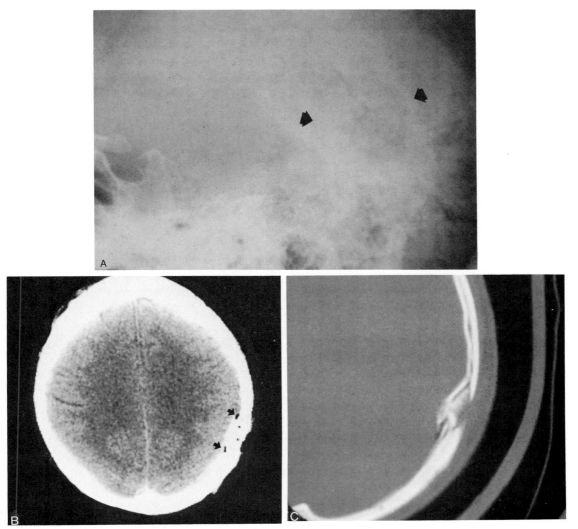

FIGURE 11–12. *A*, Plain skull examination demonstrates a stellate depressed skull fracture in the posterior parietal region (*arrows*). A tangential view may show this fracture to better advantage. Close inspection should be made for evidence of traumatic pneumocephalus.

B, CT scan at standard viewing window widths and levels reveals minor irregularity in the bony calvaria and a small amount of air beneath the inner table of the skull (*arrows*).

C, At bone window widths the nature of the abnormality—a depressed fracture—is easily appreciated. Depression of 5 mm or greater is an indication for surgical elevation.

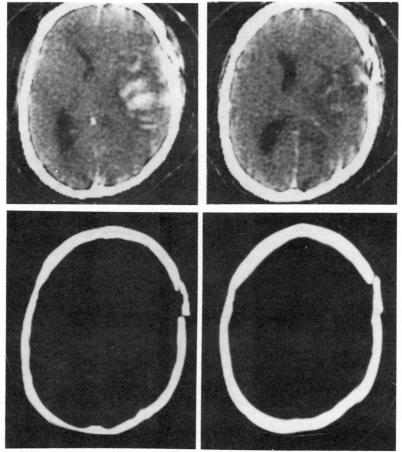

FIGURE 11–13. *Comminuted Skull Fracture with Intracranial Hematoma:* The CT on standard viewing reveals intracerebral hemorrhage and edema and some irregularity of the bony calvaria. On the measure mode the comminuted skull fracture is readily identified.

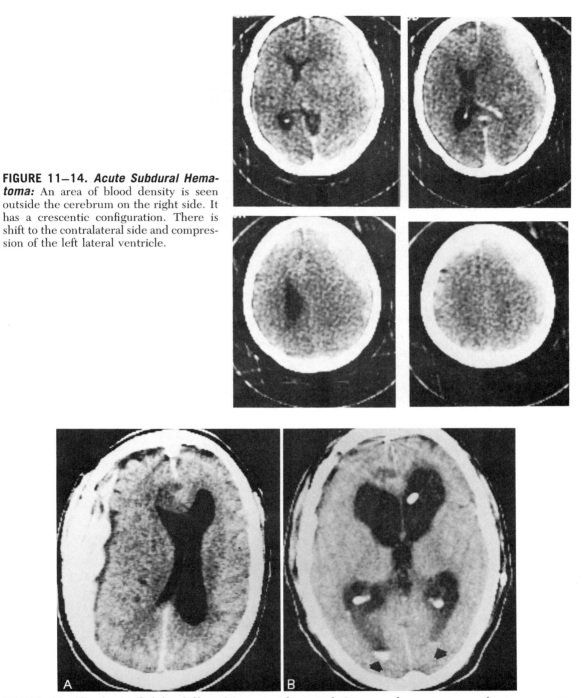

FIGURE 11–14. *Acute Subdural Hematoma:* An area of blood density is seen outside the cerebrum on the right side. It has a crescentic configuration. There is shift to the contralateral side and compression of the left lateral ventricle.

FIGURE 11–15. *Acute Subdural Hematoma:* A, The initial CT scan demonstrates a classic crescentic extracerebral collection of blood density typical of an acute subdural hematoma. There is compression of the ipsilateral lateral ventricle. There is also increased density of the interhemispheric fissure secondary to blood in the subarachnoid space.

B, The postoperative scan demonstrates enlargement of the lateral and third ventricles secondary to a communicating hemorrhage. There is also a small amount of blood in the dependent portions of the lateral ventricles (*arrows*). The hydrocephalus develops because the blood in the subarachnoid space interferes with resorption of the CSF by the pacchionian granulations. This hydrocephalus, as in this case, may require shunting, and the tip of the shunt tube projects into the frontal horn of the lateral ventricle. The subdural hematoma has been surgically removed.

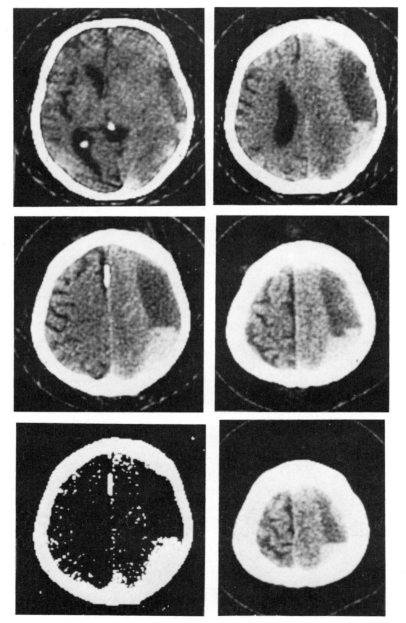

FIGURE 11–16. *Acute Subdural Hematoma with "Hematocrit" Levels:* The CT scan reveals a large left subdural hematoma, which, because the patient had been placed in the supine position for prolonged periods, has settled, giving a "hematocrit" to the blood in the hematoma. There is shift to the contralateral side and obliteration of the cortical sulci on the side of the hematoma.

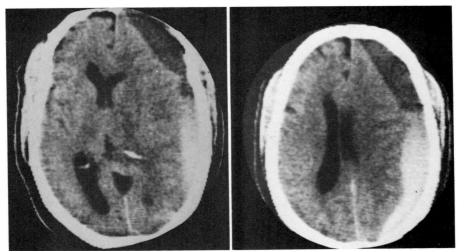

FIGURE 11–17. *Acute Subdural Hematoma:* CT examination demonstrates a classic picture of an acute subdural hematoma that has settled in a "hematocrit" level. It appears that this is a result of posterior setting of the heavier hemoglobin molecule after the patient has remained in the supine position for a prolonged period of time. If the patient has a hemoglobin level in the peripheral blood of less than 6 grams, there is insufficient hemoglobin to produce this appearance. There is shift to the contralateral side and compression of the ipsilateral lateral ventricle. The increased density of the interhemispheric fissure posteriorly is secondary to a small amount of blood in the subarachnoid space.

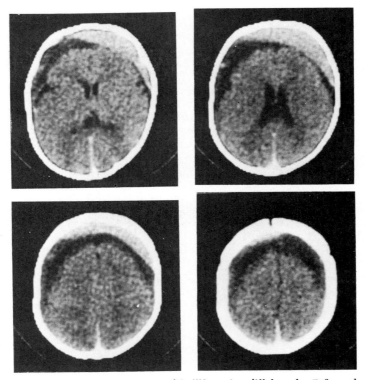

FIGURE 11–18. *Bifrontal Subdural Hematoma with "Hematocrit" Levels:* Bifrontal subdural hematomas demonstrate the "hematocrit levels" in the frontal region because the baby slept on its stomach and right frontal region of the face.

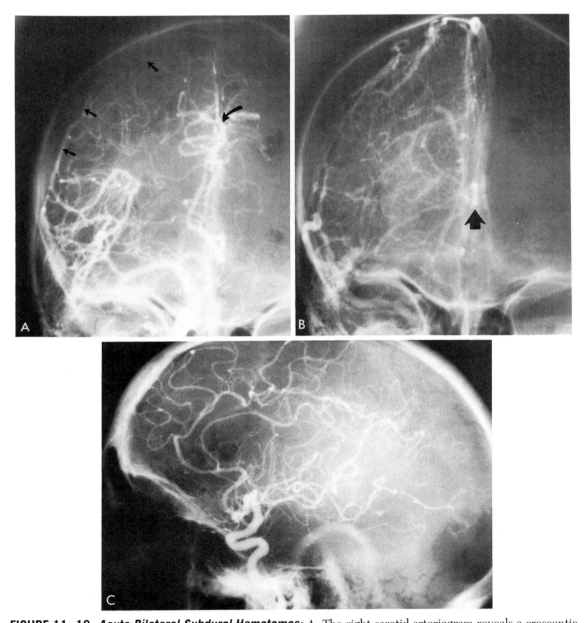

FIGURE 11–19. *Acute Bilateral Subdural Hematomas:* A, The right carotid arteriogram reveals a crescentic extracerebral accumulation of blood (*small arrows*). The branches of the middle cerebral artery are displaced by blood away from the inner table of the skull. There is slight shift of the anterior cerebral artery under the falx to the contralateral side (*curved arrow*).

B, The venous phase also shows displacement of the veins away from the inner table by the blood in the subdural space, but it does not reveal shift of the internal cerebral veins.

C, The lateral view appears essentially normal.

Illustration continued on the following page

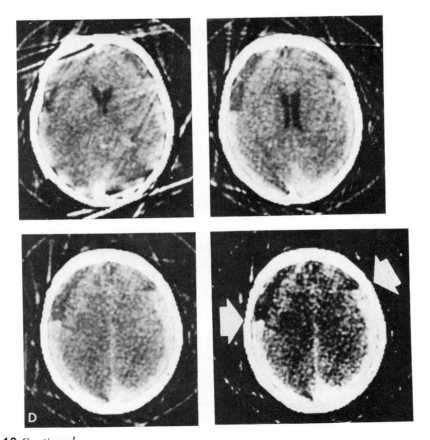

FIGURE 11–19 *Continued.*

D, The CT scan reveals bilateral crescentic subdural hematomas with "hematocrit" levels, and compression of the lateral ventricles and elongation secondary to the acute hematomas. Because of the bilateral nature of the abnormality, there is no shift of the internal cerebral vein on the arteriogram.

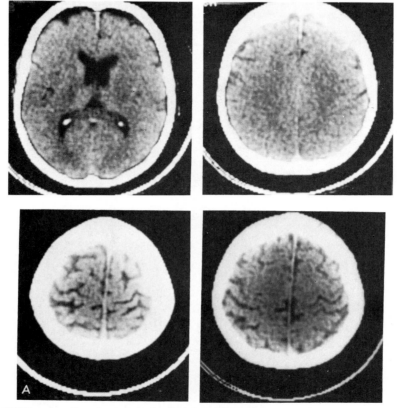

FIGURE 11–20. *CT Showing Development of a Subdural Hematoma: A,* The initial CT scan was performed because of symptoms of dizziness and right arm tingling. The scan shows mild atrophy with enlargement of the lateral ventricles and the cortical sulci.

Illustration continued on the following page

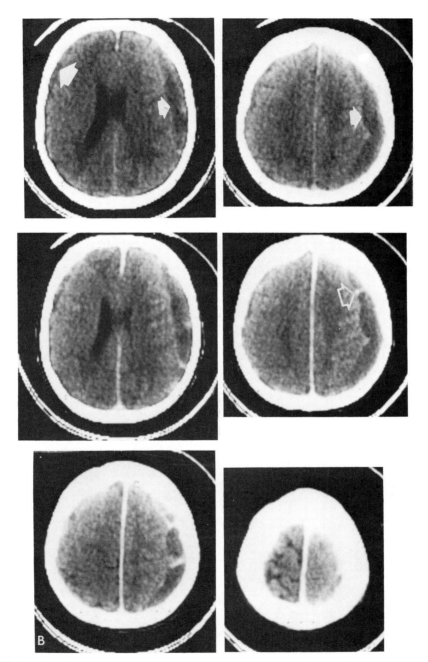

FIGURE 11–20 *Continued.*

B, The follow-up scan two months later reveals a large, chronic left subdural hematoma (*small arrowheads*) and a small, chronic right subdural hematoma (*large arrowhead*) in the right frontal region. Postinfusion, there is enhancement of a membrane around the hematoma and displacement of the cortical vein away from the inner table of the skull (*open arrow*) on the left side. Note also the obliteration of the cortical sulci on the left side as compared to the right—and compared to the initial scan performed two months earlier.

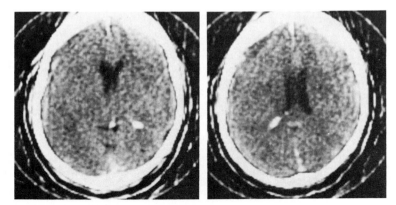

FIGURE 11–21. *Bilateral Isodense Subdural Hematomas:* The lateral ventricles are compressed toward the midline and appear elongated secondary to pressure from the bilateral subdural hematomas. There is no real shift of the midline because the accumulations are approximately equal in size. Bilateral, isodense subdural accumulations are easily overlooked on the routine CT scan.

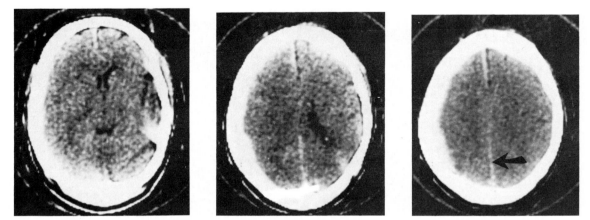

FIGURE 11–22. *Small Acute Left Subdural Hematoma:* There is a slim acute subdural hematoma on the right side. On standard viewing densities the CT scan gives the appearance of a thickened calvaria on the right side. Manipulating the window width and window level allows for better visualization of the blood accumulation. There is compression of the body of the right lateral ventricle. The falx is dense because of blood in the subarachnoid space (*arrow*).

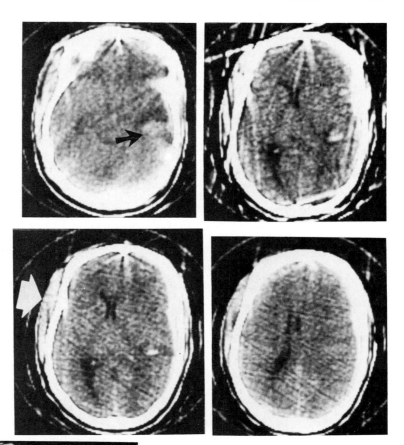

FIGURE 11–23. *Subdural Hematoma and Contusion:* A large extracranial hematoma is seen on the right side. The "contra-coup" injury has resulted in a small acute subdural hematoma on the contralateral side. In addition, a right temporal hematoma (*arrow*) and areas of contusion with small areas of hemorrhage appear on the higher cuts. There is shift of the midline to the contralateral side— more than would be present with the hematoma alone.

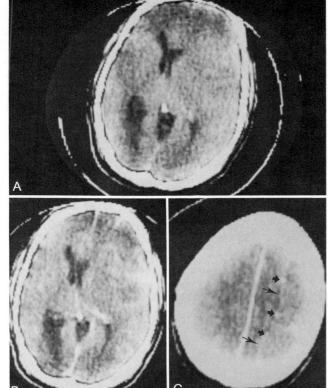

FIGURE 11–24. *Isodense Subdural Hematoma:* *A*, The preinfusion scan demonstrates shift of the midline structures away from the side of the abnormality, but no definite mass or area of abnormal density is seen.

B and *C*, The postinfusion scan does not demonstrate an enhancing mass, but there is faint enhancement of the membrane of the subdural hematoma (*arrowhead*) and the contrast-filled cortical veins (*arrows*) are displaced away from the inner table of the skull by the extracerebral collection of blood. Isodense subdural hematomas without enhancing membranes may be difficult to diagnose, and the abnormality may be mistaken for atrophy on the contralateral side. It is not uncommon that a history of trauma is not obtained on these patients until after the evacuation of the hematoma.

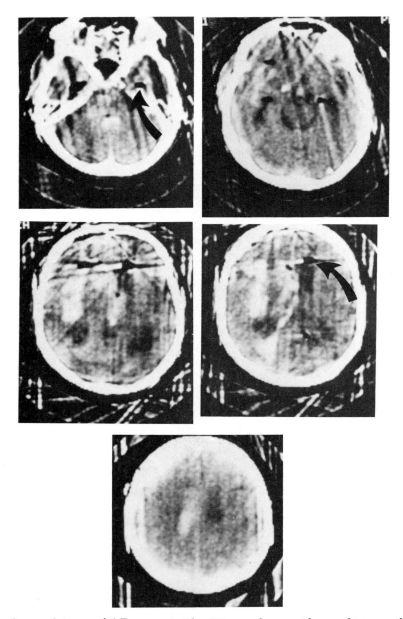

FIGURE 11–25. *Severe Intracranial Trauma:* A, The CT scan shows evidence of intracerebral hemorrhage in the right hemisphere as well as a large intraventricular hemorrhage with blood forming a cast of the right lateral ventricle. In addition, there are multiple scattered accumulations of air in the substance of the brain and within the ventricular system (*arrows*). These appear as very low density areas. The lowest cut reveals an accumulation of blood in the fourth ventricle that leads to an obstructive hydrocephalus. There is some shift to the contralateral side.

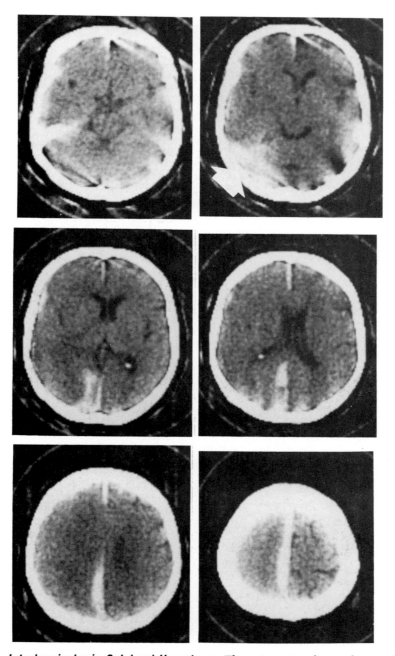

FIGURE 11–26. *Interhemispheric Subdural Hematoma:* There is an interhemispheric subdural hematoma and an accumulation of blood along the supratentorial side of the tentorium (*white arrowhead*). A very small acute subdural hematoma over the left cerebral hemisphere and a slight shift to the right side can be seen. There is obliteration of the cortical sulci of the right hemisphere.

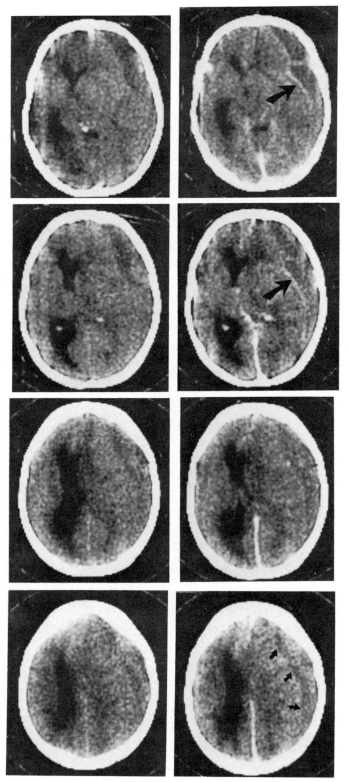

FIGURE 11–27. *Subacute Subdural Hematoma with Enhancing Membrane:* The preinfusion scans (*left column*) reveal an extracerebral accumulation of fluid that has a mottled density. There is shift to the contralateral side. After the infusion of contrast material (*right column*), there is enhancement of the membrane of the subdural hematoma (*arrows*). The demonstration of a membrane may be especially helpful when a subdural hematoma is chronic and isodense with normal brain tissue. The sign is especially helpful when there are bilateral isodense subdural hematomas and the diagnosis is obscure.

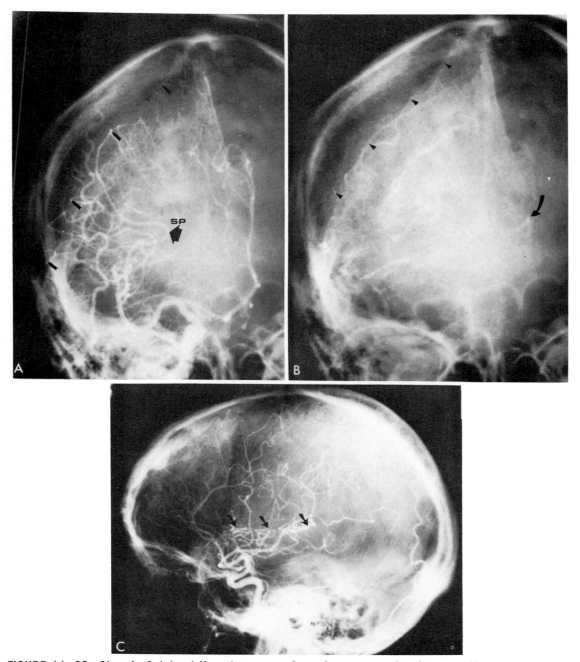

FIGURE 11–28. *Chronic Subdural Hematoma: A* and *B*, The AP arterial and venous films reveal that the branches of the middle cerebral artery are displaced away from the inner table of the skull (*arrows* in *A*), and there is a distal shift of the anterior cerebral artery under the falx cerebri and downward and medial displacement of the sylvian point (*SP*). The cortical veins are also displaced away from the inner table of the skull (*small arrows*) and there is a marked shift of the internal cerebral vein (*large arrow*). The hematoma has taken on the lentiform configuration typically seen with a chronic subdural hematoma.

C, The lateral view reveals downward displacement of the sylvian triangle by the subdural hematoma, which is suprasylvian in location.

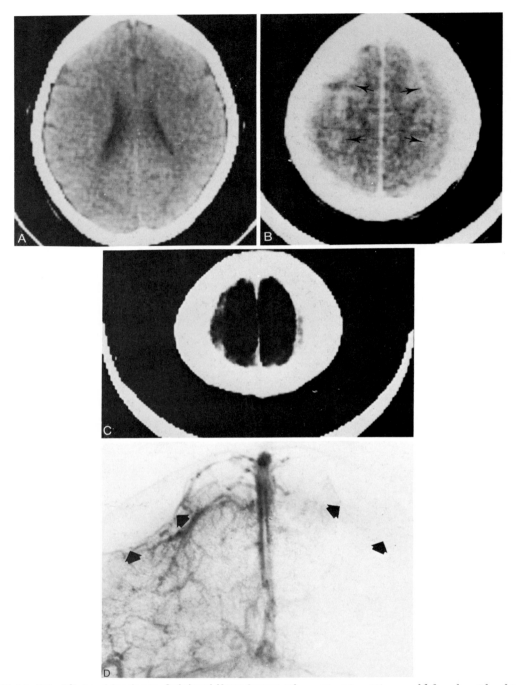

FIGURE 11–29. *Bilateral Isodense Subdural Hematomas:* The patient is a 65-year-old female with a history of TIA's. *A,* The pre-infusion scan demonstrates that the lateral ventricles are small in size for the patient's age, as are the cortical sulci. This has been termed the "hypernormal" scan for age.

B, The postinfusion CT scan reveals faint enhancement of the membranes of the bilateral isodense subdural collections (*arrows*).

C, At wide window widths, the density differences between the bilateral extracerebral collections and the brain parenchyma are more readily appreciated.

D, Angiography reveals the lentiform, chronic subdural hematomas in the convexity regions bilaterally.

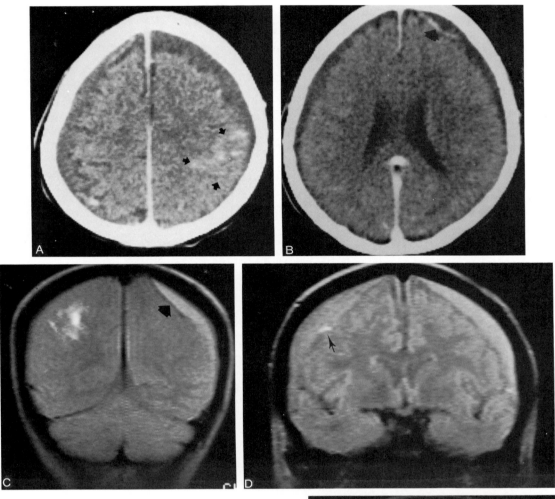

FIGURE 11–30. *Chronic Bilateral Subdural Hematomas:* *A* and *B*, The CT scan demonstrates bilateral, low-density, extracerebral collections. In *B* a contrast-filled cortical vein appears as a curvilinear structure displaced away from the inner table of the calvaria (*large arrow*). There is a poorly defined intracerebral hematoma in the parietal region.

C and *D*, The SE TR2120/TE60 image reveals the chronic extracerebral blood collection. There is no increased signal intensity on the T-1 weighted images (not shown), and the hematoma is therefore almost isodense with the normal brain. In *C* the intracerebral hematoma is seen as a poorly delineated area of increased signal intensity (*arrow* in *C*). In *D* a cortical vein appears as an oval area of high signal intensity (*arrow*) because of slow flow.

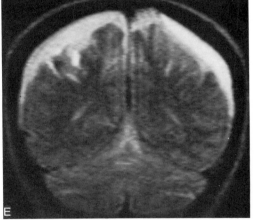

E, The SE TR3120/TE120 image reveals that the bilateral, extracerebral collections are now of increased signal intensity, as is the intracerebral hematoma.

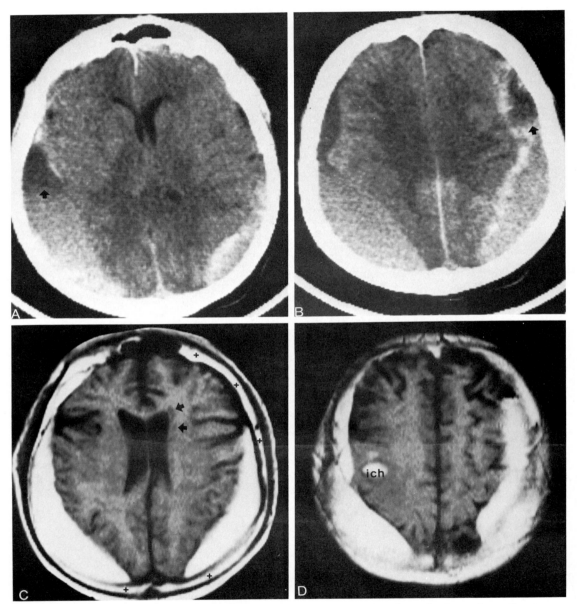

FIGURE 11–31. *Bilateral Subdural Hematomas:* Fifty-nine–year–old male studied two days after a motor vehicle accident. *A* and *B*, The CT scan reveals that the lateral ventricles are compressed and elongated and there are bilateral extracerebral collections that vary in size and density. "Hematocrit" levels can be identified bilaterally (*arrows*).

Illustration continued on the following page

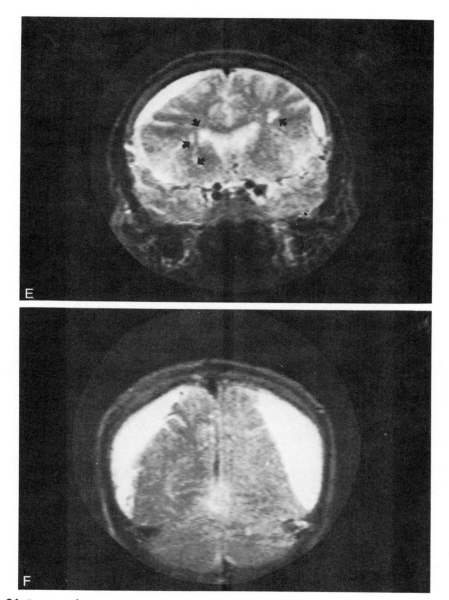

FIGURE 11–31 *Continued.*

C and *D*, The SE TR530/TE30 images demonstrate the bilateral subacute collections of blood to excellent advantage because they appear as areas of markedly increased signal intensity. An intracerebral hematoma is also identified (ich) in *D*.

E and *F*, Coronal images with SE TR3120/TE120 reveal that the blood maintains increased signal intensity, and in addition multiple periventricular infarcts (*arrows* in *E*) appear as areas of increased signal intensity. These infarcts are faintly visible as areas of low signal intensity in *C*.

Note that the fatty bone marrow shows high signal intensity and projects between the low signal intensity areas of the inner and outer tables of the bony calvaria (+ + +), in *C*.

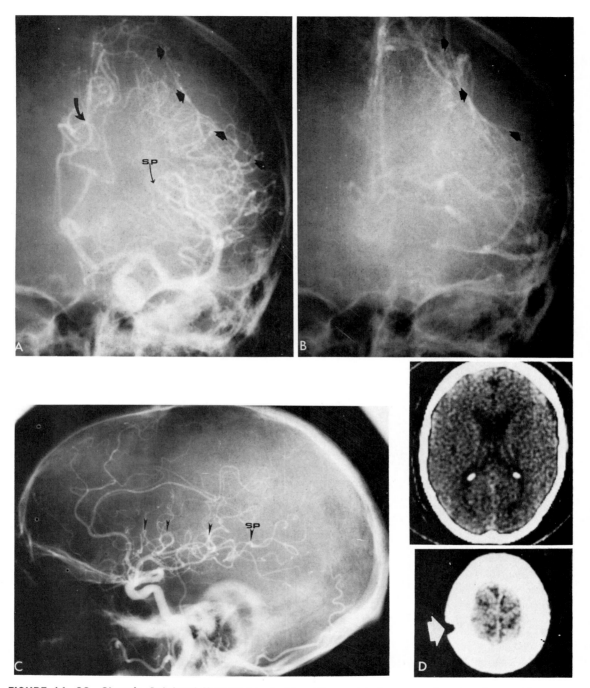

FIGURE 11–32. *Chronic Subdural Hematoma:* *A,* The AP arterial phase reveals a lentiform collection of extracerebral fluid (*arrowheads*) associated with downward and medial displacement of the sylvian point (*SP*). There is a distal shift of the anterior cerebral artery under the falx cerebri (*large arrow*).

B, The AP venous phase again demonstrates the lentiform configuration of the chronic subdural hematoma.

C, The lateral arterial view shows downward displacement of the entire sylvian triangle (*arrowheads*). The sharp angulation of the distal portion of the anterior cerebral artery represents the point where the artery shifts under the falx cerebri.

D, A CT scan obtained postoperatively reveals that the lateral ventricles are in normal position, and the bur hole used for evacuation of the hematoma (*arrow*) is visible on the high cuts. The scan is otherwise unremarkable.

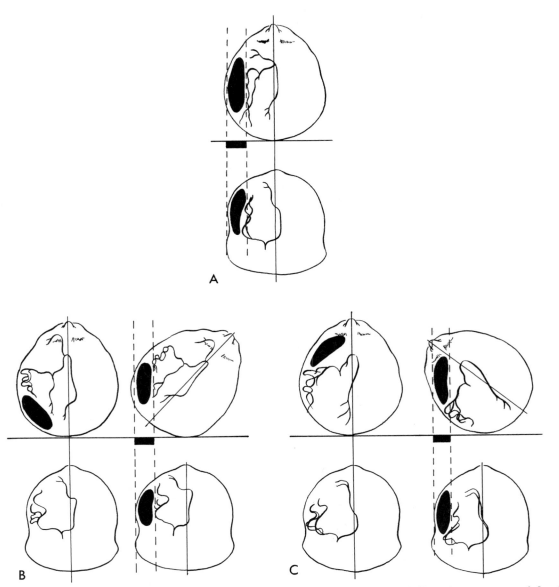

FIGURE 11–33. *Advantages of the Oblique View in Evaluating a Subdural Hematoma:* *A,* A subdural hematoma in the temporal and/or parietal area is readily visible in the standard angiographic projections.

B and *C,* Frontal and occipital subdural hematomas may not be visible in the standard projections, but are better visualized using appropriate oblique projections. (Modified with permission from Radcliffe WB, Quinto FC Jr: Semin Roentgenol 6:103-110, 1971.)

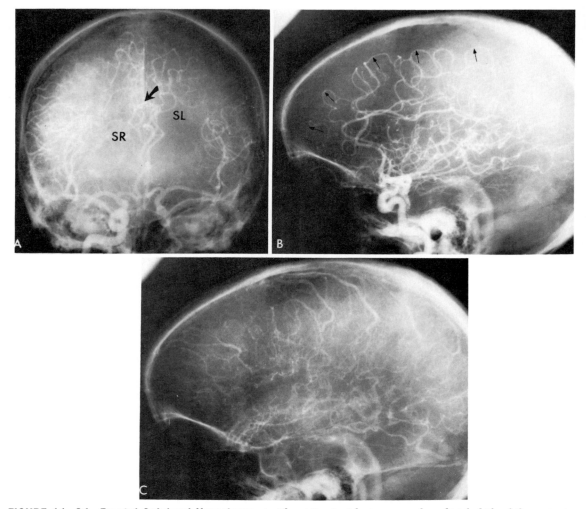

FIGURE 11–34. *Frontal Subdural Hematoma:* *A,* The AP arterial view reveals a distal shift of the anterior cerebral artery (*arrow*). This study, done with cross compression, shows that the sylvian point on the right side (SR) is displaced medially compared with the sylvian point on the normal left side (SL).

B, The lateral view reveals that the distal branch vessels of the anterior cerebral artery are displaced away from the inner table of the skull anteriorly (*arrows*). The pericallosal artery is depressed.

C, The lateral venous phase appears normal. Because the superficial cortical veins must enter the superior sagittal sinus, their actual displacement away from the inner table in the convexity region cannot be appreciated and their entrance into the superior sagittal sinus appears to be normal.

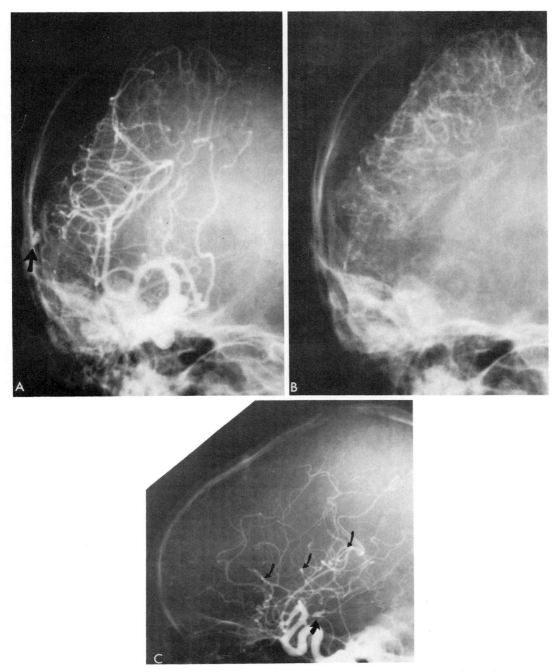

FIGURE 11–35. *Chronic Posterior Subdural Hematoma:* *A* and *B*, The AP arterial and capillary phases of the arteriogram obtained in the left posterior oblique projection reveal the lentiform configuration of a chronic subdural hematoma. The full extent is best appreciated on the oblique view. The arrowhead demonstrates an aneurysm of the middle meningeal artery—possibly post-traumatic.

C, The lateral arterial view demonstrates downward and anterior displacement of the sylvian triangle (*small arrows*) because of the posterior position of the subdural hematoma. The aneurysm of the middle meningeal artery is again demonstrated (*large arrow*).

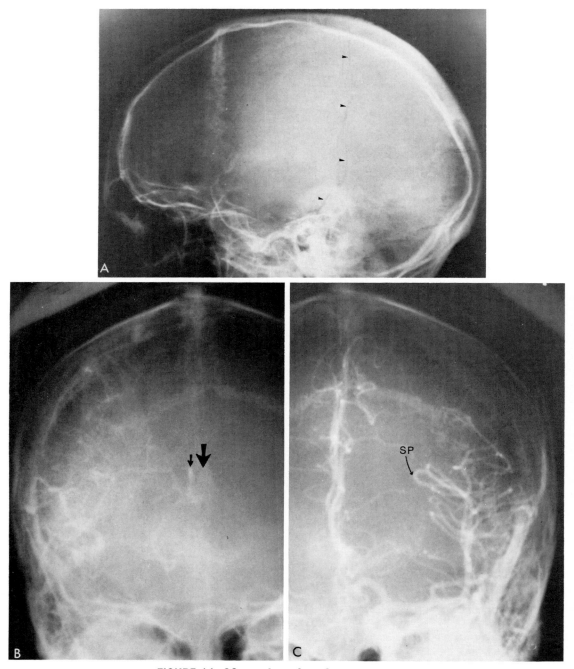

FIGURE 11–36. *See legend on the opposite page.*

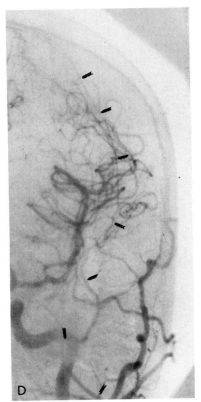

FIGURE 11–36. *Epidural Hematoma: A,* The skull film reveals a long linear skull fracture that extends from one parietal region to the other through the bregma.

B, Because of false localizing signs, a right carotid arteriogram was performed initially. The venous phase reveals shift of the internal cerebral vein (*small arrow*) to the ipsilateral side of the midline (*large arrow*).

C, The AP arterial phase of the left carotid arteriogram shows slight distal shift of the anterior cerebral artery under the falx cerebri (*arrow*) and medial and downward displacement of the sylvian point (*SP*).

D, The right posterior oblique projection of the left carotid arteriogram reveals the lentiform extracerebral accumulation of blood and, in addition, shows that the middle meningeal artery is displaced away from the inner table of the skull—confirming the presence of an *epidural* hematoma. The arrowheads trace the origin of the middle meningeal artery from the internal maxillary artery and follow its intracranial course.

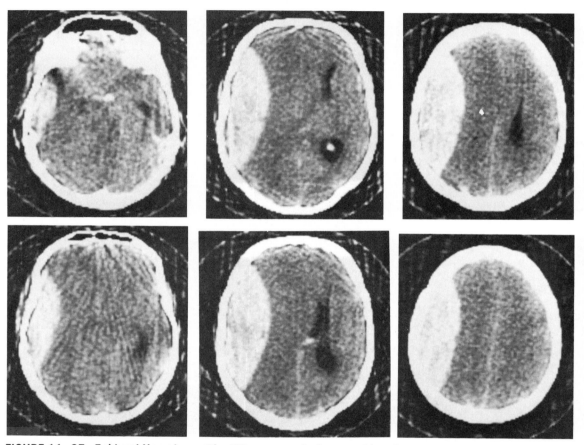

FIGURE 11–37. *Epidural Hematoma:* The CT scan reveals the typical lentiform accumulation of blood density over the left hemisphere of an acute epidural hematoma. There is marked shift to the contralateral side.

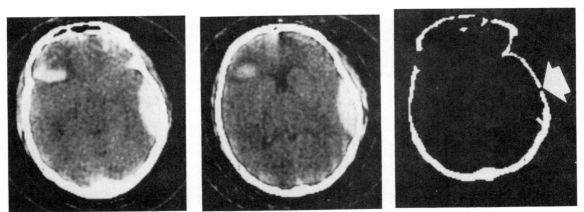

FIGURE 11–38. *Epidural Hematoma and Contra-coup Intracerebral Hematoma:* There is a biconcave epidural accumulation of blood over the left hemisphere and an intracerebral hematoma in the right posterior frontal region associated with surrounding edema. The right-sided lesion represents the coup; the right-sided lesion represents the contra-coup. Viewed on the measure mode at high window level, the linear skull fracture is demonstrated (*arrowhead*).

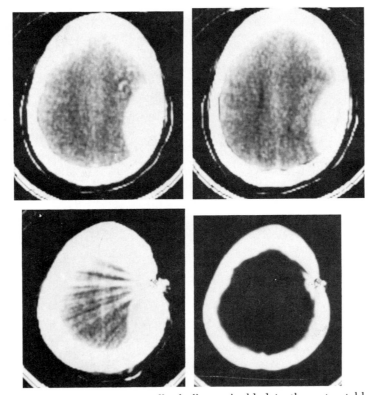

FIGURE 11–39. *Epidural Hematoma:* A metallic bullet embedded in the outer table of the skull creates computer artifacts on the upper cuts. The bullet did not enter the cranial vault, but created an epidural hematoma high in the right parietal convexity region. An additional small area of contusion can be seen just anterior to the epidural hematoma.

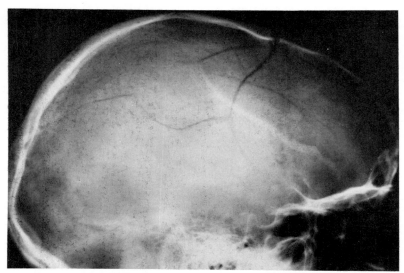

FIGURE 11–40. *Comminuted Skull Fracture:* The fracture line of this comminuted skull fracture extends across the superior sagittal sinus. This type of fracture is associated with an epidural hematoma.

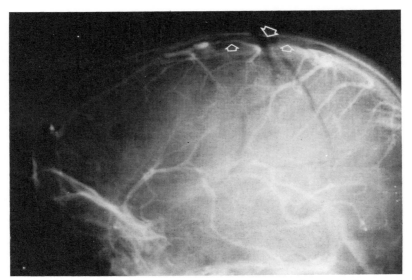

FIGURE 11–41. *Epidural Hematoma:* The comminuted fracture extends across the superior sagittal sinus, and the later venous phase of the arteriogram reveals that the superior sagittal sinus is displaced away from the inner table of the skull. In this case the epidural accumulation of blood may be venous and secondary to hemorrhage from the superior sagittal sinus.

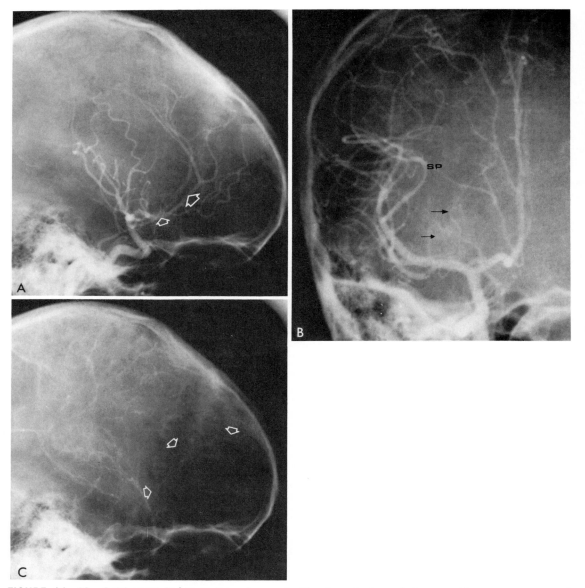

FIGURE 11–42. *Subfrontal Epidural Hematoma:* *A*, The lateral view of the carotid arteriogram reveals posterior and upward displacement of the proximal portion of the anterior cerebral artery (*open arrows*). There is a relative paucity of vessels in the frontal pole region.

B, The AP arterial view of the carotid arteriogram shows medial displacement of the sylvian point (*SP*) and lenticulostriate vessels (*arrows*). There is straightening of the anterior cerebral artery with *minimal* shift to the contralateral side.

C, In the late venous phase, an avascular region (*open arrows*) is seen in the frontal pole. The arteriographic findings are reminiscent of those seen with a subfrontal meningioma.

D, The CT scan reveals a well-defined lentiform accumulation of blood density in the left frontal region with *minimal* shift of the midline structures considering the size of the mass. There is some distortion of the frontal horns of the lateral ventricles. The higher cuts reveal a large extracranial hematoma (*arrow*) in the frontal region. The appearance is very typical of a *subfrontal epidural hematoma.*

E, The CT scan in the coronal section reveals the hematoma located just superior to the orbital roof on the left side. The extracranial hematoma is again identified (*arrow*).

Illustration continued on the opposite page

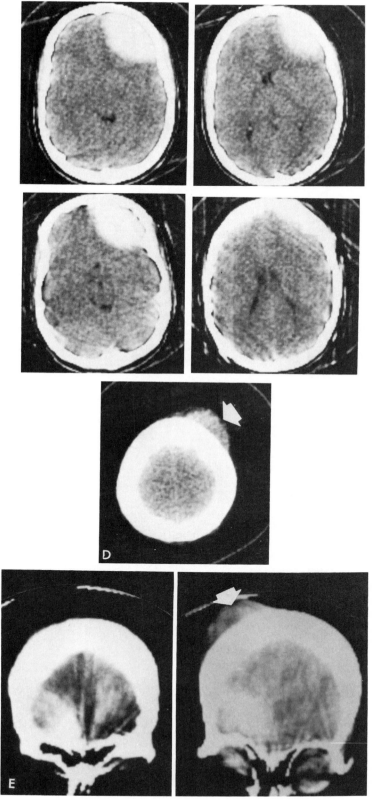

FIGURE 11–42. *See legend on the opposite page.*

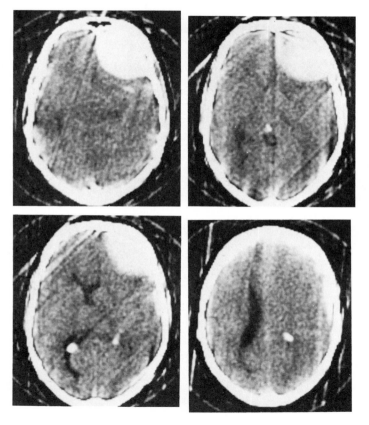

FIGURE 11–43. *Subfrontal Epidural Hematoma:* There is a biconvex accumulation of blood density in the right frontal region associated with only minimal shift of the midline relative to the size of the hematoma.

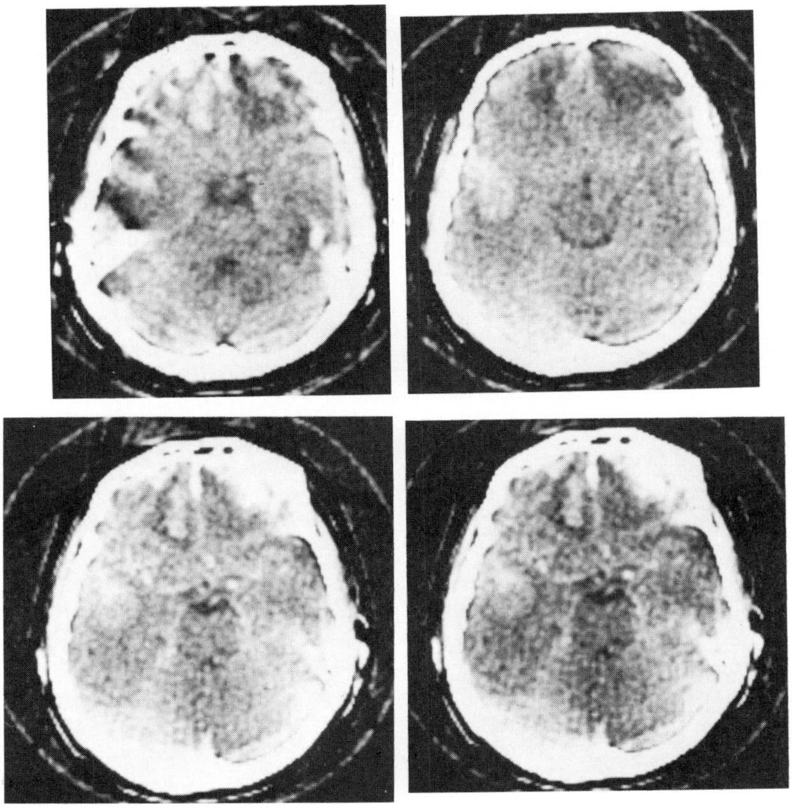

FIGURE 11–44. *Multipolar Trauma:* The CT scan shows bifrontal contusions associated with intracerebral hematomas and edema; there is also a right anterior temporal hematoma.

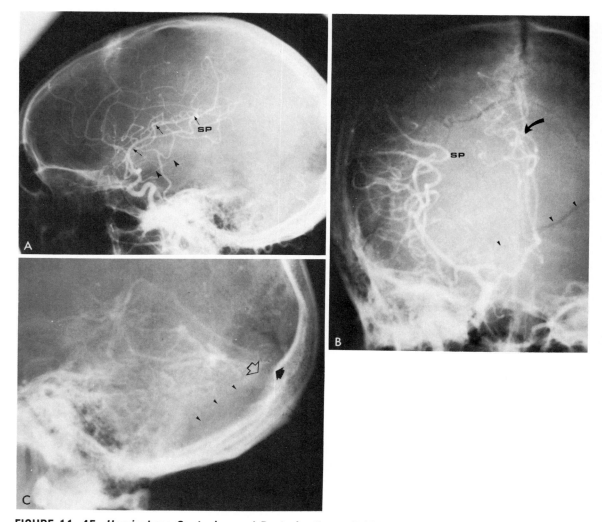

FIGURE 11–45. *Hemisphere Contusion and Posterior Fossa Epidural Hematoma:* *A,* The lateral view of the right carotid arteriogram reveals upward displacement of the branches of the middle cerebral artery and stretching of the anterior choroidal artery.

B, The AP arterial view demonstrates anterior and posterior shift of the anterior cerebral artery (*large arrow*). There is medial shift of the sylvian point (*SP*). The appearance is that of a temporal lobe mass (*arrowheads* demonstrate the occipital fracture).

C, The late venous phase of the vertebral arteriogram reveals that the torcular (*open arrow*) is displaced anterior to the point of attachment at the internal occipital protuberance (*large black arrow*), and there is anterior displacement of the inferior vermian vein (*small arrowheads*).

Illustration continued on the opposite page

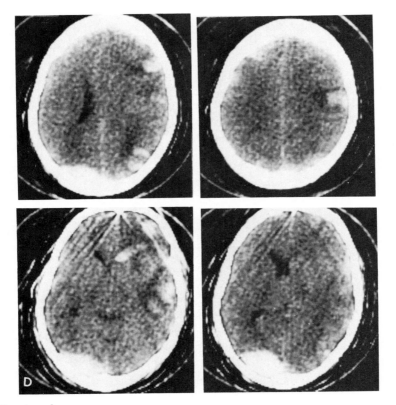

FIGURE 11–45 *Continued.*

D, The CT scan reveals the left temporal contusion and hematoma as well as scattered areas of blood density throughout the left hemisphere in the temporal, frontal, and parietal lobes. There is shift to the contralateral side with obliteration of the left lateral ventricle. In addition, a lentiform collection of blood is seen in the posterior fossa and the right occipital region—consistent with an epidural hematoma (surgically confirmed) (see Fig. 11–7).

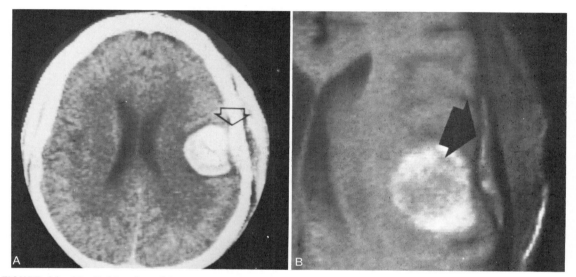

FIGURE 11–46. *Epidural and Intracerebral Hematoma: A,* The CT scan demonstrates an obvious area of post-traumatic intracerebral hematoma and slight shift of the ventricles to the contralateral side. There is a small lentiform area adjacent to the inner table of the skull that measured blood density.

B, The MR scan demonstrates that the subacute intracerebral hematoma is increased in signal intensity, there is a small epidural collection of blood of increased signal intensity, and the dura is depressed (*arrow*) by the epidural collection of blood. There is marked extracranial soft tissue swelling. Note that the dura mater remains of low signal intensity on both the T-1 and T-2 weighted images.

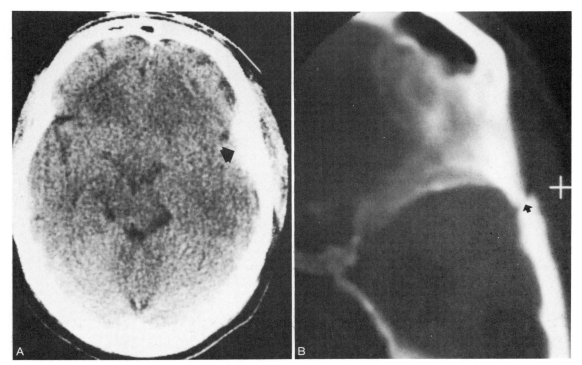

FIGURE 11–47. *Epidural Hematoma with Skull Fractures:* *A,* CT scan demonstrates a small lentiform epidural hematoma in the left temporal region (*arrow*). There is extracranial soft tissue swelling also.

B, Enlarged image of the point of impact reveals a slightly displaced linear skull fracture. The fracture was found to cross the middle meningeal artery groove; this caused tearing of the middle meningeal artery and the subsequent epidural hematoma. It is often necessary to review cases such as this, with small extracerebral collections, on the oscilloscope screen to evaluate the presence of small extracerebral collections. Wide window widths are also necessary to evaluate the presence or absence of skull fractures. (Case courtesy of Justo Rodriguez, M.D., Cook County Hospital.)

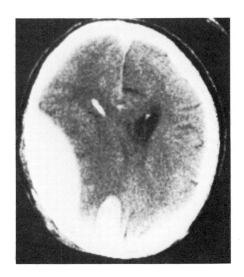

FIGURE 11–48. *Epidural and Intracerebral Hematoma:* CT scan reveals a moderate-sized epidural hematoma, shift to the contralateral side, and paradoxical dilatation of the contralateral lateral ventricle in association with transtentorial herniation. There is also an oval-shaped intracerebral hematoma in the ipsilateral frontal lobe region.

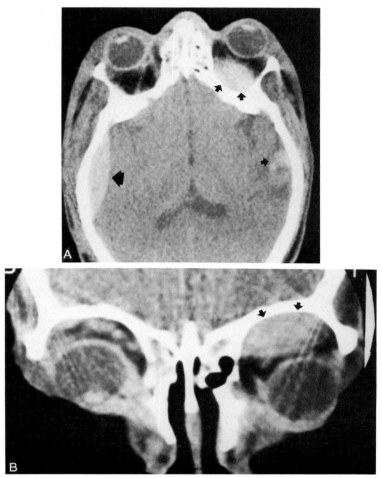

FIGURE 11–49. *Epidural and Intraorbital Hematoma:* *A,* Axial CT reveals diffuse, extracranial soft tissue swelling following a severe beating. There is a small right-sided epidural hematoma (*large arrow*), a small left temporal intracerebral hematoma (*small arrow*), and an intraorbital hematoma as well (*small arrows*). There is unilateral proptosis on the side of the orbital hematoma. There is also near complete opacification of the ethmoid sinuses bilaterally.

B, Direct coronal examination through the orbits again demonstrates the post-traumatic intraorbital hematoma in the superior portion of the orbit (*arrows*). The globe is displaced downward and outward. (Case courtesy of Justo Rodriguez, M.D., Cook County Hospital.)

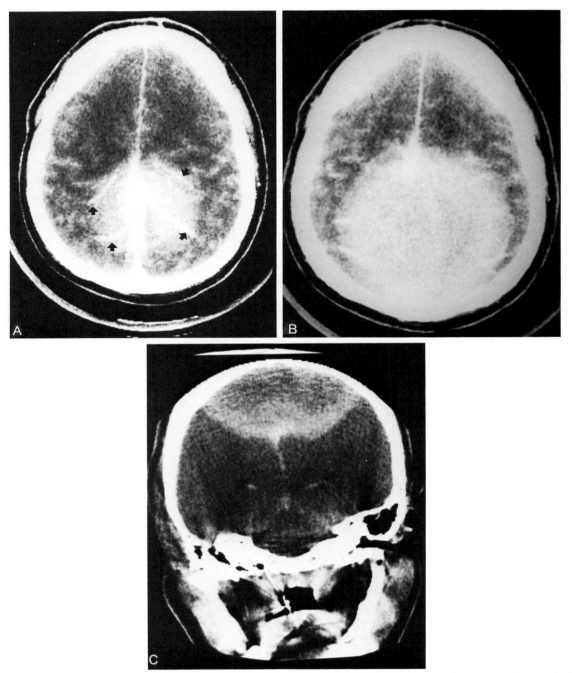

FIGURE 11–50. *Vertex Epidural Hematoma: A* and *B,* Axial CT slices obtained postinfusion reveal a rounded area of blood density in the high convexity region. The cortical veins (*arrows*) are displaced downward by the hematoma and are visible because they are opacified by contrast material. The highest slice reveals the rounded nature of this blood density mass.

C, Direct coronal CT examination reveals the high convexity extracerebral, lentiform collection. The lateral ventricles are displaced inferiorly. Surgically proved venous epidural hematoma, secondary to a tear in the superior sagittal sinus. (Case courtesy of Justo Rodriguez, M.D., Cook County Hospital.)

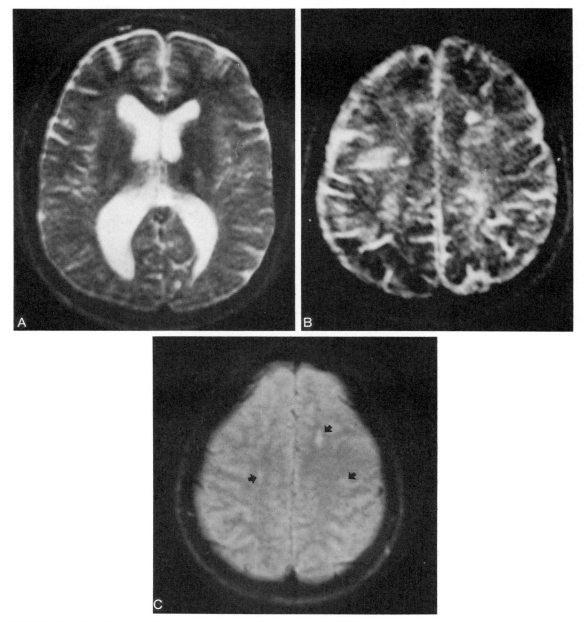

FIGURE 11–51. *Chronic Changes Following Craniocerebral Trauma:* Twenty-five–year–old female with persistent mental changes following motor vehicle accident. The CT scan (not shown) demonstrated enlarged lateral ventricles but was otherwise normal. *A,* SE TR3120/TE120 reveals enlargement of the lateral ventricles.

B, SE TR3120/TE120 reveals multiple stellate areas of increased signal intensity in both hemispheres. These abnormal areas are at the gray-white junction and are apparently secondary to old shearing injuries.

C, A slice obtained slightly higher using the SE TR3120/TE60 reveals multiple small areas of increased signal intensity (*arrowheads*), also secondary to shearing injury. The cortical sulci are not enlarged, and the appearance is otherwise that of a communicating hydrocephalus.

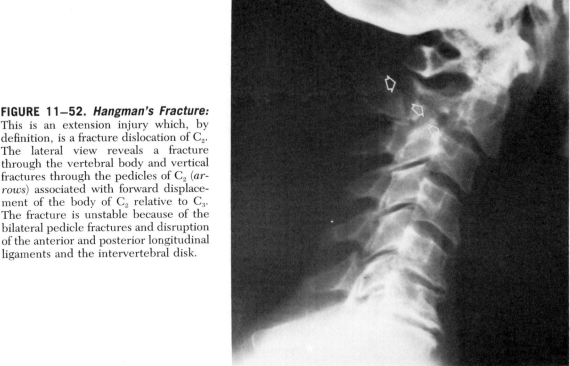

FIGURE 11–52. *Hangman's Fracture:* This is an extension injury which, by definition, is a fracture dislocation of C_2. The lateral view reveals a fracture through the vertebral body and vertical fractures through the pedicles of C_2 (*arrows*) associated with forward displacement of the body of C_2 relative to C_3. The fracture is unstable because of the bilateral pedicle fractures and disruption of the anterior and posterior longitudinal ligaments and the intervertebral disk.

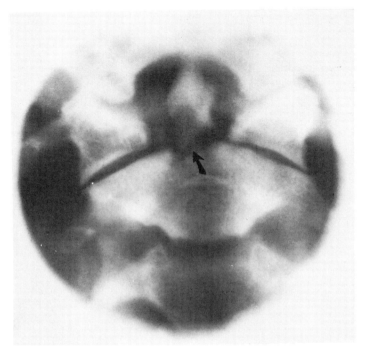

FIGURE 11–53. *Odontoid Fracture:* An oblique fracture through the base of the odontoid process is well demonstrated on the tomogram (*arrow*).

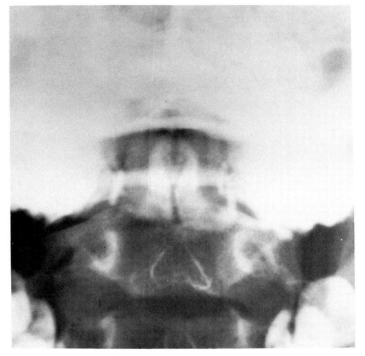

FIGURE 11–54. *Frontal Incisors Simulating an Odontoid Fracture:* The incisors may project over the odontoid process and simulate an odontoid fracture or a cleft odontoid. Close inspection of the film reveals that the "cleft" in the odontoid is actually the gap between the incisors as they insert into the maxillary gingivae.

12

THE ORBIT

Orbital pathology is better studied by CT than by any other method. Magnetic resonance, particularly with the use of surface coils, has also aided our ability to examine the orbit and, because of the lack of ionizing radiation, may ultimately replace CT for evaluation. The orbit lends itself well to CT examination (Fig. 12–1, p. 531). The bony margins of the orbit are easy to visualize and their evaluation is accurate. Direct coronal examination of axial views with coronal reconstruction provides convenient multiplanar evaluation of the orbit and its contents. The best features of CT examination are the ease and accuracy with which one can tell whether there is a retro-orbital mass in the patient with unilateral proptosis. Because the orbit is so intimately related to the paranasal sinus as well as the pituitary fossa and the parasellar region, examination of any of these anatomic areas provides evaluation of the others. CT allows a very accurate study of all these areas, usually better than any other method of evaluation. It is not uncommon that histologic type can be predicted from the appearance of lesions both in and around the orbit.

Hilal and Strohel have suggested a convenient method of classification of orbital tumors based upon their relationship to the globe of the eye and the extraocular muscle cone. This allows the various lesions to be grouped into three major categories: ocular, intraconal, and extraconal. Although at times there is crossover between these categories, in most cases an accurate evaluation of the location of origin of the abnormality can be done, and therefore a correct diagnosis can be reached. This list is adapted from Hilal and Strohel:

A. Intraocular
  1. Retinoblastoma
  2. Melanoma of choroid
  3. Carcinoma of nonpigmented layers
  4. Metastases

B. Intraconal
  1. Optic nerve glioma
  2. Optic sheath meningioma
  3. Cavernous hemangioma
  4. Lymphangioma
  5. Hemangiopericytoma
  6. Neurilemmoma
  7. Metastases
  8. Extension of extraconal lesions
  9. Hematoma

C. Extraconal
  1. Extraconal, intraorbital
     a. Lacrimal gland tumors
     b. Dermoids and epidermoids
     c. Lymphomas
     d. Rhabdomyosarcomas
     e. Hematoma
     f. Pseudotumor
  2. Extraconal, extraorbital
     a. Sphenoid wing meningioma
     b. Tumors of paranasal sinuses
     c. Tumors of nasal passages
     d. Tumors of nasopharynx

527

e. Tumors of pituitary fossa
f. Bony metastases
g. Osteomas of paranasal sinuses
h. Mucocele

TECHNIQUE OF EXAMINATION BY CT

Slices should be obtained parallel to the optic nerve, preferably with a high-resolution scanner. The maximum slice thickness should not be greater than 5 mm, and views should be enlarged for the region of interest. Examination can be performed conveniently in the axial plane using 4-mm slices overlapped by 2 mm. This allows excellent evaluation of the orbit and its contents, and the thin sections also allow excellent evaluation in the coronal plane and sagittal plane, or obliquely along the plane of the optic nerve using reformatting techniques. Other authors have suggested direct coronal examination or direct examination in both the axial and coronal planes. Any of these methods is suitable for evaluation.

CT Evaluation of Trauma

High-resolution, thin-section scanning with direct or multiple reformatted images provides excellent evaluation of fractures of the facial bones. Blow-out fractures are exceptionally well demonstrated and the accurate evaluation of the orbit, orbital contents, sinuses, and surrounding bony margins makes CT superior to any other method of evaluation. In addition, any possibility of intracranial trauma can also be evaluated conveniently and accurately with CT scanning (Figs. 12–2 and 12–3, pp. 532–533 and 534).

A foreign body is best demonstrated by CT examination of the globe using thin sections and direct or reformatted multiplanar images. The advantages of CT over other diagnostic methods include demonstration of air, soft tissues, and bony structures and the relationships between them in a direct, noninvasive, accurate, and readily reproducible fashion (Fig. 12–4, p. 535).

Associated intracranial abnormalities such as contusion, intracerebral hematoma, and subdural or epidural hematomas are also readily and accurately evaluated.

MAGNETIC RESONANCE OF THE ORBIT

MR can also be used for the evaluation of the orbit and its contents. The development and use of coils for "close-up" evaluation of the region of interest will allow convenient multiplanar evaluation of the orbit and its relationship to surrounding structures. The lack of ionizing radiation is a factor in favor of MR. MR will be sensitive to the presence of abnormalities, but its specificity remains to be determined.

Specific Abnormalities

Retinoblastoma. Seen in childhood, retinoblastoma is the most common intraocular tumor and occurs most frequently in the one- to two-year-old child. There is a sporadic as well as familial type of tumor. The tumors present clinically with leukocoria, strabismus, and hemorrhage. Usually large when first seen, the tumors are fungating, contain calcium and necrotic debris, and are associated with retinal detachment.

CT reveals a calcified tumor in the posterior portion of the globe. These tumors may or may not enhance and may be bilateral. Occasionally there is extension out of the globe.

Magnetic resonance reveals decreased signal intensity where the CT demonstrates calcification. The high signal intensity of the retroocular fat on the MR images provides excellent contrast between the globe and the surrounding structures (Fig. 12–5, pp. 536–537).

Melanoma. This is the most frequent tumor of the eye in adults and is potentially fatal. The tumor arises from the pigmented choroidal layer of the retina and may be associated with retinal detachment. This tumor is vascular and enhances after the infusion of contrast material (Fig. 12–6, p. 537).

Optic Glioma. Optic gliomas are tumors of childhood and are common in patients with neurofibromatosis. The optic canal may be enlarged if the tumor extends through the canal.

CT provides excellent evaluation of the intraorbital optic nerve where a difference of 1 mm in size is significant. There may be proptosis; contrast enhancement is variable.

Magnetic resonance provides excellent evaluation of the intracranial portions of the optic nerves, the chiasm, and the optic tracts. If MR is not available, metrizamide cisternography provides excellent evaluation of the intracranial optic pathways (Figs. 12–7 and 12–8, p. 538).

Cavernous Hemangioma. This is a common tumor of the intraconal space which is seen in approximately 12 per cent of patients with unilateral exophthalmos. This is usually a well-defined, purely intraconal mass that demonstrates dense, homogeneous enhancement after the infusion of contrast material (Fig. 12–9, p. 539).

Lymphangioma. Lymphangioma has minimal enhancement and demonstrates irregular margins.

Rhabdomyosarcoma. Although rare, this is the most common malignant orbital tumor of childhood. More common in males, rhabdomyosarcoma usually occurs before age 10. There is commonly local bone destruction by the tumor, which may be intraconal or extraconal. CT provides excellent evaluation and can be used for treatment planning (not shown).

Hematoma. Post-traumatic hematoma may be intraconal or extraconal, and its diagnosis is based upon the clinical history. Associated orbital fractures or intracranial abnormalities can also be easily evaluated (see Chapter 11).

Lacrimal Gland Tumor. The lacrimal gland is located in the superolateral portion of the orbit. Tumors are represented by a variety of cell types, including dermoids, mixed epithelial tumors, granulomas, and carcinomas. These tumors are often palpable, and CT examination is used to determine the posterior extent of the tumor as well as any evidence of bone destruction (Fig. 12–10, p. 540).

Lymphoma. Lymphoma is common in older age groups and presents with periorbital edema and proptosis. CT reveals an intraorbital, diffusely infiltrative lesion, often both intraconal and extraconal, with retroglobular increased density and inability to distinguish orbital structures. There may be bony destructive changes (Figs. 12–11 and 12–12, pp. 540 and 541).

Pseudotumor. Pseudotumor, as the name suggests, has the characteristics of a tumor but is, in fact, an inflammatory process of unknown etiology. These pseudotumors typically respond rapidly to treatment with systemic steroids such as prednisone with a decrease in the soft tissue component and increased definition of contiguous structures on follow-up CT scans. The typical clinical presentation is that of rapid onset of proptosis, lid swelling, chemosis, pain, and limitation of motion with diplopia. CT classically reveals a diffuse soft tissue mass involving the entire orbit and extending from the apex to the posterior margin of the globe. The normal fat density is obliterated and returns after treatment. There is usually enhancement of this poorly defined mass and scleral thickening with enhancement of the circumference of the globe of the eye. Less extensive, focal areas of involvement may occur. While not pathognomonic, the typical clinical presentation, CT appear-

ance, and response to treatment confirm the diagnosis and frequently obviate the need for biopsy (Figs. 12–12 and 12–13, pp. 541 and 542).

Graves' Exophthalmopathy. Patients with Graves' disease usually present with bilateral exophthalmos, but unilateral exophthalmos may also be seen. CT easily rules out the presence of a mass as the cause for exophthalmos and typically demonstrates diffuse thickening of the extraocular muscles; in severe cases, the optic nerve may also be thickened. Retro-orbital fat may also be increased (Fig. 12–14, p. 543).

Inflammatory Processes

Periorbital Cellulitis. The inflammation is confined to the area anterior to the orbital septum. There is soft tissue swelling and obliteration of the normal soft tissue and muscle planes. The clinical presentation is that of a septic course with soft tissue swelling around the eye (Fig. 12–15, p. 543).

Orbital Cellulitis. The history is that of a septic course with periorbital swelling. CT reveals not only preseptal soft tissue swelling but also an irregular mass that demonstrates enhancement and involves the extraconal and intraconal spaces and obliterates the normal soft tissue planes. Differentiation from a tumor such as lymphoma or rhabdomyosarcoma may be difficult.

Mucocele. If there is obstruction of the outlet of the sinus, there is accumulation of secretion and pus which eventually liquefy within the sinus. The accumulation eventually leads to expansion of the sinus and pressure erosion of the walls of the sinus and may exert sufficient mass effect to extend into and distort the globe of the eye, leading to proptosis. While this is a nonmalignant process, surgical treatment is occasionally unsatisfactory in terms of eliminating the process. Mucoceles are most common in the ethmoid sinuses, followed by the sphenoid and frontal sinuses, and least common in the maxillary sinuses. The presence or absence of a sinusitis as the site of origin of the inflammatory process can be easily determined (Fig. 12–16, p. 544).

ORBITAL VENOGRAM

Although it has been superseded by computed tomography in many centers, orbital venography may be used to demonstrate the cavernous sinus and, consequently, to study the size of intrasellar tumors and their lateral extent, to rule out a cavernous sinus thrombosis, and to determine vascular displacements by orbital masses.

Technique. Distention of the frontal vein is achieved by extending the head off the end of the table with the patient supine. A rubber band is then placed circumferentially around the forehead just above the eyebrows. A 19- or 21-gauge "butterfly" (scalp vein) needle is then positioned in the vein. The needle is kept patent by continuous flushing or by connecting the tubing to an intravenous infusion set. The patient is then positioned for filming in the modified Waters' and lateral projections.

The patient is instructed to press his fingers across the zygomatic bone and across the base of the nose in order to compress the facial veins and facilitate retrograde flow of the contrast into the cavernous sinus. Approximately 6 to 8 cc of Conray 60 per cent is then injected slowly to fill the veins of the forehead, the superior opthalmic veins, and the cavernous sinus. A blank film should be obtained at the start of filming so that subtraction films can also be obtained. Magnification technique also may be used. The basal veins can also be opacified by retrograde catheterization via the femoral vein (Fig. 12–17, p. 545).

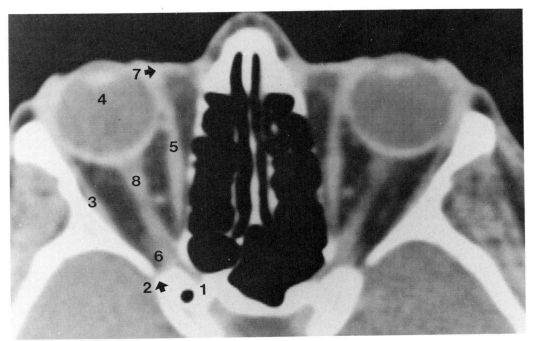

FIGURE 12–1. *Normal Orbit:* Thin-section, high-resolution CT scan through the orbit at the level of the optic nerve reveals the normal structures to excellent advantage.

1 Optic canal (just lateral to "1" is a small amount of air in the aerated anterior clinoid process).
2 Superior orbital fissure.
3 Lateral rectus muscle.
4 Globe of eye, lens projects just anterior to "4."
5 Medial rectus muscle. The ethmoid air cells project just medial to the muscle.
6 Ophthalmic artery.
7 Orbital septum.
8 Optic nerve.

The retro-orbital fat outlines the various muscles and nerves.

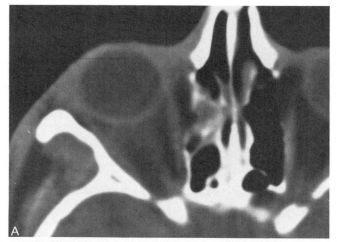

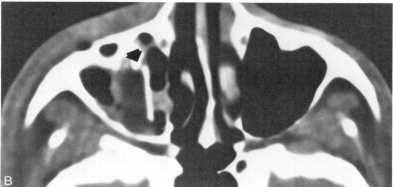

FIGURE 12–2. *Blow-out Fracture of the Floor and Medial Wall of the Orbit:* *A,* Axial CT scan reveals a fracture in the medial wall of the right orbit/lateral wall of the ethmoid sinuses and opacification of the sinus secondary to hemorrhage.

B, Section through the maxillary sinus reveals the vertical fragment of bone from the floor of the orbit (*arrow*). The fracture fragment is comminuted. There is also fat and muscle density material that has herniated from within the orbit inferiorly into the upper portion of the maxillary sinus via the defect in the floor secondary to the fracture.

Illustration continued on the opposite page

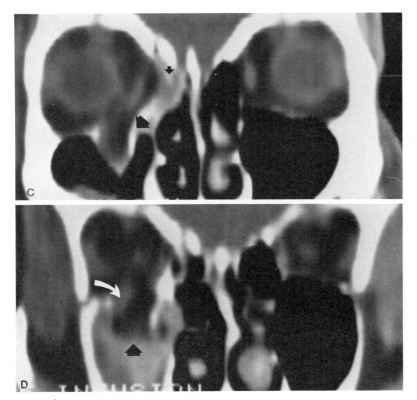

FIGURE 12–2 *Continued.*

C, Coronal reconstruction view reveals the opacification of the ethmoid sinus (*small arrow*) and the fracture of the laminae papyracea. The inferiorly displaced fracture of the floor of the orbit is also seen (*large arrow*). The intraorbital fat has been displaced inferiorly into the roof of the maxillary sinus. The inferior rectus muscle is also displaced inferiorly, and the medial rectus muscle can be seen to be displaced inferiorly and laterally as compared to the opposite side.

D, More posteriorly the coronal reformatted view reveals the inferiorly displaced medial rectus muscle (*white arrow*) and the fluid level secondary to blood in the floor of the maxillary sinus (*black arrow*).

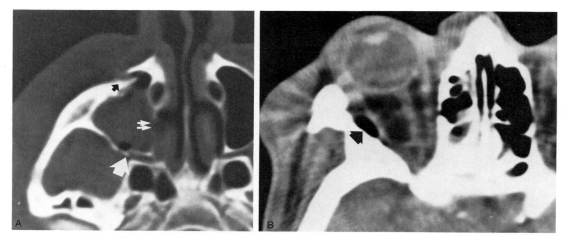

FIGURE 12–3. *Facial Bone Fracture:* *A*, Axial CT using "bone windows" reveals the fracture in the anterior wall of the maxillary sinus (*black arrow*), the opacified maxillary sinus secondary to blood, and disruption of the posterior wall of the sinus (*white arrow*). There is also a nondisplaced fracture of the medial wall of the maxillary sinus which projects just posterior to the nasolacrimal duct canal (*double arrows*).

B, At the level of the optic nerve, there is a small amount of orbital emphysema (*arrow*). Soft tissue swelling is over the orbit and the cheek. There is also irregular opacification of the ethmoid sinuses, probably secondary to hemorrhage.

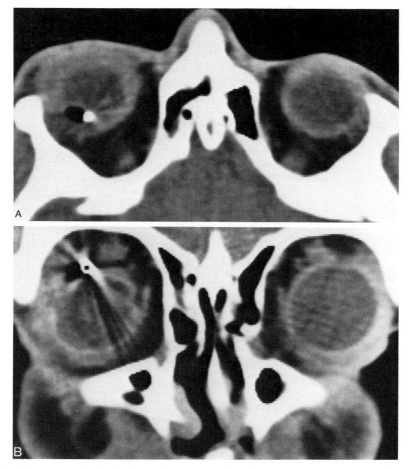

FIGURE 12–4. *Metallic Foreign Body in Globe:* *A,* Axial CT scan demonstrates a metallic foreign body in the upper portion of the right globe. The globe is ruptured and now has an irregular outline. There is a small amount of air within the globe that was introduced at the time of entrance of the foreign body.

B, The direct coronal scan reveals that the object rests just at the superior rim of the orbit. The irregular outline of the globe is better appreciated and there is a hematoma along the lateral margin of the globe.

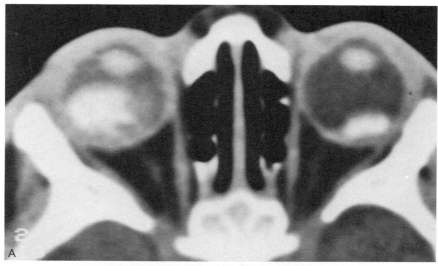

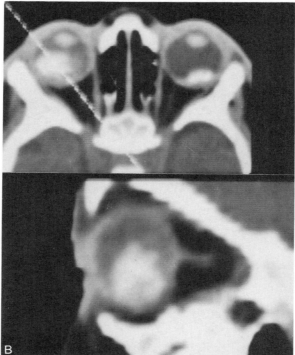

FIGURE 12–5. *Retinoblastoma:* *A*, CT scan demonstrates a large area of dense, amorphous calcification in the right globe and a similar but smaller area of calcification within the left globe.

B, Oblique reconstruction image of the right orbit better demonstrates the position of the calcification within the globe.

Illustration continued on the opposite page

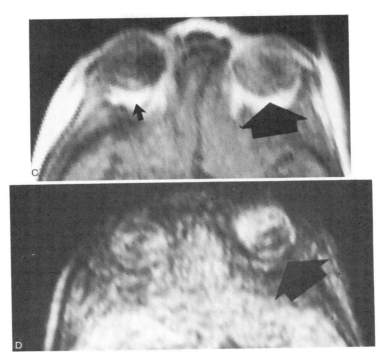

FIGURE 12–5 *Continued.*

C, MR, SE, TR530/TE30 is degraded by patient motion artifact and only faintly demonstrates the area of decreased signal intensity in the posterior portion of the globe (*large arrow*). A smaller area of decreased signal intensity is seen involving the opposite globe (*small arrow*).

D, SE, TR3120/TE120 demonstrates that the fluid within the globe becomes increased in signal intensity while the calcification remains of decreased signal intensity (*arrow*). Because of the increased sensitivity of CT to the presence of calcification, it is the diagnostic method of choice for evaluation of retinoblastoma. The addition of surface coils to MR scanning will probably aid in evaluation of the orbit, and in the future MR will be used in the evaluation of orbital pathology.

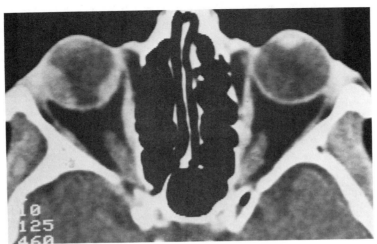

FIGURE 12–6. *Ocular Melanoma:* CT examination of the orbit reveals two biconvex areas of increased density along the posteromedial and lateral portions of the globe of the eye. These are areas of melanoma and are associated with retinal detachment. The appearance is very typical of melanoma. (As a general rule of thumb, an uncomplicated retinal detachment is not demonstrated by CT examination.)

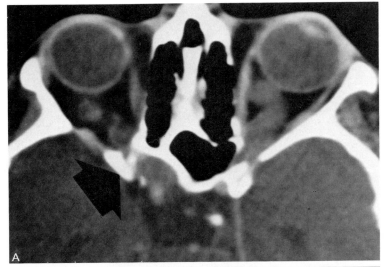

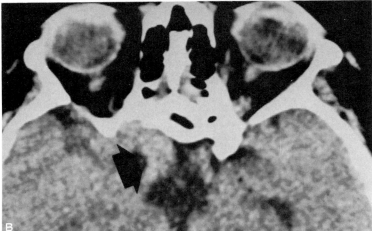

FIGURE 12–7. *Optic Glioma:* CT at the level of the optic nerve and optic canal reveals pressure erosion and enlargement of the optic canal on the right side (*arrow*). There is a "dumbbell-shaped" optic nerve glioma that extends through the optic canal. There is also involvement of the opposite optic nerve, which is seen to be greatly enlarged and serpiginous in configuration.

B, At the level of the intracranial optic nerve the intracranial portion of the tumor is seen (*arrow*). The patient has neurofibromatosis, a condition that is known to be associated with an increased incidence of optic glioma.

FIGURE 12–8. *Optic Glioma:* Midsagittal SE TR530/TE30 image reveals an optic glioma involving the optic chiasm (*arrow*). The chiasm is greatly enlarged, and there is obliteration of the suprasellar cistern. This patient is known to have neurofibromatosis and has had previous enucleation of both eyes because of involvement with intraorbital optic nerve gliomas. Also note the small area of high signal intensity of the fat in the posterior portion of the sella (*f*), a normal finding.

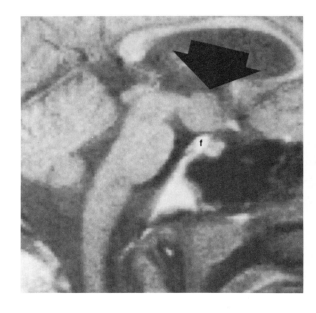

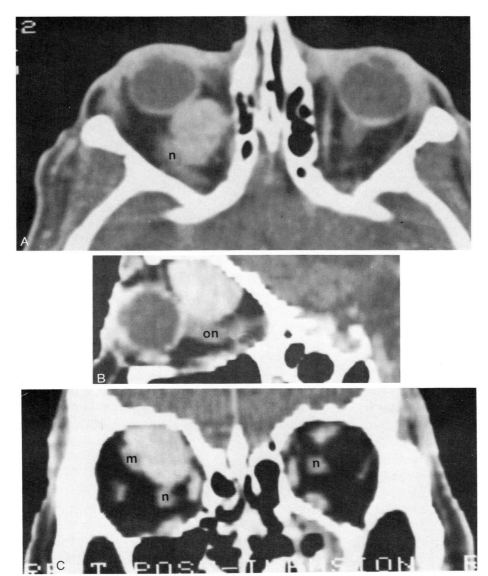

FIGURE 12–9. *Orbital Hemangioma:* *A*, Axial section through the level of the optic nerve reveals the typical appearance of a well-defined, densely enhancing intraconal mass in the right orbit. The optic nerve (*n*) is displaced laterally, and there is proptosis.

B, Oblique sagittal reconstruction image reveals that the optic nerve (*on*) is displaced inferiorly, and the hemangioma projects superiorly.

C, Coronal reformatted image better demonstrates the inferior displacement of the optic nerve (*n*) and lateral displacement of the superior oblique muscle (*m*). The mass extends superiorly beyond the muscle cone to be both intraconal and, in small part, extraconal.

FIGURE 12–10. *Lacrimal Gland Tumor:* A, Axial image reveals a mass in the upper outer portion of the orbit. The globe is displaced anteriorly and inferiorly.

B, Coronal reformatted image reveals the extraconal nature of the mass (M) displacing the globe inferiorly and medially as compared to the opposite side. Wide window widths allow evaluation of the presence or absence of bony destructive changes.

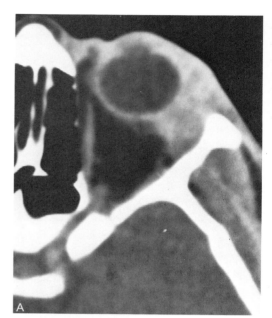

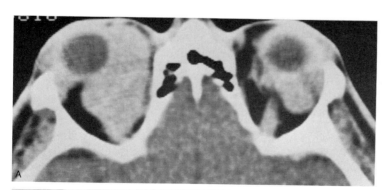

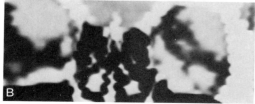

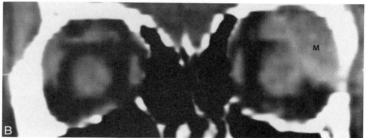

FIGURE 12–11. *Orbital Lymphoma:* A, Axial section reveals large lobulated intra- and extraconal masses in both orbits. On the right side, the medial rectus muscle and the optic nerve are no longer visible.

B, Coronal reformatted image reveals the location of the multicentric masses to better advantage. The infiltration of the extraocular muscles on the left side is also seen. There is bilateral proptosis.

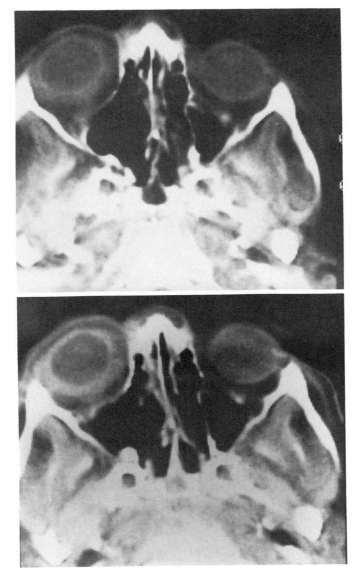

FIGURE 12–12. *Orbital Pseudotumor:* The name obviously derives from the fact that, although the abnormality has all the appearances of a tumor, biopsy demonstrates only granulomatous tissue without evidence of a tumor mass. These patients may present with unilateral exophthalmos; thus, the clinical appearance is that of a tumor mass. The CT scan demonstrates an amorphous mass behind the globe and exophthalmos. The mass enhances in a homogeneous fashion on the postinfusion scan, and not infrequently there is also enhancement of the posterior wall of the globe.

Because of the amorphous configuration of the mass and the rimlike enhancement of the posterior margin of globe, the diagnosis of pseudotumor may be suggested. The process may be bilateral.

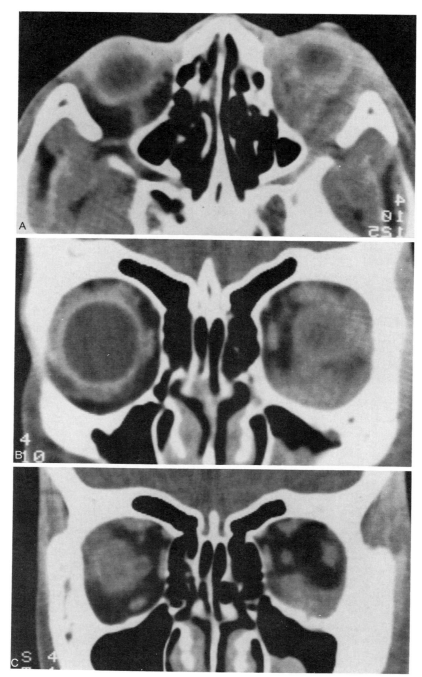

FIGURE 12–13. *Orbital Pseudotumor:* *A,* Axial image reveals the obliteration of the retro-orbital fat and thickening of the extraocular muscles by the large, poorly defined infiltrative process. Postinfusion there was enhancement of the mass and peripheral enhancement of the globe of the eye, a typical appearance of pseudotumor of the orbit.

B and *C,* Coronal reformatted images reveal the infiltrative nature of the process, with obliteration of the normal tissue planes. The intra- and extraconal nature of the process is easily appreciated.

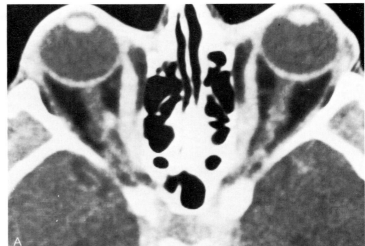

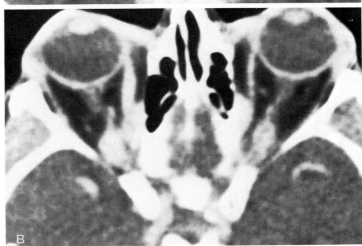

FIGURE 12–14. *Hyperthyroid Exophthalmopathy:* *A* and *B* reveal bilateral proptosis, an increase in the amount of retro-orbital fat, and thickening of the extraocular muscles of the eye. In this patient, the change is most marked in the medial rectus and superior rectus and oblique muscles, with relative sparing of the lateral rectus muscle. The findings are typical of Grave's disease.

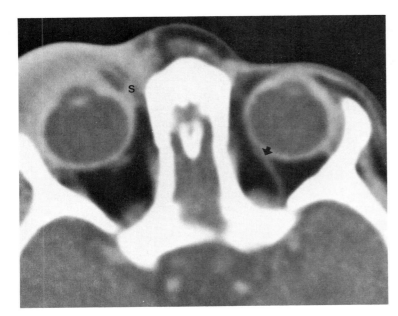

FIGURE 12–15. *Periorbital Cellulitis:* The patient is a 7-year-old male with periorbital swelling and elevated temperature. CT reveals marked soft tissue swelling over the right globe. There is obliteration of the normal soft tissue planes. The process is confined to the area anterior to the orbital septum (*S*) and therefore represents periorbital cellulitis. Orbital cellulitis extends behind the orbital septum and surrounds the globe of the eye. Incidentally, the superior ophthalmic vein (*arrow*) can be identified extending obliquely across the orbit.

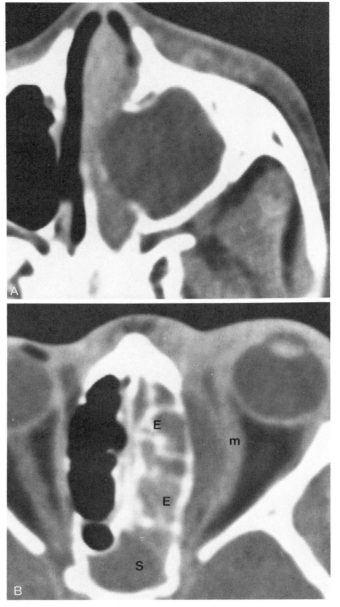

FIGURE 12–16. *Mucocele and Orbital Abscess:* A, CT section through the maxillary sinus reveals opacification of the sinus and expansion of the sinus with thinning of the medial wall and thickening of the posterolateral wall secondary to chronic infection. The sinus contains liquefied pus and the appearance is typical of a mucocele.

B, At the level of the ethmoid sinuses there is complete opacification of the ethmoid sinus (*E*) as well as the sphenoid sinus (*S*). There is expansion of the sinus, and a soft tissue mass extending into the left orbit and displacing the medial rectus muscle (*m*) laterally. There is a marginal rim of enhancement, which represents an intraorbital abscess secondary to the ethmoidal sinusitis. There is proptosis on the side of the abscess (surgically proved).

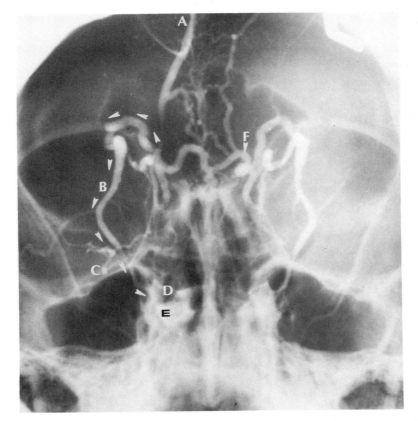

FIGURE 12–17. *Orbital Venography:* The needle is in place in the frontal vein (not shown), and approximately 6 cc of contrast has been injected. The normal study reveals: *A*, Frontal vein; *B*, Superior ophthalmic vein; *C*, Inferior ophthalmic vein; *D*, Internal carotid artery filled with unopacified blood and bathed by the contrast; *E*, Cavernous sinus; *F*, Angular vein.

At *B* the superior ophthalmic vein courses around the superior rectus muscle medially and downward to the apex of the orbit. The arrows follow the normal blood flow into the cavernous sinus (*E*).

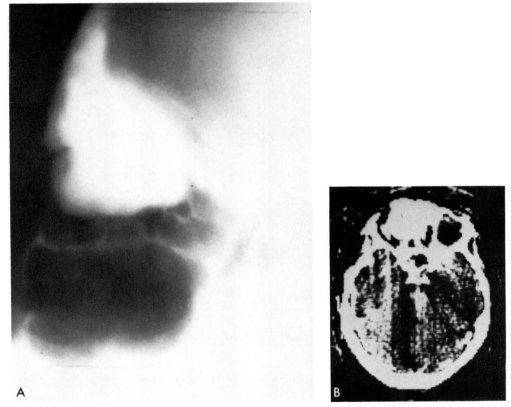

FIGURE 12–18. *Osteoma:* A, The radiographic tomogram (lateral view) demonstrates a well-defined, slightly lobulated bony mass in the region of the ethmoid sinus. The finding is consistent with a large osteoma.

B, The CT scan also demonstrates the high-density mass. The osteoma is in the region of the ethmoid sinus and extends to either side of the midline. The scan helps to delineate the posterior extent of the mass and rules out the presence of intracranial extension.

13

POSTERIOR FOSSA

This discussion of the posterior fossa will focus on the anatomic structures that are in the infratentorial space, with emphasis on the vascular structures. Included in this space are the cerebellum with its right and left hemispheres and the midline cerebellar vermis, which surrounds the fourth ventricle (see Fig. 13–1, p. 561). The pons, medulla, midbrain, quadrigeminal plate, and cerebral peduncles will be included in these discussions. The fourth ventricle and the aqueduct of Sylvius are important posterior fossa structures. In addition to these structures, several cisterns are of particular interest in the posterior fossa. Fortunately for us, as students of neuroanatomy, most of the cisterns are named for the particular area with which they are closely related. It should be pointed out that these cisterns are not individual and separate structures; rather, adjacent cisterns are simply extensions or continuations of each other but have been individually named for their related areas.

The cisterna magna is formed by the veil-like arachnoid membrane that extends down from the cerebellar hemispheres. Just anterior and inferior to the cisterna magna are the cerebellar tonsils. The tonsils are situated just off the midline on either side, and are anatomically the lowest point of the cerebellar hemispheres. More inferiorly are the medulla and the junction of the medulla with the spinal cord. Just beneath the medulla bilaterally are the vertebral arteries. These arteries join together in the midline to form the basilar artery below the mid-portion of the medulla. The vertebrobasilar system carries the blood supply to the posterior fossa structures (Fig. 13–1, p. 561).

COMPUTED TOMOGRAPHY OF THE POSTERIOR FOSSA

Before undertaking a discussion of the various structures of the posterior fossa, a few remarks are in order concerning the angiographic evaluation of posterior fossa lesions. In the supratentorial circulation, because the middle cerebral artery runs in the isle of Reil, which lies deep in the cerebral hemisphere, one is readily able to evaluate vascular displacements. Because of the relatively central location of the sylvian group of vessels, the normal vessel position usually is altered by mass lesions in various locations, whether they are presylvian, retrosylvian, supra- or infrasylvian. However, no such group of vessels runs deep through the central portion of the cerebellum; therefore, one must rely on alterations in the superficial blood vessels, even though they are rather remote from the actual mass lesions. Although some observers have had excellent success with angiographic diagnosis of posterior fossa lesions, I have found it to be less helpful than the CT scan.

The availability of CT scanning has made one appreciate the relative lack of accuracy of angiography in the diagnosis of mass lesions of the cerebellum. In addition, even when vascular alterations are demonstrated on the angiogram, the CT scan gives a more accurate concept of the anatomy of the lesion, whether cystic or solid, and whether it is or is not surrounded by edema. More important, the scan shows whether an avascular mass represents an acute hematoma. Multiple mass lesions are best demonstrated by CT scanning. The author has seen examples where the CT scan demonstrated a sizable mass lesion and the angiogram was singularly unhelpful—failing, even in retrospect, to demonstrate even the side of the abnormality.

It is becoming apparent that in some cases a definitive operative procedure can be performed on certain posterior fossa lesions without using any invasive studies after evaluation by CT scanning. In addition, the scan can tell us whether there is an associated hydrocephalus, any evidence of supratentorial extension of the mass, or an associated supratentorial mass lesion. Although obviously there is no substitute for arteriographic evaluation of such vascular lesions as aneurysms and arteriovenous malformations in the cerebellum or dura, for nearly all other lesions evaluation by CT has greatly enhanced our ability to diagnose both the type and the extent of various posterior fossa lesions with far greater accuracy than was ever possible before the development of computed tomography.

It is not unreasonable to expect that in the future angiography will no longer be used for diagnosis; instead, it will serve to demonstrate vessel landmarks and blood supply after the CT scan has revealed a mass lesion. There is, of course, no substitute for the angiogram in defining the position of arterial and venous structures.

MAGNETIC RESONANCE OF THE POSTERIOR FOSSA

Magnetic resonance has greatly aided our ability to diagnose abnormalities of the posterior fossa. Because of the fact that there is minimal signal from the bones surrounding the posterior fossa, there is also no artifact such as that seen with CT scanning of the posterior fossa. Thus MR lends itself well to study of posterior fossa structures. The ready availability of multiplanar imaging of the posterior fossa also makes evaluation of the normal anatomy, variations, and pathology very easy. The "anatomy" sequences, or the T-1 weighted images, allow ready demonstration of the various normal anatomic structures, including structures such as the red nucleus and the substantia nigra, which were previously visible only on pathologic specimens (Fig. 13–18, p. 124). It is possible to correlate each slice with the normal neuroanatomy; therefore, familiarity with the normal anatomy is a prerequisite before evaluation of the posterior fossa by MR. CT has already provided an

excellent introduction to the posterior fossa, but MR carries this evaluation even further, again without the use of ionizing radiation or the injection of contrast.

In addition to the identification of the tumor mass or other abnormality, MR has the ability to identify related changes in the intracranial contents. The exact anatomic location of the fourth ventricle can be identified with greater accuracy than with CT scanning. Localization of the fourth ventricle is facilitated by the ability to image the posterior fossa structures in the sagittal plane. The lack of degradation of the image by bone artifact, the sensitivity of MR to the densities of CSF and brain, and multislice capability make identification of the fourth ventricle relatively simple. This, of course, aids in the identification of the mass because the histologic type can often be predicted by the anatomic location. Posterior compartment masses project posterior to the fourth ventricle, whereas anterior compartment masses project anterior to the fourth ventricle. The intra-axial versus extra-axial location can also be evaluated by MR.

The displacement of the aqueduct is easy to identify, and its relationship to the third and fourth ventricles can be evaluated. Widening or narrowing of the various basilar cisterns is also related to the position of the mass and can be evaluated directly, without requiring the use of contrast material.

The presence or absence of hydrocephalus may influence the surgical approach to various posterior fossa abnormalities and influence the decision about placing a ventricular drain or ventriculoperitoneal shunt prior to surgery. The size of the ventricles and response to shunting are easy to evaluate. With obstructive hydrocephalus, there may be transependymal resorption of CSF, which results in an appearance of periventricular increased signal intensity on the T-2 weighted images. This appearance suggests that shunt placement may be advisable prior to surgery.

If a posterior fossa mass is present, there may be sufficient mass effect that the cerebellar tonsils are displaced inferiorly through the foramen magnum, below the level of the foramen magnum, and into the upper cervical region. This inferior displacement of the cerebellar tonsils is known as tonsillar herniation. While tonsillar herniation is present in the Chiari malformation, its presence in association with a mass is more significant. Lumbar puncture in the presence of tonsillar herniation may result in further compression of the brain stem and cause the patient's death. MR allows convenient evaluation of the presence of tonsillar herniation in addition to the evaluation of a mass. The sagittal plane images are best for this type of evaluation.

The normal anatomic structures are readily demonstrated, including:

- Red nucleus
- Substantia nigra
- Corticospinal tract
- Cerebral aqueduct
- Collicular plate
- Optic tracts
- Cerebellar peduncles
- Cerebellar tonsils

In addition to the normal anatomy (see Chapter 3), a variety of abnormal conditions are readily demonstrated and accurately evaluated by MR scanning.

Chiari Malformation. One of the uses of MR which became apparent very early was the ready evaluation of the presence or absence of the low cerebellar tonsils that are associated with the Chiari malformation. Several slices in the right, left, and midsagittal planes provide excellent evaluation of the presence or absence of low cerebellar tonsils. In addition, the Chiari malformation is often associated with a hydromyelia of the spinal cord, and so these same slices can also be used to determine the presence or absence of a cavity within the cervical spinal cord. With the Chiari malformation the cerebellar tonsils extend down below the level of the foramen magnum. Although an exact measurement cannot be given to define when the tonsils are "too low," it appears that some deformity of the cerebellum is often present in association with this abnormality. However, it appears that a number of individuals have low-lying tonsils even in the absence of any other abnormality. This has been called cerebellar ectopia (see Chapter 15).

Degenerative Diseases. Atrophic processes of the posterior fossa can be readily identified and are seen in patients with spinocerebellar or olivopontocerebellar degeneration. Wallerian degeneration of the cerebral peduncles is also readily appreciated with MR (see Chapter 7).

Posterior Fossa Tumors. Tumors of the posterior fossa can be located extraordinarily easily with MR. The T-1 weighted images illustrate the anatomy and any distortion of the normal anatomic structures. The T-2 weighted images demonstrate that the abnormal mass becomes increased in signal intensity when compared to the normal structures. Thus the T-2 weighted images allow for ready appreciation of the abnormality, whereas the T-1 weighted images better illustrate the distortion of the anatomy.

The multiplanar capability of MR allows the anatomic localization of mass lesions to be performed with great ease. Thus, localization into the following areas:

- posterior fossa, anterior compartment, extra-axial
- posterior fossa, posterior compartment, intra-axial
- posterior fossa, anterior compartment, intra-axial
- posterior fossa, posterior compartment, extra-axial

can be made without difficulty in most cases by examination of the various planes of section. If one can localize the point of origin of the mass, then the various other characteristics of the tumor will aid in determining the correct diagnosis. The sagittal plane of section appears to be particularly helpful in evaluation of the posterior fossa and is the best plane for initial evaluation.

Diagnostic difficulty has been encountered with calcified brain stem masses—usually proved to be slow-growing astrocytomas—which cause little deformity of the brain stem. Calcification within a mass often cannot be appreciated on the MR scan. In these cases the CT scan, with its extraordinary sensitivity to even small amounts of calcification, has proved to be more helpful than MR. Clinical history and physical findings, which lead to anatomic localization of the abnormality to the brain stem, permit the examiner to better look for and appreciate subtle alterations in the appearance of the brain stem. On the other hand, areas of hemorrhage cause an increased signal if the hemorrhage is older than approximately 48 hours. This allows excellent visualization and localization of both hemorrhagic tumors and partially thrombosed basilar artery aneurysms. In addition, the negative flow defect of the blood in the unthrombosed portion of the aneurysm can also be readily demonstrated, and the relationship of the lumen to the thrombosed aneurysm is easily defined. However, this will probably not obviate the need for angiography.

Brain Stem Glioma. MR is probably the procedure of choice for evaluation of brain stem glioma. The widening of the pons is readily demonstrated, the tumor appears increased in signal intensity on the T-2 weighted images, and the exact areas of involvement are easily appreciated. MR is also excellent for follow-up of response to treatment or for tracking tumor progression. Cystic portions of the tumor are also easily seen and appear as well-defined areas of increased signal intensity. The displaced basilar artery appears as a negative flow defect.

Areas of calcification are rare and are well-demonstrated by CT but poorly demonstrated by MR. The displacement of the fourth ventricle is easily identified, as this CSF-containing structure can be identified as a low signal intensity area on the T-1 weighted images.

Infarcts. Midbrain and brain stem infarcts, often a difficult diagnosis to make on the CT scan because of the "Hounsfield" artifact, are readily demonstrated by MR. On the T-2 weighted images, these areas of infarction appear as readily appreciable areas of increased signal intensity. Again, the multiplanar capability of the MR scanner allows exact anatomic localization and the true extent of the abnormality can be seen.

Acoustic Neuromas. These tumors themselves are best demonstrated on the T-1 weighted images in the axial and coronal planes. The effacement of the pons by the extracanalicular portion of the tumor is easily demonstrated, particularly on the coronal projections. The internal auditory canals are easily demonstrated on MR scans, and the presence of an enlarged canal can be seen because the low signal of the petrous bone provides a natural contrast with the CSF on the T-2 weighted images. The high signal intensity of the CSF on the T-2 weighted images easily outlines the normal or widened internal auditory canal (IAC), and the fluid within the cochlea and semicircular canals can also be seen. Extracanalicular tumors widen the canal and project into the cerebellopontine angle (CPA) (Fig. 13–22, p. 582). Intracanalicular tumors can also be demonstrated with MR scans.

Acoustic neuromas are readily visualized by MR. It appears that even intracanalicular tumors can be demonstrated by MR and that other diagnostic tests will be unnecessary for evaluation of acoustic neuroma. The T-1 weighted SE scans allow visualization of the tumor and also readily demonstrate the distortion of the normal anatomy. In addition, the tumors are often of higher than normal brain density and are therefore readily identified in the cerebellopontine angle (CPA), where they replace the normal low signal intensity of the CSF in the cistern. In addition, while the bony structures provide a negative signal, the T-2 weighted images cause the CSF to appear increased in signal intensity, and they are therefore of very high intensity relative to the petrous bone. Therefore, the CSF can be identified as it enters the normal-sized or dilated internal auditory canal or blends with the increased signal intensity of the cerebellopontine angle

tumor in the T-2 weighted images. It is anticipated that with additional advances in technology and thinner sections, as well as localization techniques similar to those now available with CT, the accuracy of MR should be such that it will replace other diagnostic methods.

Meningiomas. Meningiomas may not be well demonstrated because the presence of psammomatous calcification within the tumor will cause them to be poorly visualized by MR techniques. The future availability of gadolinium-DTPA will probably allow ready demonstration of these meningiomas because they will "enhance" after the injection of the gadolinium. At the present time, small meningiomas at the base or along the clivus may be overlooked. On the other hand, meningiomas that exert mass effect have thus far been fairly readily demonstrated because they distort the normal anatomy. This alteration from the normal appearance is readily demonstrated because the normal anatomic structures are easily visualized in the T-1 weighted images. In addition, the capping of the tumor by the low signal intensity of the CSF allows for localization of the tumor mass even without the aid of alterations in the signal intensity. The multiplanar capability of the MR scans also greatly aids in tumor localization. Meningiomas are fairly common, arising from the clivus and in the region of the cerebellopontine angle, where the mass replaces the CSF density, and so detection of a mass is not difficult. One densely calcified meningioma arising in the region of the tentorial notch and extending up into the middle cranial fossa was easily appreciated on both CT and MR imaging, probably because of very dense calcification (Fig. 13–47, p. 621). As a general statement, it can be said that calcified masses are much better evaluated by CT than by MR because of the high sensitivity of CT and the relative insensitivity of MR to the presence of calcification.

Chordoma. Chordomas appear as variable-density masses with mixed high and low signal intensity areas, often with areas of amorphous calcification. The exact location is readily demonstrated, and bony destruction is easily detected (Fig. 13–48, p. 622).

Cholesteatoma (Epidermoid). Also known as *pearly tumors*, cholesteatomas contain cholesterol crystals and are of epithelial origin. They are frequently located in the CPA; typically they appear as low-density masses on CT and are associated with bone erosion. Cholesteatomas may or may not enhance after the injection of contrast. They commonly demonstrate an irregular margin on CT. MR reveals a slightly higher than CSF density mass on the T-1 weighted image and an increased signal on the T-2 weighted image.

Glomus Jugulare Tumor. The area of negative flow defect in the region of the jugular bulb is abnormally prominent, and the jugular bulb is enlarged. These tumors are probably best demonstrated by CT.

Cervicomedullary and Craniocervical Junctions. MR provides excellent evaluation of the anatomy at the skull base. The medulla and spinal cord, the surrounding CSF, and the relationship between these structures and the skull base can be readily evaluated without the use of intravenous or intrathecal contrast material, awkward patient positioning, or ionizing radiation. MR is the ideal study to evaluate the Chiari malformation and the displacement of the cerebellar tonsils into the cervical spinal canal. The commonly associated syrinx of the spinal cord is also easily identified with MR.

MR can also be used to study the following:

- Basilar impression secondary to Paget's disease
- Rheumatoid arthritis—the pannus can also be seen
- Spine fractures
- Cord hematoma or swelling

Radiation Necrosis. Radiation necrosis is most commonly seen in areas remote from the original tumor bed and is usually discovered several to many years after treatment. For example, patients whose pituitary adenoma was cured with appropriate radiation may present many years later with enhancing areas in the temporal lobe regions. We had the opportunity to study one case of pathologically proven radiation necrosis of the medulla and spinal cord in a patient previously treated for neuroesthesioma of the cribriform plate region. This patient demonstrated areas of increased signal intensity on the T-2 weighted SE images. The histopathologic study demonstrated areas of demyelination in the affected regions.

It is doubtful, however, that MR will be specific for radiation necrosis. We have seen brain stem infarcts and demyelinated plaques of multiple sclerosis that have a similar appearance.

NORMAL VASCULAR ANATOMY

Before other methods such as nuclide brain scanning and computed tomography of the brain were developed, it was helpful to include the supratentorial presence of hydrocephalus, an abnormal vascular supply arising from the internal carotid system, or even evidence of additional mass lesions in the supratentorial compartment.

With the availability of femoral catheterization, selective catheterization of either the right or left vertebral artery can readily be performed in most cases with injection of contrast material directly into the vertebral artery. Using this method one hopes to fill the vertebrobasilar system; indeed, it may even "wash" the contrast material down the contralateral vertebral artery to a level below the origin of the contralateral PICA. In this fashion one can outline all the posterior fossa structures from one vertebral artery injection and include only the posterior fossa circulation. Depending on the size of the vertebral artery, 3 to 8 cc of contrast material are injected directly into the vertebral artery. With rare exceptions, do not inject more than 8 cc. We use a rate of 6 to 10 cc per second over a time period necessary to inject the amount desired; e.g., to inject 5 cc we use a rate of 10 cc/sec for 0.5 second. All injections are made with the automatic injector.

The PICA on the side of the suspected lesion should be visualized if at all possible. If the contrast material does not wash retrograde down the contralateral vertebral artery at the time of injection and evaluation of the opposite side is required, the opposite vertebral artery should be catheterized and injected for full evaluation of the vascular anatomy bilaterally. In some instances, it will be necessary to perform percutaneous brachial angiography if it is technically impossible to catheterize the vertebral arteries selectively—e.g., when there is stenosis of the vessel origin.

The right vertebral artery arises from the right subclavian artery distal to the origin of the right common carotid artery. On the left side, the vertebral artery arises directly from the subclavian artery. In 3 to 6 per cent of cases, the left vertebral artery will be seen to arise directly from the arch of the aorta as a separate vessel (see Chapter 4). In most cases, the vertebral arteries enter into the foramina transversaria of the lateral mass of the cervical vertebrae at the level of C_6. There are anatomic variations, however, and the vertebral artery may enter into the foramina transversaria at any level. The vertebral arteries then course cephalad until they reach the level of C_2. At the C_2 level the artery turns laterally and then superiorly to enter the more laterally placed foramina transversaria of the C_1 vertebral body. Following the exit from the C_1 foramina transversaria, the vertebral artery lies in a groove along the superior margin of the atlas; it then turns anteromedially and passes through the foramen magnum lying anterior to the medulla oblongata. Very shortly thereafter, the vertebral artery joins with its mate from the other side to form the basilar artery (Fig. 13–2, p. 562). In 5 to 6 per cent of cases, the vertebral artery ends in the PICA.

Three branches of the vertebral artery are of consequence to us as angiographers. In addition to these main branches, a variety of smaller branches feed the musculature of the neck and may be used to supply collateral flow to the vertebral or external carotid system (see Chapter 14). The branches that concern us are the posterior inferior cerebellar artery (PICA), the anterior spinal artery (note that at this point the spinal cord is anatomically positioned dorsal to the vertebral arteries), and the posterior meningeal artery. The posterior spinal artery may arise from the vertebral artery, but more often it arises from the PICA as it courses around the medulla. Note that a posterior spinal artery arising from the vertebral artery would have to course around the medulla to become dorsal or posterior to the cord.

To understand the normal and pathologic anatomy of the posterior fossa, one must have a thorough understanding of the anatomy of the normal pathway of the PICA (see Figs. 13–3 to 13–7, pp. 563 to 567). A simple statement, but basic to this understanding, is the fact that the PICA originates from the vertebral artery ventral to the medulla, but ultimately will supply an area that is predominantly dorsal to the medulla. As a consequence, the PICA must follow a course that will allow it to do this.

The PICA has three segments. The initial portion is known as the *anterior medullary segment* because it is still anterior to the medulla at this point. This is best appreciated on the anterior view; on the lateral view, the vessel is directed toward the observer, and its lateral course cannot be recognized because the vessel is foreshortened. This lateral direction is the first step toward this vessel's ultimate position dorsal to the medulla. The PICA then courses inferiorly for a variable distance, forms a loop by reversing its course back upon itself; it proceeds dorsally and cephalad and then courses cephalad toward the fourth ventricle. Most of this loop is lateral to the medulla; it is therefore known as the *lateral medullary segment* (Fig. 13–3, p. 563). This initial loop, which is convex caudad, is known as the *caudal loop*. When the PICA reaches its position dorsal to the medulla, that portion is known as the *pos-*

terior medullary segment (because it is dorsal or posterior to the medulla). The posterior medullary segment of the PICA then courses cephalad and anteriorly along the posterior margin of the medulla in a near midline position until it reaches the posterior margin of the fourth ventricle. At this point, the PICA gives off a small twiglike branch to the choroid plexus of the fourth ventricle. This point is known as the *choroidal point* (Figs. 13–4 and 13–5, pp. 564 and 565). The small branch to the choroid plexus is not usually visible arteriographically, but it may be seen if angiotomography or magnification and subtraction techniques are used (Fig. 13–7, p. 567).

At the choroidal point, the PICA again reverses its course, turns caudally, and bifurcates into the vermian branch and the tonsillohemispheric branches (Fig. 13–6, p. 566). This loop of the PICA is known as the *cephalic loop* (Fig. 13–5, p. 565). Note that the caudal loop and the cephalic loop of the PICA share a common limb—that portion just proximal to the choroidal point.

It should also be noted that there is a good deal of normal variation in the position of the PICA. One should be familiar with these normal variations before suggesting a mass lesion or an abnormal course of this vessel. In some cases, the PICA will initially loop upward rather than downward. Again, this is a normal variation and, in most instances, the artery will return to a more "normal" course, and the various loops such as the caudal and cephalic loops will be readily identified.

The normal point of origin of the PICA from the vertebral artery can also vary greatly. The caudal loop of the PICA may extend down to the level of the C_2 vertebral body and still be within normal limits. The fact that the PICA extends this low may suggest a posterior fossa mass lesion. If this is suspected, one should look for other correlating abnormalities. When the caudal loop of the PICA extends very low as a normal anatomic variation, it will be seen that the choroidal point is in normal position and no other vascular displacements are evident. With true tonsillar herniation secondary to a mass lesion, it is the *tonsillar branch* of the PICA that will be displaced below the level of the foramen magnum.

To measure the normal position of the choroidal point, the "T-T" line or "Twining's line" is used as an anatomic measurement (Fig. 13–2, p. 562). Twining's line extends from the tuberculum sellae (T) to the torcular Herophili (T). A line perpendicular to the midpoint of this line should fall approximately in the middle of the fourth ventricle. Therefore, the angiographic choroidal point, which is at the posterior portion of the fourth ventricle, should, in the normal individual, also lie at approximately the midportion of Twining's line.

Distal to the choroidal point, the PICA bifurcates into the tonsillohemispheric and vermian branches (Fig. 13–6, p. 566). The vermian branches course posteriorly and superiorly just adjacent to the midline and along the posterior margin of the vermis of the cerebellum. The tonsillohemispheric branches of the PICA will be seen to course laterally and then up and over the cerebellar hemispheres. The PICA forms the main blood supply to the lower portion of the cerebellum, and the vermian artery forms anastomotic connections with the superior cerebellar arteries. The tonsillar branch of the PICA *may* course along the inferior border of the tonsil, but it may also loop over or below the tonsil; therefore it is not as reliable a sign as one would like as a reflection of tonsillar herniation. The tonsillar loop *is* displaced inferiorly with tonsillar herniation, however, and this occurs when there is a lesion with enough mass effect to create downward displacement of the tonsil. It is this downward displacement of the tonsillar loop of the PICA that must be looked for when one is concerned about the possibility of a mass lesion in the posterior fossa. One should also check for the position of the choroidal point and other anatomic landmarks that will correlate with or refute the presence of a mass lesion and resulting tonsillar herniation.

Posterior Meningeal Branch of the Vertebral Artery. This vessel arises from the vertebral artery above the arch of the atlas and just below the foramen magnum. The vessel courses superiorly in the midline adjacent to the inner table of the skull. The artery may extend above the tentorium cerebelli and supply the falx cerebri and adjacent tentorium. This vessel may become enlarged with the presence of a meningioma.

Anterior Inferior Cerebellar Arteries. These originate from the basilar artery approximately 1 cm from the origin of the basilar artery. The right and left anterior inferior cerebellar arteries (AICA) are seen and usually can be visualized arteriographically. The AICA will be seen to course laterally; it then enters into and courses out of the internal auditory canal and then around the flocculus of the cerebellum. This unique course of the AICA in the region of the internal auditory canal makes it of particular value when a cerebellopontine angle mass is present. After the AICA exits from the internal auditory canal, it will be seen to course further laterally and supply the cerebellar hemisphere at the level of the great horizontal fissure. The region of the horizontal fissure of the cerebellum is a so-called "watershed" area between the distribution of the superior cerebellar arteries and the posterior inferior cerebellar arteries. There is an inverse relationship between the size of the PICA and the size of the AICA. When the PICA is small—or, in 25 per cent of cases, absent—the AICA is enlarged and supplies the distribution of the PICA.

The basilar artery gives origin to many small pontine perforating vessels; however, these cannot normally be visualized arteriographically except by magnification and subtraction techniques.

Superior Cerebellar Arteries. The next branches of the basilar artery that can be visualized arteriographically are the superior cerebellar arteries. They arise from the basilar artery just below the terminal bifurcation into the paired posterior cerebral arteries. If the posterior cerebral arteries arise directly from the carotid system, the superior cerebellar arteries then represent the terminal bifurcation of the basilar artery. This bifurcation is in the interpeduncular fossa. At this level, the superior cerebellar arteries initially course laterally in the perimesencephalic cistern (midbrain portion of the ambient cistern), then posterosuperiorly around the midbrain and then medially until they nearly touch in the midline in the region of the quadrigeminal plate cistern. The superior cerebellar artery branches then course superiorly and posteriorly up and over the vermis of the cerebellum and over the cerebellar hemisphere. Midline branches course posteriorly over the vermis until they anastomose with the vermian branches of the PICA. The superior cerebellar arteries may be either single bilaterally or double bilaterally, or they may be single on one side and double on the opposite side.

The vermian branches of the superior cerebellar artery course quite near the midline just beneath the highest point of the tentorium. The posterior cerebral arteries distribute themselves over the hemispheres more laterally at a lower, more sloping portion of the tentorium. It will be seen, therefore, that even in the normal patient the infratentorial superior cerebellar arteries may project higher than the supratentorial posterior cerebral arteries on the lateral view of a vertebral arteriogram. Review and dissection of a normal preserved anatomic specimen will be very helpful in understanding fully the course of these arteries.

In addition, it should be noted that there can be many normal variations in the course of the posterior cerebral artery. Therefore, caution should be used when interpreting an unusual course as being secondary to mass lesion.

Posterior Fossa Venous Anatomy

The venous anatomy of the posterior fossa (Figs. 13–16 and 13–17, pp. 575 and 576) is as important as the arterial anatomy in the diagnosis of space-occupying lesions in the posterior fossa. The precentral cerebellar vein outlines the anterior margin of the vermis of the cerebellum. This is a single midline vein that is curvilinear and concave posteriorly. It originates from below and drains upward initially, curving first anteriorly and then posteriorly until it joins the posterior portion of the vein of Galen.

Colliculocentral Point. The precentral cerebellar vein originates in the region of the anterior medullary vellum and courses forward until it reaches the inferior colliculi in the region of the quadrigeminal plate. The vein then courses posteriorly and superiorly in a curvilinear line along the anterior margin of the cerebellar vermis; it then proceeds posterosuperiorly where the precentral cerebellar vein joins the vein of Galen. The most anterior point of the curve of the precentral cerebellar is the *colliculocentral point*. Because the vein is situated in the midportion of the posterior fossa, it often is affected if a mass lesion is present.

A line drawn tangential to the precentral cerebellar vein at the level of the colliculocentral point and connected to the choroidal point (see Fig. 13–16, p. 575) and extending along the limb of the PICA common to both the cephalic and caudal loops falls in the midpoint of the fourth ventricle. This line divides the posterior fossa into the *anterior* and *posterior compartments* (see Fig. 13–18, p. 577). Therefore, abnormalities can be judged by measuring the deviation from the anticipated normal. With masses in the region of the pons or anterior to the fourth ventricle and the aqueduct of Sylvius—the anterior compartment—the precentral cerebellar vein is straightened and either loses its normal curvilinear course or is displaced posteriorly. On the other hand, if the mass is in the vermis of the cerebellum or

placed more posteriorly in the hemispheres of the cerebellum—the posterior compartment—the precentral vein will be displaced forward. Because of its central position, particular attention should be paid to each angiogram, making special note of the position of this vein. If mass lesions are present in the cerebellar hemispheres, a change in the position of these veins may not be detected because the veins are midline structures. If, however, the lesion is large enough to reach the midline structures, the precentral cerebellar vein will be seen to be displaced anteriorly secondary to this mass lesion. These veins are only rarely visible on the anteroposterior view.

The anterior pontomesencephalic vein lies in intimate association with the anterior inferior margin of the pons, known also as the "belly" of the pons. The origin of this vein is at the level of the posterior perforated substance in the interpeduncular fossa. Because of its intimate association with the pons, it is a more accurate representation of the actual position of the pons than is the basilar artery. This is true because the basilar artery may become tortuous secondary to arteriosclerosis and move away from the midline; also, any torsion of the pons may move the basilar artery posteriorly and away from the midline. On the lateral view of the venous phase, the anterior pontomesencephalic vein will be seen to have the shape of a squared hook, with the top of the hook lying in the interpeduncular fossa in the region of the midbrain. The vein then turns caudad to follow along the anterior margin of the pons. The remainder of the course of the vein is obscured by the overlying petrous bones; however, subtraction techniques will allow one to see this vein empty into the basilar venous plexus and ultimately drain via the internal jugular vein.

As in the supratentorial circulation, there are a large number of unnamed veins that course over the surface of the cerebellum. Except for the precentral cerebellar veins, however, there are no deep venous structures that can be used reliably to diagnose the presence or absence of mass lesions.

The *copular point* is just below and behind the fourth ventricle. It marks the beginning of the inferior vermian veins.

The basal vein of Rosenthal will be seen to course along the free edge of the tentorium and around the midbrain in the perimesencephalic cistern until it enters the vein of Galen. This vessel is discussed under the supratentorial venous structures.

The superior vermian veins lie over the upper surface of the vermis of the cerebellum just below the straight sinus. These veins drain anteriorly and superiorly into the vein of Galen. If mass lesions are present, these veins will be seen to be elevated upward and to lie much closer than normal to the straight sinus. This alteration from the normal position with elevation of the superior vermian veins is known as a "closed" or "tight" posterior fossa; it reflects the presence of a space-occupying mass in the posterior fossa.

The inferior vermian veins are paired midline veins that course along the inferior portion of the cerebellar vermis. These veins may be shifted to the contralateral side with cerebellar hemisphere lesions. The position of the patient for filming will affect the position of the vermian veins, since rotation of the head will give the impression that the vein is shifted to one side or the other—even in the absence of a true mass lesion. Therefore, it is of paramount importance that the patient be positioned in a straight anteroposterior projection. In the presence of a mass lesion, there may be poor filling of one or even both vermian veins because of localized increased intracranial pressure. If this is the case, there will usually be other signs of a mass lesion in addition to the finding of poor venous filling. It should be noted that the contralateral vermian vein may not fill well when the injection is made into one vertebral artery, thus giving the impression of a mass lesion in one cerebellar hemisphere, whereas in reality the phenomenon is due to poor filling with contrast of the vessels contralateral to the side injected.

At the base of the skull there is a large venous plexus made up of multiple interconnecting veins. Some of these veins drain into the cavernous sinus, but most drain ultimately into the petrosal sinus and then into the sigmoid sinus and out via the internal jugular vein.

Of particular interest is a group of small tributary veins also known as "brachial veins" (after the Latin word for "arms"). These all join together bilaterally in the shape of a star just above the internal auditory canals. This collection of veins is known as the *petrosal star*. It normally projects just above the internal auditory canal on the AP view. The petrosal star usually will be displaced upward—away from the internal auditory canal—when a mass lesion is present in the region of the cerebellopontine angle. Again, localized increased intracranial pressure may cause poor filling of these veins.

ANTERIOR AND POSTERIOR COMPARTMENTS

The posterior fossa can be divided into two compartments: the anterior compartment and the posterior compartment. These compartments are found by drawing a line connecting the colliculocentral point of the precentral cerebellar vein with the angiographic choroidal point. Examination of the diagram (Fig. 13–18, p. 577) reveals that this line will course through the fourth ventricle. All masses in front of this line are in the anterior compartment; masses behind the line are in the posterior compartment. One anticipates certain angiographic findings with masses in either of these compartments. Therefore, these changes should be looked for when examining a posterior fossa angiogram.

Angiographic Findings with Anterior Compartment Masses

1. The basilar artery is closely applied to the clivus.
2. There is *posterior* displacement of the precentral cerebellar vein.
3. The anterior pontomesencephalic vein is closely applied to the clivus.
4. The choroidal point is displaced posteriorly.
5. If the mass is extra-axial—e.g., a clivus meningioma, chordoma, or exophytic pontine glioma—the basilar artery is displaced *posteriorly*, as is the anterior pontomesencephalic vein.

Examples of Anterior Compartment Masses

1. Pontine glioma
2. Acoustic neuroma
3. Chordoma
4. Clivus meningioma
5. Basilar artery aneurysm
6. Metastases

Angiographic Findings of Posterior Compartment Masses

1. The basilar artery is closely applied to the clivus.
2. There is *forward* displacement of the precentral cerebellar vein.
3. The choroidal point and vermian artery are displaced to the contralateral side if the

mass is unilateral or if it arises in the midline but extends predominantly to one side.

4. The anterior pontomesencephalic vein is closely applied to the clivus.

5. There is elevation of the superior cerebellar (vermian) veins and arteries.

6. The inferior vermian veins are displaced to the contralateral side.

Examples of Posterior Compartment Masses

1. Medulloblastoma
2. Cerebellar astrocytoma
3. Metastases
4. Hemangioblastoma
5. Tentorial meningioma
6. Ependymoma

In the examples that follow, emphasis has been placed on cases that demonstrate obvious vascular displacements. Particular emphasis is placed on masses that give a "classic" appearance, and more esoteric findings have been omitted. Correlation with the CT scan has been made whenever possible. For the most part, cases with normal or nearly normal angiograms have been omitted—even though it is the author's opinion that sizable masses may be present when the angiogram shows only minor or no alterations.

The author recommends the routine use of a Towne's and lateral view, coned down for the posterior fossa, as the initial study in all cases. After review of the films, additional views may be obtained using alterations in the AP positioning—especially with a view centering the internal auditory canals through the center of the orbit. This allows an excellent demonstration of the course of the AICA. The submentovertex view is also very helpful in the diagnosis of mass lesions and aneurysms. Angiotomography is also recommended for the visualization of midline structures. Subtraction views are very helpful and, in many cases, are essential to demonstrate fully the vascular anatomy.

ANTERIOR COMPARTMENT MASSES

Chordoma

Chordomas arise from remnants of the notochordal tissues. Intracranially, they arise in the midline, often at the level of the clivus, dorsum sella, or region of the spheno-occipital synchondrosis. They may be calcified and result in destructive changes that involve the clivus. The extension and bony destructive properties of these tumors may give the appearance of a large nasopharyngeal mass. In addition to intracranial tumors, chordomas also occur in the region of the sacrum, where they result in bony destructive changes associated with a large soft tissue mass (Fig. 13–48, p. 622).

CT scans of intracranial chordomas usually reveal a large calcified midline mass.

Pontine Glioma

Pontine gliomas (brain stem gliomas, brain stem astrocytomas) arise in the brain stem and lead to diffuse enlargement of the pons—a finding referred to as "hypertrophy" of the pons. They are more common in boys than in girls and usually are noted in the first decade of life. The clinical presentation is of multiple cranial nerve palsies. These tumors appear radiographically as anterior compartment masses in the posterior fossa.

CT Scans. The preinfusion scan reveals a mass in the pons that may be radiolucent, isodense, or, rarely, of higher density than normal brain tissue. When the tumor is of sufficient size, it is possible to detect an increase in the size of the pons with posterior displacement and compression of the fourth ventricle. There is a varying degree of obstructive hydrocephalus in nearly all cases. Following the infusion of contrast material, there is marked homogeneous enhancement in some cases; however, in some cases no enhancement will be seen. The postinfusion scan also demonstrates the relationship of the mass to the surrounding edema.

Angiography. The basilar artery will be closely applied to the pons except when there is exophytic growth of the tumor. In that case, the basilar artery may actually be displaced posteriorly away from the clivus. There is posterior and downward displacement of the choroidal point and the posterior medullary segment of the PICA. The anterior pontomesencephalic vein will be closely applied to the clivus, and there is posterior displacement of the precentral cerebral vein. The tumors usually are avascular.

Ventriculography and Pneumoencephalography. These studies reveal posterior displacement of the fourth ventricle and compression of the prepontine cistern. The pons measures greater than the maximum of 4 cm in most cases. In the AP view, the fourth ventricle appears to be draped over a mass.

Acoustic Neuroma

These tumors may originate wherever Schwann cells are found. However, we are interested here in the intracranial tumors and tumors of the eighth cranial nerve in particular. Multiple schwannomas and particularly bilateral acoustic schwannomas (neuromas) are associated with von Recklinghausen's neurofibromatosis.

Histology. There is a surrounding capsule of connective tissue. Microscopic examination reveals either Antoni A or B type cells, the A type demonstrating narrow elongated bipolar cells with little cytoplasm that characteristically are arranged in palisades. In the B type there is less cellular density, and microcysts and vacuolated cells are present. There is a fine honeycombed appearance.

Reticulin fibers are present in both types.

Skull Films. Enlargement and erosion of the internal auditory meatus are evident. In general, the internal auditory canal should not be taller than 8 mm, and there should not be a difference of more than 3 mm between the two sides.

Angiography. Vertebral angiography demonstrates that the anterior inferior cerebellar artery is displaced out of the internal auditory canal by the mass. The basilar artery may be displaced to the contralateral side. The petrosal star is elevated away from the internal auditory canal. Selective external carotid angiography and the use of subtraction techniques may demonstrate a tumor blush. There may or may not be obstructive hydrocephalus.

Computed Tomography. The CT scan without and with the infusion of contrast material is the procedure of choice for the work-up of acoustic neuroma. Most tumors outside of the internal auditory canal that are larger than 1 cm are demonstrated by the postinfusion CT scan. With thin section tomography (1-mm slices), even smaller tumors may be detected. Manipulation of the window width and window level often reveals enlargement of the bony canal. The preinfusion scan frequently is entirely normal. The postinfusion scan demonstrates dense homogeneous enhancement of the tumor. These tumors may exhibit a cystic component and therefore have a central radiolucency. There may or may not be obstructive hydrocephalus. Even with a fairly sizable tumor, the fourth ventricle may not demonstrate any evidence of shift from its normal position. There may be displacement to the contralateral side or flattening of the anterior margin of the fourth ventricle.

POSTERIOR COMPARTMENT MASSES

Medulloblastoma

These tumors are usually found in the first decade of life, but may be present in the second or third decade. The lesions arise on the midline in most cases, developing from the primitive cells of the external granular layer of the cerebellum. Occasionally these primitive cells migrate away from the midline; thus, the tumor also may arise off the midline. Although the name might imply a point of origin within the medulla, medulloblastomas most frequently originate from the posterior medullary velum in its inferior portion anatomically at the base of the vermis of the cerebellum. Occasionally, the tumors invade the fourth ventricle. There is a greater than 2:1 male predominance. The medulloblastoma is a posterior compartment mass.

Skull Film. Radiographically visible calcifications are very rare, although calcifications are more frequently identified by CT scan. The skull series most commonly is normal, but it may show evidence of widening of the sutures and other changes secondary to increased intracranial pressure.

CT Scanning. The CT scan with infusion is the procedure of choice for the work-up of a patient with possible medulloblastoma. The scan reveals a varying degree of obstructive hydrocephalus in almost all cases. I have not seen a case that did not demonstrate some degree of hydrocephalus at the time when tumor was visible. The medulloblastoma itself presents as a midline posterior fossa mass. The tumor usually is slightly more dense than normal brain tissue and rarely contains calcification. Frequently there is a variable amount of edema that surrounds the tumor asymmetrically. The fourth ventricle may be obliterated or may be seen to be displaced forward in the midline or slightly to either the right or left.

The mass, at the time of presentation, usually is quite large, commonly occupying half the width of the posterior fossa on those cuts where the tumor is best seen (see Figs. 13–34 to 13–39, pp. 599 to 609).

Following the infusion of contrast material, there is marked homogeneous enhancement of the tumor. The tumor may seed the subarachnoid space; therefore, metastatic nodules may be seen in the supratentorial region. These are especially demonstrable in the supratentorial distribution on the postinfusion scan. Medulloblastomas also may metastasize to the spinal cord.

Angiography. The angiogram may be normal. These tumors may or may not show evidence of abnormal vascularity, and early draining veins are rare. The vascular displacements vary, depending on the point of origin of the tumors. Although the appearance may be similar to any other mass in the posterior fossa, in general it is that of a posterior compartment mass with anterior displacement of the precentral cerebellar vein. The PICA displacement can be in any direction, depending on the point of origin of the tumor. Because the tumor may grow in the midline or asymmetrically off the midline, the arteries and veins may be either at the midline or displaced to the contralateral side.

The arteriographic findings are not diagnostic. On the other hand, the CT appearance in most cases is very typical, and a diagnosis of medulloblastoma can be made with a high degree of certainty by CT scan.

Ependymoma

These tumors arise from the ciliated ependymoma cells that line the ventricles. In the posterior fossa the tumor arises from the ependymal lining of the fourth ventricle; therefore, it usually presents as a midline tumor in the posterior fossa. Ependymomas are posterior compartment masses.

These tumors are seen in the first two decades of life and are more common in boys than in girls.

Skull Film. Calcifications are not uncommon in ependymomas and present as areas of fine calcification. There may be signs of increased intracranial pressure with split sutures. The skull may be normal.

CT Scanning. These tumors are readily identified on the CT scan. A varying degree of obstructive hydrocephalus is present in nearly all cases. The tumor may be isodense with normal brain tissue, and its presence will be detected by the fact that there is obliteration of the fourth ventricle and obstructive hydrocephalus. Calcifications, if present in the tumor, are readily detected by the CT scan. Following the infusion of contrast material, there is marked homogeneous enhancement of the tumor (see Fig. 13–40, pp. 610–611). (The tumor arises within the fourth ventricle, which is dilated around the mass.) Ependymomas may seed into the supratentorial system or spinal regions via the cerebrospinal fluid pathways.

Angiography. These tumors are vascular with prolonged blush. Vessel displacements vary, depending on the location of the tumor. If the tumor grows inferiorly, the PICA may be splayed apart on either side of the midline. There is nothing specific that will make the angiographic diagnosis absolute.

Astrocytoma

The astrocytoma is the most common posterior fossa tumor in children. In adults, one may also find astrocytomas of the cerebellum that produce similar angiographic changes.

These tumors are typically cystic and lie in the cerebellar hemisphere; therefore, they present as posterior compartment tumors. The lesion may extend to involve the vermis of the cerebellum, or, less commonly, may arise in the midline from the vermis of the cerebellum. These tumors contain a nodule that may be located anywhere in the wall of the cyst. The cyst wall itself is benign, and the nodule is the functioning portion of the astrocytoma (Figs. 13–41 to 13–43, pp. 612–616).

Skull Film. These tumors may be slow growing and therefore may present as a long-standing process in many children. *Rarely*, there may be bowing of the occipital bone over the cystic tumor. Not infrequently there is splitting of the sutures because of the long-standing increased intracranial pressure.

CT Scanning. The CT scan reveals a cystic lesion in the cerebellar hemisphere. The border of the cyst is well-defined; there may or may not be surrounding edema. The fluid within the cyst is of higher density than CSF, reflecting its high protein content. There is always a varying degree of obstructive hydrocephalus. Following the infusion of contrast material, there may be enhancement of the nodule of tumor in the wall of the astrocytoma. Not uncommonly, however, the nodule of enhancement reflecting the vascular portion of the tumor is not seen on the CT scan. Even if no enhancing nodule is evident, a cystic lesion in the cerebellar hemisphere that is associated with obstructive hydrocephalus makes the diagnosis of cerebellar astrocytoma possible with a very high degree of certainty in a large proportion of cases.

Angiography. The angiographic findings noted in cerebellar astrocytoma are similar to those seen in any cerebellar mass. The wall of the cyst is benign and does not appear as a vascular structure; however, the nodule of tumor may appear as a vascular mass. In general, the choroidal point of the PICA will be displaced to the contralateral side. The vermian branches of the PICA also will be displaced to the contralateral side, and there is stretching of the hemispheric branches of the PICA. There may be inferior displacement of the tonsillar loops of the PICA, reflecting tonsillar herniation. The vermian branches of the superior cerebellar artery are displaced superiorly.

The superior vermian veins will be displaced close to the straight sinus. The precentral cerebellar vein is displaced anteriorly, and the choroidal point is displaced inferiorly. The basilar artery is closely applied to the clivus and may be displaced across the midline away from the tumor. There is elevation of the superior cerebellar arteries.

In those rare cases in which the tumor is particularly long-standing, upward bowing of the straight sinus may be seen—an unusual finding because the tentorium and straight sinus are rigid structures.

Hemangioblastoma

This is a vascular tumor which arises in the cerebellum from capillary endothelial cells. These tumors vary greatly in size. When the tumors are large and vascular, differentiation from an arteriovenous malformation may be difficult. Typically, the blush of a hemangioblastoma will be noted to persist well into the venous phase. These are posterior compartment masses, although they rarely may involve the brain stem (Fig. 13–45, pp. 618–619).

Hemangioblastoma associated with retinal hemangiomas and polycythemia is a syndrome known as von Hippel–Lindau's disease; it is one of the phakomatoses. These tumors may be solid or cystic.

Skull Film. Usually normal.

CT Scanning. The CT scan reveals a low-density lesion of varying size that may or may not be associated with obstructive hydrocephalus. The postinfusion scan reveals marked homogeneous enhancement of the solid portions of the tumor.

Metastases to Posterior Fossa

Metastatic lesions to the posterior fossa are fairly common. The most common source of metastasis is a primary lung tumor; however, breast carcinoma is another common source. They may be either anterior or posterior compartment masses. Metastases are the most common posterior fossa tumors in adults.

Plain Skull Film. The skull film is usually normal. The progression of the disease is too rapid to allow the changes of increased intracranial pressure to be detected in the sella. Bony metastases may be visible.

CT Scanning. The CT scan performed without and with contrast infusion affords the most accurate assessment of the presence or absence of metastatic deposits in the posterior fossa. Furthermore, the number, position, and relationship of the metastatic deposits to other anatomic structures is better defined on the CT scan than by any other diagnostic method now available.

The preinfusion scan may appear normal, or it may reveal radiolucent isodense or high-density lesions. There may or may not be displacement or distortion of the fourth ventricle. Obstructive hydrocephalus may or may not be present.

The postinfusion scan reveals a variety of patterns of enhancement. There may be a ring of enhancement, homogeneous enhancement, or a number of other varieties of enhancement.

Angiography. A variety of abnormal patterns may be seen, depending on the position of the lesions and the multiplicity of lesions.

Cerebellar Hemorrhage

Hypertensive hemorrhages occur in the cerebellum but are less frequent in the cerebellum than in the basal ganglia. If of sufficient size, the cerebellar hemorrhage leads to the rapid demise of the patient caused by mass effect with compression of the vital structures in the brain stem. Early diagnosis is therefore important so that the clot can be removed without delay. These are usually posterior compartment hemorrhages. Massive brain stem hemorrhage also may occur.

Plain Skull Film. Normal.

CT Scanning. The preinfusion scan reveals an area of blood density in the cerebellar hemisphere. There may or may not be surrounding edema; the fourth ventricle may be shifted, and there may or may not be obstructive hydrocephalus. A rapid increase in the area of hemorrhage may occur. I have seen one case in which there was a demonstrable increase in the size of the hemorrhage during the time it took to perform the CT scan. Computed tomography is the procedure of choice for diagnosis, and surgery can be undertaken without further work-up. Indeed, delay in diagnosis may lead to the patient's death.

Angiography. Vertebral angiography may demonstrate an avascular mass. The shifts of the various vascular structures will depend on the size and position of the hemorrhage.

MISCELLANEOUS POSTERIOR FOSSA LESIONS

Cerebellar Hypoplasia

The cerebellum exhibits varying degrees of aplasia and hypoplasia that are congenital and apparently developmental in origin. These variations are readily and beautifully studied by MR scanning.

Arachnoid Cyst of Posterior Fossa

Arachnoid cystic lesions of the posterior fossa are seen occasionally and have a fairly typical appearance.

Plain Skull Film. There is thinning of the occipital bone over the cystic abnormality, and there may be a bulging of the bone in the occipital region. The skull may have a dolichocephalic appearance, or that of bathrocephaly.

Angiography. The straight sinus, torcular, lateral sinuses, occipital lobes, and cerebellum are displaced anteriorly and away from the inner table of the skull by the cyst.

Pneumoencephalography. The fourth ventricle will be normal in size and configuration. The large arachnoid cyst fills with air.

MR and CT Scanning. The scans demonstrate a well-defined lesion in the posterior fossa that contains cerebrospinal fluid. The bony calvaria is thinned over the cyst; the fourth ventricle may be visualized and will be normal in size. There is usually no evidence of obstructive hydrocephalus.

Dandy-Walker Syndrome

The pathogenesis is thought to be dilatation of the fourth ventricle secondary to occlusion of the foramina of Magendae and Luschka. There is usually, but not always, dilatation of the lateral and third ventricles.

Angiography. There is upward displacement of the superior cerebellar arteries, downward displacement of the posterior inferior cerebellar artery, and a large avascular area in the posterior fossa. The torcular is displaced above the lambdoid suture.

MR and CT Scanning. There is a large CSF-containing cyst in the posterior fossa. A separate fourth ventricle cannot be demonstrated.

The Dandy-Walker cyst (malformation) is to be differentiated from arachnoid cysts of the posterior fossa that may result in enlargement of the bony posterior fossa but are separate from the fourth ventricle. Other varieties of posterior fossa hypoplasias and cerebellar hypoplasias also must be ruled out.

A normally large cisterna magna may give a similar appearance on the scan, but in this case the fourth ventricle will be seen as a separate structure that is normal in size and position. This normal anatomic variant is readily demonstrated by MR and CT scanning.

Glomus Jugulare, Glomus Intravagale, and Carotid Body Tumors

Glomus jugulare, glomus intravagale, and carotid body tumors (chemodectomas) all arise from nonchromaffin paraganglionic tissue. They are very vascular tumors and are supplied by branches of the external carotid artery. The glomus jugulare tumor may also receive blood supply from the vertebral artery. Glomus jugulare tumors may invade the bony margins around the jugular fossa and a mass lesion may be demonstrated in the jugular vein by jugular venography.

Glomus intravagale tumors displace the common carotid artery and its branches anteriorly, whereas carotid body tumors arise between the internal and external carotid arteries at the level of the bifurcation and spread them apart.

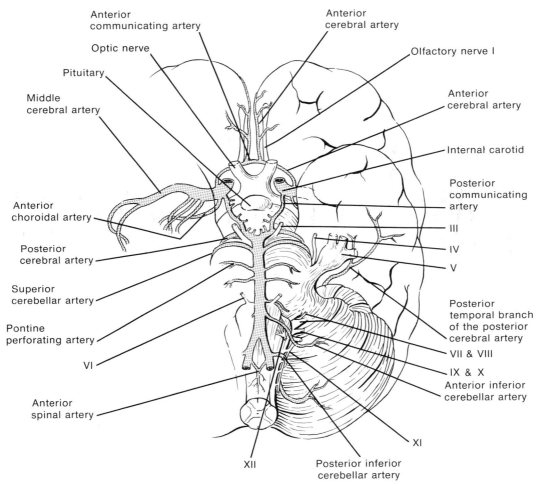

FIGURE 13–1. *Circle of Willis and Posterior Fossa Vascular Supply:* The posterior fossa structures are supplied by the vertebral and basilar arteries. The posterior fossa vessels communicate with the supratentorial circulation via the posterior communicating arteries. The surface anatomy of the base of the brain is also illustrated.

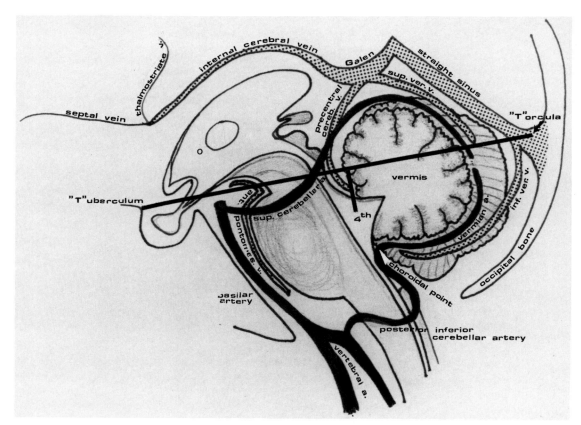

FIGURE 13—2. *Twining's Line:* The choroidal point (*white arrow*) lies at approximately the midportion of Twining's line. This line connects the *T*uberculum with the *T*orcular and is also known as the "T-T" line. Most of the important arteries and veins of the posterior fossa are also illustrated in this drawing and should be committed to memory.

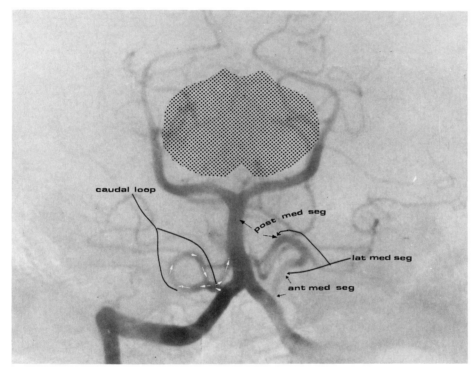

FIGURE 13–3. *Normal Anatomy of the Posterior Inferior Cerebellar Artery (PICA):* On the left side, the normal segments of the PICA are illustrated; on the right, the course of the PICA is illustrated by the white arrows. The choroidal point is in the midline and is hidden behind the basilar artery, which is filled with contrast material. The posterior cerebral arteries and the superior cerebellar arteries course around the midbrain (shaded area) and nearly meet in the midline in the region of the quadrigeminal plate cistern. (See also Figure 13–4.)

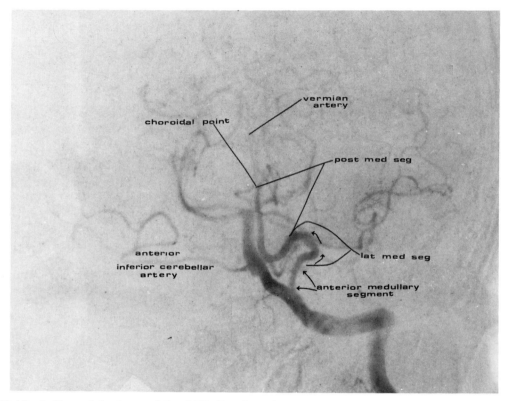

FIGURE 13–4. *Normal Anatomy of the PICA (Continued):* The contrast material has now washed out of the right vertebral artery, and this vessel is now filled with unopacified blood. The anterior inferior cerebellar artery (AICA) is well visualized on the right side but is obscured by the PICA on the left. The choroidal point is well seen, as are the vermian branches of the PICA. The various segments of the PICA again are demonstrated. (See also Figure 13–3.)

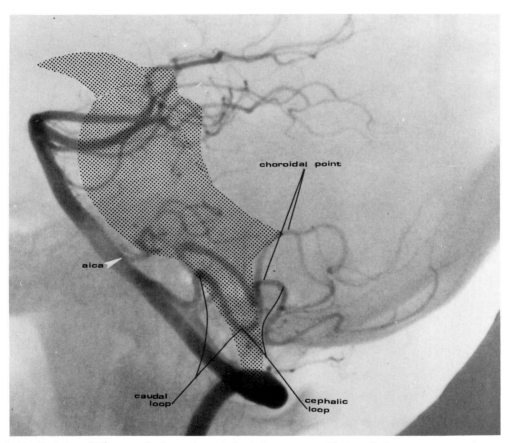

FIGURE 13–5. *Lateral View:* Both the right and the left PICA are filled, and their courses can be traced on the lateral view. The choroidal points are at different levels, but both are normal. The anterior inferior cerebellar arteries (AICA) can also be seen.

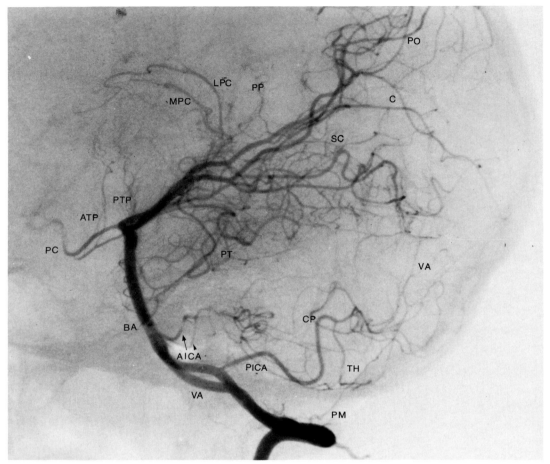

FIGURE 13–6. The lateral view of the vertebral angiogram in a normal patient using subtraction techniques demonstrates the normal arterial structures in the posterior fossa.

PC	Posterior communicating artery.
ATP	Anterior thalamoperforating arteries.
PTP	Posterior thalamoperforating arteries.
BA	Basilar artery.
VA	Vertebral artery.
AICA	Anterior inferior cerebellar artery.
PICA	Posterior inferior cerebellar artery.
CP	Choroidal point.
TH	Tonsillohemispheric branch of *PICA*.
VA	Vermian branch of PICA.
PT	Posterior temporal branch of posterior cerebral artery.
SC	Superior cerebellar arteries.
C	Calcarine branch of posterior cerebral artery.
PO	Parieto-occipital branch of posterior cerebral artery.
MPC	Medial posterior choroidal artery.
LPC	Lateral posterior choroidal artery.
PP	Posterior pericallosal artery.
PM	Posterior meningeal artery.

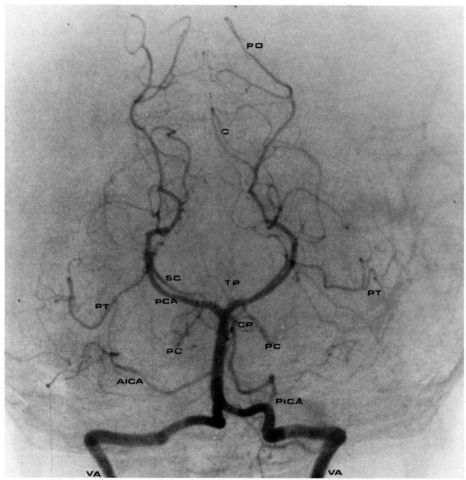

FIGURE 13–7. The AP view of the vertebral angiogram using subtraction techniques demonstrates the normal arteries in the posterior fossa. The PICA is absent on the right side, a normal anatomic variant.

VA	Vertebral artery.
PT	Posterior temporal branch of posterior cerebral artery.
PCA	Posterior cerebral artery.
SC	Superior cerebellar artery.
TP	Thalamoperforating arteries.
C	Calcarine branch of posterior cerebral artery.
AICA	Anterior inferior cerebellar artery.
PO	Parieto-occipital branch of the posterior cerebral artery.
PC	Posterior communicating artery.

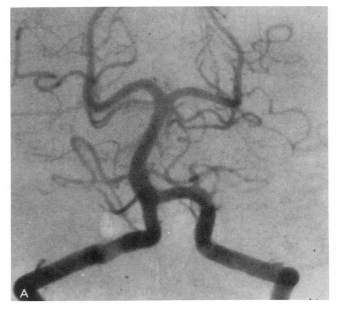

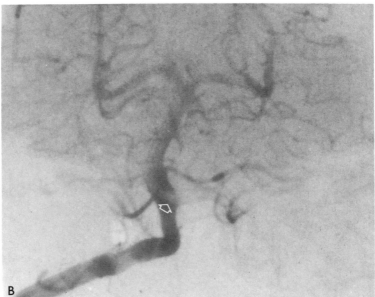

FIGURE 13–8. *Normal Vertebral Arteriogram with Wash-out:* A reveals filling of both vertebral arteries from the right vertebral injection. The left vertebral artery is filled by retrograde flow.

B, Later in the arterial phase the contrast material has been washed out of the left vertebral artery; now unopacified blood is flowing up the left vertebral artery, creating a "streaming" effect in the basilar artery. This unopacified blood creates a filling defect in the basilar artery (*white arrowhead*). This should not be mistaken for an arteriosclerotic plaque or thrombus in the basilar artery.

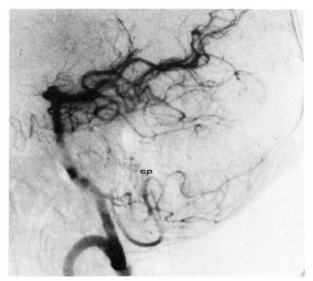

FIGURE 13–9. *Normal Low Position of the PICA:* The PICA originates in a normal position, and the caudal loop extends down below the foramen magnum. There is, however, no evidence of abnormal vascularity or vessel displacement. In addition, note that the choroidal point is in its anticipated normal position (*cp*). This is not a reflection of tonsillar herniation, but represents a normal variation.

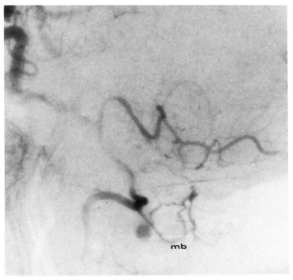

FIGURE 13–10. *Vertebral Artery Ending in PICA:* The vertebral artery ends in the PICA. This normal variation is seen in approximately 25 per cent of individuals. In these patients, the basilar artery and the remainder of the posterior fossa structures will not be filled, and it may be necessary to inject the contralateral vertebral artery. Note muscular branch (mb).

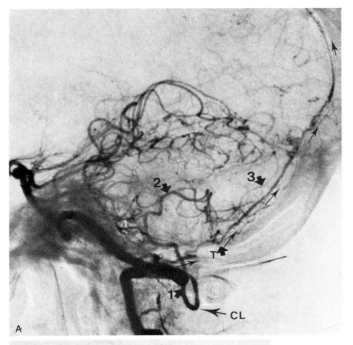

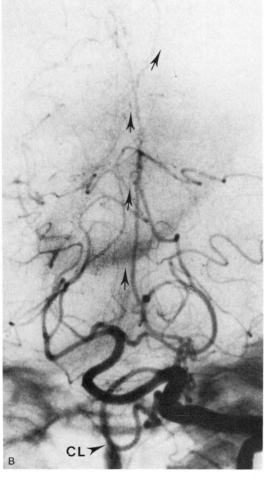

FIGURE 13–11. *Normal Posterior Meningeal Artery:* *A, 1* illustrates the origin of the PICA, *2* the choroidal point, *3* the tiny vermian branches of the PICA, and *T* the inferior loop of the tonsillar loop of the PICA. The small arrows follow the course of the posterior meningeal artery from just distal to its origin from the vertebral artery along the inner table of the calvarium to the supratentorial region. CL illustrates the caudal loop of the PICA. This is a normal anatomic variant. It is the tonsillar branch of the PICA ("*T*") that actually reflects tonsillar herniation if it is present.

B, The AP view of the vertebral angiogram again illustrates the caudal loop of the PICA (*CL*) and the course of the posterior meningeal artery (*arrows*).

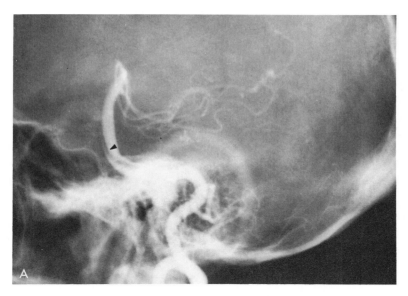

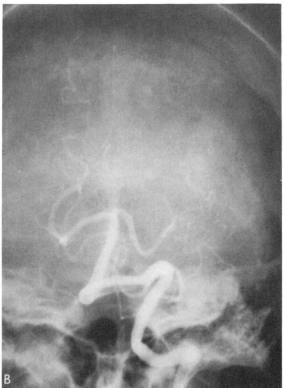

FIGURE 13–12. *Tortuous Basilar Artery:* The basilar artery is seen to be tortuous. A linear filling defect is seen on both the AP and the lateral views; this represents unopacified blood from the opposite vertebral artery (*arrowhead*). The AP view gives the false appearance that the basilar artery is narrowed because of the stream of unopacified blood. The tortuous artery may simulate a cerebellopontine angle mass, or the patient may complain of hemifacial spasms—apparently from irritation of the nerves in the cerebellopontine angle by the elongated basilar artery.

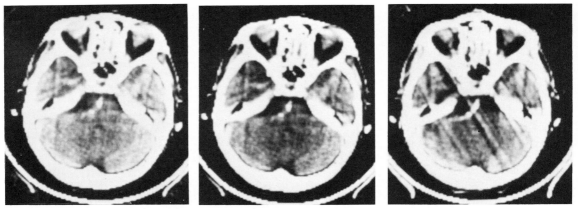

FIGURE 13–13. *CT Scan of Calcified Tortuous Basilar Artery:* The calcified basilar artery is visible on the base cut of the preinfusion scan as it extends obliquely across the pons from left to right in front of the fourth ventricle. Postinfusion, the artery is even better demonstrated.

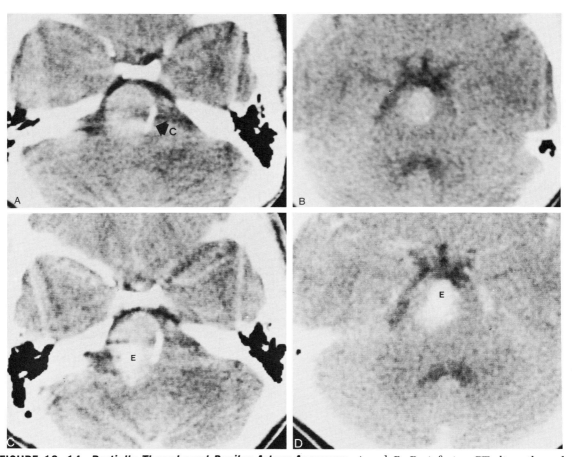

FIGURE 13–14. *Partially Thrombosed Basilar Artery Aneurysm:* A and B, Preinfusion CT slices through the posterior fossa reveal a high-density mass in the area of the pons. There is a peripheral rim of calcification along the left side of the mass (C), and faint areas of calcification are present along the periphery of the mass on B.

C and D, The postinfusion CT scan reveals central areas of enhancement (E). The fourth ventricle is visualized in B and D and is effaced along its anterior margin.

Illustration continued on the following page

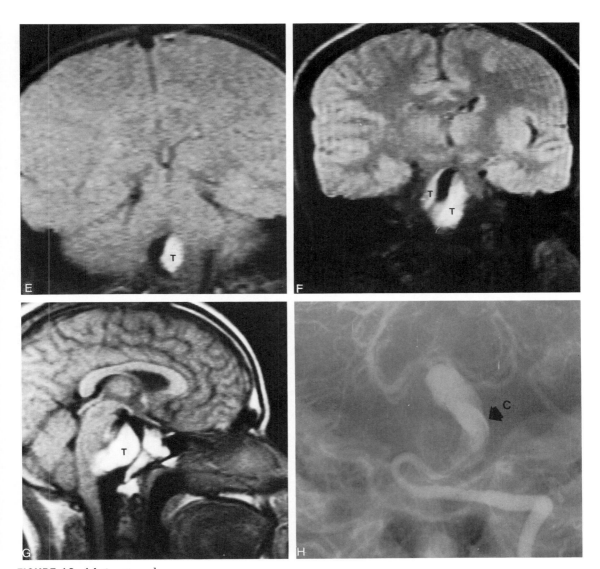

FIGURE 13–14 *Continued.*

E and *F*, Coronal SE TR530/TE30 images demonstrate the typical increased signal intensity of blood in the thrombosed portion of the basilar artery aneurysm (*T*). The curvilinear low signal intensity area along the right lateral margin of the aneurysm in *E* and between the thrombosed portions of the aneurysms in *F* represents a negative flow defect of blood in the unthrombosed portion of the aneurysm.

G, Midsagittal SE TR530/TE30 reveals the thrombosed portion of the aneurysm (*T*); the negative flow defect of the unthrombosed portion of the aneurysm projects posterior to the thrombosed portion and just anterior to the pons. There is widening of the prepontine cistern because of the extra-axial mass that displaces the brain stem structures posteriorly.

H, Vertebral angiogram demonstrates the ectatic, tortuous basilar artery with curvilinear calcification (*C*) along the left side. The aneurysm is, of course, much larger but is thrombosed and so is not visualized. This 20-year-old male presented with headache and multiple cranial nerve palsies. The CT appearance may mimic that of a brain stem mass.

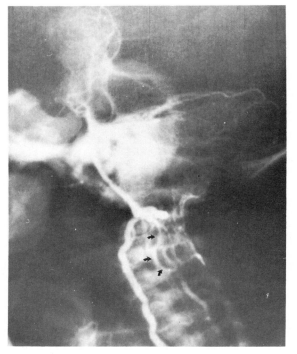

FIGURE 13–15. *Arteriogram of the Arnold-Chiari Malformation:* In the Arnold-Chiari malformation the fourth ventricle and the cerebellar tonsils are displaced inferiorly, and the vertebral arteriogram demonstrates that the PICA and the choroidal point and all the branches of the PICA are displaced far below the foramen magnum (*arrows*). This findings is typical of the Arnold-Chiari malformation.

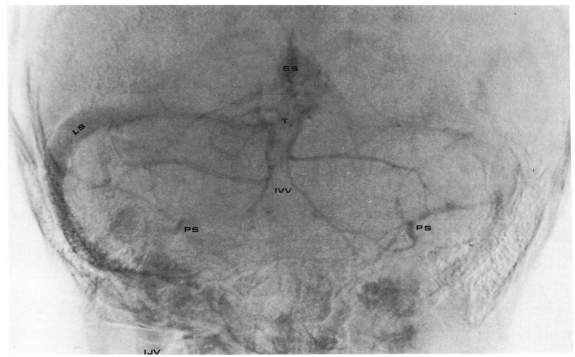

FIGURE 13–16. The AP view of the venous phase of a vertebral angiogram demonstrates the normal venous structures that one would expect to see using subtraction techniques.

LS	Lateral sinus.	*T*	Torcular.
PS	Petrosal star.	*SS*	Straight sinus.
IVV	Inferior vermian vein.	*IJV*	Internal jugular vein.

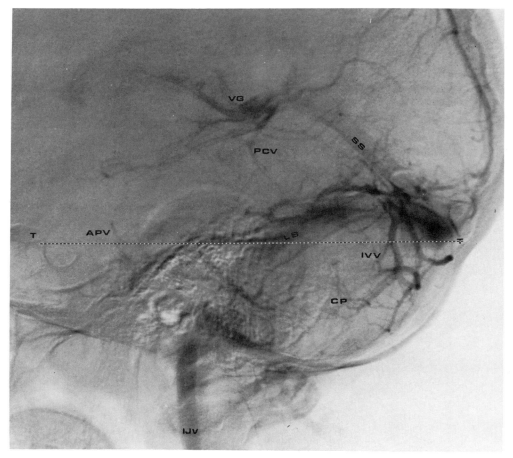

FIGURE 13–17. The lateral view of the venous phase of a vertebral angiogram demonstrates the normal vascular structures that one would expect to see using subtraction techniques.

VG	Vein of Galen.	IVV	Inferior vermian vein.
T-T	Torcular and tuberculum—Twining's line.	CP	Copular point.
PCV	Precentral cerebellar vein.	IJV	Internal jugular vein.
SS	Straight sinus.	APV	Anterior pontomesencephalic vein.

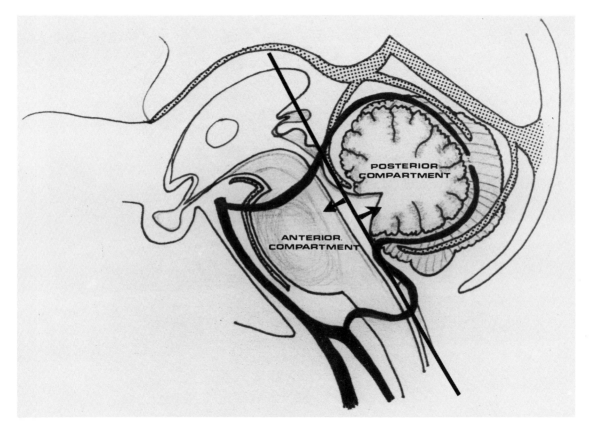

FIGURE 13–18. *Anterior and Posterior Compartments:* A line connecting the colliculocentral point of the precentral cerebellar vein with the choroidal point and running along the posterior medullary segment of the PICA divides the posterior fossa into the anterior and posterior compartments.

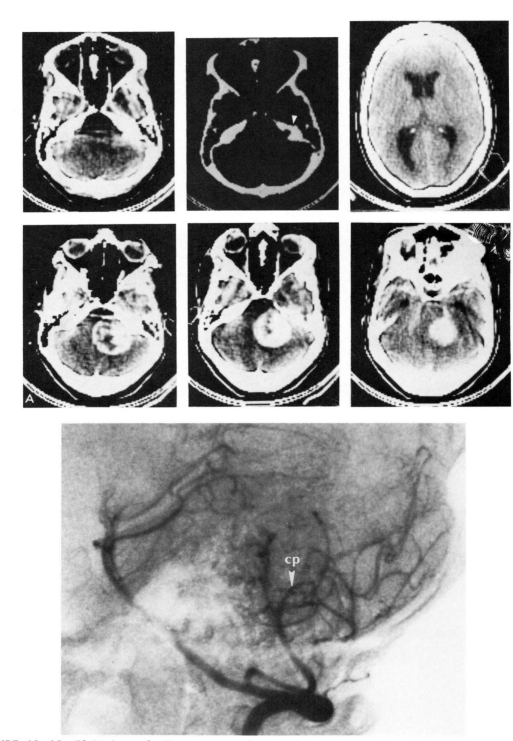

FIGURE 13–19. *Right Acoustic Neuroma:* *A,* The preinfusion scan reveals that the fourth ventricle is displaced to the left of the midline; the tumor is isodense with the normal brain. Viewed at high window width and window level, the right internal auditory canal can be seen to be greatly dilated compared to the left (*arrowhead*). There is moderate obstructive hydrocephalus. The postinfusion scan shows marked enhancement of the tumor, which is closely applied to the right internal auditory canal. There are filling defects in the tumor secondary to cystic change in the tumor or areas of necrosis.

B, The lateral view of the right vertebral arteriogram reveals that the choroidal point (*cp*) is displaced inferiorly and there is stretching of some of the branches of the PICA. The basilar artery is closely applied to the clivus.

Illustration continued on the following page

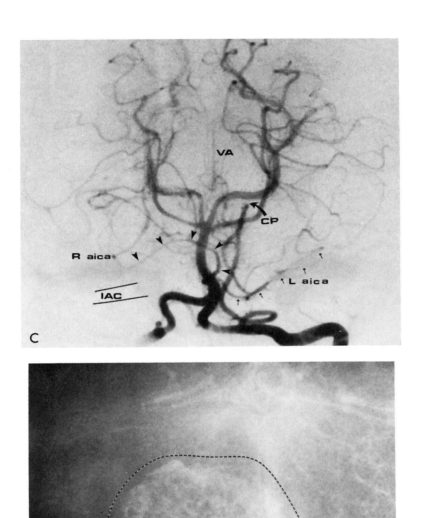

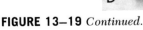

FIGURE 13–19 *Continued.*

C, The AP view of the right vertebral arteriogram reveals that the left choroidal point (*CP*) is displaced to the left of the midline. The anterior inferior cerebellar artery (*aica*) is displaced out of the right internal auditory canal (*IAC*) and courses in a curvilinear fashion around a large mass lesion in the right cerebellopontine angle (*arrows*). Left *aica* (*small arrows*) is normal. The vermian artery (*VA*) is in normal position.

D, The late arterial–early venous phase demonstrates a large area of neovascularity (*dotted line*) and some early draining views. The abnormal vessels arise from the vertebrobasilar system.

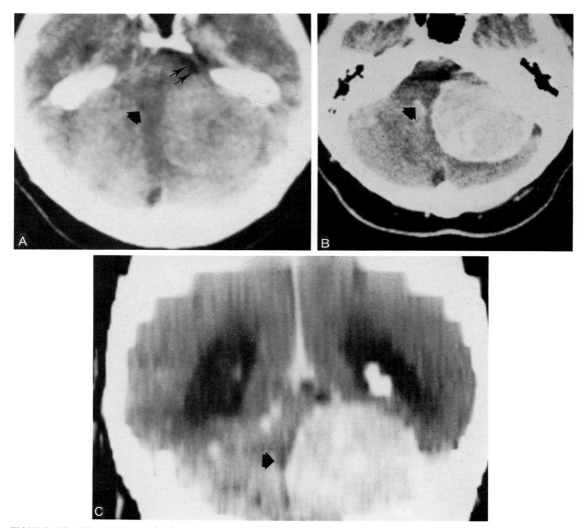

FIGURE 13–20. *CPA Meningioma:* *A,* The preinfusion CT scan demonstrates that there is a higher than normal brain density mass in the CPA that enhances densely and homogeneously *(B)* on the postinfusion portion of the examination. The fourth ventricle is displaced to the contralateral side *(arrow)* and CPA on the side of the mass is widened *(double arrows).*

C, Coronal reconstruction image better demonstrates the infratentorial position of the mass.

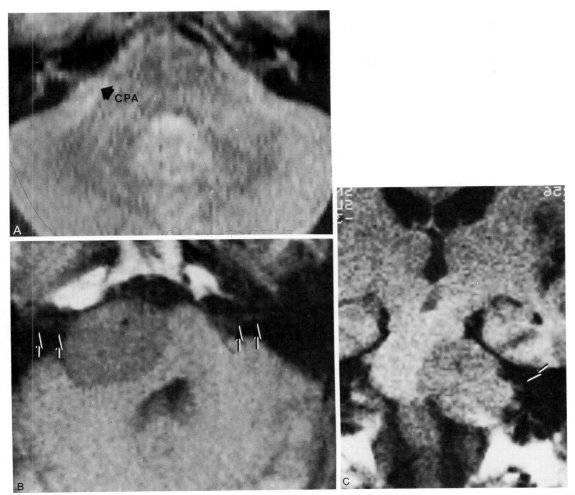

FIGURE 13–21. *Cerebellopontine Angle Meningioma:* A, MR image in another patient using SE TR3120/TE120 demonstrates that the CSF has a relatively high signal intensity. The cerebellopontine angle is filled with CSF, and the internal auditory canal courses lateral to the CPA. The cochlea projects anterior to the lateral portion of the IAC, and the semicircular canals project posterolateral to the lateral portion of the IAC.

B, Axial SE TR530/TE30 image demonstrates the lower than normal brain signal intensity mass in the right CPA. The mass obliterates the signal intensity of the CSF in the CPA and compresses the fourth ventricle and displaces it to the contralateral side. The IACs are faintly visualized (*double arrows*) and are not enlarged.

C, Coronal image SE TR530/TE30 again demonstrates the mass arising in the region of the IAC (*arrow*), pushing the brain stem and medulla to the contralateral side. The brain stem is also distorted in a curvilinear fashion around the mass, and the cerebral aqueduct, which is dilated because it is partially occluded, is also shifted to the contralateral side. The absence of widening of the IAC and the low signal intensity of the mass, which is secondary to the psammomatous calcification, suggests that this is a meningioma rather than an acoustic neuroma. Surgically proved meningioma.

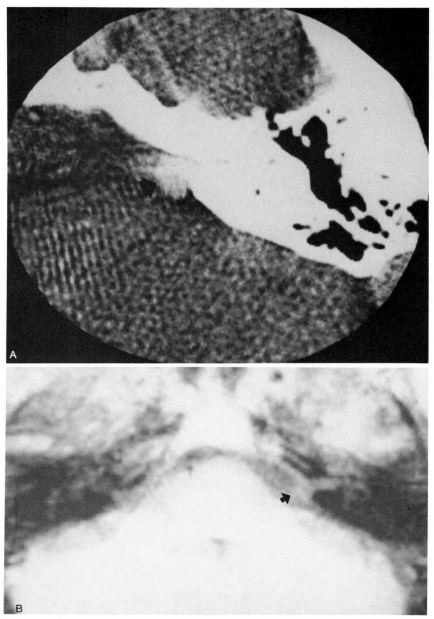

FIGURE 13–22. *Acoustic Neuroma:* *A*, Thin-section, high-resolution postinfusion CT scan through the level of the internal auditory canals reveals an enhancing mass that arises within the internal auditory canal and extends into the CPA (*arrow*).

B, The MR TR3120/TE60 scan reveals that the CSF is still of relatively low signal intensity, and the relatively higher signal intensity of the tumor can be identified projecting out of the internal auditory canal and into the CSF in the CPA (*arrow*). There is slight widening of the CPA because the tumor mass pushes the brain stem to the contralateral side. Surgically proved 1-cm acoustic neuroma.

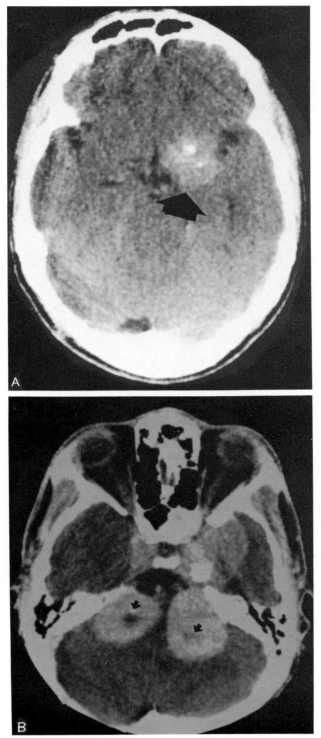

FIGURE 13–23. *Parasellar Meningioma and Bilateral Acoustic Neuromas:* The patient is a 24-year-old male with neurofibromatosis. *A,* The preinfusion CT scan demonstrates the amorphous calcification within the higher than brain density parasellar meningioma (*arrow*).

B, The postinfusion CT scan through the skull base demonstrates homogeneous enhancement of the parasellar meningioma and dense homogeneous enhancement of bilateral acoustic neuromas. The acoustic neuromas each have small cystic areas (*arrows*), a finding that is not common in acoustic tumors.

Illustration continued on the following page

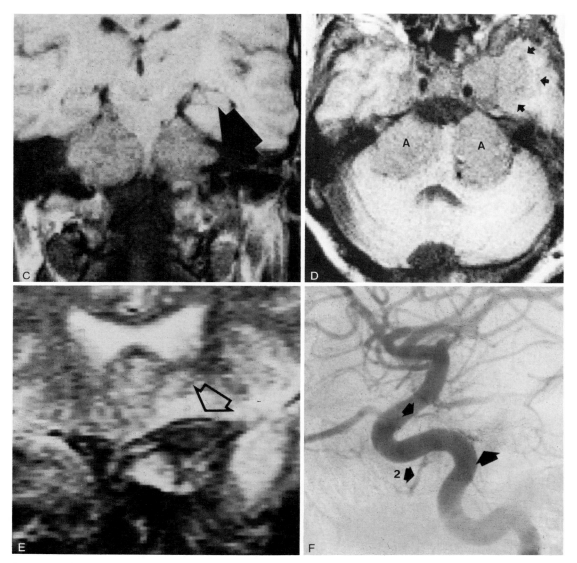

FIGURE 13–23 *Continued.*

C, Coronal T-1 image reveals bilateral CPA masses. The widened IAC is easily visible on one side (*arrow*), and the tumor can be seen extending into the CPA. The brain stem is compressed between the two tumors; interestingly, there is no hydrocephalus.

D, Axial T-1 image reveals the bilateral low signal intensity acoustic tumors (*A*). The parasellar meningioma is only very faintly seen (*arrows*).

E, T-2 weighted coronal image reveals the reactive bone formation with thickening of the lesser wing of the sphenoid bone (*arrow*).

F, Carotid angiography demonstrates an enlarged meningohypophyseal artery arising at the point where the internal carotid artery enters into the cavernous sinus (*large arrow*). The No. 2 arrow is on an enlarged meningeal artery arising in the cavernous portion of the carotid artery. The most superior arrow is on an additional enlarged meningeal vessel that supplies the meningioma.

Illustration continued on the following page

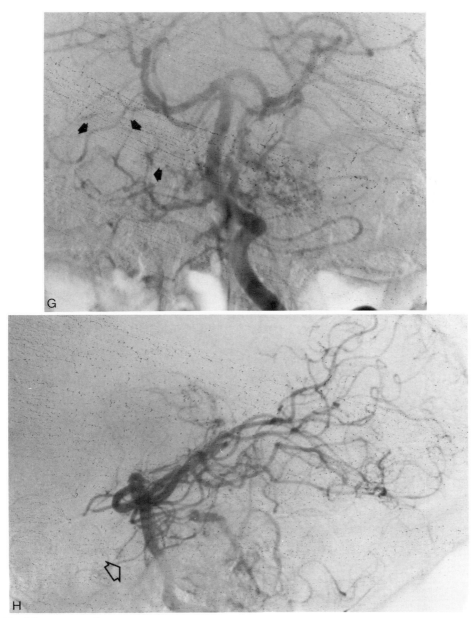

FIGURE 13–23 *Continued.*

G, AP view of the vertebral angiogram reveals the AICA displaced out of the right IAC and around the acoustic tumor in the CPA.

H, The lateral view of the vertebral angiogram reveals that the basilar artery is displaced posteriorly away from the clivus (*arrows*) by the anterior compartment extra-axial mass—the acoustic neuromas. Although there is an increase in all types of brain tumors in patients with neurofibromatosis, the finding of acoustic neuromas and meningiomas is very typical.

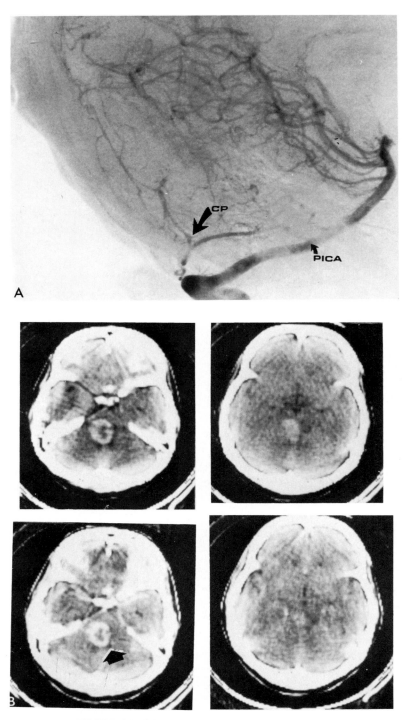

FIGURE 13–24. *See legend on the opposite page.*

Illustration continued on the following page

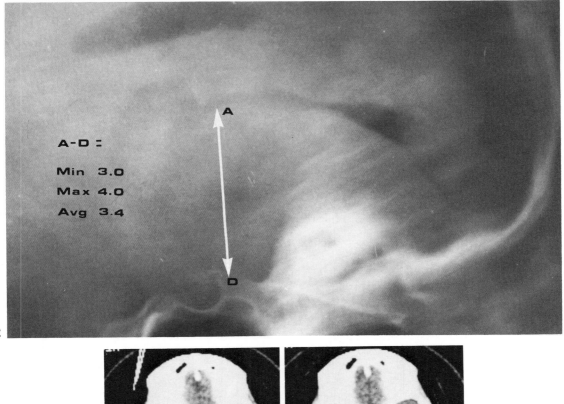

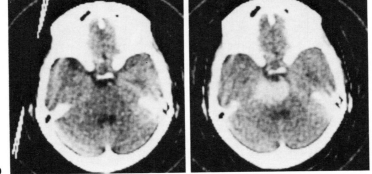

FIGURE 13–24. *Pontine Glioma:* *A,* The lateral view of the vertebral arteriogram reveals that the AICA supplies the PICA distribution as an anatomic variation. Its origin is demonstrated by the small arrowhead. The choroidal point (*large arrowhead*) is displaced inferiorly, as are the vermian branches of the PICA, which are closer to the inner table of the skull than one would normally anticipate. The basilar artery is closely applied to the clivus.

B, The CT scan demonstrates a high-density cystic lesion on the preinfusion scan. The rim of the tumor is of quite high density and perhaps contains a small amount of calcification. The fourth ventricle is flattened and displaced posteriorly. This is reflected in the arteriogram as the posterior displacement of the choroidal point and of the vermian branches of the PICA. Postinfusion, there is some enhancement of the rim of the tumor. There is no obstructive hydrocephalus.

C and *D,* In another patient, the pneumoencephalogram (*C*) demonstrates marked widening of the pons secondary to a pontine glioma. The width of the pons from the dorsum sella to the cerebral aqueduct (*A–D*) normally measures an average of 3.4 cm, with a maximum width of 4.0 cm and a minimum width of 3.0 cm.

The CT scan (*D*) also demonstrates widening of the pons, with flattening of the anterior margin of the fourth ventricle. The basilar artery is displaced to the right of the midline. The postinfusion scan demonstrates marked enhancement of the pontine glioma, which in this case is larger on the right side.

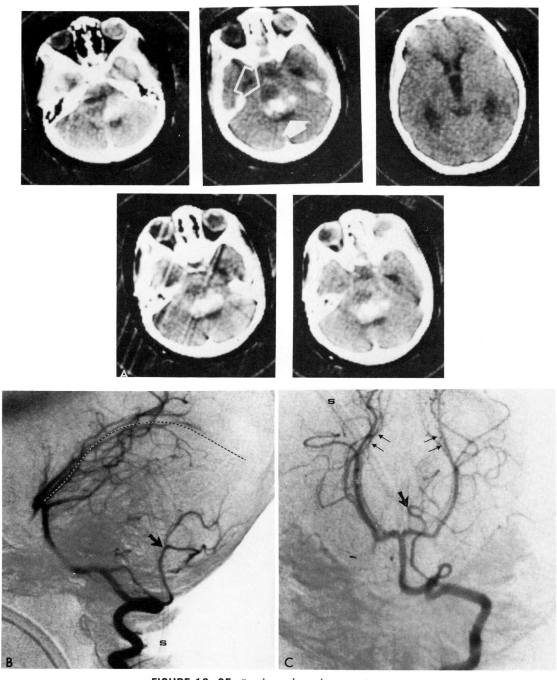

FIGURE 13–25. *See legend on the opposite page.*

Illustration continued on the following page

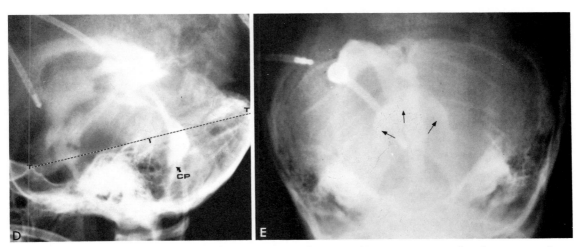

FIGURE 13–25. *Large Cystic and Calcified Pontine Glioma:* A, The CT scan reveals a large cystic (*open arrowhead*) and calcified tumor in the region of the pons which flattens the fourth ventricle and displaces it posteriorly (*white arrowhead*). There is moderate obstructive hydrocephalus. After the infusion of contrast material there is some enhancement of the tumor.

B, The lateral view of the vertebral arteriogram reveals posterior and inferior displacement of the choroidal point (*arrow*), posterior displacement of the vermian branches of the PICA, and stretching of the tonsillo-hemispheric branches of the PICA. There is superior bowing of the branches of the superior cerebellar arteries (*dotted line*). A shunt tube (S) is now in place.

C, The AP view reveals that the choroidal point (*large arrow*) is displaced slightly to the left of the midline. The branches of the superior cerebellar arteries and the posterior cerebral arteries (*small arrows*) are separated secondary to superior herniation of the posterior fossa contents. The tip of the shunt tube can be seen on the right side (S).

D, The contrast ventriculogram demonstrates marked posterior displacement of the fourth ventricle and compromise of the prepontine cistern by a very large, slightly lobulated mass in the region of the pons.

E, The fourth ventricle is flattened and distorted on the AP view by the mass lesion (*arrows*).

The calcification that was readily apparent on the CT scan could not be identified on the plain films or by other neuroradiologic studies. (Case courtesy of Dr. Justo Rodriguez.)

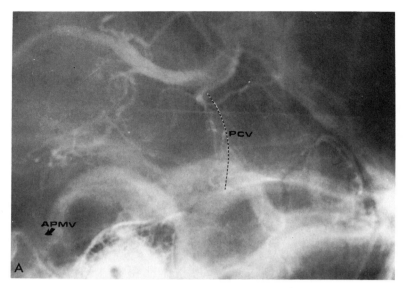

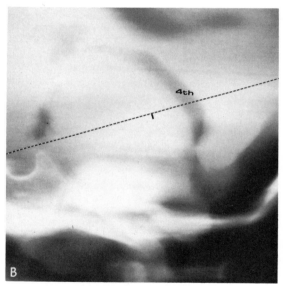

FIGURE 13–26. *Pontine Glioma with Posterior Displacement of the Precentral Cerebellar Vein:* *A,* The venous phase of the vertebral angiogram reveals reversal of the curve (*dashed line*) of the precentral cerebellar vein (*PCV*) and forward displacement of the anterior pontomesencephalic vein (*APMV*). These changes reflect the presence of a mass between the two anatomic structures.

B, The pneumoencephalogram reveals marked flattening and posterior displacement of the fourth ventricle and the cerebral aqueduct as well as compromise of the prepontine cistern. The entire pons and medulla are involved with the mass lesion.

C, The CT scan of a different patient demonstrates marked enlargement of the pons by a low-density tumor. The fourth ventricle is flattened and displaced posteriorly. The postinfusion scan reveals marked enhancement of the tumor in a homogeneous fashion. The tumor is slightly larger on the right side and displaces the basilar artery to the left of the midline (*arrow*). The appearance is typical of a pontine glioma.

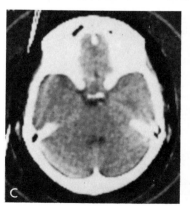

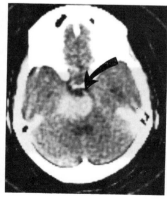

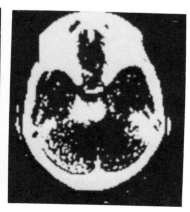

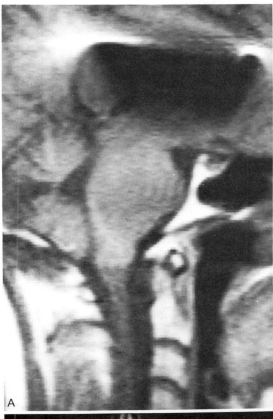

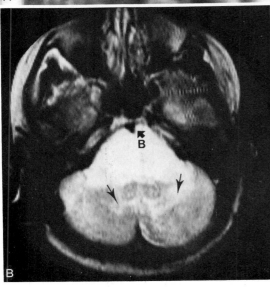

FIGURE 13–27. *Brain Stem Glioma:* Ten-year-old male with multiple cranial nerve palsies. *A,* The midsagittal TR530/TE30 SE reveals widening of the brain stem, posterior displacement of the fourth ventricle, and marked prominence of the anterior aspect of the pons with compromise of the prepontine cistern. The focal widening to the pons suggests an exophytic component of the tumor. The upper portion of the scan image is degraded by artifact from the shunt tube.

B, The axial TR3120/TE120 reveals that both the area of tumor involvement and the surrounding edema become of increased signal intensity. The basilar artery appears as a filling negative flow defect (*B*) anterior to the pons and the surrounding edema tracts posteriorly along the white matter pathway into the dentate nuclei (*arrow*). The tumor cannot be differentiated from the surrounding edema—one of the deficiencies of MR.

C, The higher slice is greatly degraded by artifact secondary to the shunt tube, making this image nondiagnostic.

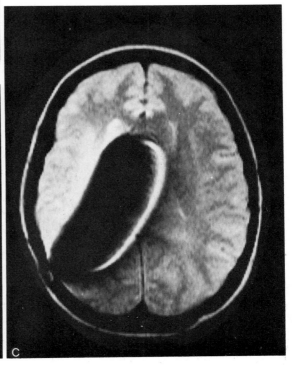

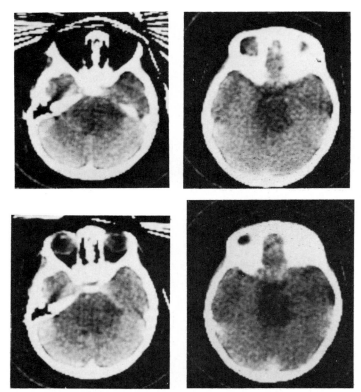

FIGURE 13–28. _Low-density Pontine Glioma That Did Not Demonstrate Contrast Enhancement:_ The preinfusion scan shows a large, low-density mass lesion in the pons that is probably surrounded by edema; it displaces the fourth ventricle posteriorly. There is no change following the infusion of contrast material. This is a large pontine glioma.

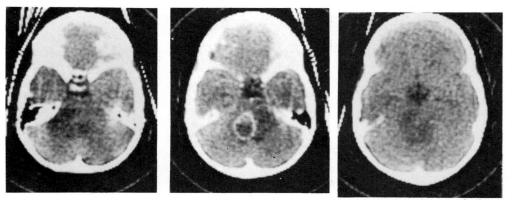

FIGURE 13–29. _Pontine Glioma with Ring Pattern of Enhancement:_ The preinfusion scan reveals a large, low-density lesion in the pons which displaces the fourth ventricle posteriorly. The area of low density is slightly irregular and appears to spare the anterior portion of the pons on the left side. The postinfusion scan reveals a ringlike oval area of enhancement to the left of the midline and extending to the midline just anterior to the fourth ventricle.

At surgery this was proved to be a pontine glioma.

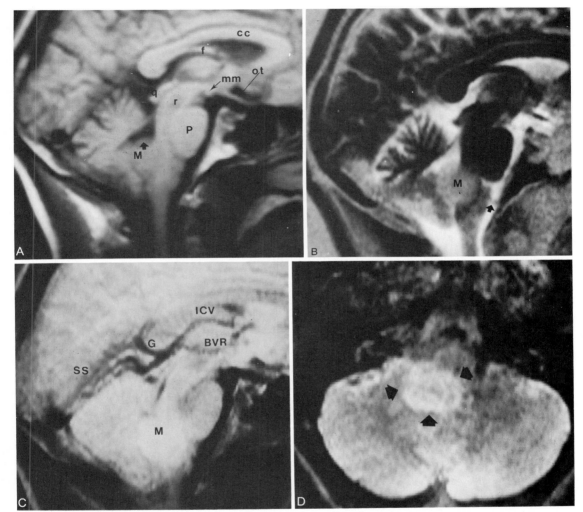

FIGURE 13–30. *Glioma of the Cerebellar Peduncle:* A, The midsagittal TR530/TE30 image reveals that there is a tumor mass arising from the dorsal aspect of the medulla that projects into the inferior portion of the fourth ventricle (arrow). The pons (*P*), the red nucleus (*r*), the quadrigeminal plate (*q*), the fornix (*f*), the corpus callosum (*cc*), the mammillary bodies (*mm*), and the optic tracts (*ot*) are all beautifully demonstrated.

B, The inversion recovery sequence reverses the colors of the various structures but reveals the tumor to better advantage (*M*). The vertebral artery or one of its branches is seen as a negative filling defect anterior to the medulla (*arrow*).

C, TR3120/TE120 reveals that the tumor is increased in signal intensity (*M*). The internal cerebral vein (*ICV*), the basal vein of Rosenthal (*BVR*), the vein of Galen (*G*), and the straight sinus (*S*) all appear as negative flow defects.

D, The axial TR3120/TE120 image demonstrates the tumor (*arrows*) in the cerebellar peduncle.

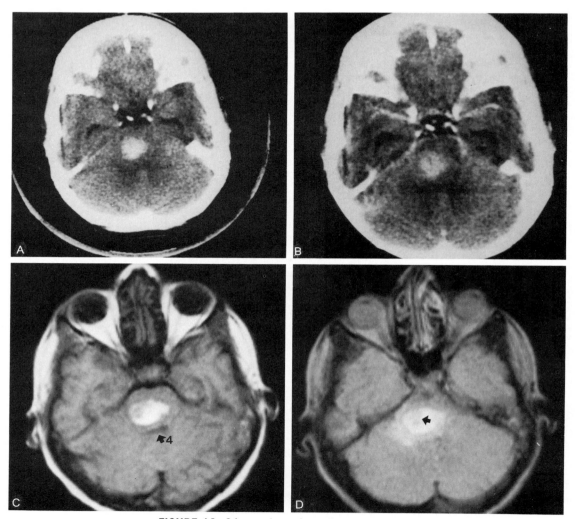

FIGURE 13–31. *See legend on the opposite page.*

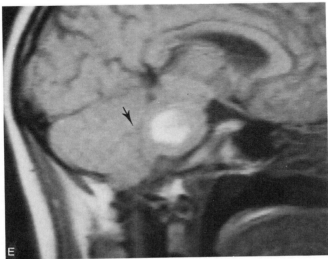

FIGURE 13–31. *Hemorrhagic Brain Stem Mass:* A 33-year-old female presented with sudden onset of quadriparesis. *A* and *B,* The pre- and postinfusion CT scans reveal a high-density mass in the pons which does not change on the postinfusion scan.

C, The SE TR530/TE30 axial image reveals that the mass is increased in signal intensity, has a slightly irregular margin, and compresses the anterior margin of the fourth ventricle (*4*). This increased density on the T-1 weighted image is typical of subacute hemorrhage.

D, The SE TR3120/TE60 reveals that the mass remains increased in signal intensity, but in addition there is an area of surrounding increased signal intensity which reflects surrounding edema. In addition, there is an area of low signal intensity in the lateral portion of the mass (*arrow*) which represents either a negative flow defect within a vascular malformation (none was identified on angiography) or an area of calcification, which, because of the partial volume effect, could not be appreciated on the CT scan.

E, Midsagittal SE TR530/TE30 localizes the intrapontine position of the mass and demonstrates the expansion of the pons. The fourth ventricle (*arrow*) is barely visible because it is compressed and because of the partial volume effect of the 1-cm thick slices. This lesion is thought to be a hemorrhage secondary to "occult arteriovenous malformation," which, because of the hemorrhage, has obliterated itself and therefore is not visible on angiography; or it may be a hemorrhage into a calcified brain stem tumor (not surgically proved).

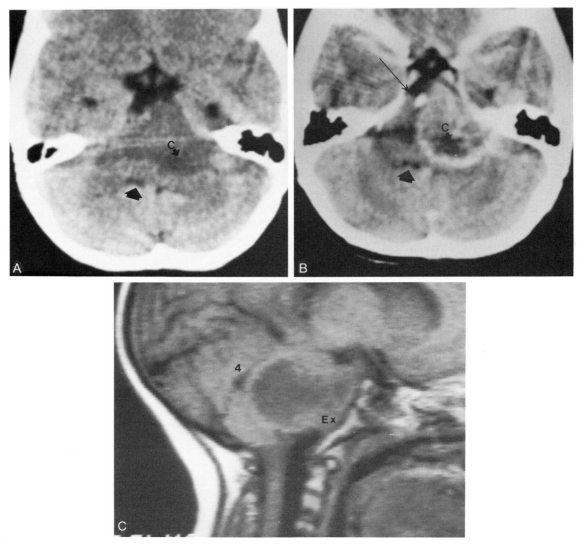

FIGURE 13–32. *Cystic and Exophytic Pontine Glioma:* The patient is a 10-year-old female with multiple cranial nerve palsies and ataxia. *A* and *B*, The pre- and postinfusion CT scans demonstrate that the fourth ventricle is displaced posteriorly and to the contralateral side *(arrow)*. There is peripheral enhancement and a low-density cystic or necrotic area posteriorly *(C)*. The basilar artery is also displaced to the contralateral side *(long arrow)* as well as posteriorly. The prepontine cistern is widened because the mass has grown in an "exophytic" or fungating fashion out of the brain stem anteriorly and into the prepontine cistern, resulting in posterior displacement of the pons and basilar artery, rather than the anterior displacement that one would usually anticipate with a pontine glioma.

C, The T-1 weighted midsagittal image demonstrates the nonhomogeneous nature of the tumor. The fourth ventricle *(4)* is compressed and displaced posteriorly. The medulla is displaced posteriorly, and the exophytic portion of the tumor distorts the appearance of the pons and can be seen occupying the prepontine cistern *(E)*.

Illustration continued on the following page

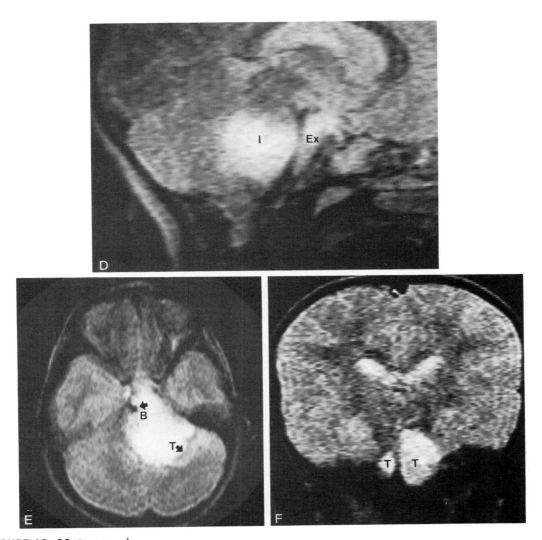

FIGURE 13–32 *Continued.*

On the T-2 weighted image (*D*) the basilar artery appears as a negative flow defect and separates the exophytic component of the tumor (*Ex*) from the intra-axial component (*I*).

E, The axial T-2 image appears similar to the CT scan. The tumor margin is demonstrated (*T*) as separate from the surrounding edema, and the basilar artery (*B*) is identified as a negative flow defect, with the exophytic component of the tumor projecting anterior to the basilar artery.

F, The coronal T-2 weighted image also reveals the tumor (*T*) wrapped around the negative flow defect of the basilar artery. There is moderate obstructive hydrocephalus.

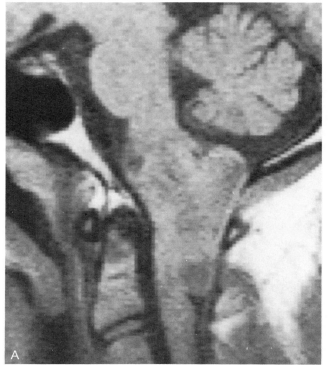

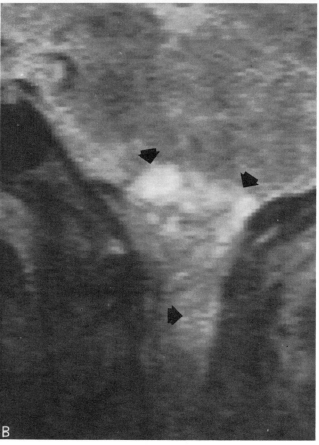

FIGURE 13–33. *Multicystic Posterior Fossa and Spinal Cord Astrocytoma:* Twenty-one–year–old male with progressive difficulty walking. *A*, Midsagittal, SE TR530/TE30 image reveals the anatomic location and multicystic nature of the mass. It involves the nodulus of the vermis as well as the vermis of the cerebellum and extends through the foramen magnum to involve the cervical spinal cord. The mass is predominantly dorsal to the cord and compresses the cord and medulla anteriorly.

B, The SE TR3120/TE120 reveals that the cystic portions of the mass become increased in signal intensity (*arrows*). In addition, the surrounding CSF also increases in signal intensity. This results in the inability to distinguish with certainty the mass, the cystic portions, and the surrounding CSF. This shows the advantage of the T-1 weighted images and the complementary nature of the imaging sequences.

The CT scan (not shown) reveals small areas of calcification that are not visualized on the MR scan, within the otherwise poorly demonstrated mass. Surgically proved multicystic glioma.

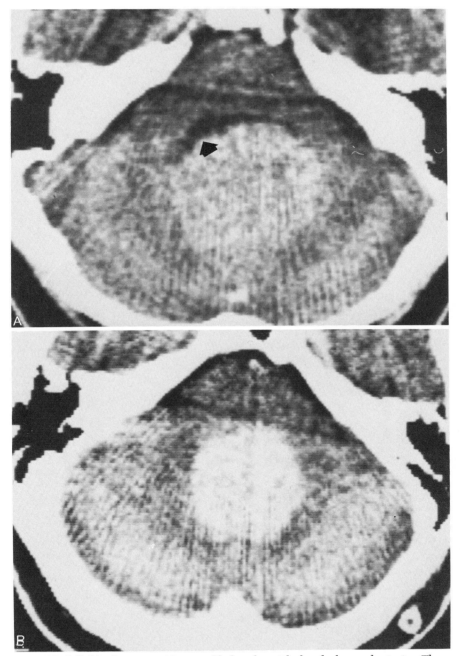

FIGURE 13–34. *Medulloblastoma:* A 32-year-old female with headache and ataxia. The pre- (A) and postinfusion (B) CT scans demonstrate a higher than normal brain density in the midline in the posterior fossa. The mass enhances homogeneously and displaces the fourth ventricle anteriorly (*arrowhead*).

Illustration continued on the following page

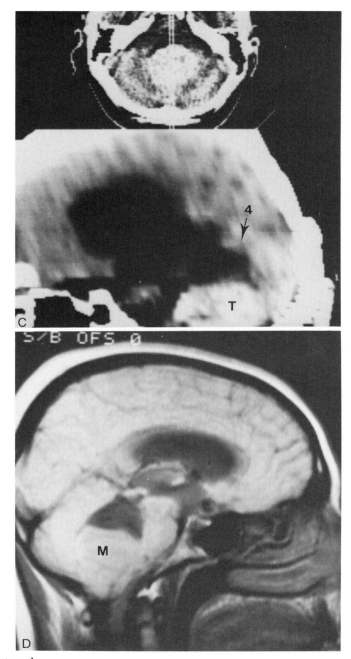

FIGURE 13–34 *Continued.*

C, The reconstruction image of the postinfusion CT scan demonstrates the tumor (*T*) in the midline with the fourth ventricle ballooning anterior to it.

D, The midsagittal T-1 SE TR530/TE30 image demonstrates the mass (*M*), which is slightly lower than the normal brain in signal intensity, and the fourth ventricle, which is ballooned and pushed anteriorly. The pons and medulla are compressed anteriorly and closely applied to the clivus. The third and lateral ventricles are also dilated secondary to the obstructive hydrocephalus.

Illustration continued on the following page

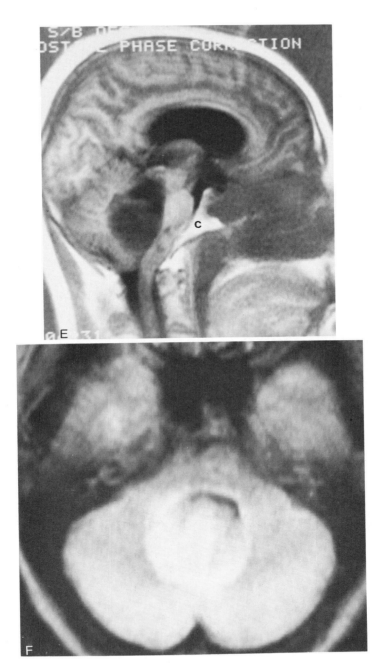

FIGURE 13–34 *Continued.*

E, The positive phase correction inversion recovery image provides excellent differentiation between the tumor and the remaining brain. The fourth ventricle is of slightly lower signal intensity. The compressed pons and medulla can be seen closely applied to the clivus.

F, The axial SE TR3120/TE60 image simulates the CT image. The appearance is very typical of the medulloblastoma that arises from the posterior medullary velum of the fourth ventricle. It would be anticipated that an ependymoma would arise within the fourth ventricle rather than displacing the fourth ventricle anteriorly. The age and sex of this patient are both atypical for medulloblastoma.

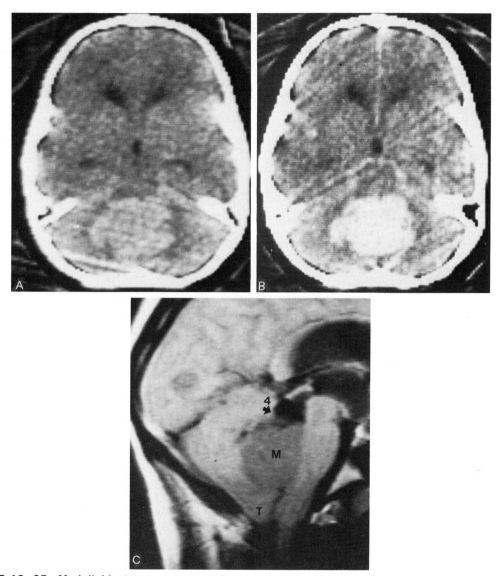

FIGURE 13–35. *Medulloblastoma:* Ten-year-old male with ataxia, nausea, and vomiting. The pre- (*A*) and postinfusion (*B*) CT scans demonstrate a slightly higher than normal brain density mass in the midline of the posterior fossa which enhances homogeneously. There is minimal surrounding edema. The slightly irregular tumor margin is atypical for medulloblastoma.

The SE TR530/TE30 image (*C*) in the midsagittal plane readily demonstrates the exact anatomic location of the tumor (*M*). The fourth ventricle is displaced superiorly (*4*), and there is cerebellar tonsillar herniation (*T*).

Illustration continued on the following page

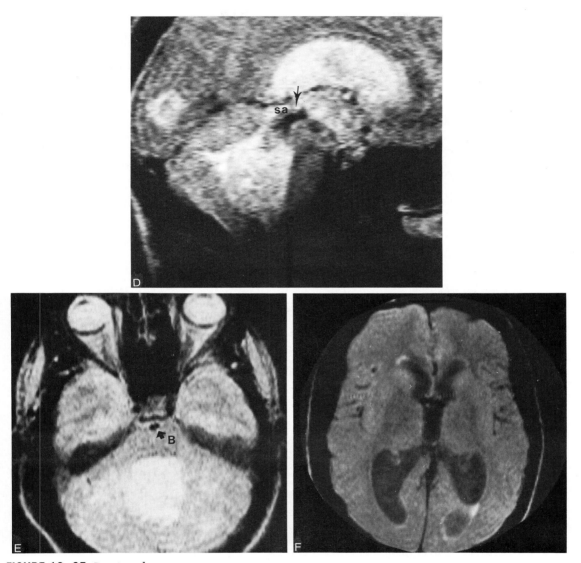

FIGURE 13–35 *Continued.*

On the TR3120/TE120 image (*D*) the tumor and surrounding edema demonstrate increased signal intensity. The sylvian aqueduct (*sa*) appears as a negative defect; this is thought to be secondary to rapid flow of the CSF through the aqueduct. Here the aqueduct is dilated.

E, The axial SE TR3120/TE120 image demonstrates the typical increased signal intensity of the tumor. The basilar artery is closely applied to the clivus and appears as a negative flow defect (*B*).

F, The SE TR3120/TE60 image demonstrates typical periventricular increased signal intensity secondary to transependymal resorption of CSF associated with obstructive hydrocephalus.

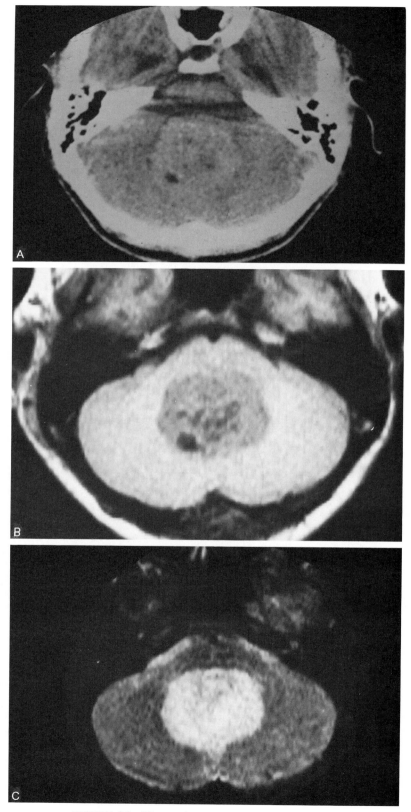

FIGURE 13–36. *See legend on the following page.*

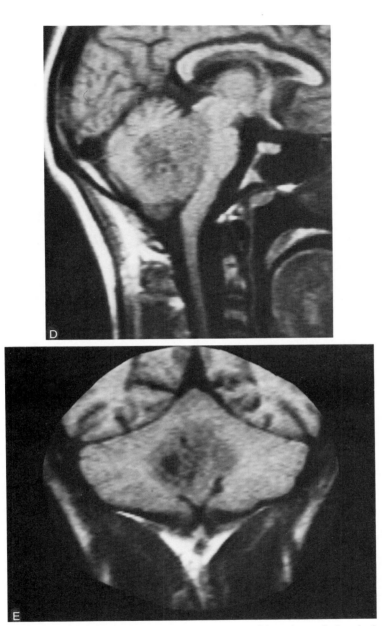

FIGURE 13–36. *Atypical Medulloblastoma:* Twenty-two–year–old male with headache and ataxia. The preinfusion CT scan (*A*) and the SE TR530/TE30 image (*B*) are remarkably similar in appearance. The tumor has a mottled appearance that is unusual and is secondary to multiple small cystic areas. The low-density areas did not enhance on the postinfusion CT scan, and the remainder of the tumor enhanced only minimally.

C, The SE TR3120/TE120 axial image demonstrates that the tumor has increased signal intensity.

D, The SE TR530/TE30 midsagittal image shows the exact location of the tumor and its relationship to the surrounding structures. The fourth ventricle is not visible, the pons and medulla are compressed, and the vermis of the cerebellum is largely replaced by the tumor mass.

E, The coronal SE TR530/TE30 image provides another perspective on the appearance of the tumor and its relationship to surrounding structures. The dura of the tentorium cerebelli is of low signal intensity.

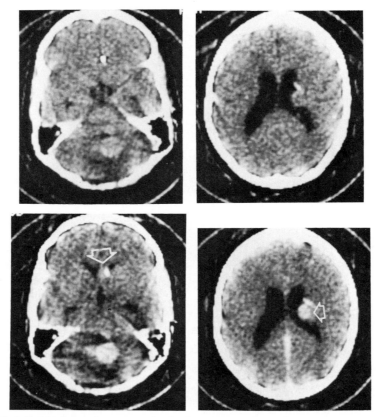

FIGURE 13–37. *Medulloblastoma Recurrent in the Posterior Fossa with Supratentorial Metastases:* The preinfusion scan reveals a craniectomy defect in the midline in the posterior fossa. Some radiolucency is visible beneath the craniectomy site. In addition, there is a well-defined mass lesion behind the fourth ventricle which flattens the fourth ventricle along its right posterior margin. The tip of the shunt tube is visible in the midline at the level of the interhemispheric fissure. There is moderate obstructive hydrocephalus and evidence of a mass lesion that indents the body of the left lateral ventricle.

The postinfusion scan reveals enhancement of the recurrent or remaining tumor in the posterior fossa behind the fourth ventricle. A second deposit of metastatic tumor in the frontal region compresses the left frontal horn. A third metastatic nodule is better seen on the postinfusion scan as it compresses the body of the left lateral ventricle.

This is an example of medulloblastoma that has metastasized to the supratentorial region. This tumor may also spread to involve the spinal cord.

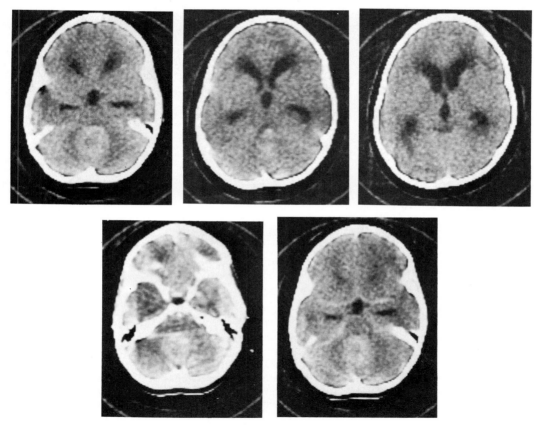

FIGURE 13–38. *Medulloblastoma:* The preinfusion scan reveals a mass lesion of higher density than the normal brain tissue that is surrounded by edema. The fourth ventricle can be seen to be displaced anteriorly and slightly to the left of the midline. There is moderate obstructive hydrocephalus. The postinfusion scan shows marked homogeneous enhancement of the tumor in the midline. This appearance is typical of a medulloblastoma.

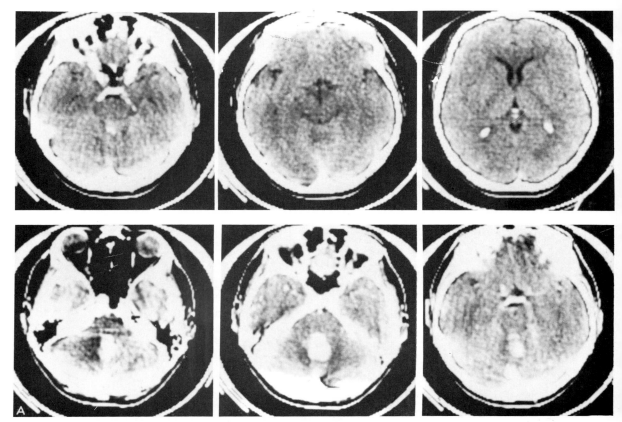

FIGURE 13–39. *Medulloblastoma Invading the Fourth Ventricle:* *A,* The preinfusion scan reveals two small punctate areas of calcification in the midline of the posterior fossa in the anticipated position of the fourth ventricle. The fourth ventricle is never well seen. Otherwise, the scan appears unremarkable, and there is no evidence of obstructive hydrocephalus. After the infusion of contrast material, there is marked homogeneous enhancement of a tumor in the midline in the posterior fossa. It appears to occupy the anticipated position of the fourth ventricle. The appearance is consistent with a medulloblastoma that has invaded the fourth ventricle. However, the appearance is certainly not typical, and the presence of the calcification argues against the diagnosis of a medulloblastoma. Ependymoma of the fourth ventricle appears more likely, and a metastatic lesion to the posterior fossa should also be considered.

B, The lateral view of the right vertebral arteriogram reveals that the choroidal points are displaced anteriorly bilaterally (*CP*). There is stretching of the tonsillohemispheric branches of the PICA anteriorly and marked posterior displacement of the vermian branches of the PICA. No abnormal vessels are seen.

C, The AP view of the arteriogram reveals that the vermian branches of the PICA are splayed apart by the growth of the tumor between the two vessels. The choroidal points (*CP*) also are splayed apart by the tumor in the fourth ventricle. At surgery this proved to be an intraventricular medulloblastoma.

D, The postoperative scan reveals an area of hemorrhage in the midline in the posterior fossa. In addition, there is a large amount of air within the cranial vault and in the suprasellar cisterns.

Illustration continued on the following page

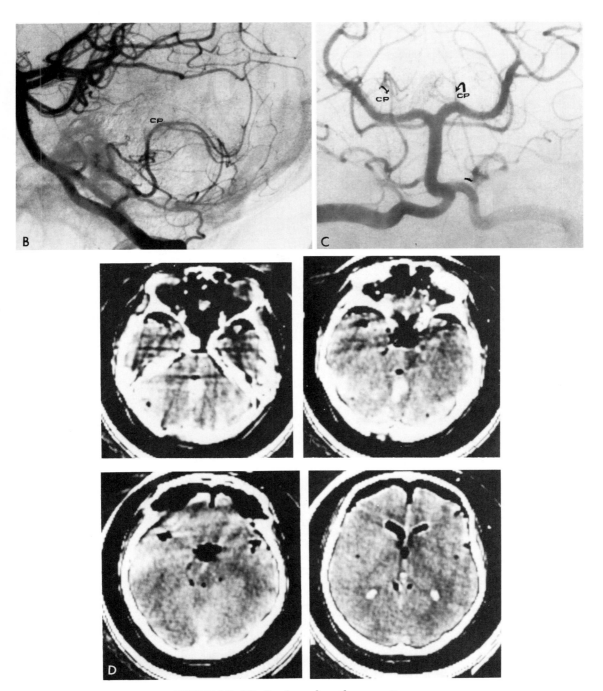

FIGURE 13–39. *See legend on the opposite page.*

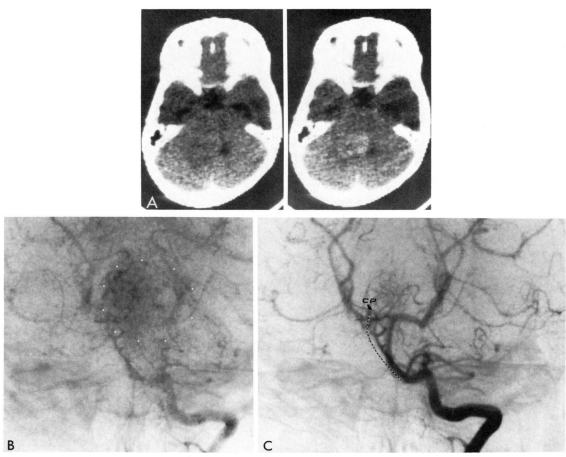

FIGURE 13–40. *Ependymoma:* *A,* The preinfusion scan (viewed from above) reveals an isodense mass in the midline in the posterior fossa. The fourth ventricle is displaced to the right of the midline around the mass. There is mild to moderate obstructive hydrocephalus. Following the infusion of contrast material, there is moderate enhancement. No calcifications could be detected. The mass is larger on the left than on the right.

B, There are myriad small tumor vessels arising from the PICA, and the later arterial phase reveals the tumor stain in the midline and extending to the left of the midline (*white dots*).

The AP view of the left vertebral arteriogram in *C* reveals that the choroidal point (*CP*) is displaced to the right of the midline, and there is curvilinear displacement of the branches of the PICA across the midline to the right side (*dashed line*).

Illustration continued on the following page

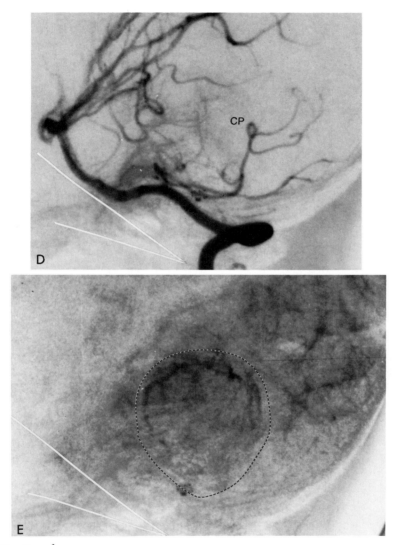

FIGURE 13–40 *Continued.*

D, The lateral view of the vertebral arteriogram reveals marked posterior displacement of the choroidal point *(CP)* and posterior displacement of the vermian branches of the PICA. The white lines outline the clivus.

E, The venous phase reveals a capsular stain of the tumor mass as it is surrounded by draining veins. This lesion was proved at surgery to be an ependymoma.

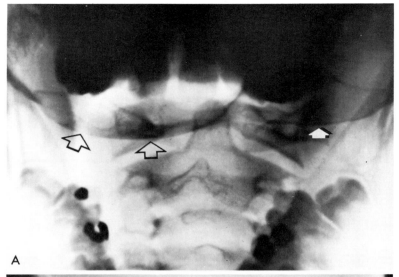

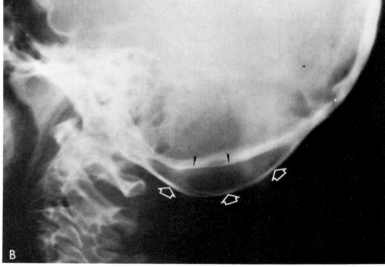

FIGURE 13–41. *Cystic Cerebellar Astrocytoma:* A, The open-mouth view of the odontoid process reveals the expansion of the bony margin of the posterior cranial fossa (*open black arrowheads*) on the side of the long-standing cystic astrocytoma. The normal left side is demonstrated by the closed white arrowhead.

B, The lateral view of the posterior fossa also demonstrates the expansion of the right side of the posterior cranial fossa (*open white arrowheads*) as compared to the left (*black arrows*). Care must be taken to be sure that this appearance is not due to an "off-lateral" technique of filming rather than to an actual bony expansion.

C, The lateral view of the arteriogram reveals that the basilar artery is closely applied to the clivus. There is upward displacement of the branches of the superior cerebellar arteries (*dashed line*), which project above the plane of the posterior cerebral arteries (*PC*); there is also posterior displacement of the choroidal point (*cp*) and vermian (*va*) branches of the PICA with marked stretching of the hemispheric branches of the PICA.

D, The lateral venous phase reveals upward bowing of the straight sinus (*ss*) because of the long-standing nature of the problem. The precentral cerebellar vein is displaced anteriorly, indicating involvement of the vermis of the cerebellum (*small arrowheads*). The anterior pontomesencephalic vein is closely applied to the clivus (*double-headed arrow*), the superior vermian veins (*svv*) are displaced close to the straight sinus (*ss*), and there is posterior displacement of the inferior vermian veins. A shunt tubing device is noted in place.

E, The AP view of the vertebral arteriogram demonstrates no filling of the right PICA (anatomic variant); the left PICA and choroidal point (*cp*) are filled and shown to be displaced markedly to the left of the midline, as are all the branches of the PICA (*double-headed arrows*). In addition there is medial and superior elevation of the posterior cerebral arteries (*long arrows*) and the superior cerebellar arteries (*arrowheads*). It is unusual for a posterior fossa tumor to affect the supratentorial posterior cerebral arteries; this reflects the long-standing relatively benign nature of the process.

F, The CT scan is one of the very earliest scans performed. It readily demonstrates the cystic lesion in the right cerebellar hemisphere. There is some artifact from the metallic shunt tubing device. No postinfusion scan is available.

G, The postmortem pathologic correlation reveals a well-defined, large cystic tumor in the right cerebellar hemisphere with a nodule of tumor that extends into the vermis of the cerebellum (*arrows*). This correlated with the forward displacement of the precentral cerebellar vein.

This is a classic example of a long-standing, rather benign cystic cerebellar astrocytoma.

Illustration continued on the following page

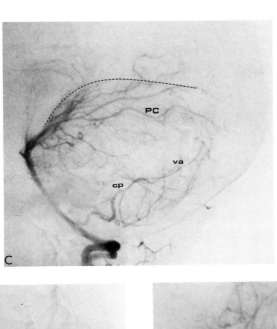

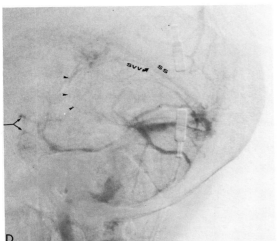

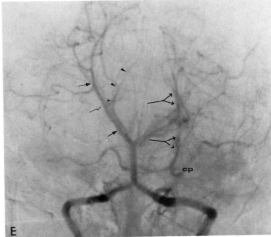

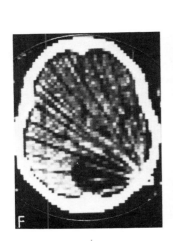

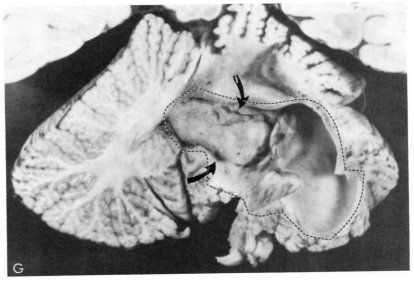

FIGURE 13–41. *See legend on the opposite page.*

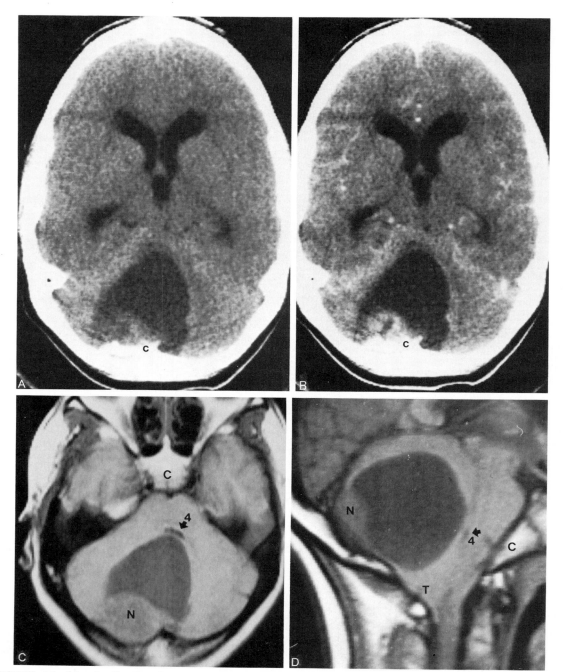

FIGURE 13–42. *Cystic Cerebellar Astrocytoma:* The patient is a 10-year-old male with a history of headaches, without other abnormal physical findings. *A,* The preinfusion CT scan demonstrates a cystic low-density mass in the right cerebellar hemisphere. The area of calcification (*C*) is atypical.

B, The postinfusion scan demonstrates the enhancing mural nodule in the wall of the tumor (*arrow*) which enhances densely on the postinfusion portion of the examination. The wall of the cyst does not enhance, and histologic examination of the wall does not reveal tumor cells.

C, The SE TR3120/TE60 axial sequence demonstrates that the nodule of tumor (*N*) has a different signal intensity than the remainder of the cystic portion of the tumor (cyst). In addition, the fluid within the cyst demonstrates a different signal intensity than the CSF within the lateral ventricle, reflecting the increased protein content of the cyst.

D, MR scan in the midsagittal section reveals the cystic tumor and the compression of the brain stem and medulla against the clivus. The fourth ventricle is compressed (*arrowhead*) and the cerebellar tonsils (*T*) have been pushed below the foramen magnum—this is "tonsillar herniation" secondary to a mass.

Illustration continued on the following page

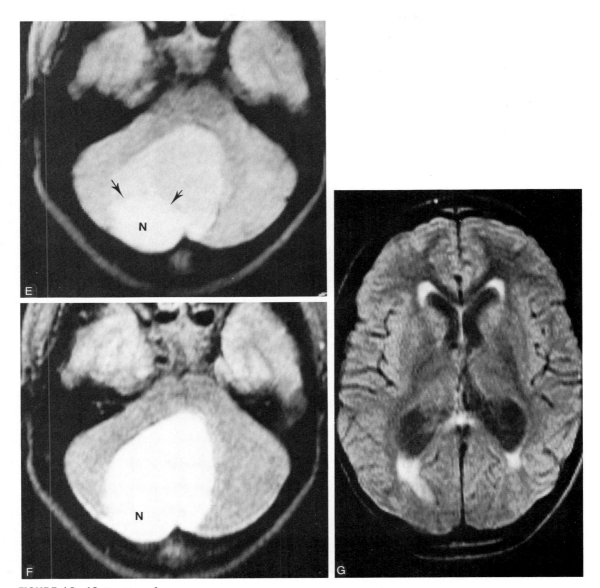

FIGURE 13–42 *Continued.*

E, The SE TR3120/TE60 image reveals the nodule (*N, arrows*) with a different signal intensity than the cystic portion of the tumor. The calcification is not seen.

F, The SE TR3120/TE120 now reveals that the nodule and fluid within the cyst all appear similar in signal intensity. If one were to perform only the longer SE sequence, the cystic and nodular appearance of the tumor would not be appreciated.

G, SE TR3120/TE60 image reveals periventricular increased signal intensity secondary to obstructive hydrocephalus.

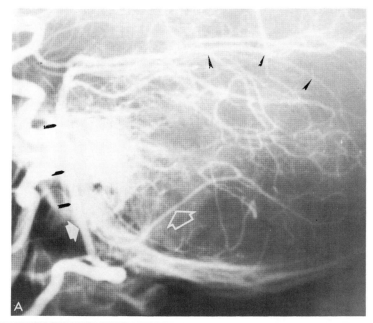

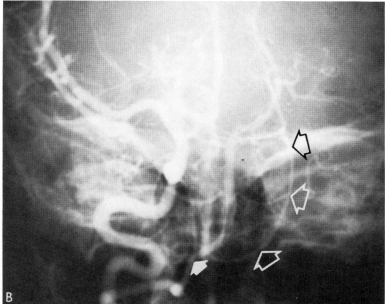

FIGURE 13–43. *Cerebellar Astrocytoma, Right Side:* *A,* The lateral view of the vertebral arteriogram reveals that the basilar artery is closely applied to the clivus (*thick dark arrowheads*). There is superior displacement of the superior cerebellar arteries (*smaller black arrowheads*). Marked stretching of the PICA and its branches (*open white arrowhead*) is evident. The origin of the PICA is illustrated by the closed white arrowhead in *A* and *B.*

B, The origin is also well seen on the AP view (*white arrowhead*). In addition, on the AP view one can see that the PICA and its branches are displaced far to the left of the midline (*open arrowheads*).

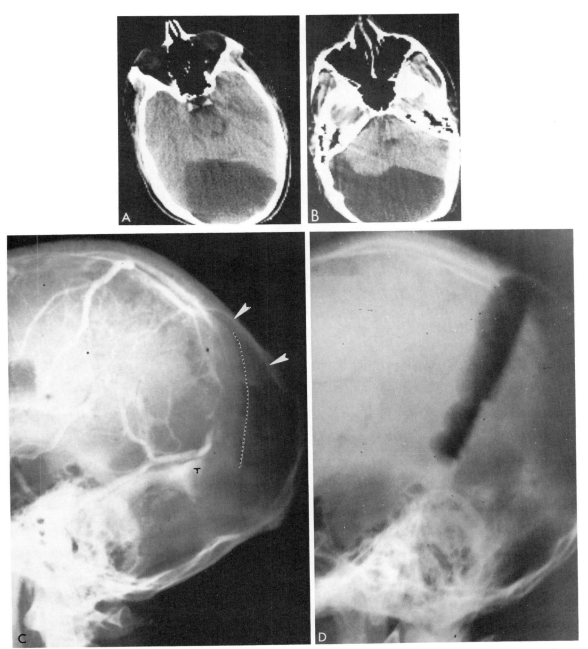

FIGURE 13–44. *Posterior Fossa Arachnoid Cyst: A* and *B*, The CT scans reveal a normal appearing fourth ventricle. There is a large CSF-containing structure in the posterior fossa that is positioned behind the lobes of the cerebellum. It thins the inner table of the occipital bone and extends up onto the supratentorial region. The lateral ventricles are within normal limits in size. The plain skull examination (not shown) demonstrated a dolichocephalic appearance of the skull and bathrocephaly.

C, The arteriogram revealed that the torcular (*T*) is displaced far forward from its anticipated position. The straight sinus is also displaced forward, and there is a large vacant area posterior to the torcular.

D, The pneumoencephalogram reveals that this arachnoid cyst fills with air, which is freely movable in the cystic cavity. The fourth ventricle could be visualized and appeared to be of normal size and in a relatively normal position.

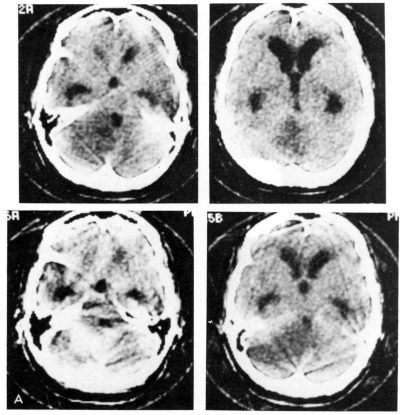

FIGURE 13–45. *Hemangioblastoma:* A, The preinfusion scan reveals a large, poorly defined area of low density in the left cerebellum. The fourth ventricle is displaced forward and to the right of the midline. In addition, there is dilatation of the aqueduct, which also is displaced to the right of the midline. After the infusion of contrast material there is marked homogeneous enhancement of a large tumor mass in the left cerebellum. There is moderate obstructive hydrocephalus.

Illustration continued on the following page

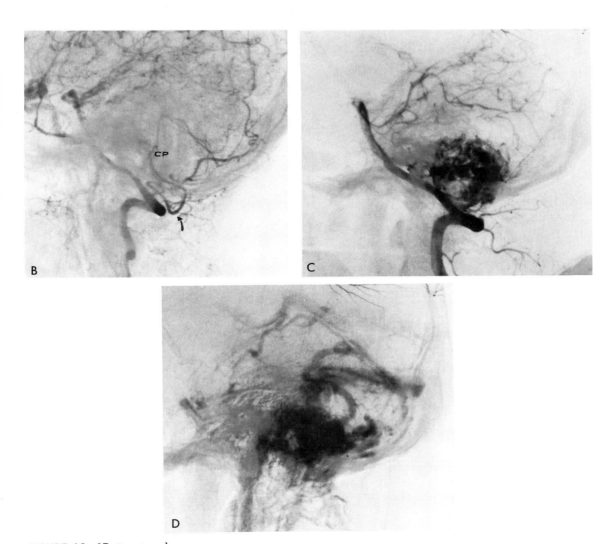

FIGURE 13–45 *Continued.*

B, The early arterial view in the lateral projection of the vertebral arteriogram reveals downward displacement of the PICA and the choroidal point (*CP*), with stretching of the vermian branches of the PICA around a large mass lesion on the posterior fossa.

C, The later arterial view reveals a large, very vascular mass in the cerebellar hemisphere that demonstrates multiple arteries and early draining veins.

D, The later venous phase reveals a prolonged tumor stain, which typically persists well into the venous phase; it again demonstrates the multiple draining veins. In this case, the veins drain predominantly superiorly up to the straight sinus and then to the lateral sinus and internal jugular. This appearance is very typical of a hemangioblastoma of the cerebellum.

This tumor may be part of a syndrome of the von Hippel–Lindau disease, where the hemangioblastoma of the cerebellum is seen in association with hemangiomas of the retina and renal tumors as well as an elevated hematocrit.

These tumors may be cystic as well as solid. If the tumor is cystic, it may be quite sizeable without creating much mass effect.

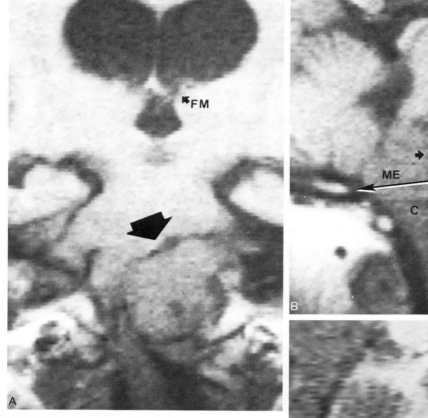

FIGURE 13–46. *Clivus Meningioma: A,* The coronal TR530/TE30 image reveals the low signal intensity mass that arises to the left of the midline and displaces the pons posteriorly and to the contralateral side. The slightly lobulated mass is outlined by the low signal intensity of the CSF (*arrow*). The frontal horns of the lateral ventricle and the third ventricle are dilated secondary to obstructive hydrocephalus. The foramen of Monro (*FM*) is seen bilaterally.

B, The TR530/TE30 image in midsagittal projection demonstrates the low signal intensity mass (*arrows*) inferior to the superiorly displaced pons (*P*), which displaces the medulla (*ME*) and spinal cord (*C*) posteriorly. The pons is displaced superiorly. The meningioma rests on the inferior portion of the clivus and extends through the foramen magnum, which is marked by a line extending from the posterior margin to the anterior margin of the foramen magnum (Chamberlain's line). Note the small irregular collection of the fat (*F*) that is also a reliable indicator of the anterior margin of the foramen magnum when the clivus is not well demonstrated.

C, The TR3120/TE120 sagittal image demonstrates that the meningioma (*arrows*) remains low in signal intensity. This is typical of meningiomas in general and is caused by the fact that these tumors contain psammomatous calcification and therefore respond similar to bone.

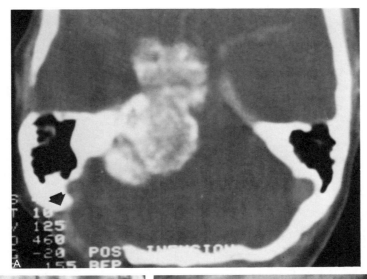

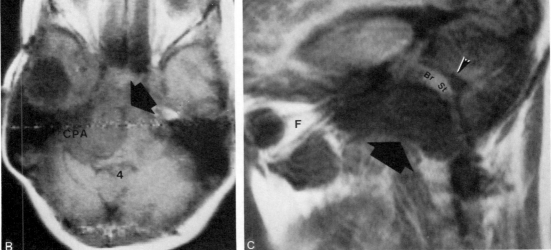

FIGURE 13–47. *Calcified Clivus Meningioma:* *A*, The CT scan photographed at high window width and window level reveals an irregularly marginated tumor arising from the clivus and extending through the tentorial notch into the parasellar region. The meningioma is densely and inhomogeneously calcified. There are postoperative changes in the posterior fossa (*arrow*) and ipsilateral temporal fossa.

B, The axial TR530/TE30 image reveals the low signal intensity mass—secondary to the calcification—in the prepontine cistern and extending into the ipsilateral CPA. The fourth ventricle is compressed along its anterior margin and displaced posteriorly (*4*).

C, The sagittal TR530/TE30 image obtained approximately 2 to 3 cm from the midline in the region of the largest portion of the mass reveals the comma-shaped low signal intensity mass (*large arrow*). The triangle-shaped fourth ventricle (*small arrow*) is displaced posteriorly, and the brain stem (*Br St*) is displaced in a curvilinear fashion around the mass. The globe of the eye appears as a low signal intensity area surrounded by the high signal intensity fat (*F*) in the orbit.

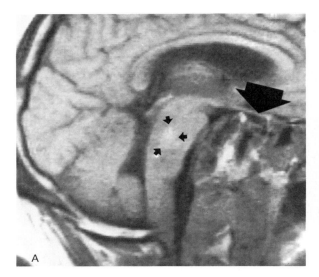

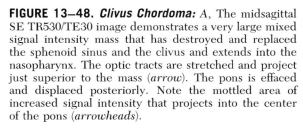

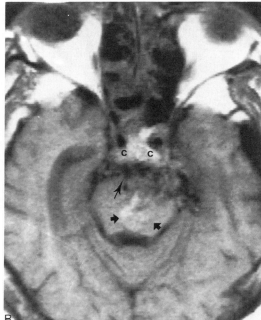

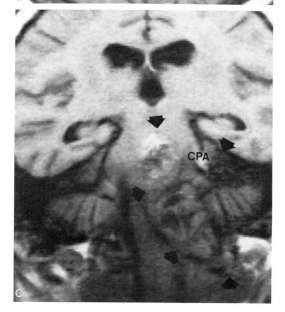

FIGURE 13–48. *Clivus Chordoma:* *A*, The midsagittal SE TR530/TE30 image demonstrates a very large mixed signal intensity mass that has destroyed and replaced the sphenoid sinus and the clivus and extends into the nasopharynx. The optic tracts are stretched and project just superior to the mass (*arrow*). The pons is effaced and displaced posteriorly. Note the mottled area of increased signal intensity that projects into the center of the pons (*arrowheads*).

B, The axial SE TR530/TE30 image demonstrates that the area of increased signal intensity within the pons on the sagittal view is actually an exophytic portion of the tumor which has invaginated into the pons (*arrows*). The carotid arteries (*C*) appear as negative flow defects surrounded by the mass, as does the basilar artery, which is displaced posteriorly by the mass (*long arrow*).

C, Coronal T-1 weighted image reveals the mottled density mass displacing the brain stem to the contralateral side and invading the CPA. The low signal intensity areas were identified as areas of calcification by CT scanning, and the areas of increased signal intensity are probably areas of the fat accumulation. There is mild obstructive hydrocephalus.

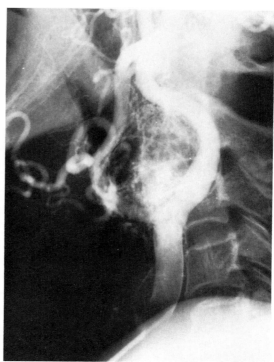

FIGURE 13–49. *Carotid Body Tumor:* The common carotid arteriogram reveals a very vascular mass lesion that is fed by branches of the external carotid artery and that splays the internal and external carotid arteries apart. This finding is both classic and consistent with a carotid body tumor. The tumors may occur bilaterally; therefore, the opposite carotid artery should be studied.

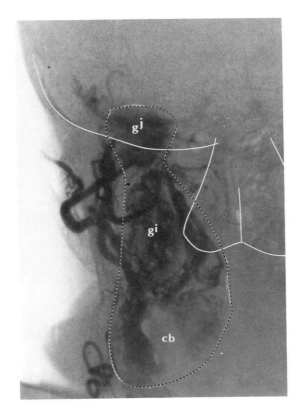

FIGURE 13–50. *Glomus Jugulare, Glomus Intravagale, and Carotid Body Tumor Associated with a Glomus Epitympanicum:* The common carotid arteriogram reveals a very vascular multilobulated tumor that is situated at the level of the jugular bulb, the vagus nerve, and the carotid bifurcation. The internal carotid artery is occluded secondary to arteriosclerosis. This tumor was discovered after examination revealed a red, pulsating mass behind the tympanic membrane of the ear.

  gj Glomus jugulare.
  gi glomus intravagale.
  cb carotid body tumor.

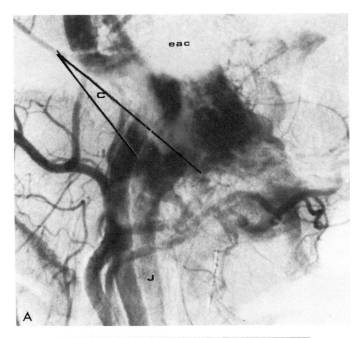

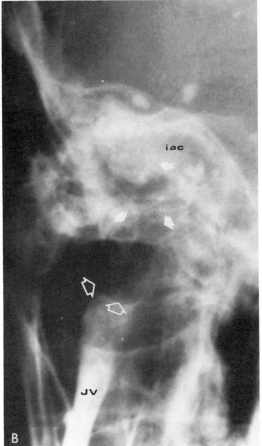

FIGURE 13–51. *See legend on the following page.*

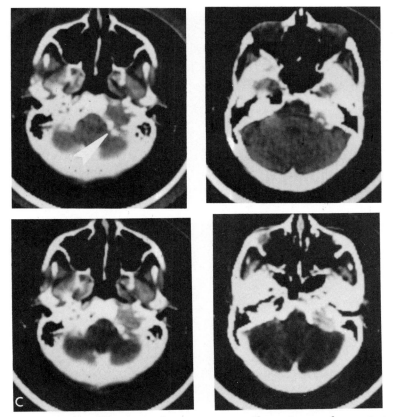

FIGURE 13–51. *Glomus Jugulare Tumor:* A, The common carotid arteriogram demonstrates a large vascular mass lesion in the region of the jugular bulb on the left that is supplied by branches of the external carotid artery. The external auditory canal (*eac*) and the clivus (*C*) are labeled, and there is early filling of the internal jugular vein (*J*) because of shunting through the tumor.

B, The jugular venogram demonstrates the tumor mass in the jugular vein (*JV*), where the tumor obstructs the retrograde flow of contrast material. The lower end of the tumor in the jugular vein is outlined by the open arrowheads; the upper end of the tumor is outlined up to its superior extent in the region of the jugular bulb by the closed arrowheads. This appearance is very typical of a glomus jugulare tumor.

C, The preinfusion scan demonstrates a greatly expanded jugular bulb (*arrow*) with erosion of the bony margin. The area of bony destruction extends to the region of the middle ear. The postinfusion scan demonstrates marked enhancement of this glomus jugulare tumor, which extends posteriorly into the left cerebellar region.

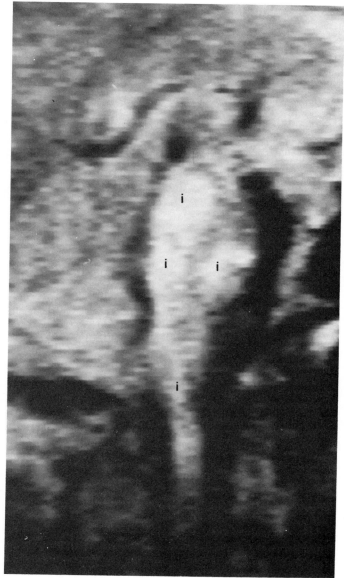

FIGURE 13–52. *Brain Stem Infarcts:* This 70-year-old female presented with sudden onset of coma and "locked in syndrome." CT and angiography were normal. MR in the midsagittal plane with SE TR3120/TE60 reveals multiple areas of increased signal intensity in the pons, medulla, and upper cervical cord. There is slight mass effect with posterior displacement of the fourth ventricle and slight expansion of the pons. Presumable multiple ischemic brain stem infarcts (*i*).

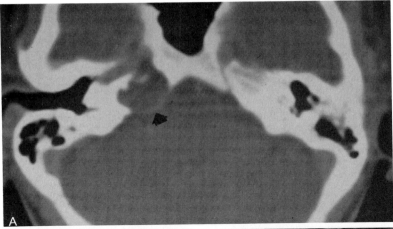

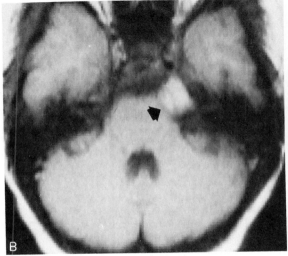

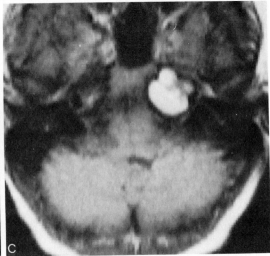

FIGURE 13–53. *Cholesteatoma of Skull Base:* A, CT scan at wide window width reveals a well-defined area of erosion of the medial end of the petrous bone that is secondary to a low density mass. The posteriorly displaced enhancing dura is faintly visualized (*arrow*). There is erosion of the lateral margin of the clivus.

B, SE TR530/TE30 reveals that the mass is slightly increased in signal intensity. Because of the extra-axial nature of the mass there is slight effacement of the left side of the pons, and the dura is visualized as an area of low signal intensity just next to the pons (*arrow*).

C, SE TR2120/TE60 reveals that the cholesteatoma becomes even more increased in signal intensity on the longer SE sequence.

D, Midsagittal SE TR530/TE30 reveals that the patient has a Chiari Type I malformation with marked elongation and inferior displacement of the cerebellar tonsils (*T*), which extend down to the level of the inferior margin of the C$_2$ vertebral body. Note also the compression of the medulla and upper cervical cord by the herniated tonsils. The fourth ventricle is enlarged slightly and elongated.

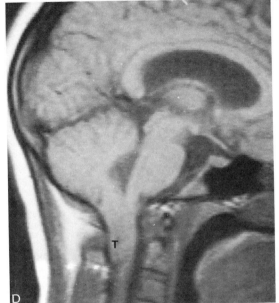

14

ATHEROSCLEROSIS

Recent advances in surgical technique have brought an ever-increasing demand for precise radiographic demonstration of the extracranial vasculature so that needed surgical repair can be undertaken. The main changes that affect these vessels can be outlined by using a variety of radiologic approaches. The method selected may in some cases be determined by the type of problem that the patient exhibits; in others, the approach may be dictated by the preference or skill of the operator or by the requirements of the referring physician.

Atherosclerosis, because of its various effects upon the cardiovascular and cerebrovascular systems, is one of the leading causes of death and disability today. Approximately 25 per cent of individuals presenting with signs and symptoms of cerebrovascular disease will have demonstrable extracranial carotid disease. Because this type of vascular change is potentially curable, there is today a greater emphasis on the precise radiologic demonstration of the lesion so that carotid endarterectomy or bypass procedure can be performed. In centers with an active cardiovascular and peripheral vascular surgical group, an increased number of patients are studied because of the possibility of surgically correctable carotid occlusive disease.

Stenosis of the carotid artery at the level of the bifurcation in the neck is quite common and is readily correctable by endarterectomy. Instead of treating these patients as another "standard work-up," each should be approached as if he were unique. Indeed, the many minor variations on the theme of atherosclerosis in each patient demand an examination tailored to the individual patient's needs. This will better serve both that patient and the referring physician.

It is obvious that surgical correction of extracranial carotid stenosis will not benefit the patient if additional areas of stenosis exist within the intracranial circulation. I feel strongly that including the neck on a nonconed view of the intracranial circulation for evaluation of extracranial carotid stenosis results in an unsatisfactory examination. It is demonstrated almost daily that biplane studies of the vessels are necessary for accurate evaluation. On one plane the vessel may appear entirely or nearly normal; on the opposite view a severe stenosis or an ulcerated lesion may be identified. Therefore, it behooves the examiner to view these vessels in at least two projections.

One must remember that more than 50 per cent narrowing of a vessel must occur to produce significant stenosis and that a stenosis greater than 70 per cent must occur to produce a hemodynamically significant decrease in the blood flow through an area. On the other hand, irregular or ulcerated lesions are more likely to accumulate such debris as fibrin or platelet clots, causing transient ischemic attacks even in the absence of significant stenosis.

A thorough examination of the intracranial circulation is needed for complete evaluation. Occasionally, a patient with a subdural hematoma or a brain tumor—particularly a meningioma, but any tumor may have this effect— may present with minimal symptoms that mimic those of a transient ischemic attack. Therefore, a study of the intracranial circulation is imperative. Finally, other disease entities, such as berry aneurysms, subdural hematomas, or unsuspected arteriovenous malformations, may be the cause of the patient's symptoms, rather than extracranial vascular occlusive disease.

FIBROMUSCULAR HYPERPLASIA

Fibromuscular hyperplasia affects the tunica media of the blood vessels, creating a variety of changes, among them fibrosis and stenosis of the vessels. This produces a "stack of coins" radiographic appearance, and often there is much more significant stenosis of the vessel than can be appreciated on the angiogram (Fig. 14–5, p. 638). A focal area of involvement may mimic the appearance of atherosclerosis, but a large area of involvement has a characteristic appearance. Fibromuscular change involves the internal carotid arteries and may be associated with similar changes in the renal arteries; it rarely involves the intracranial vessels.

STROKE SYNDROME

A variety of approaches may be used in the patient with "stroke" syndrome. Also, there are a number of different schools of thought concerning the timing of the work-up of patients with this syndrome. It is generally agreed, however, that an individual who is experiencing transient ischemic attacks—which, by definition, do not result in permanent neurologic deficit—should have angiography for diagnosis. If a surgically correctable lesion is found, an endarterectomy should be performed.

In a patient who is developing an acute stroke and who demonstrates progressive neurologic damage, angiography definitely may aggravate the condition. Therefore, the patient with a "stroke in progress" should be subjected to angiography only after utmost consideration. In an individual with a completed stroke, angiography may demonstrate the abnormality, but the patient may anticipate no benefit from surgery because of permanent neurologic damage.

Occlusive vascular disease may involve the carotid arteries in the neck, and so may be readily amenable to surgery; on the other hand, it may involve the intracranial vascular supply, which is less amenable to surgical treatment. With occlusion of the middle cerebral artery at its origin or stenosis of the horizontal portion of the middle cerebral artery, selected patients may benefit from a vascular bypass procedure. Recent advances in microsurgical techniques have made possible an anastomosis between the superficial temporal artery and the branches of the middle cerebral artery distal to the area of stenosis or occlusion. This is performed by mobilizing the superficial temporal artery and anastomosing this vessel to the middle cerebral artery. Recent research suggests that, while technically feasible, this surgery is not clinically effective and is no longer accepted.

Angiographic Findings with Stroke Syndromes

1. Over 50 per cent of the studies are normal. The involved vessel is so small that the thrombosis or embolus that has occluded the vessel cannot be visualized by angiography.

2. There may be total occlusion of the common or internal carotid artery.

3. There may be a significant (over 50 per cent) stenosis of the implicated carotid artery; or the extracranial vessel may demonstrate an ulcerated or irregular plaque, even in the absence of a significant stenosis.

4. Branch occlusions of the internal carotid artery may occur. These include occlusion of the anterior or, more commonly, the middle cerebral artery—or of any of the terminal branches of these vessels.

5. In approximately 15 per cent of acute stroke cases there will be significant mass effect, resulting in a shift of the midline to the contralateral side.

6. There may be evidence of early venous drainage.

7. There may be retrograde filling of the vessels that are occluded more proximally.

8. The areas of infarction may demonstrate early draining veins.

CT SCANNING OF ACUTE INFARCT

With an acute infarct the CT scan may have an entirely normal appearance. With time, an increasing number of infarcts will be visible on the plain CT scan. Approximately 60 to 70 per cent of acute bland infarcts will be detected by routine CT scan within the first seven days. On the other hand, a normal CT scan in a patient with an acute stroke can confirm the diagnosis by ruling out other diagnostic possibilities. Such entities as basal ganglionic hemorrhage, hemorrhagic infarct, intracerebral hematoma, subdural hematoma, and even primary or secondary brain tumors may present with the clinical appearance of an acute infarct.

The areas of infarction appear as areas of radiolucency that are variable in size. Infarcts resulting from a single small occluded vessel may be quite small. Others may be moderate in size—usually corresponding to a known vascular distribution, such as the middle cerebral artery distribution. Or the infarct may be very large, resulting in radiolucency of the entire hemisphere. Small or moderate infarcts are most common in the distribution of the middle cerebral artery. In most cases these areas of infarction will be non–space-occupying and will show no evidence of mass effect on the scan. However, in approximately 15 per cent of cases of acute infarction there will be some evidence of mass effect. This evidence may vary from a small local effect to a massive shift of the midline structures, as is seen in a total hemisphere stroke secondary to internal carotid artery occlusion. In cases of infarct that demonstrate mass effect, a postinfusion scan may help to distinguish between an infarct and a tumor with mass effect.

Hemorrhagic Infarcts. Hemorrhagic infarcts are relatively uncommon and may be difficult or impossible to differentiate from an intracerebral hematoma. Hemorrhagic infarcts, however, tend to occur in a major vascular distribution and are frequently non–space-occupying, causing only minimal, if any, shift of the midline structure.

Postinfusion Scan of Infarcts

The postinfusion scan may reveal no change in the appearance of the infarct. Sometimes the area of infarction may become less apparent; or, uncommonly, the infarct will become more apparent. Occasionally an area of infarction will become visible even though the preinfusion scan was normal. Presumably this occurs because the normal brain tissue takes up the contrast material, whereas the area of infarction does not. Thus, if the patient's clinical appearance suggests an infarct and the initial scan is negative, an infusion of contrast material may be in order for complete evaluation. On the other hand, since the postinfusion scan may reveal no change—especially soon after the acute insult—the infusion study may be academic once an area of hemorrhage has been

ruled out. A postinfusion scan gives an added risk of renal damage or allergic reaction to the contrast material.

Enhancing Infarcts. Certain infarcts will demonstrate evidence of enhancement after the infusion of contrast material. This enhancement is usually evident by one week after the stroke and persists until approximately six weeks after the stroke. Because some infarcts demonstrate enhancement sooner than one week after the infarct and some demonstrate enhancement for longer than six weeks after infarction, the exact time of infarction cannot be determined by the enhancement characteristics.

The commonly used term "luxury perfusion" has often been applied to this phenomenon. However, luxury perfusion is not really the cause of enhancement. Luxury perfusion, which occurs shortly after an ischemic infarct, is the opening of myriad vascular channels in the relatively avascular infarcted area. These are predominantly venous channels, but arterial channels open up as well. At surgery, the infarcted area thus appears to contain an increase in the number of blood vessels, which has led to the term "luxury perfusion." In reality, the vessels are not actually functioning to supply the infarcted brain, so the term is a misnomer. This luxury perfusion may be associated with the demonstration of early draining veins at the time of angiography because of arteriovenous shunting.

Approximately one week after a stroke there is breakdown of the blood-brain barrier in the region of relative anoxia. This breakdown in the blood-brain barrier is secondary to the opening up of the "tight junctions" of the endothelial lining of the capillary, which are more resistant to anoxia than the nerve cells. There is also loss of autoregulation of the blood vessels in the area of the infarction. These changes cause the accumulation of contrast material in an extravascular distribution and result in "enhancement" of the area of infarction. This enhancement usually persists for a longer period of time.

Evidence suggests that a patient who demonstrates infarct enhancement on CT does worse clinically than the patient whose ischemic infarct does not demonstrate enhancement or who does not receive an infusion of contrast material. This evidence is not clinically significant, but it is highly suggestive. Therefore, since there is really little to be gained by the infusion of contrast material, a postinfusion study is not recommended in the majority of cases. There is, of course, no way that one can predict from the preinjection scan if an area of infarction will or will not demonstrate enhancement; moreover, some authors have suggested that all infarcts demonstrate enhancement at some point. Again, while the data are not statistically significant, they do suggest that it is the contrast material itself that has a deleterious effect; for this reason, I would discourage the use of contrast material in patients who have a clinical history of infarction. Once the presence of hemorrhage, primary or secondary brain tumor, subdural hematoma, or other lesion mimicking stroke has been ruled out, there is really nothing to be gained from the infusion, and in some patients the infusion may be deleterious because of emesis with aspiration in a patient having difficulty handling secretions or even because of an adverse contrast reaction. However, in any individual case, a postinfusion scan should be performed if there is a question about the diagnosis. This is particularly true because metastatic disease may masquerade as a transient ischemic attack and the typical enhancing lesions may be visible only on the postinfusion portion of the examination. In these cases the preinfusion scan may show an area of infarction or may even have a normal appearance. An angiogram may or may not show an area of vascular occlusion with collateral flow; on the other hand, enhancement may be visible by CT scan even without evidence of major vascular occlusion on the arteriogram. As noted earlier, this enhancement can first be demonstrated approximately one week after insult and persists for approximately six weeks. This area of enhancement usually corresponds closely to the area of lucency on the preinfusion scan and often is quite dense in appearance. Occasionally this enhancement on the CT scan takes the form of dense, finger-like projections of enhancement extending into the brain from the outer convexity with intervening areas of radiolucency—a gyral pattern of enhancement. Rarely, a "ring" of enhancement similar to that seen with a tumor is seen on the postinfusion scan. Differentiation from tumor may be difficult.

Late Changes. With the passage of time the areas of infarction may disappear, but frequently they leave residual areas of lucency as evidence of their presence. The infarct may leave an area of porencephaly, or it may result in an appearance of hemiatrophy with enlargement of the lateral ventricle and cortical sulci on the side of the stroke.

The study of strokes accounts for a large percentage of patients who are examined with computed tomography. Thorough knowledge of the presentation and of the protean manifestations of infarction is mandatory for accurate interpretation of CT scans.

MAGNETIC RESONANCE OF INFARCTS

Infarcts cause an increase in the water content of the brain through vasogenic edema, resulting in an increase in both the T-1 and T-2 scans of the brain. Therefore, there is an area of low signal intensity on the short SE sequences and an area of increased signal intensity on the long SE sequences. One must rely on the usual criteria for determining if the abnormal area is an infarct: (1) clinical presentation, (2) vessel distribution, (3) involvement of the gray and white matter, with tracking of the edema along white matter pathways, (4) presence or lack of a multiplicity of lesions, and (5) lack of mass effect.

MR appears to be more sensitive than CT for the presence of abnormalities, particularly areas of edema, and infarcts are often demonstrated on MR when they are not seen on CT. Of course, in any individual case one cannot say with certainty if the infarct is recent or old unless one is fortunate enough to have an earlier study available for comparison. On the other hand, identifying an infarct may solve the clinical dilemma.

The patient with transient ischemic attacks provides a unique opportunity to evaluate the actual pathophysiology of these events. Because a number of observers believe that TIA's are actually "small strokes," then MR, with its superior sensitivity, should prove to be very helpful in the evaluation and work-up of this problem. This is particularly true in the patient who is a surgical candidate but would have surgery delayed a suitable period of time if it could be proved that an infarct had actually occurred.

The absence of bone artifact also allows ready evaluation of the region of the midbrain and brain stem, an area notoriously difficult to evaluate by CT scanning. MR allows direct, multiplanar visualization of the midbrain, brain stem, and cerebellum and readily demonstrates areas of abnormal signal intensity in these regions. This is obviously helpful for confirmation of the clinical diagnosis and also aids in treatment planning.

Because acute hemorrhage cannot be accurately evaluated by MR, and because it is necessary to differentiate an ischemic infarct from a hemorrhagic infarct, MR is not the procedure of choice for the initial evaluation. CT, on the other hand, is an excellent method to evaluate the presence or absence of hemorrhage and should be the initial examination in most patients.

COLLATERAL CIRCULATION

Subclavian Steal. A variety of "steal" circulations may exist; however, one that is seen frequently and that may result in clinical symptoms of vertebrobasilar insufficiency is the subclavian steal (Fig. 14–17, p. 648). This syndrome results from an area of narrowing or occlusion of the proximal subclavian artery—usually the left, but the right side also may exhibit this finding—proximal to the origin of the vertebral artery. This results in a deficiency of blood flow to the arm. When the arm is used, the increased demand for blood will cause retrograde blood flow down the vertebral artery and then to the subclavian artery distal to the origin of the vertebral artery. In other words, the arm will "steal" blood from the opposite side and from the vertebrobasilar system by retrograde flow down the vertebral artery on the side where there is stenosis or occlusion of the proximal subclavian artery. This obviously results in a deficient blood supply to the posterior fossa circulation, and these patients may develop syncopal attacks, dizziness, and even nystagmus (see Fig. 14–17, p. 648).

One surgical approach to this disorder is a bypass graft that extends from the carotid artery to the affected subclavian artery. This will increase the blood supply to the arm by taking blood from the carotid system. The carotid artery must be widely patent, or an endarterectomy must first be performed.

External Carotid Artery Collateral Circulation. When there is total occlusion of the internal carotid system, one of the main pathways of collateral flow is via the external carotid system. In some individuals there is opening of the collateral pathways behind the globe of the eye, with hypertrophy of the external carotid branches behind the globe that fills the ophthalmic artery and ultimately the intracranial circulation in a retrograde fashion. Clinically, these patients have an ocular bruit because of the increased blood flow through the hypertrophied retro-ocular ophthalmic collateral vessels (see Figs. 14–8 and 14–9, pp. 640 and 641). Vessels that may provide collateral flow are the facial artery, superficial temporal artery, ethmoidal arteries, and multiple small arteries and arterial branches.

External Carotid Collateral to Vertebral Artery. Another one of the more common types of collateral circulation involves the carotid and vertebral systems. With occlusion of the common carotid artery below the level of the carotid bifurcation, collateral circulation develops from muscular branches of the vertebral artery and from the thyrocervical trunk. These collateral branches anastomose with the branches of the external carotid artery. Blood then flows retrograde to the level of the carotid bifurcation and then antegrade in the internal carotid circulation or even via ophthalmic collaterals. Similarly, collateral circulation from the external carotid artery may supply a vertebral artery that is occluded or stenotic at its origin.

ANGIOGRAPHY OF COLLATERAL CIRCULATION AND THE STEAL SYNDROMES

The various collateral pathways illustrate the "imagination" of the biologic system in providing for continuous blood flow to critical areas. These collateral pathways usually demonstrate a much slower circulation than do normal anatomic pathways; therefore, when performing angiography to demonstrate abnormal circulation, a prolonged film series is necessary. The author recommends serial filming over at least eight seconds. The films may be programmed so that they demonstrate both the early arterial and late arterial phases. Films should be obtained in a biplane projection. One possible program would be two films per second for three seconds and one film per second for the next five seconds. For suspected threadlike patency of a vessel, films should be obtained at a rate of one film per second for 12 seconds. Positioning should be such that both the neck and intracranial contents can be visualized.

MOYAMOYA

This disease was originally described in children, but the author has seen cases in adults secondary to diffuse atherosclerosis. Of unknown etiology in children, it results in stenosis and progressive occlusion of multiple intracranial vessels and the proliferation of massive collateral circulation from the lenticulostriate and thalamoperforating arteries. This results in a diffuse blush at angiography, giving the appearance of the "puff of smoke" from which the Japanese name originates. I have also seen several cases having the appearance of moyamoya disease in children with sickle cell anemia (Fig. 14–15, p. 647).

The CT scans suggest atrophy. The massive collateral vessels do not demonstrate enhancement on the postinfusion scan.

DIGITAL SUBTRACTION ANGIOGRAPHY

Ziedes de Plantes originally described the technique of radiographic subtraction in 1935. The more recently developed technique of digital subtraction angiography (DSA) uses an electronic and computer method of performing the "subtraction" films, which can be generated by hand using darkroom technique. With DSA fluoroscopy and angiography, the images are produced electronically and are instantly visible on the oscilloscope screen. The standard method available on most units is known as temporal subtraction. In addition, there is also available another method that is known as dual energy subtraction, but this technique is not readily available at present and is beyond the scope of this book. Initially there was great enthusiasm for the technique of intravenous DSA (IV-DSA); more recently there has been a lessening of enthusiasm for this technique. Because of the high contrast load required with IV-DSA and because of a variety of intrinsic limitations of the technique, there has been a recent trend toward the use of intra-arterial DSA (IA-DSA), which will be discussed below.

Intravenous DSA

Indications for IV-DSA in the Patient with Atherosclerotic Disease

• To rule out carotid stenosis
• Asymptomatic carotid bruit
• Preoperative examination for coronary artery bypass
• Preoperative examination for major surgery (such as hip or gallbladder surgery in the older patient)
• Postoperative evaluation of carotid endarterectomy
• Evaluation of subclavian steal

For the patient with an asymptomatic carotid bruit, the IV-DSA may be the only examination necessary for complete evaluation, provided that it is a good quality study. However, studies have shown that most atherosclerotic plaques develop along the posterior walls of the carotid arteries; this is a major drawback of IV-DSA, because vessel overlap precludes a true lateral view. In addition, ulcerated plaques that are demonstrable using the routine cut-film angiographic techniques or using IA-DSA often cannot be demonstrated using IV-DSA techniques. This is, of course, a major deficiency of IV-DSA, because any patient who presents with a history of transient ischemic attacks could have an ulcerated plaque. These irregular plaques are the focus where small fibrin accumulations occur and where platelets may adhere and then pass intracranially, resulting in recurring symptoms—transient ischemic attacks (TIA's). Therefore the patient who presents with history of transient ischemic attacks is not a candidate for IV-DSA, but rather should be studied with standard arteriography or IA-DSA. This is because an ulcerated plaque, the source of the emboli, may not be demonstrated on the IV-DSA study, nor can the intracranial vessels be well demonstrated with this technique. I believe that all or at least most TIA's are actually little infarcts or strokes that cause small areas of permanent damage. Magnetic resonance scanning with its increased sensitivity will probably give us a better and more accurate evaluation of these small areas of ischemia or infarction.

Technique of IV-DSA

IV-DSA is readily performed as an outpatient procedure and can also be used in patients who are receiving anticoagulants. It is most convenient to use the antecubital veins, and because the cephalic vein may enter the subclavian vein at a right angle and make negotiation of this junction difficult (if not impossible), it is best to use the basilic vein. The most satisfactory technique is to use a small (4 or 5 French) catheter placed in the superior vena cava, preferably at the level of its junction with the right atrium. A straight catheter can be used (and is often easier to insert) but may result in a subintimal or extravascular injection of contrast, and so a pigtail catheter is recommended. The catheter should have multiple side holes and an end hole. If there is any difficulty with catheterization of the antecubital veins, there should be no hesitation to use the femoral veins, even for outpatient studies.

A variety of guide wires can be used, and

some wires are available with a firm, straight tip at one end and a curved tip at the opposite end so that either end may be used, or both may be used sequentially. It is not uncommon to use a variety of guide wires to complete a study. Peripheral injection with a short, end-hole catheter can also be used but is less satisfactory, and its use is discouraged. The peripheral injection results in more discomfort for the patient and provides less satisfactory demonstration of the great vessels. Peripheral injection may also result in venous reflux, particularly into the jugular vein but also into multiple smaller veins that may obscure the visualization of the carotid arteries (Fig. 14–38, p. 667).

Advantages with IV-DSA

- Easily performed, readily repeated
- Good screening technique
- Readily done on outpatient basis
- Good for follow-up examination
- May provide satisfactory image for surgical approach
- Relatively inexpensive
- Markedly decreased film cost

Disadvantages with IV-DSA

- Ulcerated plaques may be missed
- Jugular reflux may obscure the carotid arteries
- Requires a large amount of contrast material
- Poor cardiac output is a contraindication
- Renal compromise is a contraindication
- Threadlike patency may be overlooked
- Uncooperative patient is a contraindication
- True lateral view is impossible because of vessel overlap
- Only fair visualization of intracranial vessels

Other Uses for IV-DSA

- To rule out giant aneurysm
- Evaluation of pituitary adenoma and relationship to carotid arteries
- Tortuous vertebrobasilar artery
- Evaluation of superior sagittal sinus thrombosis
- Follow-up of intracranial spasm associated with subarachnoid hemorrhage
- Follow-up of intracranial arteriovenous malformations
- Rapid, easy evaluation of progress on embolization procedures
- Follow-up of superficial temporal–to–middle cerebral artery anastomosis

Guide for Standard Injection Amounts for IV-DSA

- Central injection: 76 per cent contrast, 20 cc/second
  Total, 40 cc/injection

- Peripheral injection: 76 per cent contrast, 6-8 cc/second
  Total, 36 cc/injection
- Planes and positions for imaging: RPO, LPO, AP views of carotid bifurcations in the neck, RPO arch, intracranial view

A maximum of five injections, a total of approximately 220 cc of contrast material (including test doses), is recommended.

Intra-arterial DSA

Recently there has been an interest in the performance of intra-arterial DSA (IA-DSA). IA-DSA can be performed using the same equipment that is used for IV-DSA and results in a marked decrease in the amount of contrast material necessary for the study. This is definitely advantageous in the patient with compromised renal function, and the decrease in the amount of contrast material also results in less patient discomfort. Recent economic trends encourage the performance of outpatient procedures, and IA-DSA lends itself well to this type of study. Because IA-DSA can be performed with smaller catheters (4 or 5 French) and a decreased load, it should prove to be a valuable procedure for outpatient angiography. Either the femoral or percutaneous brachial artery approach can be used.

Arterial digital techniques require the use of a more dilute contrast material. The standard Conray 60 per cent can be diluted by adding 3 to 4 cc of Conray 60 per cent to 6 cc of saline. This diluted contrast is used for direct carotid injection. For IA-DSA arch angiography one uses undiluted contrast material. As a general statement, if IA-DSA is used, it is recommended that selective studies be performed rather than arch angiography so that a more accurate evaluation can be made.

Because biplane digital equipment is not usually available, this technique does require multiple injections for each biplane examination. This may result in an amount of contrast material similar to that used with routine cut-film angiography. However, the technique does allow the demonstration of the carotid artery in the direct lateral projection, something that is usually not possible using the intravenous technique. The spatial resolution is not as good as with cut-film angiography, which remains the gold standard for evaluation of the extra- and intracranial carotid vessels; however, the studies are sufficient for diagnosis. If IA-DSA is unsatisfactory for any reason, one always has the option of returning to standard cut-film angiography, since the DSA study has been performed using an arterial puncture. Additional improvements such as finer screen images, biplane capability, larger field size, and pixel shifting capability in any plane will also aid in the improvement of DSA images of both the intravenous and intra-arterial techniques.

Advantages with IA-DSA

- May be performed on an outpatient basis
- Requires smaller amounts of contrast material than IV-DSA
- Biplane visualization of individual vessels is easily

performed, although this requires separate injections for each plane, unless biplane DSA is available
- Intracranial vessels are well demonstrated
- There is a marked decrease in film cost
- Surgical approach can be based upon IA-DSA studies, and no further studies need be performed
- Time of procedure is decreased

Disadvantages of IA-DSA

- May not be possible to selectively catheterize individual vessels, a relative disadvantage, since a standard intra-arterial study could then be performed
- Before being released, patients should be observed for four hours following study
- Requires arterial puncture

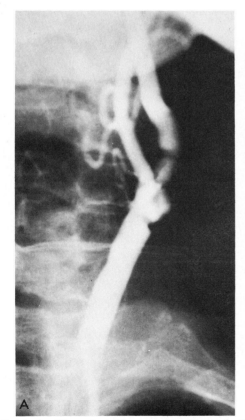 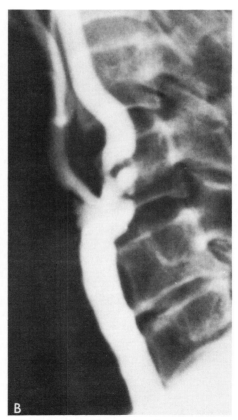

FIGURE 14—1. *Ulcerated Plaque with Stenosis Seen Well in One Plane:* *A,* The AP view reveals an irregular area of stenosis involving the distal left common carotid artery and the left internal carotid artery. On the lateral (*B*) view, however, the ulcerated plaque with a very high grade stenosis can be more readily appreciated.

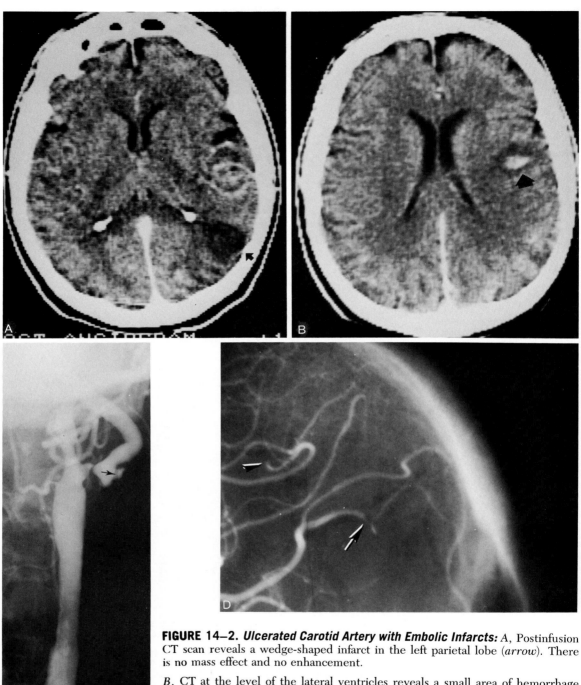

FIGURE 14–2. *Ulcerated Carotid Artery with Embolic Infarcts:* *A*, Postinfusion CT scan reveals a wedge-shaped infarct in the left parietal lobe (*arrow*). There is no mass effect and no enhancement.

B, CT at the level of the lateral ventricles reveals a small area of hemorrhage with surrounding edema. (This was also identified on the preinfusion CT scan, and without the preinfusion CT scan this area could be mistaken for an area of enhancement rather than hemorrhage.)

C, Left common carotid angiogram reveals an irregular ulcerated plaque (*arrow*) at the origin of the left internal carotid artery. This is just distal to an area of marked stenosis, and there is diffuse atherosclerotic change involving the entire left common carotid artery.

D, Magnification view of the intracranial circulation reveals an occluded vessel (*short arrow*) and a filling defect in another vessel secondary to multiple emboli (*long arrow*). This area corresponds to the area of infarction identified on the CT scan.

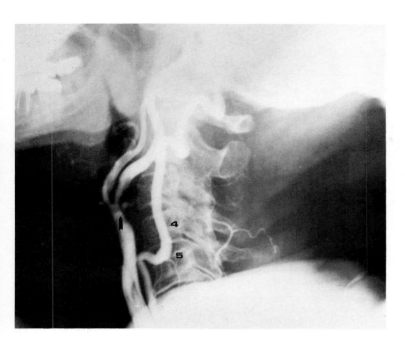

FIGURE 14–3. *Ulcerated Plaque:* The RBA demonstrates an ulcerated plaque at the origin of the right internal carotid artery (*arrow*). In addition, the vertebral artery enters into the foramina transversaria at the C_4–C_5 level rather than at the level of C_6. This is a normal anatomic variant.

FIGURE 14–4. *Carotid Stenosis, Subintimal Injection:* The percutaneous carotid arteriogram reveals a large subintimal injection (*si*) associated with areas of stenosis both proximal and distal to the area of subintimal accumulation of contrast material. There is an intraluminal collection of clotted blood in the left internal carotid artery (*ICA*) just distal to the stenosis of the internal carotid artery. In addition, there is a collection of extravasated contrast material in the soft tissues of the neck behind the carotid artery. The extravasation of contrast material probably occurs through the back wall puncture site. There is a large hematoma of the neck with forward displacement of the carotid artery in the neck.

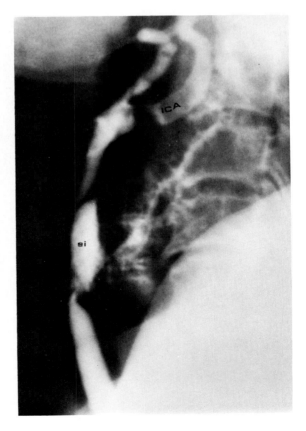

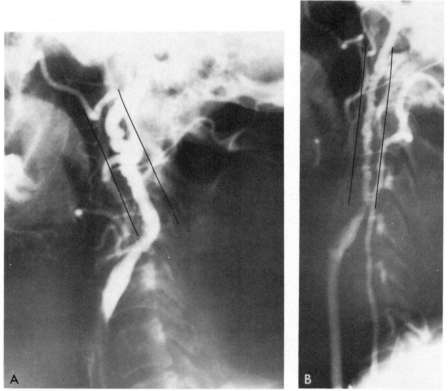

FIGURE 14—5. *Fibromuscular Hyperplasia:* A and B, Both carotid arteriograms demonstrate the "stack of coins" appearance typical of fibromuscular hyperplasia. The internal lumen of the vessel may be much more markedly narrowed than can be appreciated on the arteriogram.

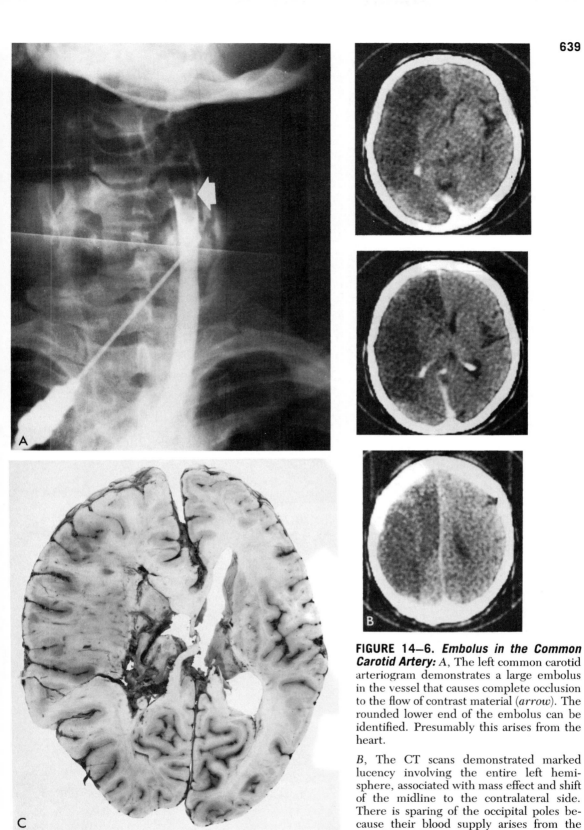

FIGURE 14–6. *Embolus in the Common Carotid Artery:* *A,* The left common carotid arteriogram demonstrates a large embolus in the vessel that causes complete occlusion to the flow of contrast material (*arrow*). The rounded lower end of the embolus can be identified. Presumably this arises from the heart.

B, The CT scans demonstrated marked lucency involving the entire left hemisphere, associated with mass effect and shift of the midline to the contralateral side. There is sparing of the occipital poles because their blood supply arises from the vertebrobasilar system, consistent with a hemisphere infarct secondary to total occlusion of the internal carotid artery.

C, The pathologic specimen demonstrates an edematous left hemisphere and shift of the midline to the contralateral side.

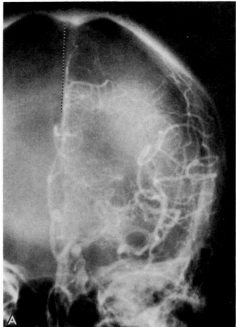

FIGURE 14–7. Acute Infarct with Mass Effect: *A,* The AP view of the common carotid arteriogram demonstrates shift of the anterior cerebral artery to the contralateral side. The dashed line indicates the anticipated position of the midline.

B, The lateral view of the arterial phase shows branch occlusions of several of the anterior branches of the middle cerebral artery *(closed arrow);* the open arrow points to an area of staining in the region of infarction.

C, The arrowheads demonstrate the occluded vessels filling in a retrograde fashion via collateral circulation. The black lines encircle an area of enhancement.

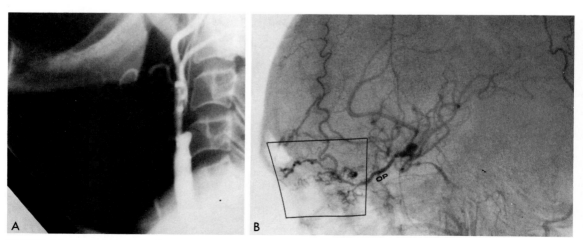

FIGURE 14–8. Ophthalmic Collateral: *A,* There is total occlusion of the internal carotid artery at its origin in the neck.

B, The external carotid artery is large, and multiple small collateral vessels *(black lines)* may be seen. These eventually fill the ophthalmic artery *(OP)* in a retrograde fashion. The ophthalmic artery then fills the internal carotid artery and the intracranial circulation.

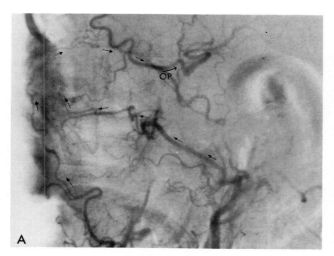

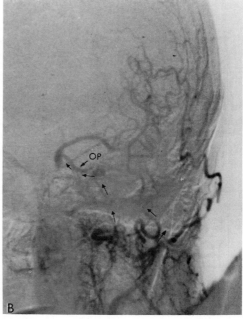

FIGURE 14–9. *Ophthalmic Collateral:* The internal carotid artery is occluded in the neck at the level of the carotid bifurcation. The branches of the external carotid artery have enlarged and demonstrate extensive collateral flow (*arrows*) through the internal maxillary and facial arteries on the lateral view (*A*) and in the facial artery on the anteroposterior view (*B*). The flow is ultimately retrograde through the ophthalmic artery (*OP*) to the internal carotid artery, which supplies the middle cerebral artery distribution. Subtraction views, as shown here, demonstrate these collateral channels to better advantage.

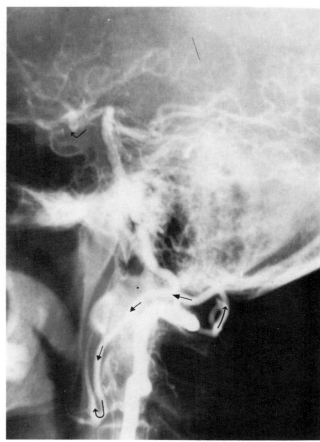

FIGURE 14–10. *Collateral Circulation:* The brachial arteriogram demonstrates a total occlusion of the internal carotid artery at its origin in the neck. The vertebral artery gives rise to a large muscular collateral vessel (*arrows*) that communicates with the external carotid artery at the level of the bifurcation, where the external carotid artery and its branches are then noted to fill via this collateral. The intracranial circulation is filling via retrograde flow through the posterior communicating artery (*curved arrow*) and then to the anterior and middle cerebral artery circulations.

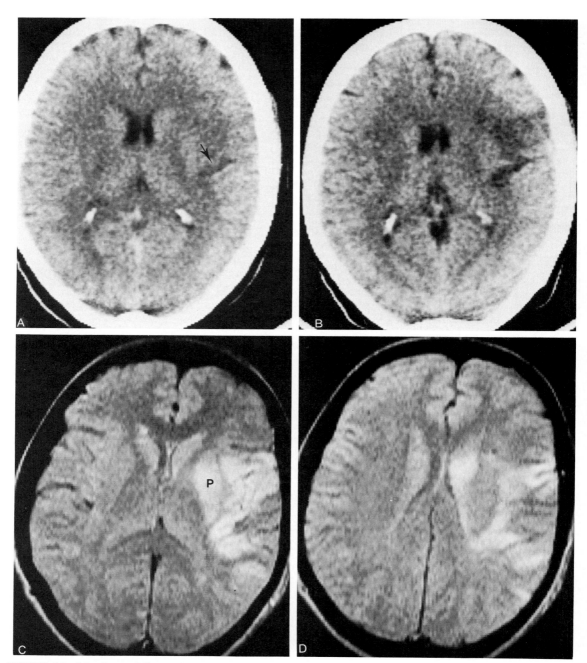

FIGURE 14–11. *Acute Middle Cerebral Artery Infarct:* A, CT scan 24 hours after the onset of acute right hemiparesis reveals a very faint linear area of lucency in the left middle cerebral artery distribution (*arrow*).

B, CT scan obtained 48 hours following ictus now clearly demonstrates a low-density area in the left middle cerebral artery distribution. There is mild mass effect with slight compression of the ipsilateral lateral ventricle.

C and D, MR, SE TR2120/TE60 reveals that the area of low density on the CT scan appears as an area of increased signal intensity. The compression of the ipsilateral lateral ventricle is better demonstrated, and, in addition, the involvement of the putamen (P) is better appreciated.

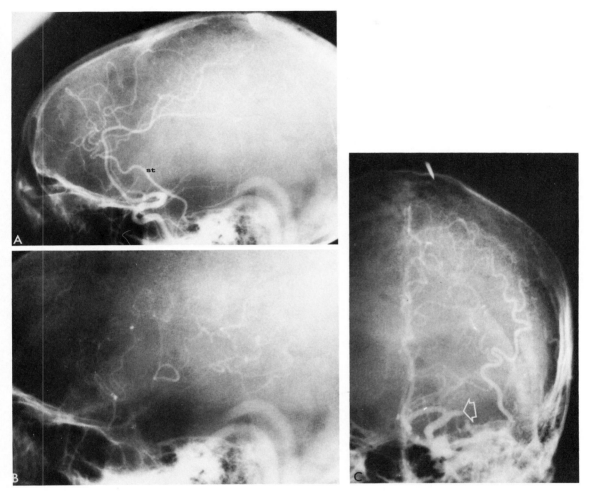

FIGURE 14–12. *Middle Cerebral Artery Occlusion:* A, The lateral view shows total occlusion of the middle cerebral artery just past the origin of the vessel from the internal carotid artery. The result, therefore, is an anterior cerebral artery arteriogram. The second large vessel seen is the superficial temporal artery (*st*).

B, The capillary phase of the arteriogram demonstrates the branches of the middle cerebral artery, which fill in a retrograde fashion.

C, On the AP view, the occluded middle cerebral artery (*arrow*) is seen. The occipital artery projects over the left side of the skull. (The broken tip of a knife blade is seen in the parietal region.)

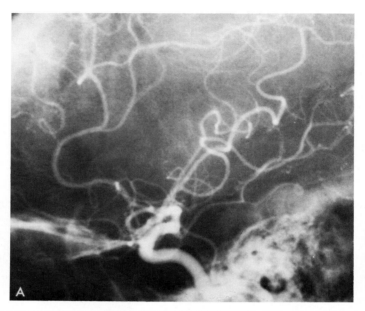

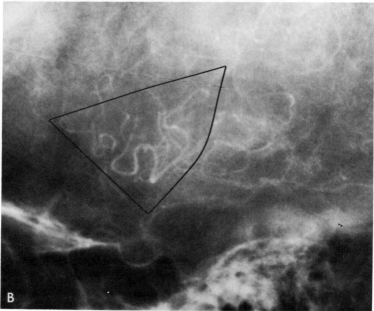

FIGURE 14–13. *Branch Occlusions of the Middle Cerebral Artery:* A, The early arterial phase demonstrates that the multiple branch occlusions involving the middle cerebral artery are present.

B, The capillary phase shows that the branches fill in a retrograde fashion via collateral circulation (*black line*). Just behind the outlined area there is a faint blush secondary to enhancement in the area of the occluded vessels.

Illustration continued on the following page

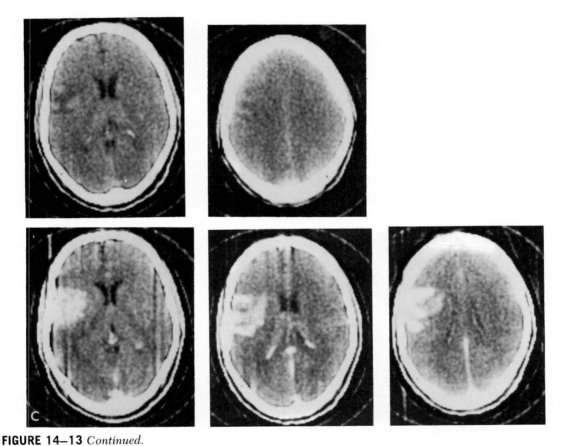

FIGURE 14–13 *Continued.*
C, CT scans reveal an area of radiolucency mixed with areas of slightly increased density; there is marked enhancement following the infusion of contrast material—a classic example of an enhancing infarct.

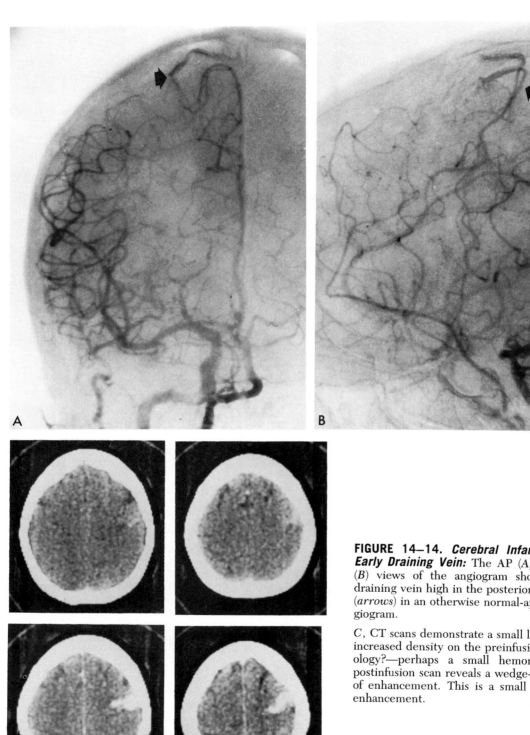

FIGURE 14–14. *Cerebral Infarct with an Early Draining Vein:* The AP (*A*) and lateral (*B*) views of the angiogram show an early draining vein high in the posterior frontal area (*arrows*) in an otherwise normal-appearing angiogram.

C, CT scans demonstrate a small linear area of increased density on the preinfusion scan (etiology?—perhaps a small hemorrhage); the postinfusion scan reveals a wedge-shaped area of enhancement. This is a small infarct with enhancement.

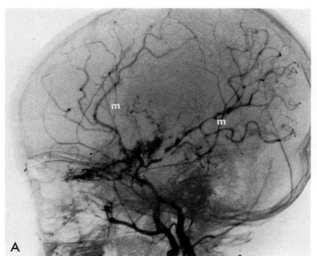

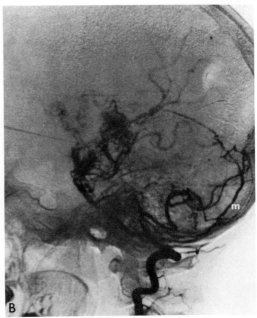

FIGURE 14–15. *Moyamoya Disease Secondary to Sickle Cell Anemia:* *A*, Occlusions and areas of narrowing involving the intracranial vessels are evident. There is marked hypertrophy of the lenticulostriate vessels and a diffuse blush in the region of the middle cerebral artery distribution. In an attempt to provide collateral flow, the meningeal arteries have hypertrophied (*m*); the ophthalmic artery also gives rise to multiple small collateral vessels.

B, The vertebral angiogram also shows the multiple vessel occlusions and dilatation of the thalamoperforate vessels with a diffuse blush in the region of the thalamus. Note the marked enlargement of the posterior meningeal artery (*m*).

C, The CT scans provide a picture of atrophy, with diffuse enlargement of the lateral ventricles (the left slightly more than the right) and enlargement of the cortical sulci over the left hemisphere. Small areas of radiolucency are also present on the right side—probably secondary to small infarcts. The blush seen on the arteriogram is not seen on the postinfusion CT scan.

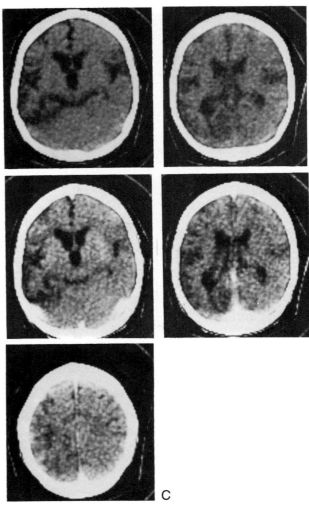

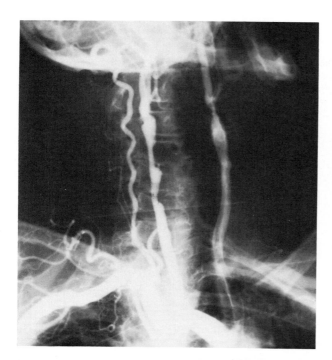

FIGURE 14–16. *Diffuse Atherosclerosis:* The arch angiogram of this patient reveals total occlusion of the left vertebral artery and marked irregularity of the carotid arteries bilaterally. The curvilinear deformity of the right vertebral artery is secondary to osteophyte formation of the cervical spine.

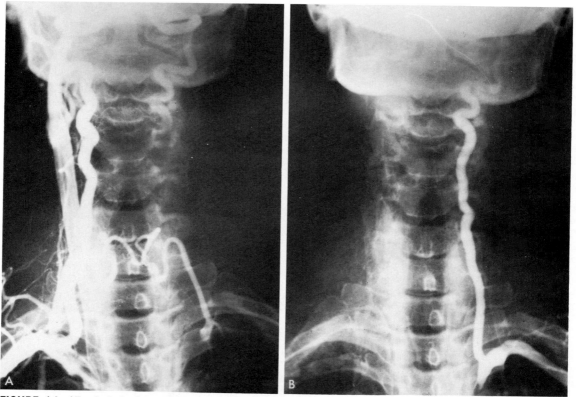

FIGURE 14–17. *Subclavian Steal:* A, The right brachial arteriogram demonstrates a large right vertebral artery and a normal-appearing right common carotid artery. The inferior thyroid artery is enlarged and extends across the midline to fill the contralateral subclavian artery distal to the origin of the left vertebral artery.

B, The late film shows retrograde flow down the left vertebral artery to fill the left subclavian artery. There is total occlusion of the proximal portion of the left subclavian artery.

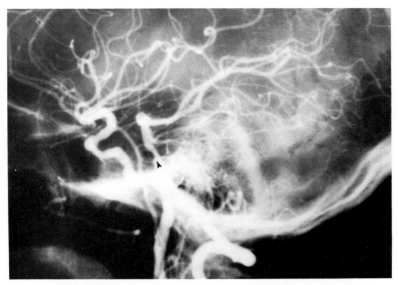

FIGURE 14–18. *Basilar Artery Plaque:* The lateral view of the right brachial arteriogram demonstrates a well-defined plaque at the distal end of the basilar artery (*arrowhead*). Small atherosclerotic plaques also are present in the cavernous portion of the carotid artery. On the AP view (not shown) this plaque of the basilar artery may give the false appearance of a fenestrated basilar artery.

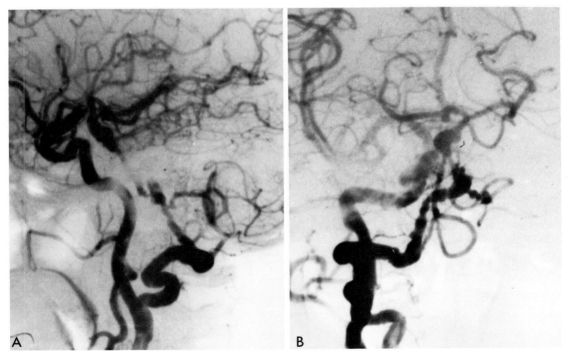

FIGURE 14–19. *Vertebrobasilar Atherosclerosis:* The entire vertebral and basilar artery demonstrates marked irregularity of the vessel walls with areas of dilatation and narrowing. The PICA also demonstrates evidence of irregularity secondary to atherosclerosis.

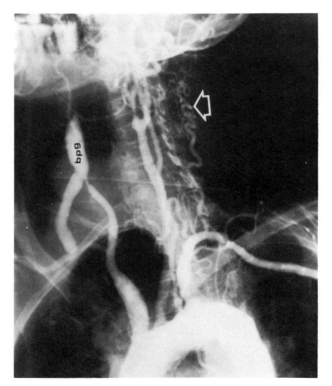

FIGURE 14–20. *Bypass Graft:* The arch angiogram with the patient in the RPO position demonstrates marked atherosclerotic change involving all the great vessels as they arise from the arch of the aorta. The right vertebral artery is totally occluded; the right internal and external carotid arteries also are totally occluded. There is stenosis of the left external carotid artery, and multiple unnamed collateral vessels arise from the thyrocervical trunk to supply the vertebrobasilar system (*arrow*). There is also a bypass graft (*bpg*) in place that extends from the right common carotid artery to the right subclavian artery. The subclavian artery has a threadlike patency in its proximal portion and is quite small, even distal to the bypass graft.

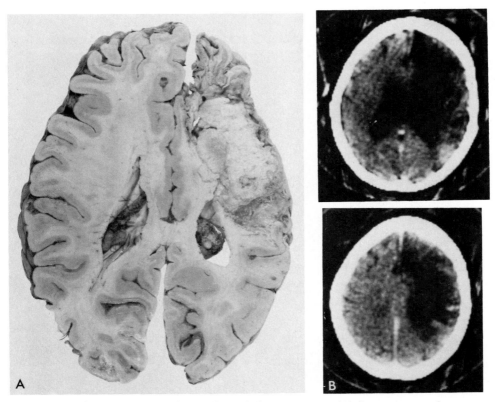

FIGURE 14–21. *Old Middle Cerebral Infarct:* The pathologic specimen (A) demonstrates a large area of cystic necrosis involving the right hemisphere. The corresponding CT scan (B) reveals a large area of porencephaly secondary to an infarct in the right hemisphere in the distribution of the right internal carotid artery (viewed from above).

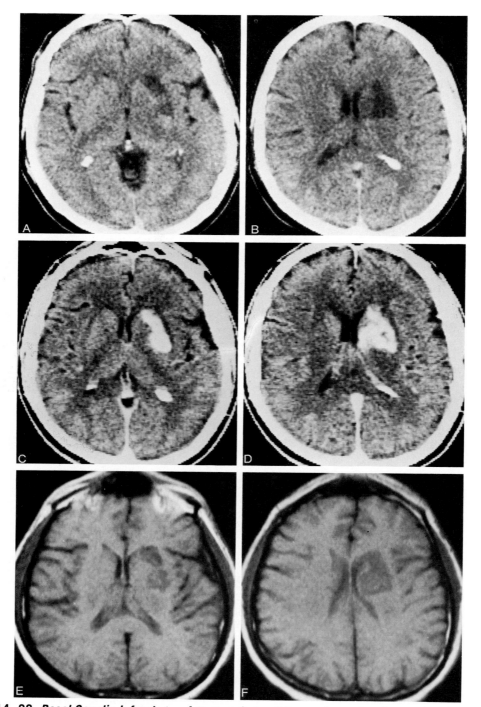

FIGURE 14–22. *Basal Ganglia Infarct:* *A* and *B*, Preinfusion CT scan obtained 24 hours after the acute onset of right hemiparesis reveals an area of lucency in the region of the basal ganglia of the left hemisphere. There is slight mass effect with compression of the frontal horn and body of the left lateral ventricle.

C and *D*, Postinfusion CT scans obtained approximately five days after *A* and *B* reveal that the mass effect has subsided, and there is now dense enhancement in the region of the previously identified infarct.

E and *F*, MR scans obtained between the pre- and postinfusion portions of the CT scan reveal that on the SE TR530/TE30 images the area of infarction appears as an area of decreased signal intensity. The minimal mass effect can be appreciated with compression of the ipsilateral lateral ventricle.

Illustration continued on the following page

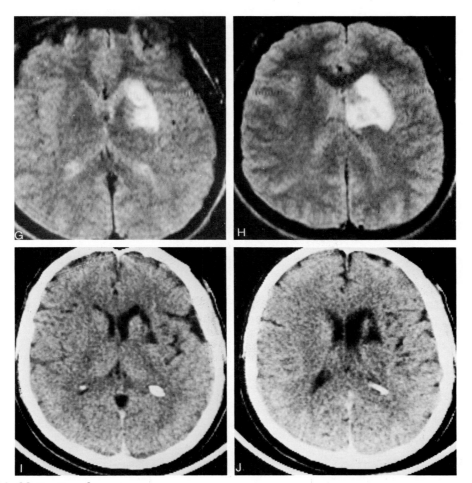

FIGURE 14–22 *Continued.*

G and *H*, The SE TR3120/TE120 images reveal that the area of infarction now appears as an area of increased signal intensity and correlates well with the appearance of the infarct on the postinfusion portion of the CT scan.

I and *J*, The CT scan obtained approximately one year after the initial examination now reveals a mature infarct in the left basal ganglia. The area of abnormality now appears smaller in size, there is no mass effect, and the infarct has progressed to an area of "closed porencephaly" which contains CSF density material.

This series of images is a nice example of the initial presentation and the progression and maturation of a typical ischemic basal ganglionic infarct.

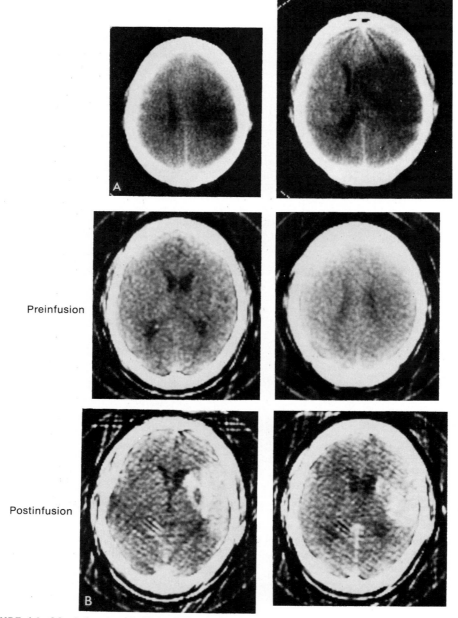

FIGURE 14–23. *Infarct with Mass Effect Followed by Enhancement:* The initial scan (*A*) obtained shortly after a stroke demonstrates a large area of radiolucency in the right hemisphere associated with shift of the midline from right to left.

B, Scans done 20 days later reveal that there is no shift of the midline and only a small area of lucency adjacent to the body of the right lateral ventricle. The postinfusion scan, however, reveals spectacular enhancement in the right hemisphere.

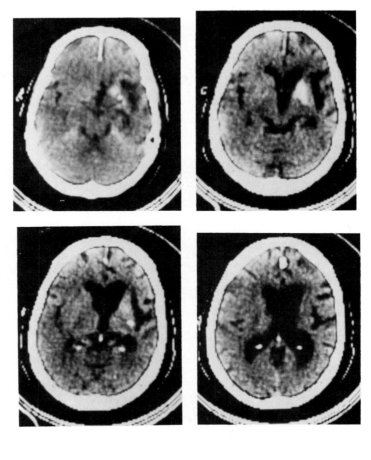

FIGURE 14–24. *Calcified Infarct, Basal Ganglia:* There is calcification in the region of the basal ganglia on the right side. In addition, there is enlargement of the sylvian fissure, the right lateral ventricle (including the right temporal horn), and the cortical sulci over the right hemisphere. The findings are consistent with an infarct in the right basal ganglia that has calcified and led to right hemiatrophy.

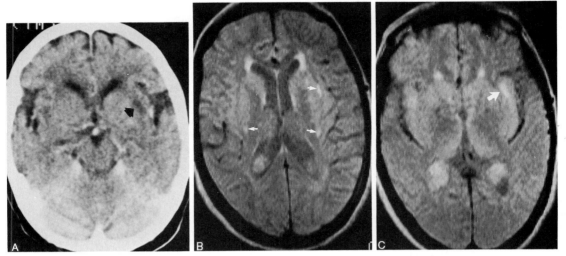

FIGURE 14–25. *Lacunar Infarcts:* Sixty-eight–year–old male with progressive dementia. *A,* CT scan demonstrates a small area of lucency in the region of the anterior portion of the left basal ganglia on the left side (*arrow*). No other areas were identified on the CT scan.

B, MR, SE TR2120/TE60 reveals multiple oval areas of increased signal intensity consistent with multiple lacunar infarcts (*arrows*).

C, MR, SE TR2120/TE120 reveals the lacunar infarct in the left putamen (*arrow*) that was identified on the CT scan. The MR scan has increased sensitivity as compared to CT in identifying these abnormalities.

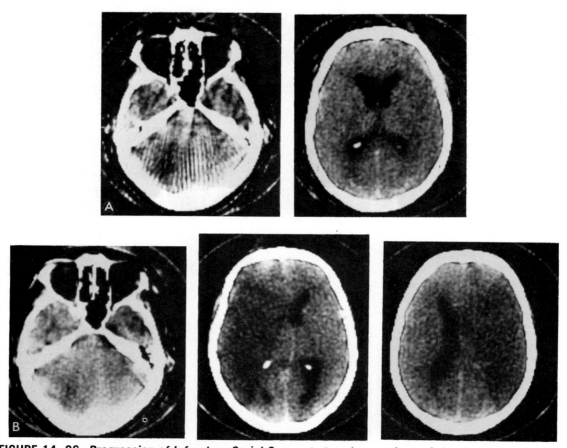

FIGURE 14–26. *Progression of Infarct on Serial Scans: A,* Initial scans obtained shortly after the onset of hemiparesis demonstrate an area of radiolucency in the right cerebellum. This probably is an infarct, although the lateral ventricles are mildly enlarged. The cerebral hemispheres are of normal density and are symmetrical.

B, The second scan, obtained two days later, reveals a large area of lucency now involving almost the entire left hemisphere. There is also mass effect, with shift of the midline to the contralateral side and obliteration of the body of the left lateral ventricle. The area of infarction is again seen in the right cerebellum. The findings are consistent with an acute infarct in the left cerebral hemisphere with mass effect.

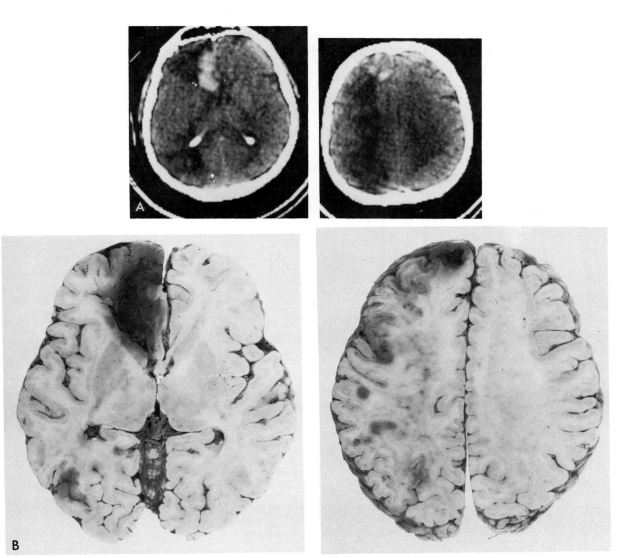

FIGURE 14–27. *Hemorrhagic Infarct:* A, The CT scan shows a hemorrhagic infarct in the distribution of the left anterior cerebral artery surrounded by an area of radiolucency secondary to edema or a surrounding bland infarct. In addition, there are scattered areas of lucency throughout the entire left hemisphere. There is a slight shift of the frontal horns to the right side.

B, The pathologic specimens demonstrated the left frontal hemorrhagic infarct and also small focal areas of hemorrhage throughout the left hemisphere, which presumably developed after the CT scan was obtained. Note the excellent correlation between the CT views and the appearance of the hemorrhage in the pathologic specimen (viewed from above).

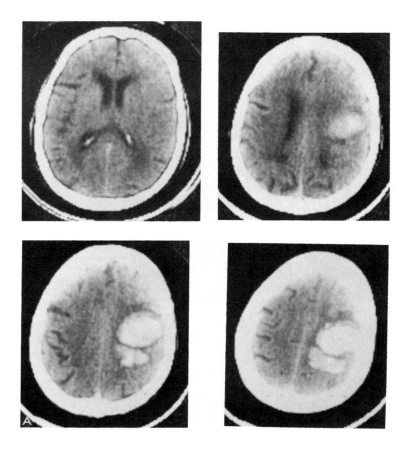

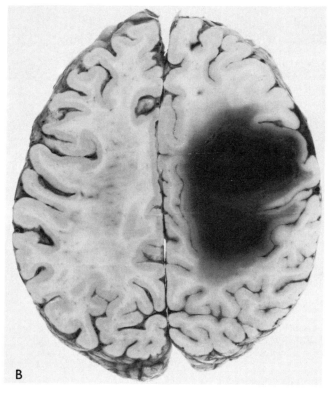

FIGURE 14–28. Hemorrhagic Infarct: *A,* A large bilobed area of hemorrhage is present in the distribution of the right middle cerebral artery. There is only minimal mass effect with mild compression of the body of the right lateral ventricle; there is focal obliteration of the cortical sulci. Although mild mass effect can be seen, there is much less than one would anticipate with an intracerebral hematoma. The findings are most consistent with a hemorrhagic infarct.

B, The pathologic specimen correlated well with the CT appearance (viewed from above).

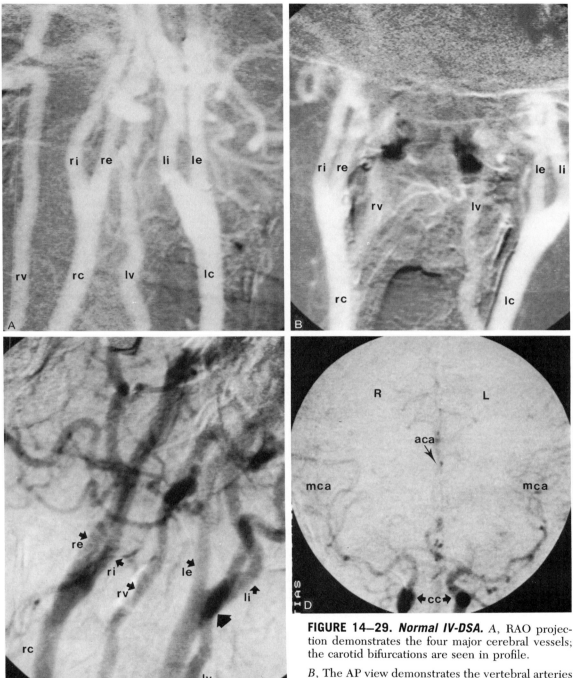

FIGURE 14–29. Normal IV-DSA. A, RAO projection demonstrates the four major cerebral vessels; the carotid bifurcations are seen in profile.

B, The AP view demonstrates the vertebral arteries medial to the carotids, the bifurcations are well seen, and the internal carotid arteries course lateral to the external carotid arteries, the usual anatomic relationship.

C, LAO projection demonstrates that there is overlap of the right internal and external carotid arteries, and the left internal carotid artery overlaps the left external carotid artery (*large arrow*).

D, The AP intracranial view demonstrates the cavernous carotid arteries and their intracranial branches very nicely.

rv	right vertebral artery.	cc	cavernous carotid: L left; R right.	ri	right internal.
rc	right common carotid artery.	mca	middle cerebral artery.	re	right external.
lv	left vertebral artery.	aca	anterior cerebral artery.	li	left internal.
lc	left common carotid artery.			le	left external.

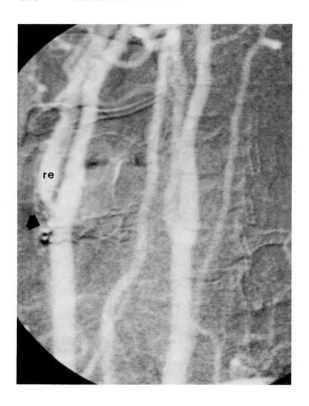

FIGURE 14–30. *External Carotid Stenosis:* Fifty-seven–year–old male with asymptomatic carotid bruit. The LAO projection of DSA reveals an approximately 60 per cent stenosis of the external carotid artery at its origin. This noncritical stenosis is the cause of the patient's bruit and therefore does not require further evaluation. The calcified cricoid cartilage causes a misregistration artifact and cannot be totally subtracted from the image (*arrow*).

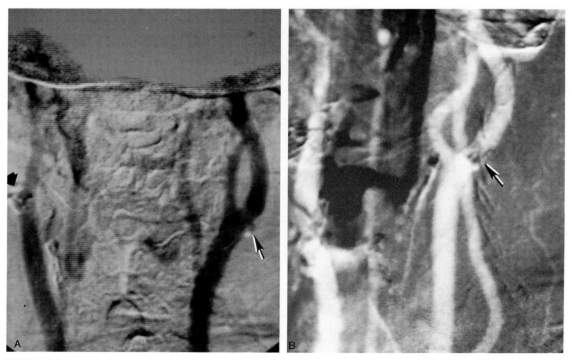

FIGURE 14–31. *Occluded RICA:* *A*, AP view demonstrates a calcified plaque and total occlusion of the right internal carotid artery at its origin (*arrow*). There is a calcified plaque at the origin of the left internal carotid (*long arrow*) that is along the lateral wall of the left internal carotid artery and creates a misregistration artifact on the LAO view (*B*), causing the mistaken appearance that there is a marked stenosis of the LICA. LAO projection reveals swallowing and motion artifact that obscures the right carotid system.

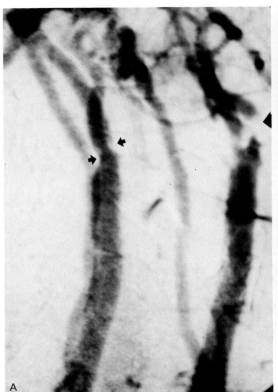

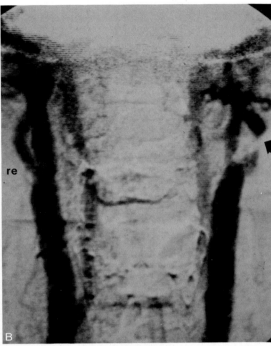

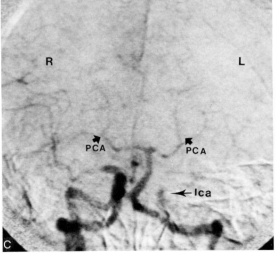

FIGURE 14–32. *Threadlike Patency of LICA:* A, RAO demonstrates overlap of the RICA and the RECA; although small plaques are identified (*arrowheads*), the exact extent of stenosis cannot be evaluated with certainty. At the level of the left carotid bifurcation, the origin of the left internal carotid artery can be seen; the internal carotid is visualized distal to what must be an area of threadlike patency (*arrow*).

B, AP view better demonstrates the threadlike patency, the mild stenosis of the external carotid (*arrow*), and the right carotid bifurcation with the anatomic variation that the external carotid artery rests lateral to the internal carotid artery. No significant stenosis of the right carotid system is seen in this view.

C, The intracranial series demonstrates that the right carotid, right vertebral, and left vertebral artery systems are well filled, but there is only slow filling of the left internal carotid artery system (*lca*), which reflects the marked stenosis of the left internal carotid artery system and results in delayed filling of the intracranial carotid artery. The posterior cerebral arteries (*PCA*) are visualized bilaterally as the terminal bifurcation of the basilar artery.

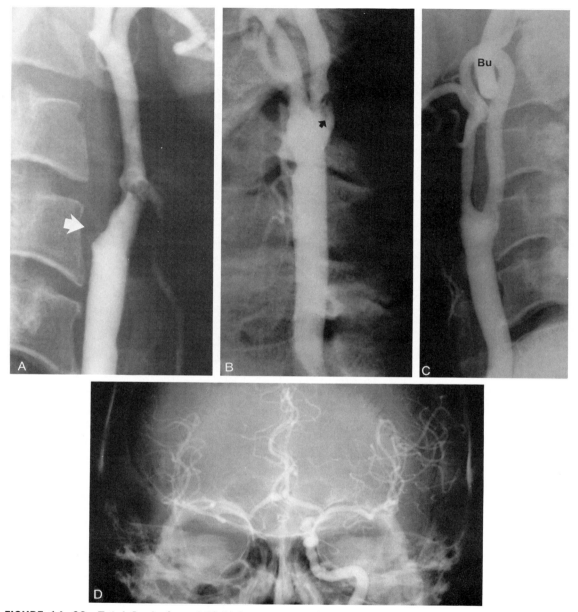

FIGURE 14–33. *Total Occlusion of Right Internal Carotid Artery: A,* Lateral view of the right common carotid angiogram reveals total occlusion of the right internal carotid artery at its origin (*white arrow*).

B and *C,* AP and lateral views of the left carotid angiogram reveal an ulcerated plaque at the origin of the left internal carotid artery—note that the ulcer (*arrow*) is demonstrated only in the AP view. The lateral view also reveals a large loop or buckle in the left internal carotid artery (*Bu*).

D, AP intracranial view demonstrates extensive filling of the right internal carotid artery system from the left common carotid injection secondary to flow via the anterior communicating artery. This type of shallow ulceration may be missed with examination by IV-DSA.

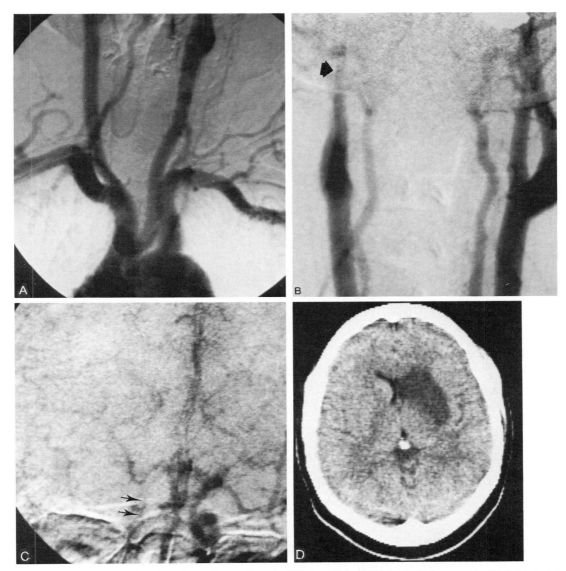

FIGURE 14–34. *Basal Ganglia Infarct Secondary to ICA Occlusion, Etiology Unknown:* A, IV-DSA in LAO projection reveals good filling of the great vessels arising from the aorta.

B, The AP neck view reveals that the RICA tapers to occlusion (*arrow*).

C, The intracranial view reveals no contrast in the anticipated position of the cavernous right internal carotid (*arrows*). On later images (not shown) the middle cerebral artery vessels on the right side were noted to fill in a retrograde fashion via collaterals from the anterior cerebral artery.

D, The CT scan demonstrates an area of lucency in the distribution of lenticulostriate arteries. The infarct is acute and therefore demonstrates mass effect with compression of the frontal horn of the ipsilateral lateral ventricle and shift of the third ventricle to the contralateral side.

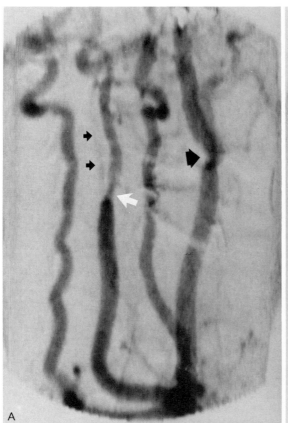

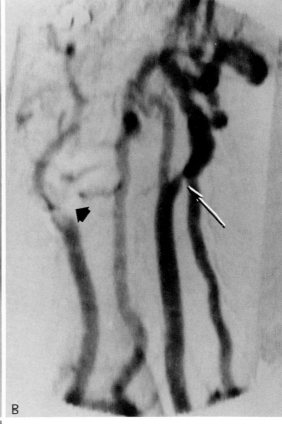

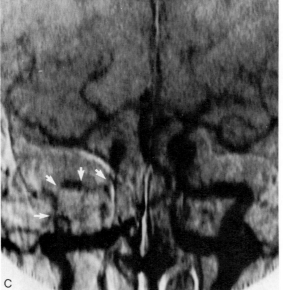

FIGURE 14–35. *Pseudo-threadlike Patency of the Right Internal Carotid Artery:* A, RAO projection demonstrates narrowing of the right external carotid artery at its origin (*white arrow*), and what appears to be a threadlike patency of the right internal carotid artery (*small black arrowheads*). There is also a 70 per cent stenosis of the left internal carotid artery at its origin (*black arrow*), which is better seen in *B*.

B, The LAO projection demonstrates the stenosis of the left internal carotid artery (*black and white arrow*) and fails to demonstrate the right internal carotid artery at its origin (*black arrowhead*).

C, The intracranial study demonstrates filling of the narrowed petrous and cavernous portions of the right internal carotid artery (*white arrows*).

Illustration continued on the opposite page

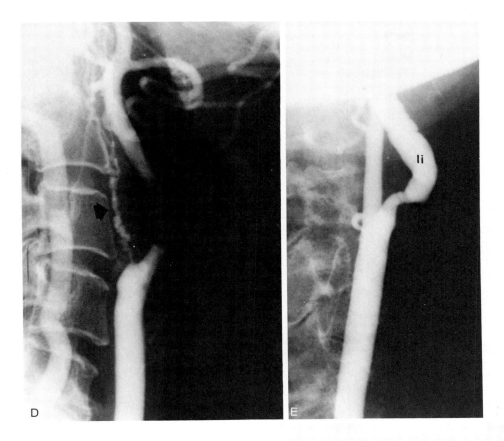

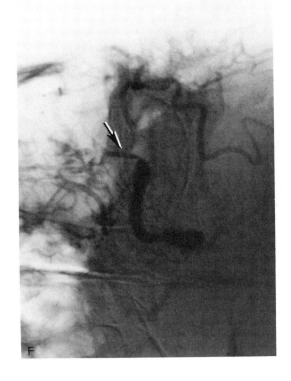

FIGURE 14–35 *Continued.*

D, Standard right carotid angiogram demonstrates that there is actually total occlusion of the right internal carotid artery at its origin and enlargement of the ascending pharyngeal artery (*arrow*). The right vertebral artery fills from contrast flowing retrograde from the right carotid artery.

E, Standard left carotid angiogram demonstrates 70 per cent stenosis of the left internal carotid (*li*) which is maximal approximately 1 cm distal to its origin and extends over 1.5 cm.

F, The intracranial series of the right common carotid angiogram reveals that the petrous portion of the right internal carotid artery actually fills via collateral vessels from the ascending pharyngeal and the right external carotid artery (*arrow*). This is an unusual pattern of collateral circulation and mimics a threadlike patency of the right internal carotid artery. Routine angiography usually requires filming over a prolonged period of time, such as one film per second for a total of 12 seconds, to identify the exact pattern of collateral flow.

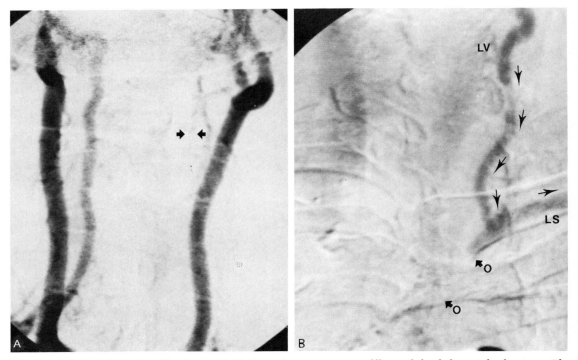

FIGURE 14–36. *Subclavian Steal: A*, AP IV-DSA demonstrates no filling of the left vertebral artery. The anticipated position of the left vertebral artery in the foramina transversaria is between the arrows.

B, Late in the filming series there is filling of the left vertebral artery in a retrograde fashion (*arrows*), which also fills the left subclavian artery (*LS*). The left subclavian artery is occluded (*O-O*) from its origin at the aortic arch to approximately 1.5 cm proximal to the origin of the left vertebral artery.

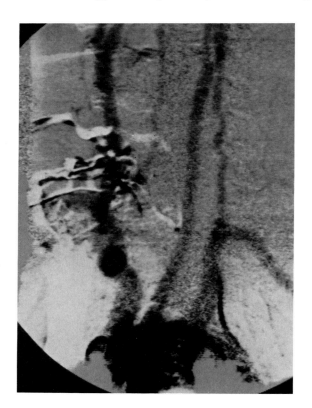

FIGURE 14–37. *IV-DSA with Peripheral Injection:* RPO view of the arch and great vessels with peripheral injection of contrast demonstrates filling of multiple small veins on the right side which obscure the midportion of the right common carotid artery. Jugular reflux may obscure the region of the bifurcations. If the peripheral injection is from the left arm, the aortic arch and origins of the great vessels are frequently obscured by contrast in multiple small veins.

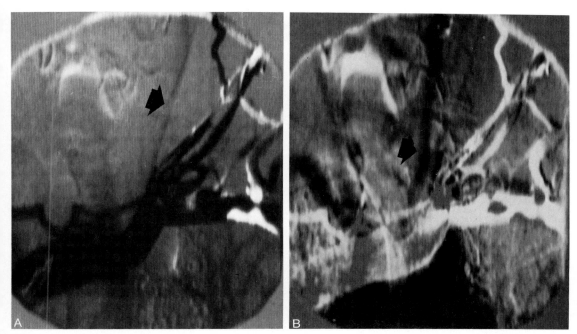

FIGURE 14–38. *IV-DSA with Peripheral Injection:* Contrast material is injected via a short catheter in a left antecubital vein. The arch of the aorta and the origins of the great vessels are obscured by the contrast material in the subclavian vein and multiple small branches. There is also retrograde flow into the left internal jugular vein (*arrow* in A). Later in the film series (*B*), the aortic arch is seen below the subclavian vein, but the origins of the great vessels continue to be obscured by contrast. The left carotid artery is poorly visualized (*arrow* in B).

Although peripheral injection is often satisfactory, central injection results in better visualization and a better bolus of contrast material.

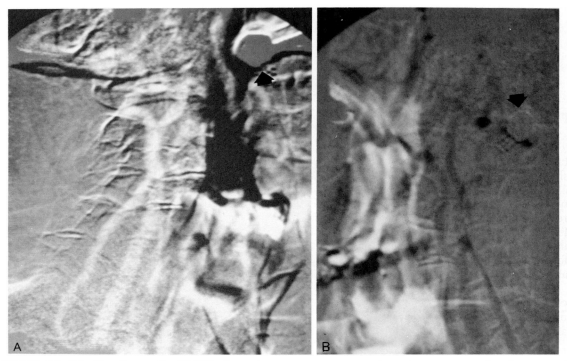

FIGURE 14–39. *Nondiagnostic IV-DSA:* Several views were attempted in this patient with a hearing aid (*arrow*), but in spite of coaching and multiple attempts the study is nondiagnostic because of poor patient cooperation and motion artifact. Whenever it is anticipated that an IV-DSA will be unsuccessful, it should not be performed. This is true whether there is poor cardiac output, inability of the patient to cooperate because of confusion, or any other reason.

15

DISORDERS OF THE SPINE AND MYELOGRAPHY

PLAIN FILM EXAMINATION

Before any myelographic procedure is undertaken, routine radiographs of the area of interest should be obtained and reviewed. Any number of disease processes may simulate those that ultimately require a myelogram, and for this reason it is important to be aware of the plain film findings. A thorough understanding of normal findings on a plain film provides the basis for identification and interpretation of any variations from normal.

In this chapter, the initial discussion is concerned with the lumbar region; the cervical and dorsal spine will be discussed later. The standard radiographic projections in the lumbar area are the anteroposterior, lateral, oblique, lateral spot of the L_5–S_1 disc space, and an additional view of L_5–S_1 space obtained in the anteroposterior view with cephalad angulation of the tube for a better view of the disc space.

The Anteroposterior View

The AP view of the entire lumbar spine (Fig. 15–1, p. 704) should be examined for alterations in vertebral body height. Certain conditions will enlarge the vertebral body or bodies; others will lead to loss of vertebral body height. Any alteration in the general contour of the vertebrae should be noted. Normally there are five lumbar vertebral bodies. Alterations in the number of vertebrae—more or fewer than five—should also be noted.

To determine the exact distribution of the vertebral bodies, it is necessary to radiograph and count the vertebral bodies in the various portions of the entire spine. In practice, the presence of six lumbar-type vertebral bodies is considered "lumbarization" of the S_1 vertebral body; the presence of four lumbar vertebral bodies is considered "sacralization" of the L_5 vertebral body.

When unilateral articulation of the lowest vertebral body with the sacrum is found, this vertebra is considered to be a "transitional segment." Also, bilateral articulation of the vertebral body at the lowest level with the sacrum is considered to be a more stable situation than unilateral articulation. This is true even when an increase or decrease in the number of vertebral bodies is seen.

A herniated nucleus pulposus (HNP) may occur at the discs between normally segmented vertebrae and between the sacrum and a transitional vertebra that articulates unilaterally. HNP does not occur between a "sacralized" vertebral body and the sacrum because the disc is hypoplastic and no motion occurs at this level.

Congenital alterations of the vertebral bodies or spinous processes may be present. Particular note should be made of spina bifida, more marked spinal dysraphia, and hemivertebrae.

The Lateral View

The lateral view (Figs. 15–2 to 15–5, pp. 705 to 708) reveals changes in vertebral body height and in the general configuration of the bone.

In addition, it affords the best view of the height of the disc spaces. Because the mechanics of positioning for radiography in the lateral view create a mild scoliosis of the spine, the lateral spot film of the L_5 disc space is angled to allow for optimal visualization of the disc space at the L_5–S_1 level. There may normally be some narrowing of the posterior aspect of the disc at the L_5–S_1 level.

A spondylolysis, or abnormal break in the pars interarticularis, can be identified on the lateral view but usually is better seen on the oblique view.

The Oblique Views

Oblique views are obtained with the patient in the prone position. It is easier for the patient to maintain the routine radiographic positions while prone rather than supine. The films are then marked so that when the right side is most dependent (RAO = right anterior oblique) the anatomic right side is marked with an "R." When the left side is most dependent (LAO = left anterior oblique), the anatomic left side is marked with an "L" marker. It is important to understand this convention, because with this positioning the pars interarticularis is viewed through the vertebral body. Consequently, in the RAO position the **left** pars interarticularis is actually displayed. Similarly, in the LAO position the **right** pars interarticularis is viewed. The oblique view best demonstrates the pars interarticularis (Fig. 15–7, p. 710). This view allows excellent visualization of the superior and inferior articulating facets and their points of articulation.

The combination of these anatomic parts and the images of the transverse processes and lamina of the spine have the appearance of a "Scottie dog" (Figs. 15–7 and 15–8, pp. 710 and 711). The neck of the dog is the pars interarticularis. A "break" in the pars interarticularis is termed *spondylolysis*. If spondylolysis is present, it appears radiographically as if the "Scottie" were wearing a collar (Fig. 15–8, p. 711). Spondylolysis may be congenital or acquired.

Areas of spondylolysis may be identified on both the AP and lateral views (Fig. 15–6, p. 709) of the spine but are best visualized on the oblique radiograph. Spondylolysis commonly leads to instability of the spine at this level and may result in forward displacement of one vertebral body on another. This displacement is termed **spondylolisthesis** (Fig. 15–9, p. 712).

Displacement of the upper vertebral body posterior to the lower vertebral bodies is considered a **reverse spondylolisthesis**.

Spondylolisthesis may also occur secondary to degenerative changes and joint space narrowing at the level of the articulation between the superior and inferior articulating facets. In this case, forward displacement of one vertebral body relative to another may occur without spondylolysis.

Conditions Demonstrated by Plain Film Examination

Vacuum Disc. Degeneration of a disc may lead to disc space narrowing with the accumulation of gas within the disc (Fig. 15–10, p. 712).

Postoperative Changes in the Spine. Plain spine radiographs reveal changes that correlate with the surgical procedure. There may be evidence of a partial or complete laminectomy, with or without bony fusion in the lumbar spine.

Hemangioma. Involvement with hemangioma causes an increase in the trabecular pattern within the vertebral body (Fig. 15–11, p. 713). These changes vary in size and may involve all or only a small portion of the vertebral body.

Lumbar Spinal Stenosis. Patients may have a congenitally small spinal canal. However, the acquired form of spinal stenosis is also of clinical importance. The diagnosis may be suspected on plain spine radiographs or by CT examination of the spine. In the presence of a congenitally small subarachnoid space, superimposed disc disease may cause a patient to become symptomatic, whereas similar changes in a patient with a large subarachnoid space may not cause symptoms. Acquired spinal stenosis may result from a spondylolisthesis, in which the posterior elements are displaced forward and impinge upon the posterior aspect of the subarachnoid space, or from hypertrophic degenerative changes associated with hypertrophy of the ligamentum flavum (Fig. 15–55, p. 749).

The following spine films illustrate a variety of diseases that can be diagnosed by plain film examination, CT, and magnetic resonance imaging.

Paget's Disease

Paget's disease (Fig. 15–12, p. 714) exhibits an increase in vertical trabeculation that involves the entire vertebral body. Although it may be monostotic, several vertebrae usually are involved. The vertebral body in Paget's disease is more dense than in hemangioma and often has a dense outer margin, giving the vertebral body a "picture-window" appearance. The vertebral body usually is enlarged as well. Paget's disease usually spares the pedicle.

Metastatic carcinoma of the prostate or breast may be considered in the differential diagnosis, but usually it does not demonstrate an increased trabecular pattern. Examination of the other bony structures will help to differentiate between the two entities. Metastatic carcinoma of the prostate—of course seen only in men—demonstrates patchy areas of osteoblastic metastatic disease, whereas Paget's disease causes an increase in the bony trabeculae in the other bones. Frequently a sclerosis of the pelvic inlet occurs in Paget's disease, and this often can be seen on routine views of the lumbar spine, helping to differentiate between the two entities.

The enlarged vertebral body of Paget's disease may completely block the flow of contrast material on myelography. The block has an extradural configuration.

Multiple Myeloma

There may be a number of small osteolytic areas, or the multiple myeloma (Fig. 15–21, p. 720) may present as diffuse osteoporosis of all the visualized bony structures. There may be multiple compression deformities of the vertebral bodies. Multiple myeloma tends to "spare" the pedicles, whereas other types of osteolytic metastatic processes usually involve the pedicles. The actual diagnosis of multiple myeloma depends on confirmatory laboratory data.

Metastatic Disease

Metastatic disease (Figs. 15–13 to 15–25, pp. 715 to 722) may be either osteolytic or osteoblastic. It may involve only a single vertebral body but usually affects multiple vertebral body segments. Because the pedicle is the most vascular portion of the vertebral body, it usually is involved early with blood-borne metastases. Metastatic disease may lead to compression deformities of the vertebral bodies; not uncommonly, it leads to the clinical syndrome of spinal cord compression, which may be seen with bony metastases or with soft tissue metastatic deposits in the absence of bony abnormalities.

Osteopetrosis

The bones, including the spine, may exhibit a "bone-within-a-bone" appearance. The increased volume of bone may cause encroachment upon the spinal canal and the foramina of the base of the skull. Encroachment upon the optic foramina may lead to blindness (Fig. 15–26, p. 722).

Enlarged Spinal Canal

In chronic obstructive hydrocephalus (Fig. 15–27, p. 723), abnormal scalloping of the backs of the vertebral bodies may occur secondary to transmission of increased intracranial pressure down the spinal canal. This is a relatively rare finding, although subtle changes may be found on close examination of the plain films of the spine. Other processes that may lead to scalloping of the posterior margin of the vertebral bodies and enlargement of the spinal canal are dural ectasia of neurofibromatosis in the absence of individual neurofibromas, multiple individual neurofibromas, achondroplasia, spinal arachnoid cysts, spinal lipomas, teratomas, astrocytomas, syringohydromyelia, and ependymomas.

Hemivertebrae

In this anomaly, one half of the vertebral body fails to develop because of lack of ossification of one lateral cartilaginous center. An isolated hemivertebra may be present and associated with an acute scoliosis. Most commonly, multiple anomalies are seen; these frequently involve several vertebral bodies and may have a counterbalancing effect. In addition, there may be more severe associated problems, such as spinal dysraphic states sometimes associated with meningocele or meningomyelocele.

NORMAL ANATOMY OF THE SPINAL CORD

The spinal cord ends, in the majority of cases, at the lower end-plate of the first or superior end-plate of the second lumbar vertebra. The cord is held by the filum terminale, which normally measures no wider than 2 mm and extends caudad from the spinal cord to the lumbar cul-de-sac. The normal cervical enlargement extends from C_3 to T_3. The lumbar enlargement, or conus medullaris, occurs from T_9

to T_{12}, where the cord tapers rapidly. The cord then branches into multiple nerve roots—the cauda equina—which exit at successive levels. The lumbar cul-de-sac ends at the mid-body of S_1 in most cases, but may end higher or lower than this. The spinal cord is sensitive to pressure damage, and compression of a few hours may create irreversible neurologic changes in the cord. Consequently, if spinal cord compression is suspected, rapid diagnosis and treatment are strongly suggested.

MYELOGRAPHY

Myelography (Gr. *myelos* = marrow, medulla; *graphe* = a drawing) is the radiographic visualization or photography of the spinal cord after the injection of a radiopaque substance into the spinal subarachnoid space. This definition of myelography suggests only a small amount of the information that actually can be gained from a myelogram. In a patient with back pain or progressive neurologic signs, demonstration of the various disease processes that affect the spinal cord is necessary for correct diagnosis and proper treatment planning.

The spinal nerves do not originate from the spinal cord at the level at which they exit the bony spinal column. This is because the cord does not continue to grow with growth of the bony spinal column but is drawn upward in the canal, leaving the nerves to exit at their proper level even though the actual level of origin of the nerve root is much higher. One should remember that a spinal cord lesion at the T_{10} level in the bony spinal column corresponds to the clinical, neurologic, and dermatome level of the umbilicus (Fig. 15–39, p. 733). With this in mind, the anatomic location of the lesion causing the patient's signs and symptoms can be roughly ascertained by moving up or down from the level of the umbilicus, or T_{10} level.

Because of the possibility of multiple lesions and because of varying biologic responses, the exact anatomic location often cannot be demonstrated by physical examination. Therefore, myelography is necessary for more accurate evaluation. Before myelography is performed, it is essential to obtain and review plain films of the areas to be studied. Review of the plain films is vital, because one must be able to account for and correlate with the plain film findings any defects seen on the myelogram. In addition, after the instillation of contrast material, bony abnormalities may be partially or totally obscured by the contrast medium. This is of particular importance in the cervical area, where one must decide whether a defect is secondary to a bone spur, to a damaged cervical disc, or to a combination of the two. In addition, one must always be alert for the possibility of metastatic carcinoma or a congenital abnormality. Evidence for metastatic disease to the bony structures or soft tissues may well alter one's approach to the myelographic study.

Contrast Materials

Through the years a variety of contrast materials have been used to outline the spinal cord and subarachnoid space. Among these are the following:

Air

Dandy reported the use of air for myelography in the 1920's, and air is still in use today as a contrast material for the study of the spinal cord. The use of air causes no long-term complications. The patient experiences some discomfort at the time of the examination but otherwise tolerates the procedure well. Air may be difficult to visualize—even with good patient positioning—and tomography is required in most cases for excellent delineation of the abnormality. In general, air myelography is not now a widely used technique, and the introduction of Amipaque and magnetic resonance has further decreased its use.

Pantopaque (Iophendylate)

Pantopaque, which was originally introduced in 1940, was a widely accepted and commonly used myelographic contrast material. It is an ester-based material with firmly bound iodine. Idiosyncratic reactions have been reported, but patients with a history of allergic reactions to intravenous iodinated contrast agents do not develop reactions to subarachnoid Pantopaque. Pantopaque is absorbed from the subarachnoid space at a rate of approximately 1 cc per year. Rarely, Pantopaque may produce arachnoiditis, which may be aggravated by surgery. Arachnoiditis is more likely to occur when the Pantopaque is mixed with blood in the subarachnoid space, and therefore Pantopaque should not be used when the CSF is bloody. When the myelographic procedure is completed, the contrast material should be removed from the subarachnoid space if at all possible. At our institution, Pantopaque has not been used since 1979.

Metrizamide (Amipaque)

In 1978 a new contrast material, metrizamide (Amipaque, Winthrop-Breon), became available for use in myelography. Amipaque is water soluble but is unique when compared to previously available materials. Earlier water-soluble contrast materials were ionic compounds, whereas Amipaque is a nonionic, molecular solution. This characteristic makes allergic reactions far less likely. Patients who have been allergic to intravenous contrast material do not react to Amipaque. The water-soluble compound is resorbed from the CSF and excreted by the kidneys, with approximately 75 per cent removed after 24 hours. Therefore, Amipaque need not be removed from the subarachnoid space. At the time of this writing, no **clinically significant** cases of arachnoiditis have been reported following the use of Amipaque. It has low neurotoxicity, but grand mal seizures may develop if the intracranial contents are flooded with Amipaque.

As an added benefit, this contrast material is of significant help in diagnosis when used in conjunction with CT scanning of the spine and the intracranial structures.

Amipaque is packaged as a crystalline material that is reconstituted just before injection. The solution is mixed in a concentration appropriate to each individual patient (see below). Amipaque is light-sensitive and is stable for 12 hours after reconstitution.

Iohexol

Iohexol (Omnipaque, Winthrop-Breon) is a nonionic, stable, aqueous radiopaque contrast medium that was introduced in 1986 for intravascular as well as intrathecal use. As with Amipaque, Omnipaque should not be allowed to enter the cranial vault in large quantities, as generalized motor seizures may result. A total dose of 3060 mg of iodine, or a concentration of 240 mg I/ml, should not be exceeded in a single myelographic examination.

The usual recommended total doses for lumbar and thoracic myelography are 1.70 to 3.06 gm of iodine:

Omnipaque 180 (180 mg I/ml) 10 to 17 ml; 1.8 to 3.06 gm I
Omnipaque 240 (240 mg I/ml) 7 to 12.5 ml; 1.7 to 3.00 gm I

The patient should remain in the 30-degree head-up position and under close observation for 12 hours following the procedure.

At the time of this writing, Omnipaque is approved for use in lumbar and thoracic myelography, but not for cervical myelography.

Iopamidol

Iopamidol (Isovue-M, Squibb Diagnostics) is a nonionic, stable, aqueous, radiopaque contrast medium that was introduced in 1986 for use as both an intravascular and an intrathecal contrast agent. As with Amipaque, the contrast material should not be allowed to enter intracranially in large amounts, because iopamidol has been reported to cause generalized motor seizures. The reader is referred to the package insert for further information. A total dose in excess of 4500 mg iodine, and iopamidol formulated to contain more than 300 mg I/ml should *not* be used intrathecally. Isovue-M is approved for use with cervical, thoracic, and lumbar myelography. The adult dosage schedule listed in the insert is as follows:

Dosage Table for Iopamidol (Isovue-M)

Procedure	Concentration of Solution (mg I/ml)	Usual Recommended Dose (ml)
Lumbar myelogram	200	10 to 15
Thoracic myelogram	200	10 to 15
Cervical myelogram (via lumbar injection)	200 or 300	10 to 15
Cervical myelogram (via lateral cervical injection)	200	10
Total columnar myelography	300	10
CT cisternography (via lumbar injection)	200	4 to 6

Postmyelography orders are similar to those recommended with Amipaque. Specifically the head should be elevated for the first 12 to 24 hours following myelography and the patient should remain under close observation for the first 24 hours.

Indications

Myelograms are performed for a variety of reasons. Most often patients undergoing myelography suffer from either acute or chronic back pain and are referred for myelography to rule out the presence of a herniated nucleus pulposus (HNP, "ruptured disc"). Other patients suffer from multiple sclerosis but have atypical symptoms that require a contrast study to rule out another disease process or a surgically treatable lesion. Metastatic disease often involves both the bony spine and the spinal cord. A syringohydromyelia may involve the lumbar, thoracic, or cervical spine. Meningioma and neurofibroma are other possible causes of back pain. Primary spinal cord tumors, such as ependymomas and astrocytomas, as well as intramedullary metastases are also seen. Arteriovenous malformations that involve the spinal cord also occur. The patient's symptoms may sometimes help in differentiating one lesion from another but in many cases are not helpful.

Classes of Lesions

Three major classes of lesions are seen at myelography (Fig. 15–28, p. 724). The more common types of abnormalities are listed below; however, many other less common lesions may be seen.

1. Extradural lesions
   A. Herniated disc
   B. Metastases
   C. Postoperative change
   D. Neurofibroma (may also be intradural)
   E. Hematoma
   F. Spondylosis
   G. Epidural abscess
   H. Paget's disease or other vertebral body processes such as hemangioma, myeloma, chondroma

2. Intradural lesions
   A. Neurofibroma
   B. Meningioma
   C. Metastases—"seeding"
   D. Arachnoid cyst
   E. Dermoid
   F. Ependymoma
   G. Lipoma

3. Intramedullary lesions
   A. Ependymoma (most common)
   B. Astrocytoma
   C. Syringohydromyelia
   D. Dermoid
   E. Hematoma or swollen cord

4. Miscellaneous lesions
   A. Spinal cord arteriovenous malformations
   B. Epidermoid cyst secondary to multiple spinal taps

Should any of these lesions reach such a size that it completely blocks the flow of contrast, the typical myelographic appearance may be lost. Obviously myelography can no longer be relied upon for exact diagnosis in such patients.

Patient Preparation

Before the myelographic study, it is helpful if the individual who is to perform it greets the patient at the bedside and discusses the procedure in some detail. Patients are much more cooperative if they understand what the goals of the study will be. In addition, acquaintance with the procedure relieves much of the fear of the unknown, helping the patient to be more relaxed. Not uncommonly, patients have the misconception that a myelogram can lead to lower extremity paralysis. It should be emphasized that patients with neurologic problems often have myelographic procedures, but that the myelographic procedure itself does not lead to paralysis or neurologic difficulty. In addition, I have found it helpful if the patient is told in some detail about the steps that precede the myelogram.

Patients should be told (1) whether or not they will receive premedication before the study; (2) that they will be sent to the radiology department on a cart; (3) that they should empty their bladder before leaving for the study; and (4) that they should take nothing by mouth before the study. This is to avoid aspiration of gastric contents should nausea and emesis develop during the procedure. However, patients having myelograms with water-soluble contrast material should be well-hydrated and may be given fluids either by mouth or intravenously.

It is reassuring to the patient to be told that he will be met in the department of radiology by the physician performing the study. Telling the patient that the contrast is heavier (or lighter, in the case of air myelography) than cerebrospinal fluid and that manipulation of the radiography table will be done in order to allow the contrast to flow to the areas of interest allows the patient to understand and tolerate better the sometimes uncomfortable positions that must be assumed and held for certain periods of time. The patient also should be informed that he will be requested to remain flat in bed for 8 hours following a Pantopaque myelogram and to sit up at a 30- to 45-degree angle for 12 hours following a myelogram with water-soluble contrast. Then he must rest in bed for an additional 12 hours.

Outpatient Myelography

Myelography can be safely performed on an outpatient basis. Usually the patient requires no premedication, and the examination is performed in the standard fashion. The contrast material can be removed from the subarachnoid space at the end of the examination. These patients should be accompanied by another individual who can be responsible for the patient's care. The companion can also report any adverse reaction to the contrast material.

Typical Premyelogram Orders

1. Nothing by mouth on day of procedure (except that patients having myelograms with water-soluble contrast material should be well hydrated either orally or intravenously)
2. 100 mg Nembutal IM on call to radiology
3. 0.4 mg atropine IM on call to radiology
4. Have patient void before coming to radiology
5. Sign consent

Typical Postmyelogram Orders Following Pantopaque Myelography

1. Flat in bed for 8 hours
2. Bed rest for 24 hours
3. Cerebrospinal fluid to be sent for routine and special studies
4. Push oral fluids
5. Resume previous diet
6. Vital signs every 2 hours, then per routine

Typical Postmyelogram Orders Following Myelography with Water-Soluble Contrast Material

1. Patient to sit up at 30- to 45-degree angle for 12 hours; then sitting or flat for an additional 12 hours
2. Push oral fluids
3. Vital signs every 30 minutes for 2 hours, every 60 minutes for 2 hours, and every 3 hours for 24 hours
4. Resume previous diet
5. Cerebrospinal fluid to be sent for routine and special studies

Needles

Many different types of needles are available for myelography. A 22-gauge, short beveled needle is recommended for water-soluble contrast material.

It should be emphasized that meticulous technique is important when performing myelography. In addition to precise needle puncture technique, which of course greatly facilitates the performance of the myelogram, rigorous attention to detail is desirable throughout the procedure. Sterile technique should be used throughout. At the time of instillation of contrast material, it is necessary to fill the plastic tubing and syringe full of contrast without allowing any air bubbles to form in the system. If this is not done, small amounts of air will enter the subarachnoid space at the time of contrast instillation. In fact, with fluoroscopic control, one can occasionally see a small amount of air rise upward while the contrast flows to the dependent portion of the canal. This air, even though small in amount, may be one reason for the vasovagal response that may develop early in the course of study. (A similar reaction is also seen during pneumoencephalography.) However, even before the procedure is begun, some patients develop a vasovagal reaction with diaphoresis, nausea, hypotension, and vomiting. If these reactions occur, it is wise to interrupt the procedure, start an IV solution of dextrose and saline, and wait until the patient stabilizes before continuing the examination.

Technique of Myelography

In our department, lumbar puncture is performed with the patient in the prone position. A pillow is placed under the abdomen in order to round the back and allow for easier needle placement between the spinous processes. Several types of prepackaged and presterilized myelogram trays are available commercially, or a specific tray set-up can be made.

Needle placement is always performed under fluoroscopic control. If we are interested in the lumbar area, puncture is performed in the midline at the L_2–L_3 interspace, unless, of course, this is the level of interest. In this way, since disc disease is most common in the lower lumbar area, we will avoid the levels most likely to be involved. We use one of two approaches for the initial lumbar tap. If a *midline* lumbar puncture is to be performed (Fig. 15–29, p. 725), the L_2–L_3 interspace is identified under fluoroscopic control, and local anesthetic is instilled along the needle tract. A generous amount of local anesthetic is recommended to make the procedure as pain-free as possible. Transitional vertebrae will have been identified by preliminary perusal of the plain films; if there is a variation from normal in the number of vertebrae, the first non–rib-bearing vertebral body should be considered the number one lumbar vertebra. The spinous processes angle inferiorly in the lumbar region, and this must be taken into account when performing the puncture. It may be necessary to angle the needle cephalad.

Again, the needle is advanced under fluoroscopic control in the midline until one feels the slight resistance of the ligamentum flavum, followed by the slight resistance of the dura. Entrance is then made into the subarachnoid space. It is best to elevate the patient's head just before puncture of the subarachnoid space to allow hydrostatic pressure to expand the subarachnoid space. As the needle is advanced, but before entering the subarachnoid space, it is wise to remove the inner cannula periodically to check for flow of CSF, as it is not always possible to be sure of the exact moment of entrance into the subarachnoid space. After flow has been established, the patient's head is kept elevated to ensure flow of CSF, and a sample of fluid is collected and sent to the appropriate laboratories for routine study.

For the beginning myelographer, it is wise to obtain a cross-table lateral radiograph both to check for radiographic technique and to be certain that the tip of the needle is well centered in the subarachnoid space.

Oblique Puncture Technique

A second—and in many ways preferable—method of lumbar puncture is the oblique approach (Fig. 15–30, p. 725). When using this method, local anesthetic is placed between the pedicle and the spinous process at the level where lumbar puncture is to be performed. Local anesthetic is then infiltrated along a line directed at the midline and slightly cephalad to the starting point. The puncture needle is then advanced along this oblique line, passing over the lamina of the vertebral body until the "give" of the ligamentum flavum and dura is felt. The needle is then advanced slightly farther until the bevel is well within the subarachnoid space. Again, for the beginning myelographer it is wise to obtain a localization film to check radiographic technique and to confirm the needle position in the lateral projection. This method has the advantage of avoiding any calcified longitudinal ligaments and any midline scarring that may be present from previous surgery. It is also possible to direct the needle tip easily so that when the subarachnoid space is entered the tip is at the mid or upper vertebral body level rather than at the disc space. This is important because the needle placement may result in a "needle defect" that occasionally is difficult to differentiate from an organic defect.

When using the midline puncture technique, the needle often must be directed cephalad, necessitating entrance into the subarachnoid space at the disc space level. This is suboptimal because entrance at this level, if it has resulted in a "needle defect," can mimic the appearance of a defect secondary to a bulging or herniated disc. The needle defect is secondary to the puncture—not an anatomic abnormality. When the needle has entered at the vertebral body level, even if a needle defect occurs, confusion with a disc defect is less likely. Furthermore, when using the oblique technique the only bony structure in the direct line to the subarachnoid space is the lamina of the vertebral body. Merely by directing it slightly cephalad, the needle tip will drop over the lamina and into the subarachnoid space. A detailed study of the anatomic skeleton in addition to radiographs is helpful before undertaking myelographic procedures.

It should be added that when using a sharp, small-caliber needle, the point at which the tip passes through the dura and into the subarachnoid space is less obvious. This is particularly true when a 20- or 22-gauge needle is used for instillation of water-soluble contrast material.

Lumbar Myelography

Following removal of a sample of CSF, usually about 5 to 6 ml, contrast is instilled into the subarachnoid space. Varying amounts of contrast material are used, depending on the level of the spine being studied. In the lumbar region, 9 to 12 ml of contrast is usually adequate to cover the areas of interest. A general rule of thumb is to instill enough contrast to outline two disc spaces very well when the patient is in the upright position. There is a good deal of variation from one patient to the next. Although 6 ml may be all that is needed in one patient, 18 ml might be required in another. These recommended amounts should be used only as guidelines, and in any individual case the amount actually used may vary. Each myelogram should be "tailored" to fit the patient.

In addition to the anatomic variations seen from patient to patient, infrequently arachnoid cysts in the lumbar region will hold several milliliters of contrast material (Fig. 15–36, p. 730). Obviously, these must be filled before one can proceed with the myelogram. I have seen one case in which a small occult lumbar meningocele required the instillation of 18 ml of contrast material to reach the L_5–S_1 level. The recommended amount of water-soluble contrast material should not be exceeded.

Both a standard puncture technique and a standard filming technique should be used for each patient. The resulting myelograms are not only more pleasing esthetically, but there is also less likelihood that a particular area will be inadequately evaluated. Parenthetically, at a future date this also will help to determine whether any films are missing (Fig. 15–37, p. 731).

Suggested routine filming sequence:

1. PA vertical-beam upright and prone films that cover the lower lumbar area.

2. Horizontal-beam lateral films "cross-table lateral" in the upright and prone positions which cover the lower lumbar area.

3. PA 45-degree oblique films with the patient in the upright position (vertical beam) and in the prone RAO and LAO positions (if needed) to cover all areas of interest in the lumbar region.

4. Horizontal-beam RAO and LAO "cross-table" projections with the patient upright and prone as needed. These are also done if the myelogram appears normal or to further substantiate findings noted on other views.

5. PA vertical-beam spot films in the dorsal and cervical areas are also taken while the contrast material is allowed to flow up to the cervical region.

A brief or, if necessary, an extensive examination of the cervical region is suggested in **all** patients with low back pain. A single PA film with the contrast centered in the cervical region may suffice. This dorsal and cervical examination is particularly important if the examination of the lower lumbar region is normal; however, it is also important in others, because the visualized lumbar lesion may not be the actual cause of the patient's clinical problem. The author has seen many patients who have had a recent myelogram limited to the lumbar region—only to have a high thoracic or low cervical lesion demonstrated when a second examination was performed because of persistent or progressive symptoms.

After the myelographic study, the patient is returned to his room on a cart. Following myelography with water-soluble contrast material, the patient should sit up at a 30- to 45-degree angle for 12 hours (see below). After this period, a clinical evaluation must be done to determine how much activity the patient is to be allowed. Also, the patient is advised to drink additional fluids but is otherwise returned to his previous diet.

If there is any question of total or even high-grade block to the flow of contrast material, it is wisest to be very cautious during the procedure. If a block is suspected and a lumbar puncture performed, only one drop of CSF should be removed—and this is only to make certain that the needle is in the subarachnoid space. Then only a small amount of contrast material—1 to 2 ml should be instilled. The contrast is then allowed to flow up to the level of the block, where the site is marked with a lead dot or paper clip to facilitate surgery or radiotherapy. If excessive fluid is removed below the level of a block, a "vacuum" effect may be created which causes further cord compromise secondary to interruption of vascular supply. Worsening of the patient's symptoms may follow, including paraplegia—a neurosurgical emergency.

If no block is encountered, one may then pool the contrast below the level of the needle, remove the desired amount of fluid for routine study, and proceed with the study without fear of complication. If this lumbar puncture technique is followed closely—even in those patients in whom suspicion of block is remote—one will not encounter any grave difficulties secondary to excess CSF removal.

Subdural Injection (Figs. 15–31 and 15–32, pp. 726 and 727)

Because of its bevel, the myelogram needle tip may be only partly in the subarachnoid space and still provide excellent flow of CSF (Fig. 15–31, p. 726). However, when one attempts to instill contrast material, it will be seen that the contrast enters the subdural and epidural spaces before going into the subarachnoid space (Figs. 15–32 to 15–34, pp. 727 to 729). These potential spaces allow easy entrance of contrast even under the gentlest of pressure. At times, some of the contrast will simultaneously enter both the subarachnoid and subdural spaces. This, of course, usually results in an unsatisfactory examination. The study sometimes can be salvaged by advancing the needle deeper into the subarachnoid space and continuing the injection of contrast or by attempting puncture at another level. If an anterior subdural injection has occurred, the needle should be withdrawn slightly and repositioned in the subarachnoid space.

One should also attempt to place the short beveled spinal needle well into the subarachnoid space so that the contrast does not accumulate in the subdural area. It is suggested that rather than slowly inserting the needle, the needle should be advanced using short, 1- to 2-mm "jabs." This technique will pierce the dura and arachnoid rather than merely indent them. The position of the needle tip in the vertebral canal is easily evaluated by lateral fluoroscopy or cross-table lateral radiography. This will accurately localize the needle tip, and adjustments can then be made prior to continuing the myelographic study. This precaution markedly reduces the possibility of subdural injection.

If contrast is injected into the subdural space, it usually will be noted at fluoroscopy that the material collects under the tip of the needle and does not drop readily into the lumbar cul-de-sac (Fig. 15–31, p. 726). The contrast may enter the subdural or epidural space even with apparently adequate needle positioning if the dura has thickened following previous surgery or an inflammatory process. Another possibility is that the tip of the myelographic needle has been dulled by multiple use, and the dura is carried forward rather than punctured by the needle.

The top of the column of contrast material in the subdural space does not oscillate up and down with changes in respiration and the transmitted pulsation of heart beat as does contrast in the subarachnoid space. Also, coughing will cause contrast material in the subarachnoid space to "jump" because of transmitted changes of pressure. When contrast material is in the subdural space, there is usually little or no

fluoroscopic evidence of changes with transmitted pressure differences, or changes may be less pronounced than when the material is in the subarachnoid space. In addition, any contrast material that is in the subdural space will not flow **readily** up to the cervical subarachnoid space.

At times, however, it may be very difficult to identify subdural contrast material. I have witnessed one case in which contrast flowed up to the cervical region without difficulty (Fig. 15–32, p. 727). Lateral views may be helpful for further evaluation and may demonstrate that contrast has accumulated in the subdural space either ventrally or dorsally. With subdural accumulation of the contrast, the spinal cord cannot be visualized.

If an injection of contrast does occur subdurally, removal should be attempted by pooling the material under the tip of the needle and aspirating as much as possible. If the needle cannot be repositioned, the patient may be retapped at another level and the procedure continued. A better approach is to discontinue the examination and attempt it again 10 days to 2 weeks later. In an emergency, the contrast material should be instilled via a C_1–C_2 tap.

Removal of Water-Soluble Contrast Material

Although aspiration of water-soluble contrast material is not necessary, this author recommends removal of a portion of the contrast material at the end of the myelogram. This removal decreases the total contrast load and also allows the patient to have CT evaluation of the spine immediately after the myelogram, whereas a four-hour delay is usually recommended to decrease the contrast load if none is aspirated.

The contrast material is pooled under the tip of the needle using fluoroscopic guidance. Approximately 10 ml of contrast material admixed with CSF is then aspirated from the subarachnoid space.

Technique of Cervical Tap

With lateral fluoroscopy with the patient in the supine or prone position, local anesthesia is administered and the needle is positioned in the posterior portion of the cervical subarachnoid space anterior to the posterior limit of the subarachnoid space (Fig. 15–73, p. 763).

The needle is advanced until the "give" of

the dura is felt and then slightly farther until the tip is well into the cervical subarachnoid space. The needle position can be readily checked by fluoroscopy in the anteroposterior position if desired.

If lateral or biplane fluoroscopy is not available, a C_1–C_2 tap may be performed after the patient is placed in the lateral position with the head level and the chin flexed upon the chest. After instillation of local anesthetic, the spinal needle is again placed in position in the cervical subarachnoid space. When the stylet is removed, CSF will be noted to "well up" into the hub of the needle, even with the patient in a horizontal position. If desired, the patient may be placed in a modified Trendelenburg position to promote flow of CSF. After fluid removal, contrast material may be instilled under fluoroscopic control with the patient in the lateral decubitus position, or the patient may be placed either prone or supine.

If no obstruction is encountered, contrast will accumulate in the lumbar subarachnoid space. We have used this method quite frequently in patients in whom a complete block to flow seems likely. It is especially useful in patients with metastatic disease, in whom outlining the upper border of the lesion is often all that is necessary before treatment.

Cervical Myelography with Amipaque

Amipaque may be used for cervical myelography using the lumbar approach. With this method, a standard lumbar puncture is performed and 10 ml of 250 to 300 mg I/ml is instilled. The contrast is then placed, under fluoroscopic guidance, in the cervical subarachnoid space without further delay. The patient should be kept in the head-down position during the instillation. The contrast material admixes with CSF and becomes more dilute than when it is instilled directly into the cervical region; however, if performed without delay, the procedure allows for adequate visualization of the cervical region. Again, care must be taken to prevent the inadvertent entrance of excess contrast material into the cranial vault. If there is accentuation of the thoracic kyphosis, the contrast should be allowed to flow cephalad with the patient in the oblique or lateral decubitus position. When the contrast accumulates in the cervical region, the patient is placed prone with the chin extended.

It is also possible to instill the contrast material directly into the cervical subarachnoid space via a C_1–C_2 lateral cervical tap with the patient in the prone position. With this technique the needle is placed in the cervical subarachnoid space (Fig. 15–73, p. 763), a CSF sample is collected, and 10 ml of 220 mg I/ml contrast is instilled under fluoroscopic guidance. The normal cervical lordosis holds the contrast material in the cervical region. PA lateral and oblique films are then obtained, preferably with angulation of the tube.

If the dorsal aspect of the cervical subarachnoid space does not fill satisfactorily, the patient may be placed supine and the contrast allowed to bathe the posterior margin of the foramen magnum. Do **not** allow the contrast material to flood the intracranial system.

Lateral tomograms may be helpful for complete evaluation and may be obtained with the patient either prone or supine, depending on the clinical situation. A CT scan may also be obtained following myelography.

Thoracic Myelography with Amipaque

A lumbar puncture is performed, 3 to 5 ml of CSF is removed, and approximately 12 ml of 220 to 250 mg I/ml is instilled. The patient is then placed in the lateral decubitus position with the head cocked toward the ceiling. The head of the table is then tipped slowly down, and the contrast is allowed to flow into the dorsal region. Films are then obtained in the lateral- and horizontal-beam AP positions. The table is tilted head-up to reaccumulate the contrast in the lumbar region, and the same procedure is repeated in the opposite lateral decubitus position. All motion should be made slowly to prevent admixing and consequent dilution of the contrast material.

At the end of the procedure the contrast is accumulated in the lumbar subarachnoid space, and the patient is returned to his room in a sitting position.

Computed Tomography

Computed tomography of the spine can be performed at any level after the instillation of water-soluble contrast material.

Tips on Water-Soluble Myelography

1. Use fluoroscopic control to determine the amount of contrast material.
2. The patient should remain as immobile as

possible to minimize the amount of admixing of the contrast with CSF both during and after the myelogram.

3. Do not allow the contrast to flood the intracranial region because a grand mal seizure may result.

4. The presence of blood in the subarachnoid space has **not** been shown to complicate a myelographic procedure performed with Amipaque.

5. Patients should be kept well hydrated before and after the procedure.

6. Radiographs should be obtained immediately after the instillation of contrast.

Complications of Myelography

Pantopaque

1. Headache
2. Coccygodynia
3. Traumatic herniated intervertebral disc secondary to puncture technique with traumatic perforation of the anulus fibrosus
4. Transection of nerve filament
5. Confusion
6. Iatrogenic intraspinal epidermoid
7. Arachnoiditis
8. Intravenous injection of contrast
9. Vasovagal reaction with hypotension, nausea, vomiting, dizziness, diaphoresis, and lightheadedness or even fainting

Water-Soluble Contrast

1. Grand mal seizures if an excessive amount of contrast material enters the intracranial area
2. Severe nausea and vomiting
3. Severe headache

Arachnoiditis (Fig. 15–35, p. 729)

Arachnoiditis can be seen following trauma and for unknown reasons. However, postsurgical arachnoiditis and the arachnoiditis seen after myelography are far more common and of greater interest and concern to those involved in the diagnosis and treatment of low back pain. The entity appears to be rare, although its exact incidence is unknown.

The myelogram in a patient with mild arachnoiditis reveals radiographic changes consisting of matting of the nerve roots (which appear thickened and clumped) and obliteration of the nerve root sleeves. More extensive radiographic changes reveal irregular lacy interruption of filling of the entire lumbar subarachnoid space.

In its most severe form, there may be a complete block to the flow of contrast material.

Pantopaque alone has been shown to produce arachnoiditis in some cases. The risk appears to be potentiated by blood in the subarachnoid space; thus, if blood is admixed with CSF at the time of myelography, Pantopaque should not be instilled. In addition, Pantopaque myelography followed by surgery may also aggravate arachnoiditis. The **exact** causes have not yet been identified. No known treatment has been shown to be truly effective with arachnoiditis. There have not yet been any proven clinically significant cases of arachnoiditis when Amipaque is used in the recommended doses. This is apparently true even when contrast material is admixed with blood.

Amipaque (Metrizamide) Cisternography with Computed Tomography

A lumbar puncture is performed, and 4 to 6 ml of 180 mg I/ml Amipaque is instilled in the lumbar subarachnoid space. The patient is then placed in the 45-degree head-down position for five minutes. The contrast may be allowed to flow cephalad with the patient either prone or supine; the patient may be rotated 360 degrees several times to facilitate the entrance of Amipaque into the lateral ventricles. Initially, the contrast should be kept below the puncture site and then allowed to flow rapidly cephalad to prevent leakage out of the puncture site.

The CT scan is then performed either immediately or up to several hours after instillation. The contrast outlines the basilar cisterns, the fourth ventricle, the lateral ventricles, and the cortical sulci. Mass lesions appear as areas of negative contrast bathed by the high density of the Amipaque. This technique is especially helpful for use with mass lesions in the region of the sella turcica. MR has essentially eliminated the need for cisternography.

Discography (Fig. 15–45, p. 737)

Discography is another method used to evaluate the presence or absence of disc disease. A needle is inserted into the disc, and contrast material is instilled to demonstrate that the needle is in the disc and to evaluate the quality of the disc. A normal disc will accommodate only 1 to 2 ml of contrast, and the material will remain in a central location within the nucleus pulposus. If there is a break in the anulus fibrosus of the disc, the contrast will be noted to run out of the disc at the point of break. In a posteriorly herniated nucleus pulposus, the contrast will run out posteriorly into the spinal canal. Discography can be used to diagnose an abnormal disc when the myelogram is normal or equivocal.

With a large extradural space at the disc space level, a herniated nucleus pulposus not visualized at myelography may be demonstrated at discography. This is especially true at the L_5-S_1 level. On the other hand, a normal discogram may further substantiate the normal findings of other examinations. Discography can be used in either the lumbar or cervical region. The injection of contrast and disc puncture should be done with care so as not to create a break in the anulus fibrosus and perhaps cause herniation of the nucleus pulposus.

The use of discography alone for diagnosis is to be discouraged. Neoplasms of the cauda equina may present with signs and symptoms similar to those seen with a herniated nucleus pulposus and would be missed if myelography were not performed.

Pitfalls and Accuracy

Discography usually is performed under general anesthesia because it may be quite painful. At times, it may be technically impossible to position the needle in the disc space. It is theoretically possible to precipitate a herniated nucleus pulposus by puncturing the anulus fibrosus. With increasing age, an intervertebral disc undergoes normal degeneration; the disc may appear to be abnormal, but this appearance is not clinically significant.

Although discography has its limitations, a normal myelogram and a normal discogram can obviate unnecessary surgery.

Radiographic Diagnosis of Lumbar Disc Disease

By far the most common type of extradural lesion demonstrated by myelography is the abnormal disc, which usually is seen at the disc space level and which creates a smooth extradural type of indentation on the contrast column. Occasionally the nucleus pulposus may be extruded out of the disc space and displaced either cephalad, or more commonly, caudad, creating an extradural defect not at the disc space level. This results in an appearance more suggestive of metastatic disease than disc disease. The history may help one differentiate between the two entities.

With lumbar disc disease, the symmetry or lack of symmetry of the subarachnoid space is of great importance when one attempts to make a diagnosis of an abnormal lumbar disc (Fig. 15–37, p. 731). Very small defects at the disc space levels may be considered to be protruding discs; larger defects may be considered to be bulging discs; and the largest defects, or those with a complete block to the flow of contrast material, may be considered to be herniated discs or, more accurately, herniated nucleus pulposus (HNP) (Figs. 15–47 to 15–54, pp. 739 to 748).

Symmetry or lack of symmetry of the nerve root sleeves as they extend down along the nerve should be noted in particular. If the HNP is laterally placed, elevation of the affected nerve root sleeve and an edematous nerve root will be seen. The swelling of the nerve is secondary to irritation and/or mechanical compression. One should compare the appearance of the root sleeves from one side to the other on all views obtained. If the disc is not lateralized, the elevation will be symmetric. There will also be a ventral defect on the contrast column in the lateral films. With a laterally placed disc, there is often a prominent "double density" shadow on the cross-table lateral films. This finding confirms what is seen on the other views. This radiographic appearance is created by the laterally placed disc elevating one side of the subarachnoid space more than the other.

When in doubt about the presence of a disc, the oblique views obtained with the horizontal beam (cross-table) are sometimes helpful in establishing the presence of a small, laterally placed disc. In complete block secondary to a herniated nucleus pulposus, the obstruction usually is at the level of the disc space, arising from the ventral aspect of the subarachnoid space. With this type of complete block, the contrast column will have a "brush border" appearance similar to the end of a paint brush. This is most prominent in the cauda equina region, where the nerve roots are compressed together. This appearance is quite characteristic—nearly pathognomonic—of an extradural defect. In addition, close inspection of the preliminary films may show the rare finding of a calcified degenerated disc fragment that has been extruded into the spinal canal. Having the patient flex and extend or turn over to the supine position often allows the contrast to flow below the level of a block that is secondary to a herniated disc.

Abnormal discs are most common at the L$_4$–L$_5$ and L$_5$–S$_1$ levels. They also may occur at higher levels. These changes may be seen at multiple levels and in 8 to 10 per cent of individuals are present at both L$_4$–L$_5$ and L$_5$–S$_1$.

In adults one will very rarely encounter a lipoma or arachnoid cyst in the lumbar canal. While destruction of the vertebral pedicles may provide evidence of metastatic disease, pressure erosion or undercutting of the pedicles may be seen with slow-growing tumors, such as neurofibromas, lipomas, and arachnoid cysts. Scalloping of the backs of the vertebral bodies may be seen with long-standing increased intracranial pressure (Fig. 15–27, p. 723), with dural ectasia of neurofibromatosis, in the presence of individual neurofibromas or with a lipoma or other spine tumors such as a dermoid of the spine (Fig. 15–83, p. 773).

The subarachnoid space may be closely applied to the posterior aspect of the vertebral bodies. If this is the case, a protruding, bulging, or herniated disc will produce a ventral indentation on the contrast column. These defects in the contrast column can be readily identified. However, a certain percentage of patients will demonstrate a large extradural space; the contrast column is then displaced away from the posterior aspect of the vertebral bodies. If this is the case, protruding or bulging discs may not produce an indentation on the contrast column. Indeed, if this extradural space is large enough, even the presence of a herniated disc may not be appreciated because the contrast column is displaced so far from the disc. The large extradural space is seen most commonly at the L$_5$–S$_1$ level but sometimes extends up to the L$_4$–L$_5$ level.

Accuracy of the Myelogram in Lumbar Disc Disease

Even in the presence of a herniated nucleus pulposus, the myelogram may be normal. The myelogram will be accurate in 80 to 85 per cent of cases. In most patients with normal myelograms, surgery will reveal the herniated disc at L$_5$–S$_1$. Far laterally placed discs may not be visualized by myelography, and a large extradural space also may interfere with visualization of an abnormal disc.

Postoperative Myelogram

Dorsal and lateral defects on the contrast column may be secondary to scar formation from a surgical procedure. A ventral defect should, however, be viewed with the same suspicion as a ventral defect noted on the preoperative myelogram (Figs. 15–56 and 15–57, p. 750).

COMPUTED TOMOGRAPHY OF THE LUMBAR SPINE

Computed tomography (CT) of the lumbar spine, with a high-resolution later-generation scanner, is a practical, useful, and dependable method for the evaluation of herniated disc in the lumbar region. CT is performed following examination by routine radiography. Although digital examination of the lumbar spine can be performed prior to examination by CT, more accurate evaluation is made with routine spine radiographs. Because it is vital to identify the precise level of any abnormality, accurate evaluation is required. CT examination is usually obtained prior to myelography and provides an accurate and readily reproducible method of evaluating the vertebral bodies and discs in a noninvasive manner. If the clinical setting is convincing, surgery for a herniated disc may be performed without the need for further evaluation, although many surgeons still prefer a myelogram prior to surgery.

Spine radiographs should be evaluated for the presence of a number of vertebral bodies, vertebral body height, disc space height, bony destructive changes, spondylolysis, and spondylolisthesis.

Alterations or anatomic variations in the plain spine examination allow ready evaluation of the spine for any specialized approaches to the examination by CT. Routine spine radiographs include AP, lateral, and cone down views of the lowest lumbar disc space; oblique views are helpful for complete evaluation.

Computed tomography has greatly expanded our diagnostic abilities in the evaluation of the spine. Any level of the spine can be conveniently evaluated with a minimum of discomfort for the patient and with only a minor amount of movement of the patient; this latter fact is of importance when one is considering the acutely injured patient. CT of the spine can be performed both with and without water-soluble contrast material in the subarachnoid space. In some cases, the study may be performed both before and after the addition of contrast material to the subarachnoid space.

Routine Lumbar Spine Scan

For evaluation of the patient with a possible herniated lumbar disc, the lowest three disc space levels are routinely scanned. Prior to scanning, preliminary radiographs should be obtained to evaluate the number and configuration of lumbar-type vertebral bodies. This also aids in ruling out the presence of a process such as discitis or metastatic disease which may masquerade as low back pain secondary to disc disease. As a general rule, the author suggests incorporating these plain spine radiographic findings into the CT report.

At the time of each scan, a "topogram" or "scout view" (Fig. 15–40, p. 734) or some type of initializing film should be obtained so that each scan slice location can be marked numerically and identified easily. The initial series of images is then obtained using approximately 4-mm slices that begin at the level of the mid-body of the third lumbar-type vertebral body segment (assuming five lumbar-type vertebral body segments). The slices are obtained perpendicular to the vertebral canal and are contiguous down approximately to the level of the mid-body of the first sacral segment. Following this, additional slices are obtained which are angled through the individual disc spaces. The angled slices may be only one single slice, but three contiguous slices are preferable.

The scan slices are contiguous rather than just at the disc levels, because a herniated disc may migrate away from its disc space and not be identified unless slices are obtained above and below this level. Although most herniated discs that migrate away from the disc level move inferiorly, occasionally the disc may migrate superiorly.

At the lowest lumbar level, there may be such an accentuation of the normal lumbar lordosis that the slices cannot be angled directly through the disc level. This occurs because the gantry or carriage opening of the scanner is mechanically limited to angles of 20 degrees forward and backward. However, the best possible angled cuts should be obtained. If there are additional areas of interest, such as the upper lumbar region, these additional areas of interest should also be scanned.

With the later-generation scanners, reconstruction views or reformatted views can be obtained so that the spine can be evaluated in a variety of planes. This can be particularly helpful when evaluating the neural foramina at any of multiple levels.

Technique of Needle Placement

It is recommended that a 22-gauge or smaller needle be used for the examination. This creates a smaller puncture hole, reducing the chances that there will be a leakage of the contrast from the subarachnoid space following the myelogram. The author also recommends an oblique approach to the puncture because this facilitates the needle placement and because the tip of the needle can then be directed toward the back of the vertebral body rather than toward the disc space. This serves two purposes: (1) it prevents the possibility of a needle defect at the puncture site, i.e., an iatrogenic defect that might be confused with an abnormal disc or posterior degenerative changes, and (2) the tip of the needle will then be prevented from passing through the subarachnoid space and into the disc—this has been reported as a cause of traumatically herniated disc. The so-called needle defect is thought to be secondary to an accumulation of CSF in the subdural space.

The Normal Scan

The L_3–L_4 disc is usually concave posteriorly and follows closely the posterior margin of the L_3 vertebral body (Fig. 15–40, p. 734).

The L_4–L_5 disc may be concave posteriorly, similar to the L_3–L_4 level, but more commonly it is more or less straight across its posterior margin.

The L_5–S_1 disc is usually straight across its posterior margin. In addition, the L_5 vertebral body is usually "lemon"-shaped and therefore can be identified by its typical configuration.

Computed Tomography of the Lumbar Spine

Muliple hard copy images are obtained using two different window widths and window levels. One emphasizes the bony structures while the other emphasizes the soft tissues. These are best evaluated when presented in a side-by-side fashion. In addition to the routine viewing levels, it is important at times to examine the studies using varying window widths and window levels. Subtle abnormalities may be visible only after evaluation on the oscilloscope screen. This is particularly true with a disc that is isodense, or nearly isodense, with the subarachnoid space. The normal disc measures 40 to 80 Hounsfield units (HU), but occasionally, probably because of the partial volume phenomenon, a very large herniated disc is difficult to appreciate.

The Abnormal Scan

A "bulging" disc extends circumferentially beyond the bony margin of the vertebral body. While usually considered to be a variation of normal, when coupled with hypertrophic degenerative changes of the interfacet joint, this type of bulging disc may be symptomatic (Fig. 15–45, p. 737).

A "herniated" disc is present when there is a tear in the anulus fibrosus and a portion of the nucleus pulposus extends through this tear and out of its normal position. Note that a herniated disc may occur in any direction, including anteriorly, but is clinically significant when the nucleus extends posteriorly or laterally and compresses the nerve roots in the canal or at the level of the neural foramen.

A "sequestered" disc is one that has not only extended through the tear in the anulus but has migrated away from the disc and is no longer contiguous with the remainder of the nucleus pulposus. While this diagnosis may be suggested when the disc fragment is identified remote from the actual disc level, diagnosis frequently cannot be made with absolute certainty. The normal disc measures 40 to 80 HU, and so this disc-density material can usually be identified, but in the vast majority of cases it is difficult to say with certainty that the fragment is no longer contiguous with the remainder of the disc (Fig. 15–48, pp. 740 and 741).

The significance of the sequestered disc is the fact that this type of disc will not respond to the injection of chymopapaine, because the enzyme is injected into the nucleus pulposus and would therefore not communicate with the fragment of disc that has migrated away from the disc space.

Isodense Disc

At times a very large herniated disc will occupy almost the entire spinal canal at the level of the disc. If this is a midline herniated disc, it is possible that the appearance is similar to the normal subarachnoid space of the vertebral canal and that this very large disc will not be appreciated. Obviously, the density of the disc is between 40 and 80 HU, which is much higher than the density of the subarachnoid space. Therefore, if a herniated disc is a clinical consideration, density measurements should be taken (Fig. 15–49, p. 742).

Laterally Herniated Disc

If the disc is placed far laterally, the myelogram may be normal. This laterally placed herniated disc will still cause pain for the patient because it impinges upon the nerve distal to the ganglion. In these cases CT is particularly helpful because the herniated portion of the disc can be readily identified, and any encroachment upon the nerve and the surrounding perineural fat can also be seen (Fig. 15–50, p. 743).

In these cases CT can be performed either prior to or after the instillation of contrast material. At times, subtle effacement of the nerve root sleeve or lumbar subarachnoid space can be appreciated on the CT scan when it is not visible on the myelogram.

CT is also helpful when there is a large extradural space posterior to the disc space or with a laterally herniated disc. The presence of a herniated disc may not be appreciated on the myelogram, and so CT becomes the diagnostic procedure of choice. This can be performed either before or after the instillation of water-soluble contrast material. The signs to look for are:

1. Irregular margin of the disc outline
2. Focal protrusion of the disc into the vertebral canal or neural foramen
3. Distortion of the subarachnoid space by the herniated disc
4. Compromise of the periganglionic or perineural fat
5. Displacement of a gaseous degenerated disc into the canal
6. Disc space narrowing on the digital preliminary study

Postmyelography CT Scanning

Indications

1. Nondiagnostic myelogram or need for more information
2. Symptomatic patient with normal myelogram or poor visualization of an area of interest
3. The presence of a cord tumor
4. To demonstrate the area below or above a nearly complete block

Technique

The scan may be performed using the same technique as that used for a study without the instillation of contrast material. If there is a more limited area of interest, the scan may be tailored to incorporate only that specific area. No special patient preparation is necessary, and the scan may be performed at any time within 6 hours following the myelogram. It is helpful to have the patient rotate 360 degrees on the cart one or two times after the myelogram and before the CT scan so that the contrast material is well mixed with the CSF. If this is not done, there may be layering of the contrast material or the contrast material may all accumulate in the lumbar cul-de-sac and not be visible at the area of interest.

With a CT scan obtained immediately following the myelogram, the contrast may be so dense that it causes artifact and degradation of the image. While some authors recommend delaying the scan for 1 or 2 hours after the myelogram, it is expeditious to remove a portion of the contrast material immediately after the completion of the myelogram and before the CT scan is obtained.

Advantages

When the myelogram is equivocal or nondiagnostic, CT may be helpful in identifying subtle changes or subtle effacement of the contrast material not visible on the myelogram. Postmyelographic CT may also be helpful when noncontrast CT is not diagnostic.

The myelogram may be normal when there is a far laterally placed disc that compresses the nerve distal to its exit from the foramen. CT with contrast may be particularly helpful in these patients, particularly if the patient is convincingly symptomatic and the myelogram is nondiagnostic or normal.

The Postoperative Spine

The postoperative patient presents some unique problems that often cannot be totally evaluated by computed tomography. Although in many cases CT can differentiate between recurrent herniated disc and postoperative scar, this is not always the case. Scar tissue usually forms posteriorly at the surgical site but may also be found in the anticipated position of a recurrent herniated disc. The literature is controversial on whether or not scar can be differentiated from disc when one compares a pre- and postinfusion CT scan of the spine. In theory, one would anticipate that scar tissue would demonstrate enhancement following infusion, while a herniated disc would not. As a general

rule, scar tissue is lower in density than a herniated disc, but this finding is also variable, and so one cannot rely on Hounsfield numbers for absolute diagnosis.

In addition to the problem of differentiating scar from herniated disc, the presence of arachnoiditis cannot be determined with CT without the instillation of water-soluble contrast material prior to scanning. Therefore, in the postoperative patient with recurrent back pain, complete evaluation may require pre- and postinfusion CT scan, myelography, and possibly postmyelographic CT. This author has rarely used the postinfusion CT scan of the lumbar spine to aid in the differentiation of scar versus recurrent herniated disc. MR can also be used for evaluation of the postoperative patient (Figs. 15–56 and 15–57, p. 750).

As a general rule, even in the presence of arachnoiditis and/or scar formation, reoperation is indicated if a herniated disc is identified.

Interfacet Degenerative Changes

Interfacet degenerative changes are easily evaluated by CT examination. Although facet joint space narrowing and sclerosis are visible on routine radiographic examination, the changes are much more readily appreciated by CT examination. A number of changes can be seen: narrowing of the interfacet joints, small cystic changes in the facets, hypertrophic changes in the facets, "vacuum" changes involving the facet joints, and thickening of the ligamentum flavum.

The bony overgrowth is particularly easy to evaluate by CT examination, as is the presence of encroachment upon the neural foramen. The axial plane of examination also readily allows evaluation of the configuration of the vertebral canal and the presence of congenital spinal stenosis. In addition, some normal anatomic variations in the configuration of the canal may result in a smaller canal than others. If this is the case, then even small amounts of degenerative bony overgrowth may compromise the canal.

Interfacet degenerative changes result in narrowing of the facet joints and a variable amount of forward displacement of one vertebral body on the next. This causes a spondylolisthesis that is not associated with a spondylolysis. With this alteration in the normal relationship of the vertebral bodies, there is almost always loss of intervertebral disc height. The combination of these facet changes causes other changes, such as thickening of the ligamentum flavum and an acquired spinal stenosis. In addition, there are usually hypertrophic degenerative changes involving the facets, and this bony overgrowth creates specific areas of stenosis. These areas may encroach upon the vertebral canal or the neural foramina. The combination of hypertrophic facet changes and a bulging disc may cause radicular pain even in the absence of a herniated disc (Fig. 15–55, p. 749).

There are four different developmental configurations to the normal vertebral canal: (1) triangular, (2) round, (3) diamond, and (4) trifoil. These configurations are variable in their susceptibility to encroachment by hypertrophic spurs. In some cases, specifically the trifoil canal, the canal is congenitally small in size, so any encroachment is likely to cause symptoms earlier than in a patient without a small canal.

These congenital and acquired changes are best appreciated by altering the window widths and levels so that the encroachment can be demonstrated to best advantage.

Conjoined Root

In the usual case each nerve root exits separately and is surrounded by the nerve root sleeve. This results in a symmetric appearance of the lumbar subarachnoid space. In the presence of a conjoined root, two nerves exit at one level, and there is no nerve exiting at the next lower level. This results in an asymmetric appearance to the lumbar subarachnoid space which can be mistaken for a herniated disc at myelography. To further complicate this diagnosis, the CT appearance without contrast may not allow differentiation of a conjoined root from a herniated disc. The conjoined root sleeves can give a similar appearance to a herniated disc, and while theoretically it is possible to differentiate the two on the basis of Hounsfield numbers, in actuality this is not always possible. The fluid in the lumbar subarachnoid space measures between 7 and 15 Hounsfield units, and theoretically the fluid in the nerve root sleeve should have a similar density. However, the partial volume effect results in inclusion of both the nerve and the fluid in the nerve root sleeve, producing a density higher than that of the CSF in the density measurement pixel. This density measurement may be similar to the 40 to 80 HU of normal disc material. At times, it may be necessary to proceed to myelography for complete evaluation. The myelogram will demonstrate the conjoined nerve rootlets and surrounding sleeves, which also

can be evaluated by CT. In addition, CT following the instillation of water-soluble contrast also differentiates between a simple conjoined root and the additional presence of a herniated disc, which would be almost impossible to demonstrate on the myelogram (Fig. 15–39, p. 733) without the use of complementary CT scanning.

Nerve Root Meningoceles (Tarlove Cyst)

This cystic dilatation of the nerve root sleeve is probably not a pathologic condition but rather a normal anatomic variant (Fig. 15–36, p. 730). These cysts may also be demonstrated on the CT scan and may cause pressure erosion of the surrounding bone space.

Spinal Cord Tumors

Extradural

Second only to disc disease, metastatic disease is the most common type of extradural defect seen in an active clinical neuroradiology service. The size of the defect depends on the size of the metastatic lesion, which often is associated with abnormalities of the bony structures at the level of involvement (Fig. 15–72, p. 762). When metastases are suspected, a close inspection of the preliminary films will be rewarding in many cases. If multiple abnormal levels are found, the patient will more likely be a candidate for radiation therapy rather than surgical treatment.

In metastatic disease, the contrast column is compressed at a level other than that of the disc space; not infrequently, multiple lesions can be demonstrated (Figs. 15–15 to 15–25, pp. 716 to 722). Myelographic abnormalities secondary to metastatic disease may or may not be associated with a detectable bony abnormality. Careful examination of the plain films may reveal a productive or, more commonly, a destructive lesion. Look carefully for a destroyed pedicle, since the pedicle is often the first area involved by metastatic disease.

A complete extradural block to the flow of contrast material will have a "paint brush border" appearance and may demonstrate what appears to be a circumferential narrowing of the subarachnoid space (Figs. 15–43 and 15–44, pp. 736 and 737).

Primary tumors that commonly metastasize to the spine or its soft tissues are (1) breast tumor, (2) lung tumor, (3) multiple myeloma, and (4) lymphoma.

Intradural Extramedullary

Neurofibromas (Figs. 15–73 to 15–83, pp. 763 to 773) and meningiomas are the most common tumors in this category. In neurofibroma, the patient may be known to have neurofibromatosis, and the plain film of the spine may reveal widening of one or even several of the neural foramina at the level of the neurofibromas. This enlargement is secondary to the dumbbell configuration of the neurofibroma (Figs. 15–74 and 15–76 to 15–82, pp. 764 and 766 to 772). In these cases there is frequently a rather small intradural spinal component and a relatively large extradural soft tissue component that may be palpable in some cases.

Rarely, meningiomas may demonstrate a similar appearance, with widened neural foramina because of bilobed development of the tumor. There is marked predominance of meningiomas in women—about 80 to 85 per cent occur in women. Meningiomas occur most often in the thoracic spine.

The myelographic appearance of an intradural lesion is quite typical. At the point of origin of the tumor the cord will be displaced to the contralateral side—away from the tumor. The contrast column will form an acute angle with the tumor at its point of attachment to the dura and then bathe the tumor, creating a curvilinear line that has the appearance of a meniscus. If the tumor is of sufficient size, the spinal cord will not only be displaced away from the tumor but will also be flattened by the mass. Because the cord is flattened against the dura on the side away from the tumor, the contrast column on that side will be noted to form an acute angle with the spinal cord and the dura. This appearance is typical of an intradural extramedullary tumor. If the spinal cord is viewed as one is looking directly at the tumor, it may appear that the cord is merely widened, with the contrast column thinned on either side. The appearance, because of the widening of the cord, is similar to that seen with a purely intramedullary mass. Great care must be taken to obtain and examine closely views that are at 90-degree angles to one another. Failure to do so will result in errors of diagnosis. This is important because intradural lesions are surgically curable, whereas intramedullary tumors usually are not.

Intradural Intramedullary

As the name implies, these lesions arise from within the substance of the spinal cord. The most common tumor of the intramedullary type is the ependymoma; the second most common is the astrocytoma, followed by syringohydromyelic abnormalities and a variety of less common lesions. The myelographic abnormality demonstrates widening of the spinal cord in all views. This results in narrowing of the contrast column at the point of the mass lesion. If there is a complete block to the flow of contrast material, the contrast column will be widened and the contrast will form an acute angle with the mass at the level of the tumor (Figs. 15–84 to 15–90, pp. 774 to 779). In all projections the appearance of the contrast column and its relationship to the spinal cord will be the same. If the widening of the cord is secondary to a tumor, the area of cord widening usually will be limited; if the cord widening is secondary to a syringohydromyelia, the cord will appear to be widened over a much longer segment.

Summary

Each of the three classes of spinal cord tumors may mimic the appearance of another if examined in only one view. Therefore, it cannot be overemphasized that the abnormality should be viewed in multiple projections for a more accurate diagnosis.

In addition, if any of the abnormalities reaches sufficient size to cause a complete block to the flow of contrast material, the diagnostic characteristics are often obscured or take on an appearance consistent with two different classes of tumors, preventing an accurate diagnosis. In some cases, additional information can be gained by instilling contrast material both above and below the level of the block in order to characterize the abnormality better. With a complete block, surgical decompression is usually performed; therefore, the information to be gained by both myelographic studies must be weighed against the risks involved.

Computed Tomography of Cord Tumors

Computed tomography of cord tumors is not particularly helpful when there is no contrast material in the subarachnoid space. Occasionally, a calcified meningioma may be demonstrated to be encroaching upon the vertebral canal. Neurofibromas of sufficient size may also be visualized in the neural foramina or in the paraspinal area; however, their extent and particularly the intracanalicular component are best demonstrated by myelography or by CT obtained following myelography.

Occasionally, the cord tumor creates a sufficient block to the contrast material that the upper or lower margin cannot be adequately evaluated. In a large number of cases, a sufficient amount of contrast material can move past even a relatively high grade block to permit evaluation of the size, configuration, and position of the tumor. CT is also helpful if the lesion is small or questionable, as the greater sensitivity of CT allows more accurate evaluation. This is particularly true in cases of multiple small neurofibromas, multiple intradural metastases, or drop metastases from a tumor such as a pinealoma, medulloblastoma, or ependymoma.

CT is also helpful in determining the exact relationship of the cord to the tumor and the surrounding vertebral canal. This author has found CT to be the most helpful in lesions around the foramen magnum and/or masses that extend from the cervical spinal canal into the intracranial region. Before the availability of MR, or in its absence, postmyelographic CT with thin slices is the method of choice for evaluation of this region.

Occasionally a specific mass cannot be categorized into anatomic location without the use of CT. Again, this technique is helpful in those rare intradural-intramedullary tumors in which there is an exophytic component that may mimic the appearance of a purely intradural mass.

Subtle areas of calcification may also be seen on the CT scan when they are not identified by any other method.

Magnetic resonance will probably replace myelography and CT myelography in a large number of cases (see below).

CERVICAL SPINE RADIOGRAPHIC ANATOMY

Radiography of the cervical spine includes anteroposterior, lateral, and oblique views as well as an AP view of the odontoid process (Fig. 15–60, p. 753). C_2 through C_7 will be considered together in this section; C_1 will be considered separately.

The cervical spine vertebrae are unique when compared with those of the remainder of the spine. A well-developed "lateral mass" is present on each of the cervical vertebral bodies. The pedicles of the cervical vertebrae project more posterolaterally than elsewhere in the spine and so are less well seen in the AP projection. The lateral mass is made up of (1)

transverse process, (2) foramina transversaria, (3) articulating facets, and (4) apophyseal joints.

The foramina transversaria at the C_1 level are more lateral in position than at other levels of the cervical spine. The vertebral artery normally enters the foramina transversaria at C_6 but may enter at any level. The vertebral artery exits above C_2; it courses laterally and then superiorly, where it re-enters the foramina transversaria of C_1 and turns 90 degrees posteriorly to lie in a groove along the top of the C_1 vertebral body. It then courses anteromedially to enter the skull through the foramen magnum.

The odontoid process is in close relationship to the anterior arch of C_1 and should not be displaced posteriorly more than 3 mm in the adult. The odontoid is held in position by the transverse and cruciate ligaments. Following soft tissue trauma or in rheumatoid arthritis (which causes relaxation of the ligaments), there may be subluxation of the odontoid from the atlas (Figs. 15–61 and 15–62, pp. 754 and 755). Trauma also may cause fractures (Fig. 15–64, p. 756), but a discussion of this subject is beyond the scope of this book.

Unlike studies of the lumbar spine, positioning for oblique views does not reveal the areas of interest "through" the vertebral bodies. When the patient is in the RAO position, we view the lateral masses and the right neural foramina. The anatomic right marker will indicate the right side, which is the side of interest. Similarly, with the patient in the LAO position we view the left neural foramina and left lateral mass. This radiographic projection in the cervical region occurs because the lateral mass is nearly lateral to the vertebral body. The articulation of each lateral mass with the adjacent lateral mass is the apophyseal joint. This is a synovial joint, and degenerative changes may occur at this level and encroach posteriorly upon the neural foramina.

Each cervical vertebral body contains a small, thin piece of bone that projects superiorly along the lateral and superior edge of each vertebra. This is the uncinate process. Each higher vertebral body is consequently beveled along its inferior lateral margin in a corresponding fashion so that it articulates with the uncinate process to form the joints of Luschka (Fig. 15–64, p. 756). The joints of Luschka are not true synovial joints, but they do develop degenerative osteophytes. The normal uncinate process should not be mistaken for osteophytes.

The normal cervical spinal cord itself measures 10 mm in its anteroposterior dimension.

The cervical subarachnoid space is limited anteriorly by the back of the vertebral bodies and posteriorly by the level where the laminae of each side fuse together to form the dorsal spinous process. Where they fuse appears as a white line—the spinal laminar line—on the lateral view because the point of bony union is viewed tangentially. The anteroposterior dimension of the bony subarachnoid space normally measures approximately 17 mm, with a range from 14 to 20 mm.

In general, the indications for cervical myelography are similar to those for lumbar myelography. If the study is being performed with particular reference to the cervical area, the lumbar tap for contrast instillation can theoretically be performed at any level in the lumbar region. It should be noted that if the study is being done for possible cervical disc disease, there is often symptomatic or asymptomatic lumbar disc disease as well. Thus it is best to perform the puncture at L_2–L_3, away from the most common levels of lumbar disc disease.

Following instillation, the contrast material is allowed to flow cephalad while the patient extends the neck and elevates the head, assisted by a pillow under the chin. At the same time, the table is tilted with the patient's head down until the contrast reaches the cervical region. The head should be kept straight. Once the contrast is in the cervical region, the patient may be returned to the horizontal position, and the normal cervical lordosis will hold the contrast in the cervical regions. Films should be obtained in the PA and lateral projections, with the contrast covering all levels of the cervical spine, including the clivus. (Note that since the advent of computed tomography of the head most of the intracranial portion of the study will be covered by a routine head scan.) In addition, films may be obtained in both the PA prone vertical-beam oblique projections as well as in the lateral horizontal (cross-table) oblique projections. Again, the radiographic filming should be altered to aid and facilitate diagnosis in each indiviual case (Figs. 15–66 to 15–68, pp. 758 to 760).

Because of variations in radiographic equipment and myelographic filming, it is difficult to speak of cervical cord size in terms of absolutes; rather, it must be discussed in terms of its relationship to the bony cervical spine. The cord can be seen outlined in the pool of contrast as the gray shadow in the middle of the contrast pool.

The cervical spinal cord normally has an area of widening in its mid-portion that is largest at the C_6 level but extends from C_3 to T_3. This normal widening should not be mistaken for an intramedullary lesion. The normal thoracic cord is smaller than the cervical cord and is approximately the size of the smallest digit of the hand. This normal localized area of widening of the cord serves to accommodate the increased numbers of nerve cell bodies at these levels that supply the upper extremity.

The cervical cord in its widest dimension should be no wider than two thirds of the interpeduncular distance. This distance is measured from the medial side of each peduncle as seen on the PA radiograph. Also, the cord should be no wider than three fourths of the width of the subarachnoid space measured from one side of the contrast column to the other.

The nerve root pouches also can be seen readily as they exit through each neural foramen. Several small nerves can be seen at each level. In addition, the anterior spinal artery often can be readily visualized along the ventral aspect of the cord as it is outlined by the contrast. Again, any defects detected on the myelogram should be correlated with the routine cervical spine radiographs. With the patient's neck well extended and not rotated, the contrast material can be pooled in such a way that both the ventral and dorsal aspects of the cervical subarachnoid space can be covered by the contrast column. In this way, mass lesions and other filling defects can be ruled out in either the dorsal or ventral aspect of the cord. In some cases, however, it may be necessary to remove the lumbar puncture needle and turn the patient on his back. If Pantopaque is used, it can then be run up to the cervical region to the level of the cisterna magna and even into the fourth ventricle to evaluate the presence of a mass lesion around the posterior margin of the foramen magnum. In this case, lumbar tap can be repeated at the termination of the procedure and the contrast material removed, or the patient may be brought back to the department for contrast removal at a later date. The same procedure can be followed when Amipaque is used or CT is obtained postmyelographically.

The cervical nerve roots arise from the cervical cord and course anteroventrally to their point of exit via the neural foramina. Each root will be seen to be made up of several small rootlets. The right cervical nerves are best demonstrated by oblique views with the patient in a gentle LAO position. Likewise, the left cervical nerves are best demonstrated in the RAO projection. An excessively oblique positioning will cause the heavier-than-CSF contrast to flow away from the area of interest. Ideally, and if the equipment allows, the oblique views should be obtained by angulation of the tube and appropriate film positioning without moving the patient. This is particularly true if water-soluble contrast material is used, because patient motion causes dilution of the contrast material.

On the lateral view, there is often a prominent ventral bulge on the subarachnoid space at the cervical level behind the odontoid process. This, however, is due to ligaments, not to a tumor. Care must be taken to avoid calling this normal finding a pathologic process. In addition, the dentate ligament may be seen on the lateral projections as a lucent line in the mid-portion of the contrast column (Fig. 15–65, p. 757).

Myelography in Cervical Spondylosis

Spondylosis

This all-inclusive term implies a general degenerative process in the cervical spine. The process includes a variety of changes that occur in the cervical spine: osteophyte formation around the joints of Luschka, bulging or herniated cervical discs (which would not be visible on plain films of the spine), degenerative changes of the facets, and disc space narrowing.

Trauma has been implicated as a cause, but spondylosis appears to be more prevalent with increasing age and unrelated to overt trauma. The changes seen with age may be related to the multiple small "traumas" of daily living. It does appear that trauma may be a factor in some cases, and constitutional factors may be incriminated in others.

The uncovertebral "joints" will be considered to be true joints and therefore susceptible to arthritic changes. Plain films will reveal the formation of bony osteophytes at a single or multiple levels. These changes are most common at C_5–C_6 and next most common at C_6–C_7. These uncovertebral osteophytes may be seen to impinge on the neural foramina in the oblique views and to project posteriorly in the midline, where the osteophytes may reach to the ventral aspect of the spinal cord.

The myelogram will reveal changes reflecting the findings seen on routine plain film examination. Osteophytes around the joints of Luschka and lateral in position will obliterate the nerve roots and produce small triangular defects in the contrast column. Midline osteophytes will indent the contrast column and produce one or more ventral bars in the cervical region. In the absence of a cervical disc, the contrast column will be closely applied to the posterior margin of the osteophyte.

The vast majority of cases with or without herniated disc—95 per cent—occur at C_5–C_6 or C_6–C_7. Again, review of the preliminary films usually reveals degenerative changes with osteophytes that can be seen to impinge on the neural foramina, particularly in the oblique projections (Figs. 15–66 and 15–70, pp. 758 and 761).

If bony osteophytes encroach upon the cervical subarachnoid space and the ventral aspect of the spinal cord, there can be clinical evidence of the spinal cord compression and pyramidal tract signs. Lower extremity symptoms also may result from pressure on the anterior spinal artery, resulting in interference with the blood supply to the cord. By inspection of the lateral view of the cervical spine one can actually measure from the most posterior extent of the osteophyte to the spinal laminar line, which marks the posterior extent of the cervical subarachnoid space, to obtain the **bony** width of the cervical canal. If this measures 11 mm or less, there is definite evidence of bony compromise of the cervical cord. This is true because at least 1 mm must be allowed for accommodation of the posterior spinal ligament connecting the vertebral bodies and the ligamentum flavum dorsally connecting the vertebral laminae in addition to the meningeal coverings of the spinal cord. Therefore, a measurement of 12 mm might be considered suspicious for cord compression by bony encroachment. In a congenitally small or stenotic cervical canal, these osteophytes will produce symptoms sooner than in a patient with a large anteroposterior spinal canal diameter.

In cases of cervical disc disease, there is thinning of the contrast column at the levels of the disc in the PA views; interruption of nerve root filling at the abnormal levels is best shown on the oblique views. These findings should always be confirmed by cross-table lateral projections of the mid and upper cervical spine and a swimmer's view to include the lower cervical and upper thoracic spine levels.

At myelography, there may be complete obstruction to flow at the level of the large cervical osteophytes and/or discs. This obstruction to flow is most commonly seen with the patient in the extended position. Indeed, when the neck is flexed and the chin is placed on the chest, contrast will often flow beyond the level of the block. This maneuver should certainly be attempted in order to evaluate the abnormal levels fully and accurately. It may become necessary to instill contrast above the block via a C_1–C_2 tap in order to outline the upper border of the block more accurately. With impingement on the cord from a ventral disc, one can at times actually see widening of the cord. This widening is due to a flattening of the cord in the anteroposterior dimension, and this finding will be confirmed on the lateral views. It should not be mistaken for an intramedullary tumor. All abnormal levels should be studied in at least two projections—ideally obtained at 90-degree angles to one another.

If there is herniation of the nucleus pulposus in the cervical region in addition to bony osteophytes, there may be compromise of the cord by soft tissue abnormalities not visible on plain film radiograph of the spine. These disc defects will be identified on the myelographic study when the contrast column is displaced farther than can be accounted for by the bony osteophyte alone (Figs. 15–66 to 15–70, pp. 758 to 761).

It is not always possible to be certain whether myelographic changes are secondary to a cervical disc or to bony osteophytes. Patients with myelographic changes secondary to spondylosis are a common problem in an active clinical practice. Their management can be challenging and difficult.

Meningiomas and Neurofibromas

Neurofibromas of the cervical region may be associated with widening of the neural foramina secondary to pressure erosion. Neurofibromas and meningiomas represent most of the intradural-extramedullary tumors seen in the cervical region. With intradural lesions, there will be a sharp angle made with the contrast column, a rounded defect of the tumor itself, and displacement of the cord away from the mass. Again, it is advisable to obtain views of the abnormal levels in two projections. If only one view is obtained, it may appear that there is cord displacement similar to that seen with an extradural lesion. In the upper cervical level, the low-lying cerebellar tonsils should not be mistaken for a mass lesion along the dorsal aspect of the cord. Similarly, the dura and ligamentum flavum may be noted to form a corrugated pattern with the patient's head in the extended position—a normal finding (Figs. 15–73 to 15–83, pp. 763 to 773).

Syringohydromyelia

Syringohydromyelia is seen most commonly in the cervical cord region (Figs. 15–91 to 15–100 and 15–103, pp. 780 to 786 and 790), although a post-traumatic syrinx may be located at any level in the spinal cord. In these cases the patient may have minimal symptoms but usually will have a history of long duration and may have Charcot joints involving the upper extremity (Fig. 15–91, p. 780). Plain films of the cervical spine usually reveal a widened AP and lateral diameter of the spinal canal.

In syringohydromyelia, the cord will be noted to be widened over multiple vertebral body segments. The widened cord usually extends into the region of the thoracic cord. The wide cervical cord associated with a syrinx and demonstrated with standard myelography usually will collapse with air myelography. The collapse of the syrinx with air myelography also rules out the presence of a spinal cord tumor. This occurs because the air flows cephalad when the head is raised, while the fluid within the syringohydromyelia sac flows caudally in the enlarged canal by the force of gravity.

Cervical myelography is performed in the usual fashion, usually following lumbar puncture. If a Chiari malformation is present, there will be low tonsils in the cervical region; a cervical tap may enter close to the low tonsils. When the patient is studied in the supine, head-down position, the resulting enlargement of the cervical cord makes the diagnosis of a syrinx easier. In this position, the thoracic spinal cord and conus medullaris usually appear normal in size, although they may be involved with the syrinx. Any additional areas of focal enlargement of the cord that may suggest a tumor should also be noted. Approximately 6 hours after the myelogram with water-soluble contrast material, the patient should be returned to the radiology department and a CT scan obtained of the area of interest. The CT slices may be either 4 or 8 mm in thickness and may be either contiguous or interrupted throughout the area of interest. If a syrinx cavity is present, the contrast material accumulates in the central portion of the cord. Therefore, the cavity is high in density, the spinal cord is relatively low in density, and the contrast material in the subarachnoid space is high in density and surrounds and outlines the spinal cord. This demonstration of the cavity is possible even up to 24 hours following the procedure and rarely is visible only after a delay of longer than 6 hours.

If a spinal cord tumor is present, visualization of the cord cavity is interrupted and a mass causing focal expansion of the cord and interruption of the syrinx cavity is evident.

The postmyelographic CT scan will allow demonstration of the true length of the syrinx cavity, which not uncommonly involves the entire length of the spinal cord. Magnetic resonance, particularly with surface coil images, should replace CT as the diagnostic method of choice.

Thoracic (Dorsal) Spine

Anteroposterior and lateral views of the dorsal spine are obtained routinely. Inspection of the vertebrae should be performed in a manner similar to that described for the corresponding views of the lumbar spine. Diastematomyelia (Fig. 15–104, p. 791), if present, is associated with congenitally abnormal vertebral bodies and is usually found in the lower dorsal or upper lumbar region. Herniated discs are uncommon in the thoracic region.

Ivory Vertebra

The single white vertebra or "ivory vertebra" is seen most commonly with Hodgkin's disease or the non-Hodgkin's lymphoma. The ivory vertebra also may be seen with osteoblastic metastatic disease, myeloid metaplasia, Paget's disease, fluorosis, and osteopetrosis.

Myelography of the Dorsal Cord

The dorsal spinal cord may be studied by filling the entire column with contrast material. More commonly, approximately 18 to 24 ml of Pantopaque is used. After removal of 10 to 12 ml of CSF, the contrast is instilled very slowly into the lumbar subarachnoid space. The patient is then placed in the lateral decubitus position, and the contrast is allowed to flow cephalad by tilting the table in the Trendelenburg position until the entire dependent side of the dorsal spine is outlined by contrast. With the patient in the true lateral position, films are then obtained in the lateral and AP projections.

Care should be taken to make sure that the patient holds his head tipped upward with his ear resting on his upper shoulder. This will ensure that contrast material is held in the cervical region and does not flow into the cranial vault. After the necessary films have been obtained, the patient is returned to a prone, head-up position. The contrast is again pooled in the lumbar subarachnoid space and then allowed to flow cephalad, with the patient positioned in the opposite lateral decubitus position. A similar technique is used with water-soluble contrast material and is described under the discussion on Amipaque myelography. Radiographic tomograms or CT may be necessary for complete evaluation after study with water-soluble contrast material.

Spinal Cord Arteriovenous Malformations

Spinal cord arteriovenous malformations (Fig. 15–105, p. 792) are seen infrequently. They do, however, have a rather characteristic appearance on myelography. Most commonly, they appear as wormlike accumulations of dilated vascular channels upon the dorsal aspect of the cord. If this diagnosis is suspected, it is necessary to remove the needle and place the patient in the supine position, allowing the contrast to flow into the dorsal region of the cord. In addition, it may become necessary to study these abnormalities by spinal arteriography. Arteriovenous malformations of the cord may be suspected in patients who have had subarachnoid hemorrhage and when no intracranial source of bleeding has been identified in spite of multiple arteriographic examinations.

Spinal cord arteriography is a lengthy procedure, requiring selective catheterization of the artery of Adamkiewicz and as many lumbar arteries as possible, with serial filming after injection of contrast. The use of magnification and subtraction techniques and digital subtraction angiography allows better visualization of any vascular malformations of the cord. There are dangers inherent in spinal cord arteriography, including the possibility of paralysis of the lower extremities because of occlusion of the blood supply to the cord and because of a direct toxic reaction of the cord to the contrast material. Therefore, caution should be used when performing the procedure. Because of its meticulous nature, this procedure is of necessity quite prolonged and physically taxing for both the patient and the individuals performing the study. Intra-arterial digital subtraction angiography greatly facilitates this type of study (see Chapter 14).

Nerve Root Avulsion

A severe injury to either the brachial plexus or more rarely the lumbar plexus may result in an avulsion of the nerve root at its attachment to the spinal cord (Fig. 15–71, p. 762). This injury appears to be secondary to a stretching of the nerve beyond its endurance, as when the patient suffers a harsh traction injury on an arm or leg. This type of damage to the brachial plexus is irreversible and generally results in a partially or totally flail upper extremity.

The myelographic appearance is very characteristic. The cord appears intrinsically normal, but the contrast material readily enters a sac of the arachnoid layer of the meninges that formed when the cervical nerve was pulled from the spinal cord at its point of attachment. The severed end of the nerve will be found at the distal end of the sac, where it retracts after being pulled from the cord. Although the contrast material readily **enters** this sac, its egress is often not seen, even after returning the patient to the upright position. Surgical attempts to anastomose this avulsed nerve to the cord have not met with success. Similar damage to the lumbar plexus is rare and is associated with extensive soft tissue and bone damage.

Epidural Abscess and Spinal Tuberculosis

Abscesses in the epidural space are not common but may be seen—particularly in drug addicts with a history of intravenous drug abuse. They also may develop following dental procedures. Epidural abscesses may or may not be associated with a bony abnormality. The patient often experiences severe pain, and the extradural block to the flow of contrast material typically extends over a long length of spinal column.

Tuberculosis is most common in the thoracic spine. Typically, tuberculosis affects two vertebral bodies and the intervening intervertebral disc space (Fig. 15–58, p. 751). There is commonly an acute kyphosis at the level of the abnormality.

Epidural Venography

Selective catheterization of the ascending lumbar veins is performed, using the Seldinger technique. Failure to fill the anterior internal vertebral veins is significant, as is posterior displacement of these veins. Venography is of no help in the postoperative patient and should not be performed in the patient allergic to contrast material.

Epidural venography is helpful in patients with a normal myelogram and in those with a wide epidural space.

Because of anatomic variations in the venous system, some feel that venography is not helpful. Others find the accuracy similar to that of myelography. The author has not been impressed with the value of epidural venography.

CEREBELLOPONTINE ANGLE CISTERNOGRAPHY

CT Cisternography

Cerebellopontine angle cisternography was and is a popular procedure for the diagnosis of space-occupying lesions in the cerebellopontine angle. One begins by following the identical procedures used for myelography. Lumbar tap under fluoroscopic control is performed with the patient in the prone position. When studying the cerebellopontine angle, one needs to use only a small amount of contrast material. Approximately 5 ml of 190 mg I/ml concentration Amipaque is instilled and allowed to flow intracranially. The patient is then placed in the CT scanner, and multiple and thin or overlapping cuts are obtained.

The eighth and seventh cranial nerves exit from the internal auditory canal, and the usual clinical history is that of involvement of these two nerves. Involvement of the fifth cranial nerve suggests that the tumor has reached a certain size. The fifth cranial nerve and its trigeminal ganglion rest in Meckel's cavity, which is an outpouching of the dura along the top of the petrous bone 1.5 cm from the internal auditory canal. Therefore, involvement of the fifth as well as the seventh and eighth cranial nerves implies that the tumor is at least 1.5 cm in size. This can be readily appreciated at myelography. In the normal study, the shadow of the trigeminal ganglion occasionally can be seen along the top of the petrous ridge (see Chapter 13).

Amipaque and/or air cisternography used with computed tomography and more recently MR scanning have replaced Pantopaque cisternography.

AIR MYELOGRAPHY

In addition to positive contrast materials, it is also possible to use air as a myelographic contrast agent. This method is useful in the acutely injured patient to rule out the presence of cord edema resulting in complete block to the flow of contrast. When the diagnosis of syringomyelia is suspected, the procedure is performed using the C_1–C_2 approach with the patient in the supine Trendelenburg position. Initially, a large amount of CSF is removed from the cervical subarachnoid space and air is instilled. The patient is placed in the Trendelenburg position to allow the air to rise into the lumbar region. Then further CSF is removed, and the procedure is continued until the CSF has been replaced by air in the subarachnoid space. Radiographs are then obtained. It is vital that tomographic studies be available for complete evaluation. Without tomography it is impossible to evaluate thoroughly the relationship between the cord and the subarachnoid space.

COMPUTED TOMOGRAPHY OF SPINAL TRAUMA

As mentioned earlier, CT is an ideal method of evaluating anatomic deformities of the vertebral column caused by spinal trauma. CT does not require manipulation of the patient other than positioning the patient in the supine position on the CT table, thus making it superior to radiographic tomography. Images can then be obtained at any level of the spine in the axial plane without further movement of the patient. The rapid scanning speed of CT makes it a convenient, fast, accurate, and noninvasive method of evaluating the spine. For bony abnormalities, the study can be performed without the use of water-soluble contrast material. If desired, or necessary for diagnosis, the study can be performed following myelography (see below). The presence of contrast material in the subarachnoid space allows evaluation of the spinal cord as well as the vertebral column and provides accurate evaluation of the relationships among the various structures.

If a myelogram is necessary for identification of spinal cord abnormalities, it should be performed with minimal manipulation of the patient. Ideally, lateral fluoroscopy provides easy and convenient evaluation of the instillation of the contrast via a cervical spinal tap at the C_1–C_2 level. The patient is therefore allowed to remain in the supine position, and under fluoroscopic guidance the needle is placed in the cervical subarachnoid space and CSF removed for evaluation. Following this, an adequate amount of water-soluble contrast material is instilled in the subarachnoid space. The patient is simultaneously tilted head up, and the contrast is allowed to flow caudad. Once the contrast material is positioned at the level of interest, films are obtained in the AP, lateral, and oblique positions so that the level of the abnormality can be identified. Following this, the patient is taken to the CT scanner where additional studies are performed as necessary. In Figure 15–102 (pp. 788 to 789) the fractures of the posterior elements are well demonstrated as is the fact that the Amipaque does not accumulate in the lower subarachnoid space.

In the usual appearance of a fracture of the lumbar vertebral bodies, the superior end-plate of the vertebra is displaced posteriorly into the vertebral body as a triangular fragment. The fractures are usually comminuted. The exact extent of involvement is readily and much more accurately evaluated by CT than by any other method. CT, particularly with the aid of reconstruction views, can readily evaluate the encroachment upon the vertebral canal, the presence or absence of involvement of the posterior elements and transverse processes, the presence and extent of encroachment upon the subarachnoid space, and the presence of a paraspinal hematoma.

MAGNETIC RESONANCE OF THE SPINE

Magnetic resonance (MR) is an ideal method of evaluating the spine for a variety of diseases. MR provides a readily reproducible, noninvasive method of evaluating the spinal column and its contents. No adverse biologic effects have been identified, and the method does not require the use of ionizing radiation or the injection of contrast material. There is also the advantage that MR provides a more direct evaluation of the spinal cord than other methods such as CT, which also requires the injection of contrast material, or myelography, which gives an indirect evaluation of the spinal cord. MR can be used for evaluation of the presence or absence of metastatic disease involving the vertebral bodies, spinal cord tumors, disc disease, syringohydromyelia, and a variety of miscellaneous processes. Evaluation of the upper cervical region is usually accomplished by the use of a head coil and can be particularly helpful when a patient has multiple sclerosis; the examination of the craniovertebral junction rules out the presence of an organic disease process such as a foramen magnum meningioma. The remainder of the spine can then be evaluated with the use of the body coil, although for complete evaluation it is necessary to use surface coils. (Note that surface coils do not actually "coil" around the patient's body, but have an appearance similar to that of a heating pad, on which the patient reclines. The "coil" is positioned below or adjacent to the area of interest for the best visualization and evaluation.)

Magnetic Resonance of Disc Disease

Magnetic resonance is an easy method of establishing the presence of a degenerated lumbar disc. It is possible that MR could be used as the initial screening procedure in a patient with possible disc disease. If the disc is normal by MR evaluation, then one can consider other possible causes of the patient's back pain. On the other hand, if the tentative diagnosis is spinal stenosis, then CT is probably the diagnostic procedure of choice.

Technique of MR Examination

The mid and right and left slices are the best images to use to initiate the evaluation of the spinal column in general, and the lumbar spine is no exception. The initial evaluation can be performed using the T-1 weighted SE sequences to evaluate the general configuration of the vertebral bodies and also the possible presence of metastatic disease, which can occasionally masquerade as lumbar disc disease. The initial slices are made using the T-1 weighted SE sequences (TR530/TE30) with the multislice technique. With this technique an odd number of slices contiguous with one another and 1 cm in thickness can be obtained with one pulsing sequence. This initial series of slices allows ready evaluation of the vertebral body and disc space heights. With this SE sequence the CSF is low in signal intensity, and the marrow within the vertebral bodies is relatively high in signal intensity because of its high fat content. The cortical margin of the vertebral bodies is of very low signal intensity, as is the anulus fibrosus, which forms a continuous line with the cortical margin of the vertebrae. The nucleus pulposus is of relatively low signal intensity but is more gray than the anulus fibrosus or the cortical bone. Any replacement of the fatty bone marrow with tumor tissue appears as areas of low signal intensity. This tumor replacement is easy to appreciate in most cases (Figs. 15–15 to 15–25, pp. 716 to 722).

The second scan series is a T-2 weighted series also using multiple slices. The best technique is a TR3120/TE60-120 SE sequence. This is sufficiently to the right of the cross-over point of CSF that the CSF within the vertebral canal is now of very high signal intensity and the normal nucleus pulposus is also of very high signal intensity if the disc is normal. On the other hand, a disc that remains low in signal intensity is a degenerated disc. This low signal intensity of the degenerated disc on the T-2 weighted images appears to be secondary to loss of water within the disc. This alteration is also easy to appreciate, and the abnormal discs can be readily demonstrated. Since the images can be somewhat degraded at either end of the magnetic gradient, the anatomic areas of interest should be placed in the middle of the field gradient. The low signal intensity of the degenerated discs does not mean that there is an associated herniated disc at this level. In fact, while some herniated discs can be demonstrated by MR, the presence of a herniation is best demonstrated by CT at the present state of the technology. On the other hand, most herniated discs do show evidence of degeneration. The herniated discs that are demonstrable by MR are usually those discs that are in the midline; on the T-2 weighted images, with CSF of very high signal intensity, the low signal intensity of the degenerated disc is readily seen protruding into the high signal intensity of the CSF (Figs. 15–53 and 15–54, pp. 746 to 747 and 748).

The Surface Coils

With the development of surface coils, the presence of herniated discs is much more readily demonstrated. In addition to slices obtained in the sagittal plane, slices in the axial plane with T-1 weighted TR530/TE30 SE sequences which are made beginning with one normal disc and progressing through the abnormal discs readily demonstrates the abnormal disc. The presence of compromise of the low signal intensity CSF is easy to appreciate. The perineural fat in the neural foramina is easy to demonstrate on the MR scans, and the presence of a laterally placed herniated disc that is of low signal intensity will obliterate the fat in the neural foramen.

Uses of MR in Disc Disease

Since MR is so sensitive in detecting disc degeneration, MR may well be used in the future for the initial screening of the patient with back pain or sciatica. If the disc is normal with the MR scan, then one may look elsewhere for the cause of the patient's pain.

Surface Coil Imaging

Technique:
TR530/TE30: three to seven sagittal sections
TR3120/TE120: three to seven sagittal sections
TR530/TE30: axial sections through abnormal disc levels

Magnetic Resonance of Metastatic Disease

Magnetic resonance is an ideal way to evaluate the spinal column for the presence or absence of metastatic disease. MR is very efficient for visualization of the replacement of the normal fatty bone marrow with low signal intensity tumor cells, and it is likely that MR will replace radionuclide bone scanning for the evaluation of vertebral column metastases (Figs. 15–15 to 15–25, pp. 716 to 722).

Technique

The TR530/TE30 SE is the most efficient method of evaluating the spine for metastases. With this SE scan the normal high signal intensity of the bone marrow is replaced by low signal intensity tumor, which is easily detected on the MR scans. In the majority of cases this is the only sequence that is necessary for complete evaluation. The entire vertebral column can be evaluated in approximately one-half hour. Scans are performed in the mid and right and left parasagittal slices. The number of slices depends upon the presence or absence of a scoliosis. If a physiologic or pathologic scoliosis is present secondary to a pathologic fracture of a vertebral body, then a larger number of contiguous slices must be generated. The slices are obtained from left to right in the body part examined, and therefore the exact location of the tumor replacement can be easily determined. Since the pedicles and facets are usually well demonstrated, the anatomic location of the abnormal signal intensity can be easily determined. In addition, the presence or absence of a paraspinal mass can also be readily determined. These paraspinal masses secondary to extension of tumor outside of the vertebral body, or secondary to hematoma caused by recent pathologic fracture, can be easily identified. Coronal plane slices may be helpful for evaluation of a paraspinal mass.

The TR3120/TE120 SE scans may reveal that the low signal intensity areas on the T-1 weighted scans become increased in signal intensity on the T-2 weighted scans; however, most commonly the abnormal areas are less well visualized on the T-2 weighted scans. Other areas of involvement such as the sternum can also be readily demonstrated. The T-2 weighted images cause the CSF to be of very high signal intensity, so that subtle areas of encroachment can be readily demonstrated on these images when they cannot be seen on the T-1 weighted images.

Areas of cord compression can also be readily identified in most cases, as can areas of spinal cord widening or narrowing. Inability to visualize the CSF surrounding the spinal cord may also imply cord compression or at least encroachment upon the subarachnoid space without frank cord compression. These changes correlate very well with the myelographic findings in patients with possible cord compression, and the author believes that even at the present stage of technology, MR can replace myelography for the diagnosis of cord compression in the majority of cases. Difficulty is encountered in those patients with diffuse osteolytic or osteoblastic metastatic disease, in whom the vertebral bodies are homogeneously involved and therefore a comparison between vertebral bodies cannot be made. In most cases a comparison with plain spine radiography will be helpful for complete evaluation.

Technique:
TR530/TE 30 SE: three to seven sagittal sections (most important sequence)
TR3120/TR120-60 SE: three to seven sagittal sections (may be omitted for metastatic workup)
TR530/TE30: axial or coronal sections allow excellent evaluation of possible paraspinal mass

MR provides relatively rapid, convenient, and easily reproducible evaluation of the spinal column for the detection of metastatic disease. It is likely that MR will replace nuclide scanning for the evaluation of metastases. MR not only identifies the presence of abnormal signal from the vertebral body but also evaluates the presence of a paraspinal mass, pathologic fracture, or partial or complete spinal cord compression. When a vertebral body is involved with metastatic disease, it appears lower in signal intensity than the normal vertebral body. The presence of a scoliosis, either physiologic or secondary to a pathologic fracture may compromise the examination with body coils, but this is usually overcome with the use of surface coils. This replacement of the vertebral bodies with tumor is best evaluated on the T-1 weighted images (TR530/TE30). The planar multislice technique of MR also allows one to localize any abnormality to one or the other of the vertebral bodies. The T-2 weighted images have not been particularly helpful for the evaluation of metastatic disease, but they have occasionally been helpful in evaluating the presence of compromise of the subarachnoid space. This evaluation is possible because the CSF becomes increased in signal intensity on the T-2 weighted images, and therefore areas of encroachment may be more easily identified.

For evaluation of the entire spine as a screening procedure, the spinal column is first evaluated using the body coil. This may be performed using 1-cm or 0.75-cm thick slices in the sagittal plane. This initial study is performed using the TR530/TE30 SE sequences. The entire spine can be evaluated in two scanning sequences using this method and allows an overlap of the field of view in the lower thoracic region. This entire procedure requires approximately 30 minutes of table time. If there is an additional area of interest, then surface images can also be obtained, and these can be performed in the sagittal or another plane.

Typical Appearance of Metastatic Disease

Osteolytic metastases cause the vertebral bodies to appear decreased in signal intensity.

Osteoblastic metastases cause the vertebral bodies to appear decreased in signal intensity, both because of replacement by tumor cells and because the blastic lesions respond like bone in other areas, i.e., low in signal intensity.

Primary marrow processes such as lymphocytic leukemia also appear of decreased signal intensity because of replacement of the normal fatty bone marrow with tumor cells.

Because of the similar appearance of different types of metastatic disease, it is important to compare the MR scan with the plain spine radiographs for complete evaluation.

Magnetic Resonance Appearance After Radiation Therapy

Following radiation treatment there is an alteration in the appearance of the vertebral bodies. In the region of the treatment port, there is an increase in the signal intensity within the vertebral bodies relative to the remainder of the vertebral bodies. This increase in signal intensity occurs because there is a relative increase in the amount of deposition of adipose tissue. This area of increased signal intensity corresponds exactly to the treatment port. The exact time of its initial appearance has not yet been determined, but the increase in signal intensity probably lasts indefinitely.

This alteration in signal intensity following radiation treatment can be used for treatment planning and also for evaluation of patients who have received radiation treatment but in whom the exact port is unknown (Figs. 15–16 to 15–18, pp. 716 to 717).

Magnetic Resonance of Cord Compression

In the patient with metastatic disease MR provides an excellent method of evaluating the presence of metastases to the vertebral column. As noted above, MR also allows one to determine the presence of a pathologic fracture, scoliosis secondary to fracture, or a paraspinal mass. The abnormal vertebral body is readily identified by body coil imaging in the sagittal plane. Following this, surface coil images should be obtained of any areas that are suspicious for cord compression. If no area of suspicion is identified by body coil examination, then the surface coil images should be obtained of the clinical level of suspicion. The surface coil images can be performed in the sagittal plane or in the coronal or axial planes.

Signs of cord compression include (1) compromise of the CSF surrounding the cord, (2) paraspinal mass extending into the vertebral canal, (3) compromise or compression of the spinal cord, and (4) soft tissue metastases in the epidural space.

The changes noted above may be isolated to a single vertebral body or may affect multiple levels. MR readily identifies these levels and can be used to direct appropriate therapy. Obviously, response to treatment can also be readily evaluated with this noninvasive procedure.

It appears that even small interruptions in the CSF should be closely evaluated for early cord impingement and surface coil images obtained of any suspicious areas. There is excellent correlation with myelographic findings, and it is anticipated that MR will replace myelography for evaluation of cord compression. One of the advantages of MR is the fact that the areas between a widespread block to the flow of contrast, such as might be seen following instillation of contrast via lumbar tap and cervical tap, is readily evaluated. Whereas by myelography alone only the extreme ends of the abnormality are identified, by MR the central portion of the cord, between areas of block, is also evaluated without the injection of contrast material and any risks that this may entail.

In addition to the involvement of the vertebral bodies with metastatic disease, other areas of soft tissue metastases to the epidural space can also be identified. This is particularly easy to appreciate when there is replacement of the fat in the epidural space by the decreased signal intensity tumor. The index of suspicion must be high to appreciate these changes in some cases, while in others the change is very easy to detect. Because there is normally a great deal of variation in the amount of fat in the epidural space, replacement of fat by tumor may be difficult to detect in areas where the amount of fat is scarce. The multiplanar capability of MR is very helpful for this type of evaluation.

Because of the readily reproducible and noninvasive nature of MR and because of its accuracy, MR will probably replace radionuclide and other diagnostic methods for evaluation of metastatic disease.

The CSF that normally surrounds the cord is easily identified as an area of low signal intensity on the T-1 weighted images. This circumferential area of CSF density is relatively generous in the upper cervical region but becomes progressively smaller in the lower cervical region and smaller yet in the thoracic region. There is an area of focal expansion in the lower cord known as the conus medullaris that begins at T_9 and ends at approximately T_{12} to L_1. The cord tapers rapidly below the conus and gives rise to multiple nerve roots of the cauda equina, and the cord itself ends at the level of the lower end-plate of L_1 or upper end-plate of L_2 in the majority of cases. Below the level of the cord, there is a definite increase in the amount of CSF space relative to the neural tissue. When there is cord compression, there is interruption or compromise of the CSF density material that surrounds the cord. This change is most obvious on surface coil images but can also be identified on body coil images. In fact, it is the presence of these subtle changes in the appearance of the CSF that allows one to identify and therefore better study the levels of abnormality.

The presence of epidural metastases with compromise of the surrounding CSF may vary from a subtle compromise to total lack of visualization of CSF over a multilevel segment. Associated with this compromise of the CSF, there is often mechanical compression of the spinal cord which appears as an area of either cord widening or cord narrowing. The appearance of widening occurs because there is cord compression in the orthogonal plane. All of these changes are similar to those identified on the myelogram, but they are now identified on the MR scan with direct visualization of the spinal cord. In fact, MR allows the most direct visualization of the cord and the least interference with visualization by the surrounding bony artifacts. The MR scan of metastatic disease and cord compromise should be read with attention to small detail and slight interruption of the CSF so that early and/or subtle areas of abnormality will not be overlooked.

In the case of one abnormal vertebral body, a pathologic fracture, and posterior displacement of the abnormal vertebrae into the vertebral column, the changes are not difficult to appreciate. This, however, is only occasionally the case. Further progression of metastatic disease reveals involvement of multiple vertebral bodies with replacement of the normally high signal marrow with low signal intensity tumor, pathologic fractures, paraspinal masses, and multiple levels of partial or complete cord compression. When all the vertebrae are involved, change is sometimes difficult to appreciate because there are no normal vertebrae remaining to provide a basis for comparison. One convenient feature is the fact that in the normal patient the disc is lower in signal intensity than the vertebral body, while in the pathologic case the vertebral body is lower in signal intensity than the intervertebral disc. In any case, it is best to compare MR scans with plain films.

Another class of metastatic disease is the presence of involvement with osteoblastic metastatic disease. In most instances, the MR appearance is very similar to that of involvement by osteolytic metastatic disease. As a general rule, bone has a low signal intensity because of the relative lack of mobile protons. Therefore, osteoblastic metastatic deposits similarly give a decreased signal intensity appearance. This change is most commonly seen in the patient with metastatic prostatic carcinoma. Because metastatic disease is easily amenable to surgical treatment or radiation therapy, it is important to make the correct diagnosis, and therefore it is again vital to compare the MR image to plain spine films. It is not uncommon that osteoblastic metastases involve vertebral bodies, resulting in multiple levels of abnormality. If radiation therapy is the chosen method of treatment, then MR is probably sufficient for evaluation. When surgery is contemplated, myelography may be necessary if MR does not correlate with the physical findings.

Orthogonal plane, or 90-degree opposite view, may demonstrate cord compression; again, these reflect the same findings that are seen on a myelogram. An additional advantage of MR is the fact that at the level of an epidural mass with compromise of the cord or simply the CSF, there is usually an associated abnormal vertebral body. This obviously makes the identification and diagnosis of an abnormality significantly easier.

Magnetic Resonance of Spinal Cord Tumors

Magnetic resonance provides for direct imaging of the spinal cord. Other methods of evaluation provide only indirect evidence that an abnormality of the cord is present. Plain spine films are usually not helpful for detecting the presence of a spinal cord abnormality. If an abnormality is present, it is usually an area of destruction or erosion of the spinal canal or vertebral column; rarely there may be an area of calcification within the cord or tumor which is visible on plain film examination. This, of course, provides direct evidence of an abnormality, but the full extent of the abnormality is often not visible. CT does allow visualization of a calcified spinal cord tumor, but this lesion is very rare and CT must usually be performed after the introduction of water-soluble contrast material to allow demonstration of the abnormality. Myelography, of course, demonstrates the cord, but only indirectly, as it is surrounded by the contrast in the subarachnoid space. Magnetic resonance, particularly the T-1 weighted images, allows direct visualization of the spinal cord and its relationship to the surrounding structures. The TR530/TE30 SE images using five sagittal cuts usually allows optimal visualization of the spinal cord. The five 1-cm slices are sufficiently wide to demonstrate the cord except in those cases in which there is a very severe scoliosis. Areas of expansion of the cord can usually be demonstrated directly if there is an intramedullary tumor, and in addition to the cord widening, the compromise of the CSF surrounding the cord can also be demonstrated. This allows both direct and indirect evidence of the presence of an abnormality. With the 1-cm slice technique, focal displacement of the cord can also be readily appreciated when the cord is demonstrated well except in one focal area. If this is the case, then additional images can be obtained in other planes.

The standard myelographic classification of the images is, of course, unchanged, but the CSF, rather than water-soluble contrast material, provides the "contrast agent" surrounding the spinal cord which is used for classifying the tumor abnormality.

Technique

The TR530/TE30 SE images provide the best images of the anatomy of the spinal cord and its surroundings. The entire spinal cord can be demonstrated in two imaging sequences. The base of the skull and the cervical and upper thoracic spine can all be visualized on one series. The patient is then brought out of the scanner and the TR530/TE30 SE sequence is repeated to include the remainder of the thoracic spine and the entire lumbar spine. Following this the same sagittal cuts are obtained using the T-2 weighted TR3120/TE120 multiecho SE sequence of the slice that provides the best image.

The T-2 weighted image causes the CSF to become high in signal intensity, so any areas of encroachment can be readily identified. In addition, any abnormal discs can be visualized. The patient is then moved back to the starting position, and the initial slices are repeated using the longer SE sequences. If close attention is paid to the original table and scanner position, then the T-1 and T-2 weighted images can be easily compared and any areas of abnormal signal intensity easily identified.

It appears that most abnormalities are demonstrated on the T-1 weighted images. In fact, the T-2 weighted images may obliterate any abnormal area and should not be used as the only scanning sequence. As in the brain, abnormal tissue—tumors—becomes increased in signal intensity when examined with T-2 SE techniques. However, while the tumors become increased in signal intensity, the signal intensity of the surrounding CSF also becomes increased, obliterating the abnormal signal from the tumor. Surface coil images are obtained of any area of interest.

Technique
Summary: TR530/TE30 SE with five sagittal slices

TR3120/TE120 SE with five sagittal slices
or
Single-slice, multiecho SE in plane of interest

One single-slice, multiecho sequence available on the Teslacon is the TR2240/TE30-60-90-120-150-180-210-240 SE.

Magnetic Resonance of the Cervicomedullary Junction

Magnetic resonance is a very useful method of evaluating the cervicomedullary junction. MR allows direct visualization of the spinal cord without the artifact seen with CT scanning, without the injection of contrast materials, and without manipulation of the patient. The cervicomedullary junction can be visualized using either the head coil or the surface coil. The anterior margin of the foramen magnum is identified by noting the inferior margin of the clivus; the clivus is usually easily identified by the high signal intensity fatty bone marrow. In those cases in which the clivus is poorly visualized, one may also rely on a small, irregular collection of high signal intensity fat that is located just above the odontoid process, just below the clivus, and just at the level of the anterior margin of the foramen magnum (Figs. 15–61 and 15–62, pp. 754 and 755).

The posterior margin of the foramen magnum is less well visualized but can usually be identified by the point where the inner and outer table of the calvarium meet. This point is characterized by the high signal intensity fatty marrow of the diploe of the skull separating the two tables. The odontoid process is also easily identified because the fatty bone marrow of the odontoid allows it to be easily seen even though the low signal intensity of the cortical margin is frequently difficult to see. Therefore, the various anatomic margins of the foramen magnum are easily identified and any alterations in the relationships easily noted.

Magnetic Resonance of the Chiari Malformation

Associated with the Chiari malformation is downward displacement of the cerebellar tonsils (Figs. 15–92, 15–93, 15–97, and 15–98, pp. 781, 782, 784, and 785). This downward displacement of the tonsils is easily identified by MR examination, as is any associated syrinx. With the Chiari Type II malformation there is deformity of the brain stem in addition to the downward displacement of the tonsils. These changes are also easily appreciated. Other deformities, such as beaking of the midbrain, an enlarged massa intermedia, alterations in the cerebral aqueduct, and hydrocephalus, are also easily identified and evaluated. This tonsillar herniation is not uncommonly seen even in asymptomatic patients. The mild degree of varying downward displacement of the tonsils is sometimes considered "tonsilar ectopia" rather than a pathologic condition.

In some cases the cystic area within the central portion of the cord extends superiorly to the level of the medulla, a condition known as syringobulbia. At times the communication between the medullary cyst and the cervical cord cavity can be easily identified.

Magnetic Resonance of Rheumatoid Arthritis

Patients with rheumatoid arthritis may develop basilar invagination (basilar impression) with upward mobility of the odontoid process relative to the foramen magnum. This basilar impression occurs because of the laxity of the ligaments around the odontoid process, resulting in movement of the odontoid process from its normal position. One can identify the relationship between the spinal cord and the surrounding soft tissue and bony structures (Fig. 15–61, p. 754), as well as the position of the odontoid process.

With basilar impression the odontoid process is upwardly mobile and compresses the intracranial medulla. This abnormal relationship is easily identified and evaluated by MR. Because there is a relatively generous amount of space around the odontoid process at the C_1–C_2 level, the cervical spinal cord can be displaced to one side or the other. This displacement produces a curvilinear configuration of the spinal cord and inability to visualize the cord on a single slice of the multiplaner images. Therefore, the anatomic location and configuration of the spinal cord must be evaluated on multiple contiguous sections and at times is best evaluated on the axial images.

There may be marked erosion and destructive changes of the odontoid process with rheumatoid arthritis. Although the exact cortical margin may be difficult to identify at times, the resulting displacement usually allows accurate evaluation of these changes. There may also be overgrowth of the pannus, which results in destruction of the odontoid process. This pannus appears of low signal intensity on the T-1 weighted images and at times may be quite large in size. This large mass of pannus may cause distortion of the cervical spinal cord, posterior displacement of the spinal cord, and marked compromise of the subarachnoid space as well as erosion of the odontoid process. One of the valuable assets of MR is the ability to evaluate all of these changes without manipulation of the patient, thus obviating the possibility of serious injury. MR is superior to CT because contrast injection is unnecessary. The bony structures may be better visualized by CT, but superior visualization of the soft tissues makes MR the procedure of choice.

Technique of Examination

Sagittal images using the TR530/TE30 SE may be all that is necessary. In some cases T-1 weighted images in the axial plane may also be required. The entire evaluation can be performed in approximately 10 minutes of scanning time.

Magnetic Resonance of Spinal Trauma

Acute Trauma

Because the patient who presents with acute spinal trauma is often a victim of multiorgan injury, this individual is often not a candidate for evaluation acutely with MR. Multiple life support systems usually cannot be brought into the room with the magnet, and the acutely injured patient is unable to cooperate for the relatively long period of time required for MR scan. On the other hand, if only the spinal column and spinal cord are of interest and the patient is not on life support systems and is able to cooperate, then MR is probably the ideal method of evaluation. MR allows direct visualization of the spinal cord, and changes such as might be seen with cord swelling or acute cord hematoma can be readily identified. It can be stated with a fair degree of certainty that hematomas in the first 48 hours are of low signal intensity, and therefore very acutely one cannot differentiate between swelling and acute hematoma; after the first 48 hours, areas of acute hemorrhage become increased in signal intensity and therefore are easily identified and diagnosed. However, this delay of 48 hours may be critical in the treatment of the patient. Again, as with metastatic disease, areas of encroachment resulting from swelling or epidural hematoma are also identified because of compromise of the surrounding CSF or because of narrowing or widening of the cord. In addition, the ready availability of multiplanar imaging is obviously a great advantage.

One of the criticisms of MR is that it provides rather poor visualization of bone, particularly the cortical bone, because of its low signal intensity. This does not, however, appear to be a real problem. The marrow within the vertebral body appears high in signal intensity and is easily identified; therefore, the surrounding cortical margin is easily seen. The presence or absence of abnormalities of the vertebral body is easily determined. Loss of vertebral body height is easily identified, and again the multiplanar capability allows detection of any accentuation of scoliosis or kyphosis secondary to these fractures. The axial images provide noninvasive evaluation of the relationship of the spinal cord, surrounding CSF, and vertebral body. MR may provide the initial and best method of evaluating the patient with acute spine trauma.

Once injury to the spinal cord has been ruled out, it is then possible to proceed to other types of examination, such as CT of the spine and metrizamide myelography, if additional evaluation is required.

Old Trauma

MR is the method of choice for evaluation of the patient with a history of old spinal injury. The sequelae of spinal cord injury lend themselves well to examination by MR. Early in the course of an injury—up to six weeks or two months—the presence of hemorrhage is easily identified as an area of increased signal intensity. Cord edema is also easily seen, as are areas of compromise of the CSF. Even later in the course of the injury there may be cord atrophy. This may be focal or involve multiple vertebral body segments. Again, the ease with which these changes can be identified with MR is remarkable.

Ancient trauma may lead to the development of a cavity or syrinx within the spinal cord. The presence of this type of syrinx does not imply that that was a definite cord hematoma. A syrinx can also be seen following cord edema. The latter produces an area of myelomalacia that can ultimately progress to a syrinx cavity. The syrinx cavity may be focal or involve a large length of the cord. A syrinx cavity is best evaluated with surface coil imaging and may not be visualized with body coil studies (Fig. 15–102, pp. 788 to 789).

Because MR is a planar type of examination, the presence of scoliosis or even acute kyphosis may interfere with the visualization of a cavity within the cord. If a cavity is strongly suspected, then imaging in the axial plane is suggested as the best method of evaluating the cord. In addition, a syrinx does not definitely enlarge the spinal cord, so a cavity may be present even in the normal or atrophic cord.

Magnetic Resonance of Syringohydromyelia

When there is a syrinx or cavity within the cord, the spinal cord may be normal in size, more commonly enlarged, and rarely small in size. In addition, there is an increased incidence of spinal cord tumor in the presence of a syrinx. Therefore, if a syrinx is identified, then it is necessary to rule out a spinal cord tumor. The syrinx cavity is most commonly identified in the cervical region, although a post-traumatic syrinx may be located at any level in the spinal cord (Fig. 15–92, p. 781).

At the time of this writing, MR is the procedure of choice for the evaluation of syringohydromyelia. The syrinx is best demonstrated on the T-1 weighted images using surface coil technique. The syrinx appears as an area of low (CSF) signal intensity, a cystic cavity of varying size within the spinal cord. The cord containing a syrinx cavity is usually enlarged; however, at times the cord is normal or even small in size. The sagittal plane is the most satisfactory; however, the axial plane may best demonstrate a syrinx cavity, particularly if there is a marked scoliosis.

Because the Chiari malformation is frequently associated with a syrinx, MR also serves the purpose of evaluating this developmental deformity. If the syrinx is associated with a tumor, the fluid within the syrinx cavity may contain a high protein content and therefore appear similar in signal intensity to the spinal cord. The tumor itself may or may not be visible by MR, although the secondary changes of cord widening are readily apparent. While the T-2 weighted images may be helpful, it is not uncommon that the increased signal intensity of the CSF obscures the spinal cord, syrinx cavity, and/or tumor.

Magnetic Resonance of a Syrinx

In the usual case, the involved area of the spinal cord is enlarged. There is a decrease in the normal amount of cerebrospinal fluid that surrounds the cord, and the CSF signal intensity area within the central portion of the cord is of variable size. Because of the partial volume phenomenon that is seen with MR, if the cavity is not centered in the middle of the slice or if the cavity is not of sufficient size, then the signal intensity of the syrinx cavity is averaged with that of the adjacent tissue and appears higher than the signal intensity of CSF. At times, with a high-resolution scanner, the appearance of the gray matter and white matter may falsely suggest a syrinx cavity. A cavity filled with fluid that has an increased protein content may appear to be of the same signal intensity as the spinal cord, and differentiation between the cavity and cord may be difficult or impossible (Figs. 15–93 to 15–100 and 15–103, pp. 782 to 786, and 790).

A syrinx is best demonstrated on the T-1 weighted images; in fact, it is not uncommon on T-2 weighted images that the cord and surrounding structures increase in signal intensity and obliterate any difference in signal intensity between the two. Therefore, it is vital to use the T-1 weighted images if a syrinx is suspected. The syrinx cavity may be homogeneous or variable in size throughout its length or it may be multiseptated. A syrinx cavity may be focal or involve a variable number of vertebral body segments; it is not uncommon to see the entire spinal cord involved.

A syrinx is associated with an increased incidence of spinal cord tumor; therefore, a filling defect within the syrinx should be assumed to be a tumor until proved otherwise. Syringohydromyelia is also common in patients with the Chiari malformation. In fact, since the development of MR, both the Chiari malformation and syringohydromelia have been seen with markedly increased frequency, probably owing to the ease with which the abnormality is diagnosed even in the relatively asymptomatic patient. However, if a syrinx is identified, then the cervicomedullary junction should be evaluated for the presence of the Chiari malformation.

Magnetic Resonance of Discitis

For the diagnosis of discitis, magnetic resonance is probably the procedure of choice. The T-1 weighted image does not aid significantly in the diagnosis, but the T-2 weighted images reveal a typical "bright" disc in the presence of discitis. In addition, the "brightness" on the T-2 weighted image extends into the adjacent vertebral body end-plates. This increased signal intensity is probably related to increased water content and resultant increased proton density (Fig. 15–58, p. 751). This appearance is quite typical and is helpful in the differential diagnosis of back pain, because the degenerated disc appears decreased in signal intensity on the T-2 weighted images. Therefore, differentiation between discitis and degenerated disc is easily made. This appearance of discitis on MR image is also helpful because the CT appearance is usually not pathognomonic, but rather usually demonstrates a bulging disc without other identifying signs.

Magnetic Resonance After Chymopapaine Injection

The injection of the enzyme chymopapaine results in degeneration of a disc. Therefore, following the injection of this enzyme there is decreased signal intensity of the disc similar to that seen in a disc that has undergone degeneration even in the absence of the use of chymopapaine injection.

Magnetic Resonance of Spinal Cord Arteriovenous Malformations

Spinal cord arteriovenous malformations are rare lesions. Because flowing blood causes a negative flow defect on the MR scan in both the T-1 and T-2 weighted images, it is possible to detect an arteriovenous malformation by MR imaging. Typically the vessels appear as serpiginous structures in or surrounding the spinal cord (Fig. 15–105, pp. 792 to 793). It is not uncommon to identify the enlarged draining vein that flows away from the malformation. Although the diagnosis may be suggested by the appearance of the MR scan, angiography is necessary for complete evaluation. The spinal cord is usually enlarged at the level of the malformation, but the appearance may be similar to that of an intramedullary tumor.

These patients may present with a catastrophic event that reflects either a subarachnoid hemorrhage or a hemorrhage into the spinal cord. Other patients may present with progressive extremity weakness.

DIASTEMATOMYELIA

This uncommon lesion consists of a fibrous or bony band that extends from front to back in the spinal canal at the lower thoracic level. This structural abnormality sometimes can be seen on the plain radiograph or by tomography, but more commonly it is detected only by myelography. In addition to any physical symptoms that the patient may have, this abnormality is often associated with spinal dysraphism. Tomograms of the body structures reveal a developmental abnormality in all cases. Because of the bone spur that divides the subarachnoid space, the cord is also split or divided in some fashion. This splitting and tethering of the cord by the bony spicule is the cause of the patient's symptoms and may lead to scoliosis. Myelography reveals that the contrast material flows around the bony defect, creating a double shadow where the dorsal cord is divided. Because this abnormality is often fibrous rather than bony, myelography may be the only procedure that outlines the diastematomyelia.

Computed tomographic body scanning of the spinal column is helpful in the diagnosis of diastematomyelia. The technique is of particular value after the instillation of Amipaque, when the CT scan may be the only procedure necessary to outline the abnormal anatomy (Fig. 15–104, p. 791).

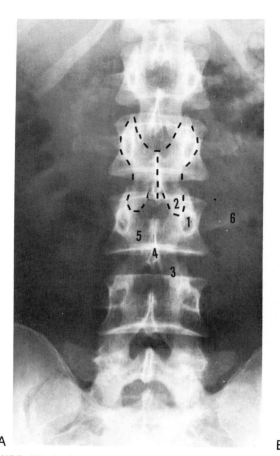

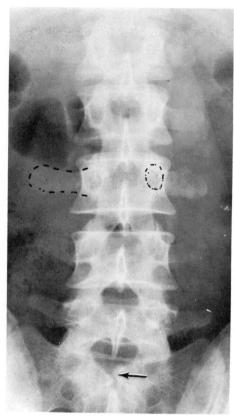

A   B

FIGURE 15–1. *Lumbar Spine:* *A,* On the AP view the pedicles appear as oval areas with a dense cortical margin (*1*). The pedicles project directly posteriorly in the lumbar region and join with the superior and inferior articulating facets (*2* and *3*). The bone between the superior and inferior facets is the pars interarticularis. The laminae (*5*) then extend medially and posteriorly and join in the midline to form the spinous process (*4*). The spinous process projects inferiorly in the lumbar region. The transverse process extends laterally (*6*). The curved dased lines in the illustration follow the superior and inferior articulating facets. The straight dashed line is on the spinous process.

If a total laminectomy is performed, both laminae are cut and the spinous process is removed. However, more commonly a small portion of the lamina is removed, leaving a small crescentic defect in the lamina. This approach often provides sufficient exposure to a herniated disc.

B, Normal anteroposterior view. The oval dotted line outlines the pedicle. The larger dotted line illustrates the transverse process.

There is also a spina bifida (failure of fusion) of the spinous process of S_1 (*arrow*).

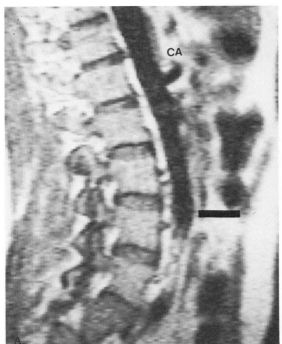

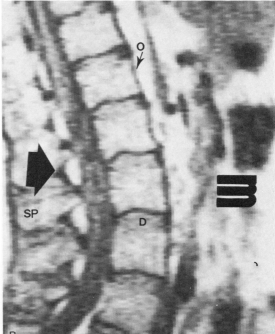

FIGURE 15–2. *Normal MR of the Lumbar Spine:*
The Teslacon scanner generates the scan slices from left to right; therefore, as one reviews the multiple image slices, the sequence of the scans is such that (with standard patient positioning), the left side is visualized first, then the midline, and then the right side. *A,* The image to the left of the midline demonstrates the interfacet joints and neural foramina on the left. The aorta appears as a negative flow defect, and the celiac artery is also seen (*CA*) as it arises from the abdominal aorta.

B, The midline slice reveals the high signal intensity fat in the dorsal epidural space (*large arrow*). The CSF is of low signal intensity on this short SE sequence.

C, This image to the right of the midline demonstrates the interfacet joints (*large arrow*) and the neural foramina on the right side. This right-sided image also demonstrates the negative flow defect of the inferior vena cava.

Other structures that can be seen in *B* and *C* are:

D = intervertebral disc
M = relatively high signal intensity in the bone marrow
O = low signal intensity of the cortical margin of the bone
P = vertebral pedicle
I = inferior articulating facet
S = superior articulating facet
G = nerve ganglion projecting below the level of the pedicle
SP = spinous process of the vertebral body

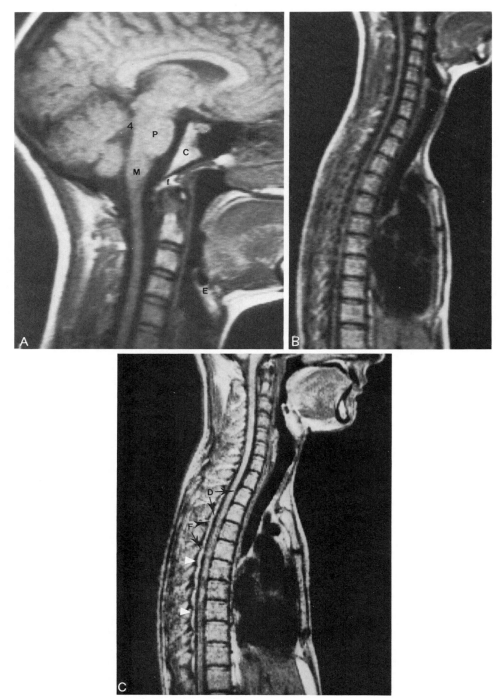

FIGURE 15–3. *Normal Cervical and Thoracic Spine:* All images are TR530/TE30 SE. *A*, The cervicomedullary region is visualized accurately and without the use of contrast material. Normal structures that are seen on nearly all studies are (*C*) clivus, (*P*) pons, (*M*) medulla, (*4*) fourth ventricle, (*f*) fat—this small irregular collection of fat marks the anterior margin of the foramen magnum, and (*E*) epiglottis. The cervical vertebrae are well visualized and can be easily counted.

B, The cervical and thoracic vertebrae are easily seen and counted.

C, A different patient also demonstrates the normal cord and vertebral bodies. There is slight prominence of the dorsal epidural fat (*F*) that appears as increased signal intensity. The posterior spinal laminar line is cortical bone of low signal intensity which projects posterior to the epidural fat (*white arrowheads*). The dura (*D*) and CSF surround the relatively higher signal intensity of the cord and appear as low signal intensity.

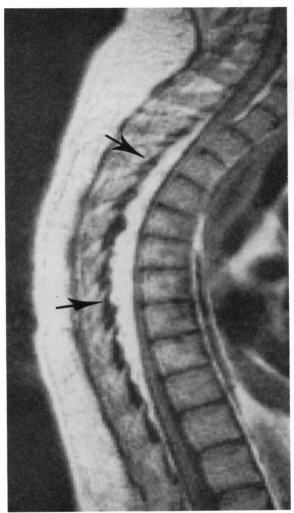

FIGURE 15–4. *Increased Dorsal Epidural Fat:* The T-1 weighted TR530/TE30 SE image reveals an increase in the amount of dorsal epidural fat (*arrows*) in the thoracic region. The spinal cord is compressed and displaced anteriorly. This change may possibly also be related to a process such as cord atrophy, with a resulting increase in the amount of epidural fat. There is also accentuation of the dorsal kyphosis.

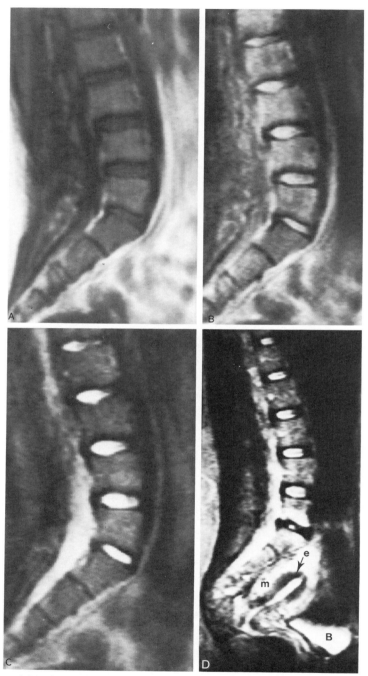

FIGURE 15–5. *Normal Lumbar MR, the Effect of Changing TR/TE Intervals:* *A,* SE TR530/TE30. *B,* SE TR2120/TE60. *C,* SE TR2120/TE120. *D,* SE TR3120/TE120. With increasing TE and TR intervals, the normally low-signal-intensity CSF gradually increases in signal intensity until, with a very prolonged TE and TR interval, the CSF displays high signal intensity. This increased signal intensity of the CSF provides an excellent "contrast" to any abnormal, degenerated, bulging, or herniated disc that might extend posteriorly into the vertebral canal. The normal disc also increases in signal intensity with the increasing TE and TR intervals. Note that in *D* the fluid-filled urinary bladder also increases in signal intensity (*B*). The uterus is also demonstrated, and one can identify the myometrium (*m*) and the endometrium (*e*).

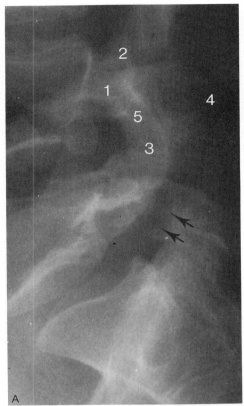

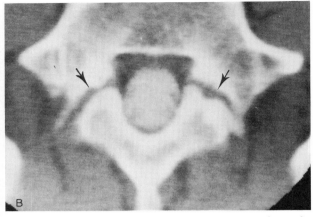

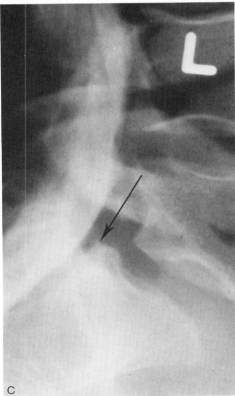

FIGURE 15–6. *Spondylolysis with Spondylolisthesis:*
A, Plain spine examination reveals a break—spondylolysis—in the pars interarticularis (*arrows*). There is a grade one spondylolisthesis with forward displacement of L_5 on S_1.

B, CT scan following myelogram reveals the bilateral spondylolysis (*arrows*).

C, Lateral view of the myelogram reveals the spondylolisthesis with forward displacement of L_5 on S_1. The arrow marks the top of the S_1 vertebral body. Note the widened extradural space behind the vertebral body of L_5.

D, T-1 weighted MR image in a different patient reveals that the widened extradural space fills with high-signal-intensity fat (*arrow*). Note the slight prominence of the anulus fibrosus of the L_5-S_1 intervertebral disc. Close inspection of the MR scan at the level of the facet joint often demonstrates the spondylolysis.

The lateral view (*A*) provides the best evaluation of the heights of the vertebral bodies and the disc spaces. The anatomic structures identified on the AP view also can be seen on the lateral view: (*1*) pedicle, (*2*) superior articulating facet, (*3*) inferior articulating facet, (*4*) spinous process, (*5*) pars interarticularis.

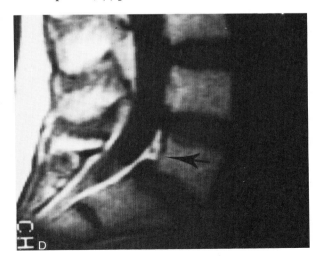

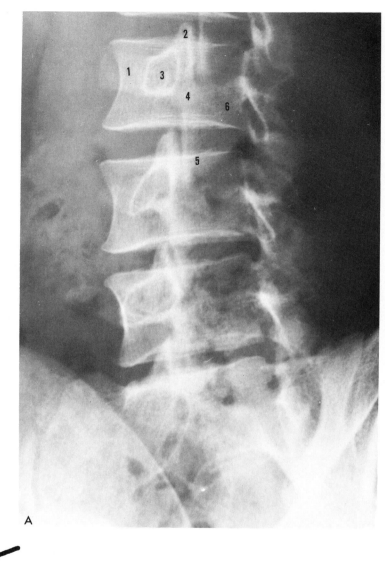

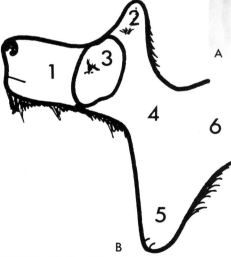

FIGURE 15–7. *The Oblique View:* A, This view provides the best means for evaluation of the pars interarticularis. The oblique view with its combination of structures forms the image of a "Scottie dog" (*B*). The transverse process is the dog's "nose" and also contributes to the anterior margin of the "eye." The pedicle contributes the posterior margin. The superior articulating facet forms the "ear," and the inferior articulating facet forms the "front leg." The "body" of the dog is formed by the lamina of the vertebral body. (*1*) Transverse process. (*2*) Superior articulating facet. (*3*) Pedicle (the transverse process forms the anterior margin). (*4*) Pars interarticularis. (*5*) Inferior articulating facet. (*6*) Lamina.

The articulation between the superior and inferior articulating facets is well demonstrated. The pars interarticularis forms the neck of the Scottie in the oblique view. Although a pars defect may be visualized on other views, it is best demonstrated on the oblique view.

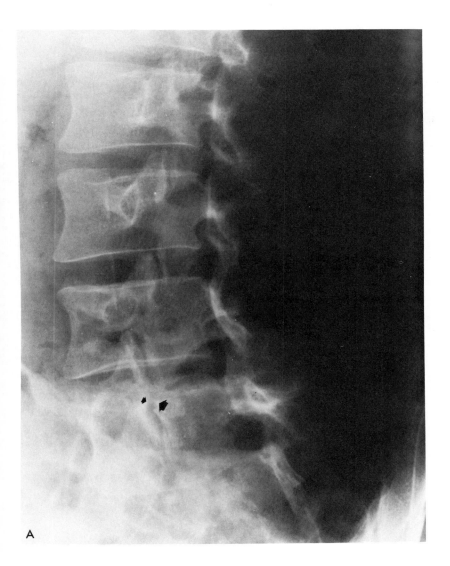

A

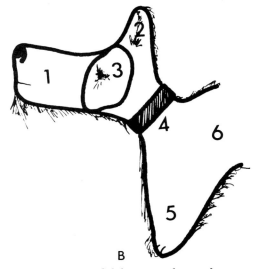

B

FIGURE 15–8. *Oblique View with Spondylolysis at L₅:* There is a spondylolysis involving the pars interarticularis at the L$_5$ level (*arrows*). This break appears as a radiolucent line—as if the Scottie were wearing a collar.

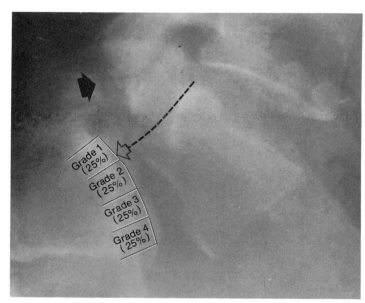

FIGURE 15–9. *Spondylolisthesis:* One method of grading is pictured above. The superior end-plate of the vertebral bodies is divided into four equal parts. A line is drawn along the posterior margin of the vertebral body above (*dotted line*) and extended down to a point on the end-plate of the reference vertebral body (*open arrow*). If displacement of the end-plate is 25 per cent or less, it is a Grade 1 spondylolisthesis; 25 per cent to 50 per cent is a Grade 2; 50 to 75 per cent is a Grade 3; 75 per cent or greater is a Grade 4 spondylolisthesis.

The spondylolysis is visible (*closed black arrow*) at the L_5 level.

Spondylolisthesis also can occur in the absence of a spondylolysis. In such a case there is interfacet degenerative change and joint space narrowing that allows forward slippage.

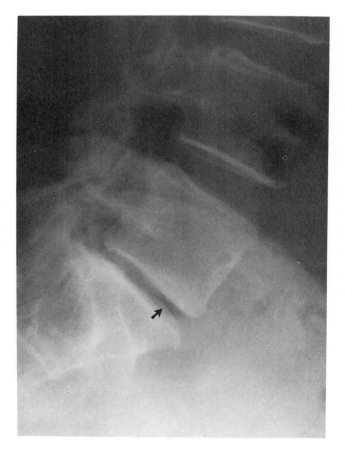

FIGURE 15–10. *"Vacuum Disc":* The L_5-S_1 disc is abnormal, resulting in a vacuum sign. The radiolucent area is not actually a vacuum but reflects the presence of nitrogen in a degenerated disc.

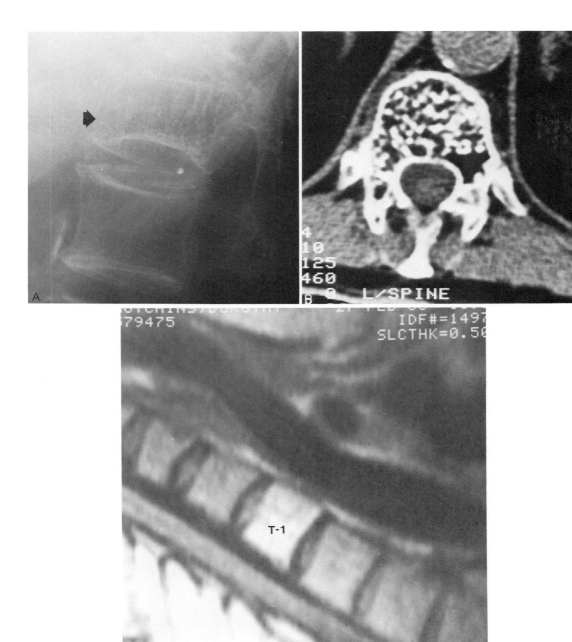

FIGURE 15–11. *Hemangioma of T$_{12}$:* *A,* Plain spine examination reveals the typical appearance of a hemangioma of the vertebral body. There is an increase in the trabecular pattern of the vertebral body, a finding that is typical of a hemangioma.

B, CT scan of the involved vertebral body reveals the increased trabeculae as dotlike areas of bone. Note that there is no destructive change of the vertebral body, and the appearance is quite typical of a hemangioma.

C, MR scan of another patient reveals a hemangioma of the first thoracic vertebral body. The vertebral body is bright because there is slow or turbulent flow within the hemangioma.

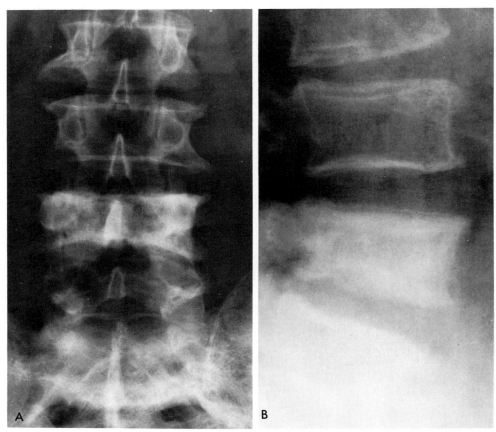

FIGURE 15–12. *Paget's Disease of Lumbar Spine:* The L$_4$ vertebral body is particularly involved. It is larger than the adjacent vertebral bodies, yet has sustained a compression fracture because it is actually weaker than the normal bone. The pelvis also demonstrates an increased trabecular pattern. The L$_4$ vertebral body exhibits a "picture window" appearance with a dense peripheral margin typical of Paget's disease.

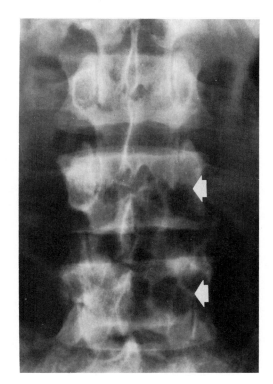

FIGURE 15–13. *Metastatic Disease:* There is lytic destructive metastatic disease involving the left pedicles at L₄ and L₅ (*arrows*). This is the "absent pedicle sign" of metastatic disease.

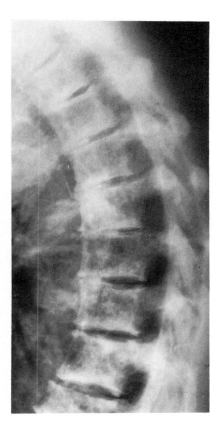

FIGURE 15–14. *Mixed Osteolytic and Osteoblastic Disease:* The bony structures are diffusely abnormal in appearance. Areas of increased and decreased density occur in a mixed pattern. The pattern is typical of metastatic disease with destructive and reparative bony changes.

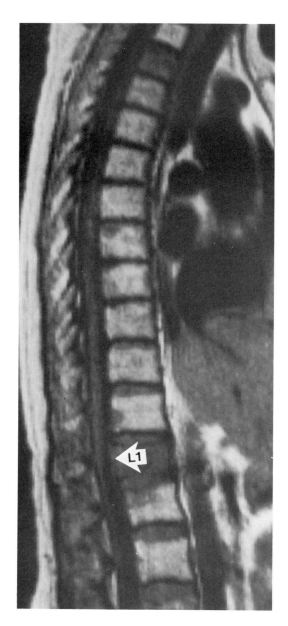

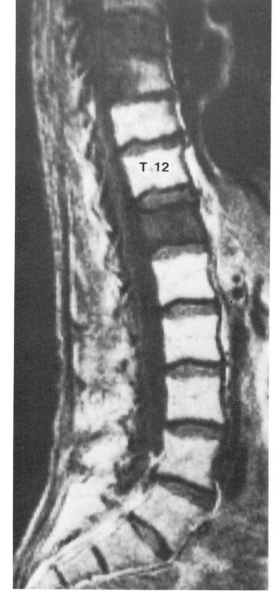

FIGURE 15–15. *Spinal Column Metastases:* TR530/TE30 SE of the thoracic spine reveals multiple low signal intensity areas involving the vertebral column. These low signal intensity areas represent areas of metastatic disease. There is replacement of the normally high signal intensity of the fatty bone marrow by tumor cells, resulting in this alteration of the signal intensity. There is essentially complete replacement of the L_1 vertebral body (*L1*), which also demonstrates loss of vertebral body height because of a pathologic fracture. The posterior margin of the vertebral body is displaced posteriorly into the vertebral canal (*arrow*); there is compromise of the anterior subarachnoid space and posterior displacement of the spinal cord by the L_1 vertebral body. This MR appearance correlates with an extradural indentation upon the contrast column seen on a myelographic study.

FIGURE 15–16. *Spinal Column Metastases:* A 47-year-old male with known lung cancer. TR530/TE30 SE demonstrates complete replacement of the L_1 vertebral body with metastatic disease. The posterior half of the T_{10} and entire vertebral body of T_9 are also involved with metastatic disease. There is no pathologic fracture at any level, and there is no compromise of the subarachnoid space. Incidentally, the vertebral bodies of the spinal column are diffusely increased in signal intensity secondary to previous radiation treatment.

FIGURE 15–17. *Metastatic Lung Cancer:* This 32-year-old male had partial surgical removal of a primary lung tumor three months prior to this study. Postsurgically, the patient received radiation therapy to the remaining tumor and the mediastinum, including the spine. The mid-sagittal T_1, TR530/TE30 SE image reveals invasion of the T_2 and T_4 vertebral bodies, which exhibit decreased signal intensity (*black arrows*). The C_7 and T_1, as well as the T_5-T_7 vertebral bodies, demonstrate increased signal intensity secondary to the previous radiation treatment and a relative increase in the amount of adipose tissue within the vertebral bodies (*white arrows*). Note also the anterior paraspinal mass at the level of T_2-T_4, with tumor invasion of the esophagus. There is no evidence of cord compression.

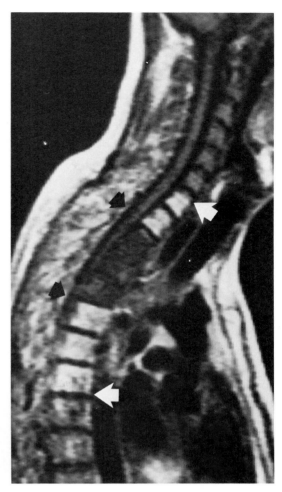

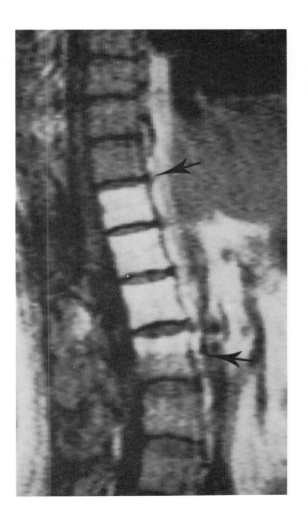

FIGURE 15–18. *Radiation Change:* This 36-year-old male had previous surgical resection of an astrocytoma at the level of the conus medullaris and radiation to the surgical site. There is increased signal intensity of the T_{10} to T_{12} vertebral bodies, as well as of the upper half of the L_1 vertebral body (*arrows*). This increased signal intensity is secondary to a relative increase in adipose tissue following radiation and corresponds precisely to the treatment port.

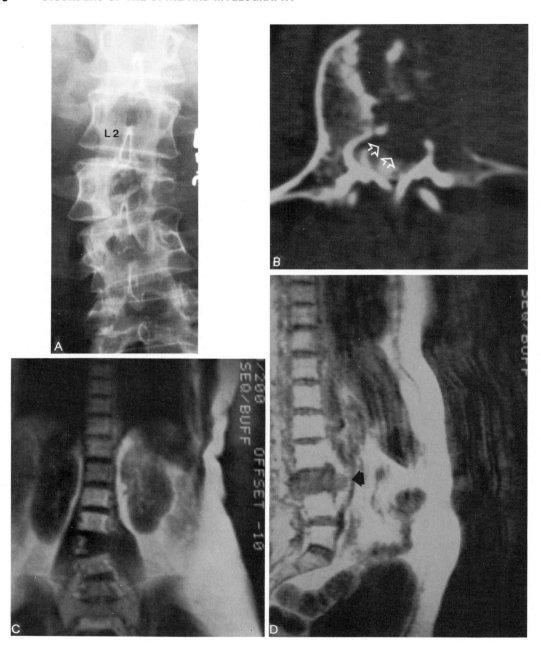

FIGURE 15–19. *Metastatic Leiomyosarcoma:* *A*, Plain spine examination reveals a pathologic fracture of the L_3 vertebral body. There are marked destructive bone changes involving the left side of the L_3 vertebral body and accentuation of the scoliosis secondary to the pathologic fracture.

B, CT examination at this same level reveals the marked destructive bone change. There is also a large paraspinal mass and encroachment upon the anterior aspect of the subarachnoid space (*arrows*) by the tumor. The spinous process is also involved with metastatic disease.

C, Coronal T-1 weighted image obtained with the body coil reveals the tumor replacement of the majority of the L_3 vertebral body with low signal intensity tumor. There are a left lateral paraspinal mass and distortion of the psoas shadow.

D, The sagittal SE TR3120/TE60 image reveals the tumor replacement of L_3, a paraspinal mass extending anterior to the vertebral body (*arrow*), and posterior extension into the vertebral column as well. Note the distended bladder, secondary to acute cord compression.

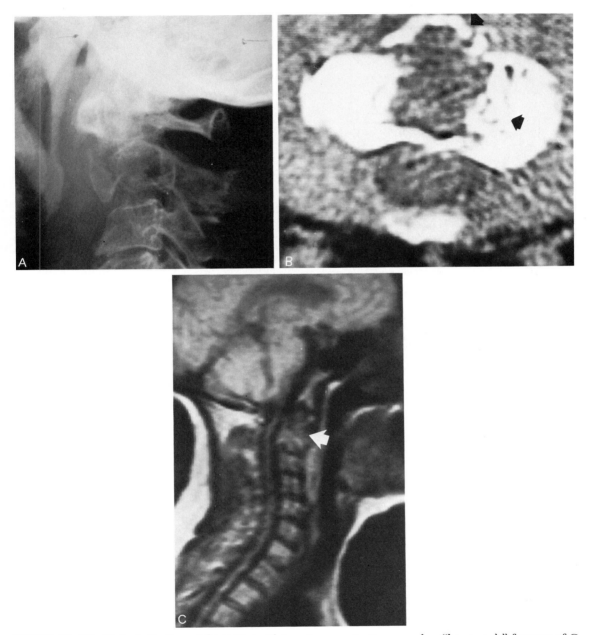

FIGURE 15–20. *Metastatic Breast Cancer:* A, Plain spine examination reveals a "hangman's" fracture of C_2 with the associated forward subluxation of C_2 on C_3.

B, Axial CT scan at the level of the C_1 vertebral body reveals that there is actually extensive destructive bone change of the vertebral body of C_1 as well as a pathologic fracture of the anterior margin and lateral mass of the vertebra (*arrows*).

C, MR TR530/TE30 SE reveals low signal intensity of the odontoid process (*arrow*) and superior portion of the C_2 vertebral body secondary to metastatic disease. There is an acute kyphosis at this level, and curvilinear distortion of the medulla and upper cervical cord without actual cord compression. MR provided the ideal method for evaluation of this patient, as it obviated the possibility of permanent neurologic deficit following myelography.

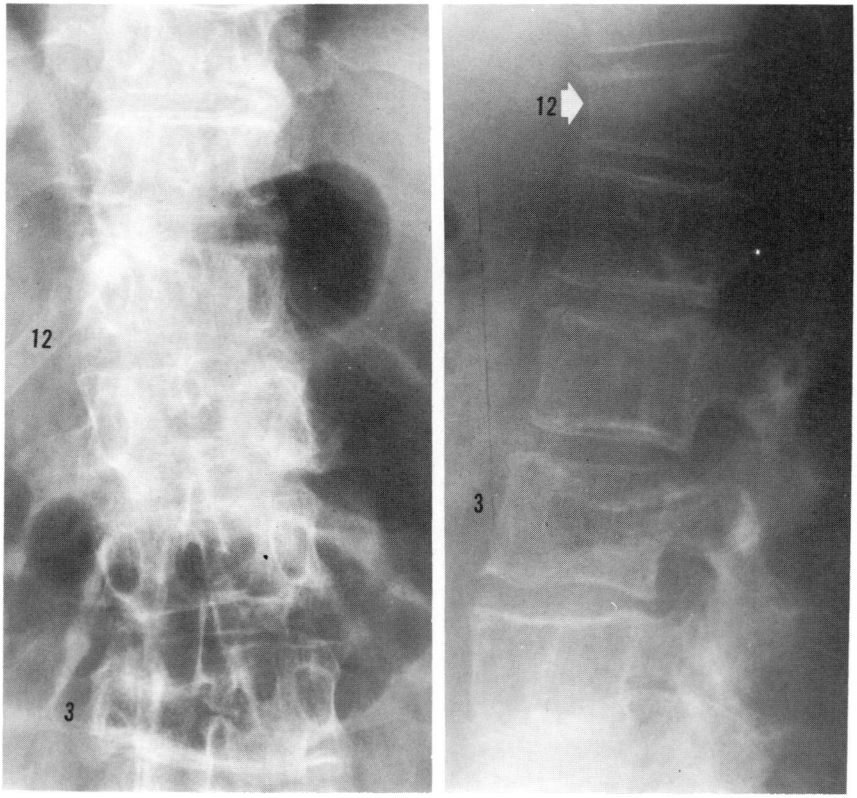

FIGURE 15–21. *Multiple Myeloma:* There is diffuse deossification of the bony structures. The pedicles are spared. There are compression deformities of the T_{12} and L_3 vertebral bodies.

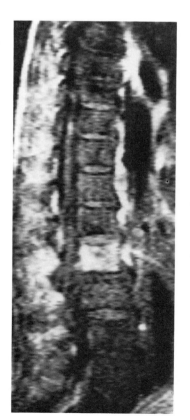

FIGURE 15–22. *Chronic Lymphocytic Leukemia:* Mid-sagittal T-1 weighted TR530/TE30 SE image reveals decreased signal intensity of all the vertebral bodies secondary to replacement of the marrow by tumor cells. There is increased signal intensity from the L_3 vertebral body, probably because of involvement by a hemangioma.

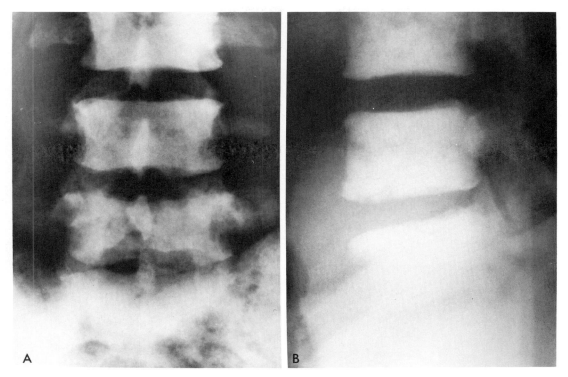

FIGURE 15–23. *Osteoblastic Metastatic Disease:* All of the visualized bony structures demonstrate increased density that is somewhat irregular in its distribution. This is characteristic of osteoblastic metastatic disease. It is differentiated from Paget's disease by the absence of prominent trabeculae.

FIGURE 15–24. *Spinal Column Metastases:* A 67-year-old male with known metastatic prostate cancer. *A*, AP view of the myelogram reveals osteoblastic metastatic disease involving all the visualized vertebral bodies. There are multiple areas of extradural encroachment upon the subarachnoid space from the expanded vertebral bodies involved with metastatic disease.

B, TR530/TE30 SE demonstrates that all the vertebral bodies are involved with metastatic disease and appear to be of very low signal intensity because of the blastic or bony nature of the metastatic deposits. Without the mandatory comparison with plain films, such diffuse involvement may not be appreciated and may, in fact, be considered normal.

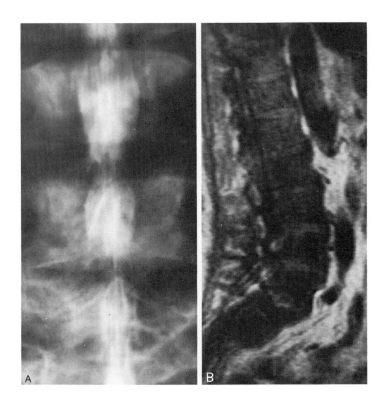

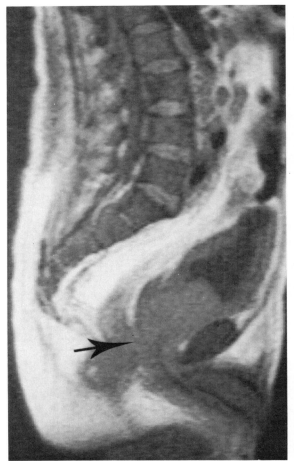

FIGURE 15–25. *Metastatic Prostatic Carcinoma:* The mid-sagittal, T-1 weighted image reveals that all the vertebral bodies are replaced by osteoblastic tumor of decreased signal intensity. Note that the intervertebral discs are higher in signal intensity than the vertebral bodies, while in the normal patient the reverse is true. The prostatic carcinoma (*arrow*) is seen at the base of the bladder. The bladder is greatly distended, and there is marked thickening of the wall of the bladder secondary to chronic obstruction.

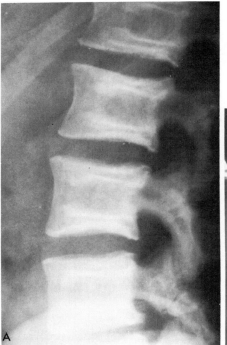

FIGURE 15–26. *Osteopetrosis:* The bony structures are of diffusely increased density and exhibit a typical "bone-within-a-bone" appearance.

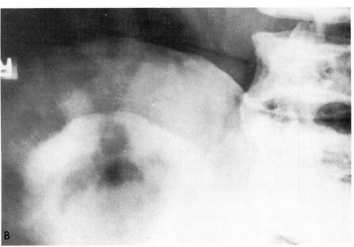

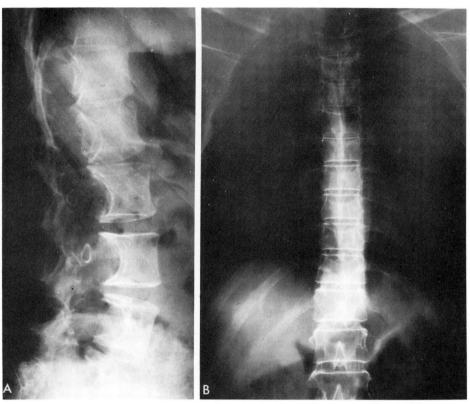

FIGURE 15–27. *Chronic Increased Intracranial Pressure:* The patient had an astrocytoma of the posterior fossa. Because of chronic increased intracranial pressure transmitted to the spine—without tumor actually being present in the spinal canal—there is marked widening of the interpedicular space in the thoracic region. There is also a marked increase in the AP diameter of the spinal canal in the lumbar region, with marked scalloping of the posterior bodies of all the lumbar vertebrae. (Case courtesy of Drs. Oscar Sugar and Glen Dobben.)

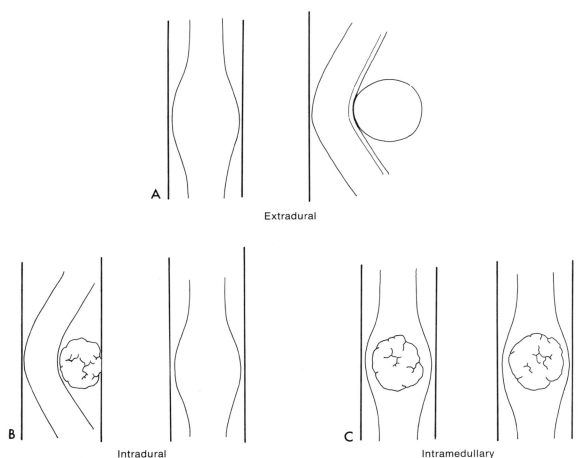

FIGURE 15–28. These three illustrations demonstrate graphically the roentgenographic changes seen with the three classes of spine tumors. Note that if only one view is obtained any one of the three varieties may resemble another class: the cord will appear widened and the contrast column will be thinned on either side of the cord. However, it is the view *perpendicular* to this view that more accurately evaluates the true nature of the mass.

A, With an *extradural* mass, such as a herniated disc, both the dura and the subarachnoid space will be pushed, and the contrast will course smoothly over the mass. The cord will be displaced away from the mass and widened by pressure from the mass. The contrast material will be thinned on both sides of the cord.

B, With an *intradural* mass, the contrast will form an acute angle with the tumor at its attachment with the dura. There will be a meniscus going around the mass and a widened contrast column between the mass and the compressed cord. The contrast column on the side of the cord opposite the tumor will be thinned.

C, With an *intramedullary* tumor the cord will appear widened in all views, and the contrast column will be thinned on all sides of the cord in all views.

It is, of course, unusual in radiologic practice to see any of the classic appearances in one standard projection. Therefore, multiple views must be obtained and the patient placed in oblique projection if necessary. All attempts should be made to define the lesion and the class of the abnormality so that proper treatment can be planned. Also, a mass may be of such size as to create a complete block to the flow of contrast material. If this is the case, standard criteria for diagnosis may no longer be helpful. On the other hand, even smaller lesions may take on the characteristics of masses in more than one class, making preoperative diagnosis difficult or impossible.

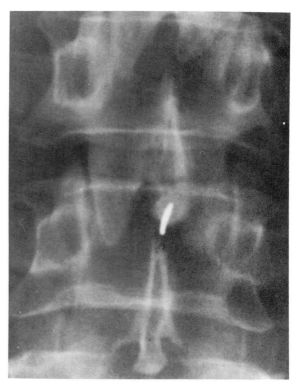

FIGURE 15–29. *Midline Needle Puncture Technique:* The plastic hubbed needle projects directly in the midline. The tip of the needle is at the mid-portion of the back of the vertebral body. Skin puncture is made just below the spinous process of the superior vertebral body.

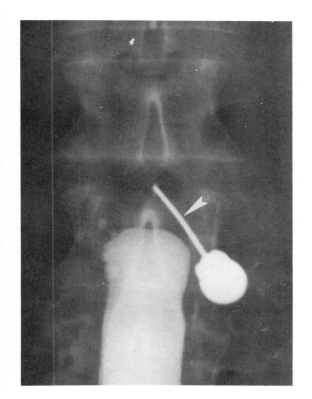

FIGURE 15–30. *Oblique Needle Puncture Technique:* Skin puncture is made at a level between the vertebral pedicle and the top of the spinous process of the same vertebral body. The needle is then slanted down and forward until lumbar puncture is performed in the midline. The arrowhead marks the skin puncture site.

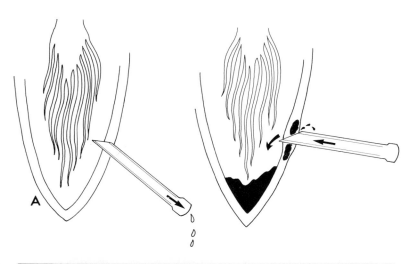

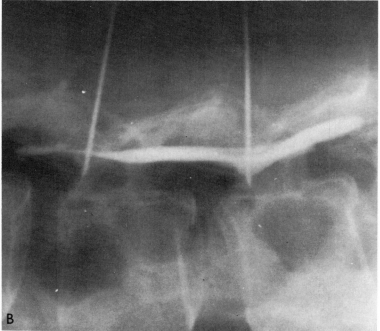

FIGURE 15–31. *Subdural Injection of Contrast Material: A,* These drawings illustrate the cause of entrance into the subdural space. The use of a long beveled needle should be avoided because of this phenomenon. Note that there will be flow of CSF but that contrast will enter the extradural and subdural spaces.

B, Lumbar puncture was performed without difficulty at the upper level, but there was poor flow of CSF. For this reason a second puncture was performed at the lower level. Flow of CSF was again felt to be adequate; however, after injection of contrast material, it was noted that the contrast had accumulated dorsal to the anticipated position of the subarachnoid space—i.e., in the subdural space. Usually most of this contrast material can be aspirated from the subdural space.

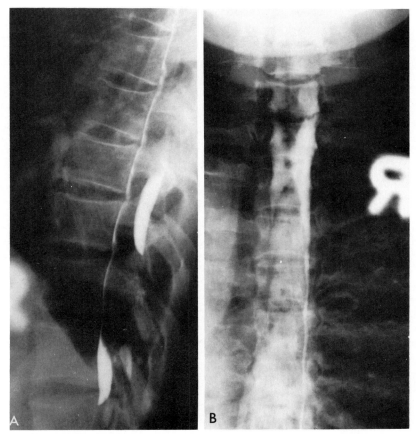

FIGURE 15–32. *Subdural Contrast:* A large amount of contrast material has entered into the ventral subdural space, and a small accumulation of subdural contrast material is present in the dorsal subarachnoid space. Notice that the dorsal spinal cord cannot be visualized. This subdural contrast flowed freely up into the cervical region. Generally speaking, subdural contrast material does not flow readily but tends to move slowly and over only one or two vertebral body segments.

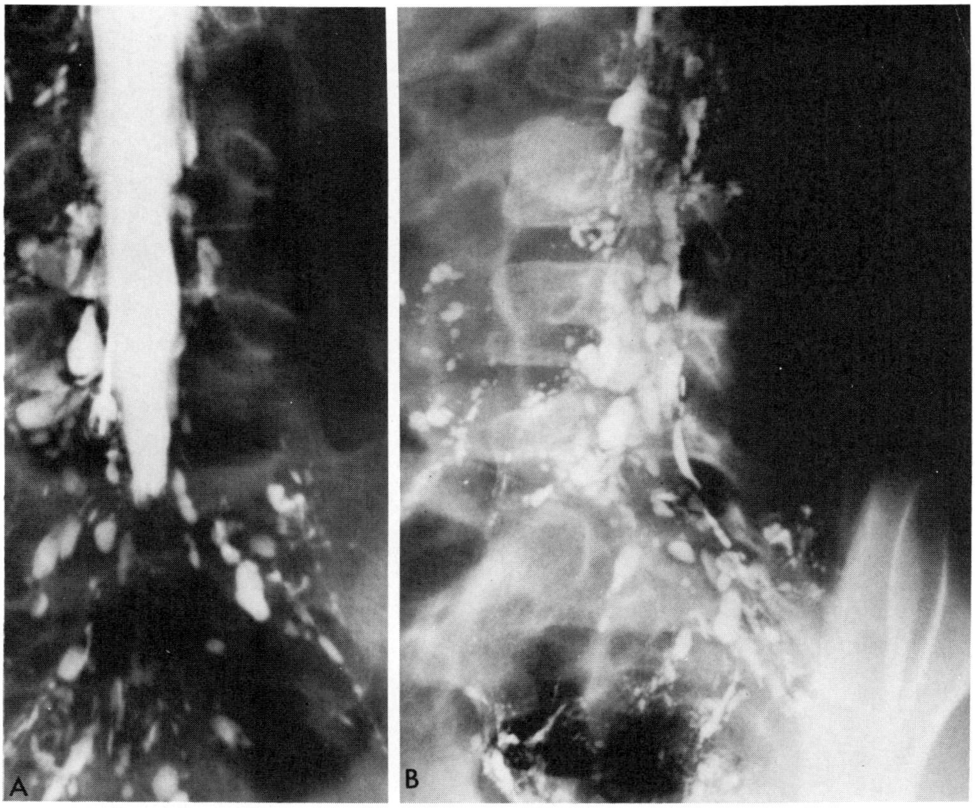

FIGURE 15–33. *Extradural Pantopaque:* *A*, A large amount of Pantopaque is noted in the extradural space. This contrast tracks peripherally along the nerve pathways. There is also a large amount of contrast material in the subarachnoid space. Fluoroscopy should be performed intermittently during the instillation of contrast material to avoid this large accumulation of contrast in the extradural space.

B, Following the aspiration of contrast material from the subarachnoid space, a moderate amount of contrast is also noted in the subdural space, forming a linear pattern that outlines the lumbar spinal column.

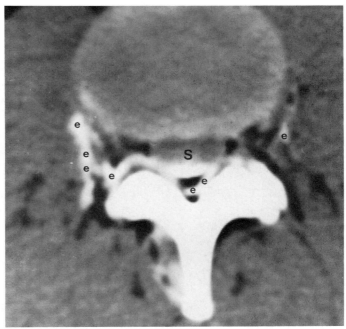

FIGURE 15–34. *Extravasation of Water-soluble Myelographic Contrast Material:* There is high density contrast material layered in the posterior aspect of the subarachnoid space (*s*). There is also leakage of the contrast material into the extradural space (*e*). The contrast material apparently leaked out of the lumbar puncture site into the soft tissues.

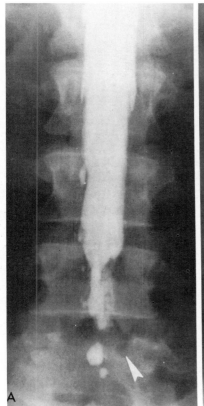
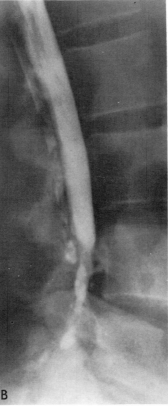

FIGURE 15–35. *Postoperative Arachnoiditis:* A, Instillation of contrast material was performed via a C_1–C_2 tap because there was no flow of CSF following several attempts at lumbar tap. There is failure of filling of the lumbar cul-de-sac below the L_4 level, with irregular globular accumulations of contrast material. There is obliteration of the nerve rootlets at L_2 and L_3. The partial laminectomy site is noted at L_5 on the left side (*arrowhead*).

B, The lateral view reveals that the nerve rootlets of the cauda equina are matted together to form an almost solid structure, which is placed dorsally in the lumbar subarachnoid space. The appearance is typical of arachnoiditis.

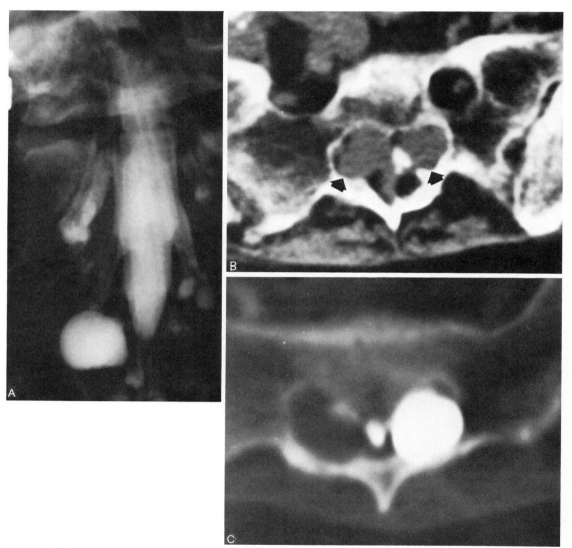

FIGURE 15–36. *Normal Tarlov's Cysts (Perineural Cysts):* Multiple cystic accumulations are noted along the extensions of the nerve root sleeves. These are normal anatomic variants that occur in different sizes and may be single or multiple.

A, Myelogram reveals contrast accumulation in multiple cystic areas.

B, CT scan demonstrates the typical erosion that may be seen with these nerve root cysts (*arrows*), particularly when they are large in size.

C, Following myelography there is accumulation of the contrast material in the cyst. These have also been called nerve root meningoceles.

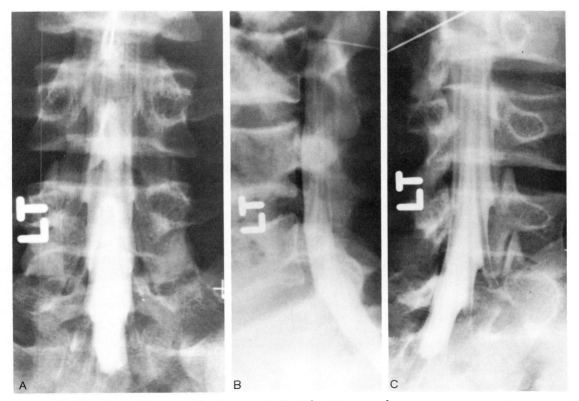

FIGURE 15–37. *Normal Lumbar Myelogram:* A, Upright, PA view demonstrates symmetric nerve root sleeve filling at all levels.

B, Upright, lateral view demonstrates good needle position in the subarachnoid space. The contrast column follows the posterior margin of the vertebral bodies and the nerve roots of the cauda equina can be seen in the subarachnoid space.

C, Upright, oblique view demonstrates the nerve roots surrounded by the contrast-filled nerve root sleeve.

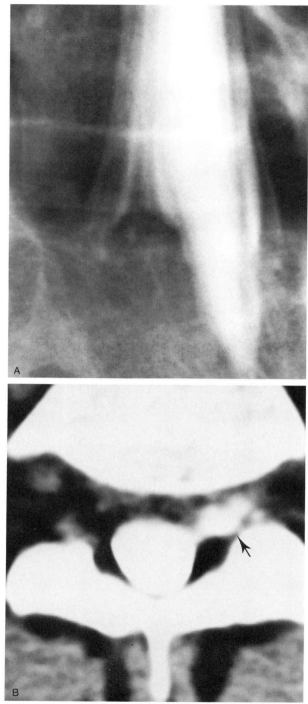

FIGURE 15–38. *Conjoined Root:* *A,* Myelogram with water-soluble contrast material reveals that at the L$_5$–S$_1$ level two nerve rootlets exit in a single nerve root sleeve. This is a normal anatomic variation and is known as a conjoined nerve root. This also results in an asymmetric appearance on the myelogram because of the fact that there is one less nerve root sleeve to fill on one side.

B, CT scan following myelography is helpful in differentiating between a conjoined nerve root and a herniated disc. Before myelography, the CT appearance of a conjoined nerve root (*arrow*) may mimic a herniated disc, as the figure-8 appearance demonstrated here may have the appearance of an abnormal disc. Even the density within the conjoined nerve root sleeve may measure disc density, because the partial volume phenomenon of the nerve within the nerve root sleeve may raise the Hounsfield number into the range of disc density material.

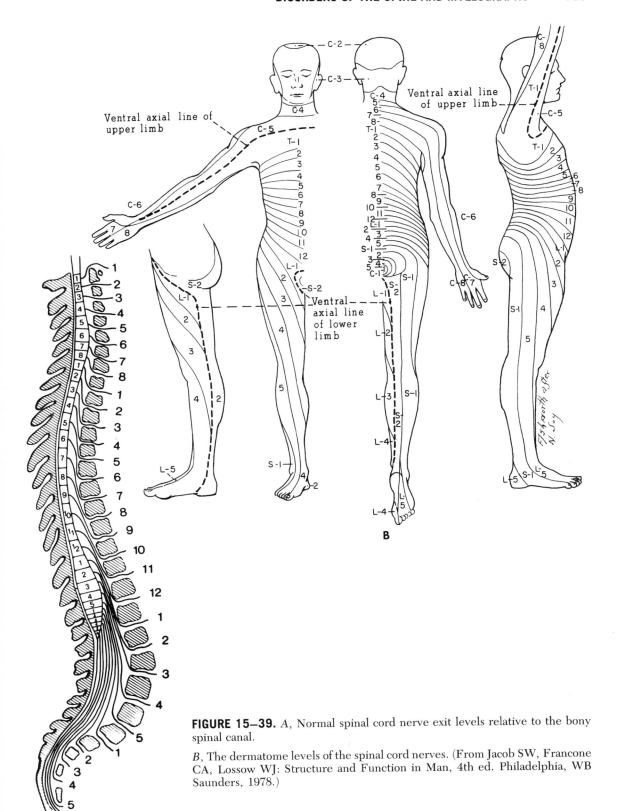

FIGURE 15–39. *A*, Normal spinal cord nerve exit levels relative to the bony spinal canal.

B, The dermatome levels of the spinal cord nerves. (From Jacob SW, Francone CA, Lossow WJ: Structure and Function in Man, 4th ed. Philadelphia, WB Saunders, 1978.)

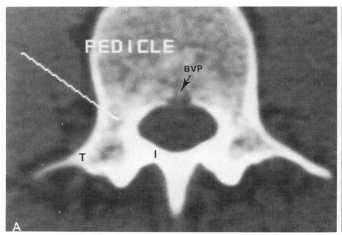

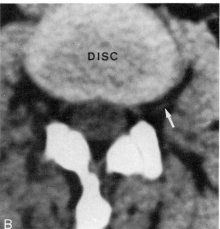

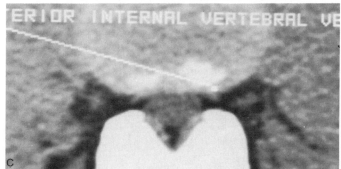

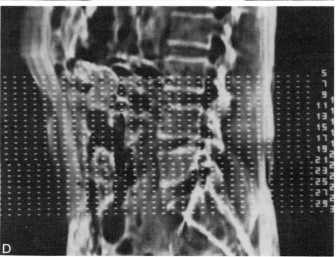

FIGURE 15–40. *Normal Slices in the Lumbar Region:* *A,* At the level of the pedicle, one also identifies the lamina (*l*), the transverse process (*T*), and the small defect in the posterior margin of the vertebral body that gives entrance to the basivertebral venous plexus (*BVP*).

B, Below the level of the nerve root and ganglion, one comes to the level of the intervertebral disc. Lateral to the position of the nerve root ganglion, one can identify the nerve as it is surrounded by the low density fat (*white arrow*).

C, The anterior internal vertebral vein can be seen as it rests along the posterior margin of the disc.

D, Initialized preliminary film for CT of the lumbar spine: Four mm, parallel, contiguous slices are obtained from the level of the midbody of L3 through the sacrum. Each slice level is clearly labeled.

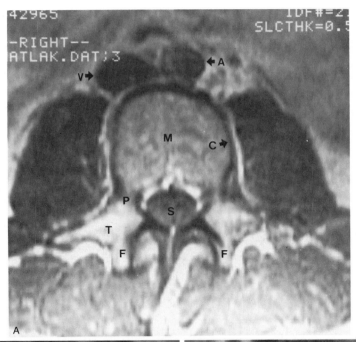

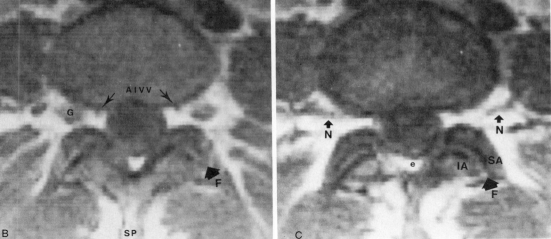

FIGURE 15–41. *Normal Axial MR Scan of the Lumbar Spine:* Three sequential scans of the lumbar spine obtained with 0.5-cm slice thickness reveal a number of normal structures and are very similar to CT scans through similar regions.

P = pedicle
S = subarachnoid space
F = facet joint—SA = superior articulating facet; IA = inferior articulating facet
T = transverse process
V = inferior vena cava
A = aorta
G = nerve root ganglion
N = nerve
M = marrow within the vertebral body
C = cortical bone of the vertebral body
SP = spinous process
AIVV = negative flow defect in the anterior internal vertebral veins
e = dorsal epidural fat

Note that the nerve root ganglion and nerve distal to the ganglion are both surrounded by high signal intensity fat.

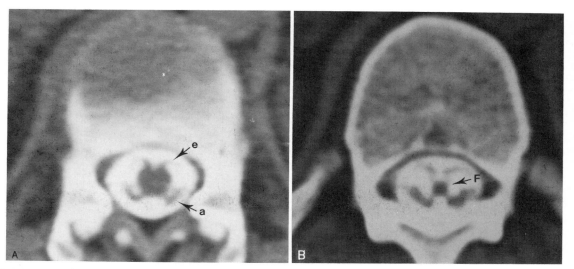

FIGURE 15–42. Normal Conus Medullaris: A, CT scan following myelogram reveals the water-soluble contrast material surrounding the conus medullaris at the level of the "lumbar enlargement." The afferent (a) and efferent (e) nerve rootlets can be seen outlined by the contrast material.

B, At the very bottom of the conus medullaris the filum terminale (F) is seen. Below this level, the spinal cord breaks up into the nerve rootlets of the cauda equina.

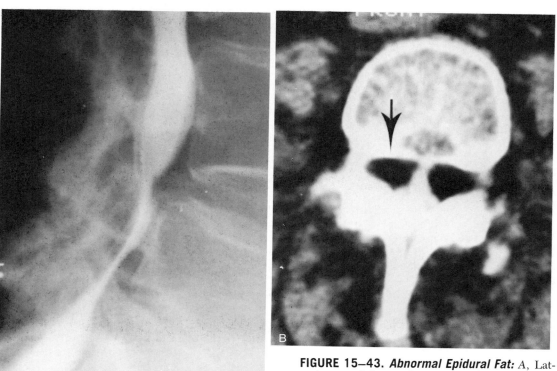

FIGURE 15–43. Abnormal Epidural Fat: A, Lateral view of the myelogram reveals circumferential narrowing of the subarachnoid space. The encroachment is along the dorsal aspect of the contrast column but also extends anteriorly.

B, A CT scan reveals the nature of the abnormality to be an increase in the amount of epidural fat (arrow), with compression of the contrast material in the lumbar subarachnoid space. This may be idiopathic or may be seen following the administration of exogenous steroids.

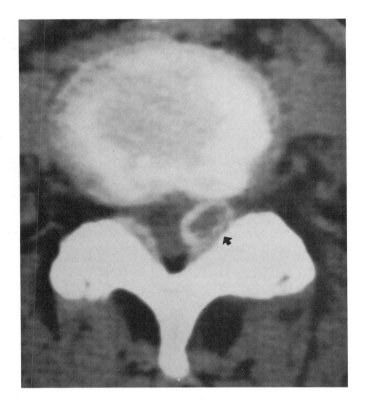

FIGURE 15–44. *Synovial Cyst:* There is a cystic lesion (*arrow*) within the spinal canal. The lesion has a low density central portion and a high density peripheral margin. The appearance is typical of a synovial cyst. These have been shown to arise from the joint space of the interfacet joints as an evagination of the synovial lining.

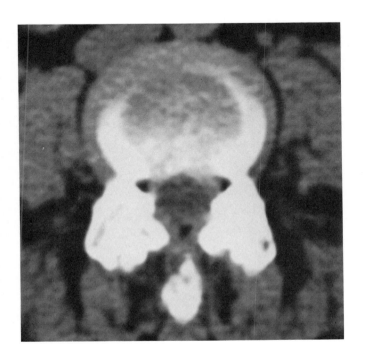

FIGURE 15–45. *Bulging Disc:* The disc extends beyond the margin of the vertebral body in a circumferential fashion. This type of bulging disc may be considered a variation of normal. However, a bulging disc in conjunction with hypertrophic interfacet degenerative changes may cause compromise of the neural foramen (as seen in this example), leading to compromise of the perineural fat and nerve root compression. The resulting pain mimics that of a herniated disc.

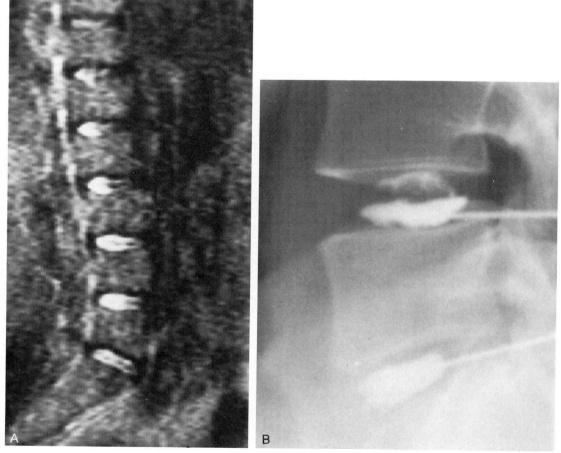

FIGURE 15–46. *Normal Intervertebral Disc: A,* The T-2 weighted TR3120/TE120 SE image reveals that all of the normal discs become increased in signal intensity, and the normal cleft is also demonstrated. Note that the T-2 weighted MR image simulates the image obtained with discography.

B, The discogram reveals contrast material in the intervertebral disc. There is no leakage of the contrast out of the disc, as would be seen with a herniation. There is a normal-appearing upper and lower locule with an intervening cleft that has been shown histologically to represent an invagination of the anulus fibrosus.

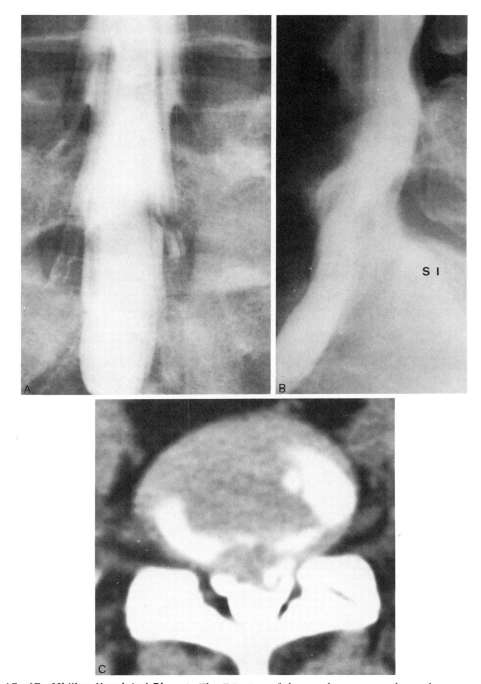

FIGURE 15–47. *Midline Herniated Disc:* A, The PA view of the myelogram reveals good nerve root sleeve filling at all levels.

B, The lateral view reveals a large ventral defect upon the contrast column at the L_5–S_1 level. The myelographic defect extends both above and below the level of the disc space. This appearance is secondary to the posterior displacement of the dura by the herniated disc, a change that is well demonstrated by MR (See Fig. 15–51). There is also minimal disc space narrowing at the L_4–L_5 level, with a bulging anulus fibrosus resulting in a minimal myelographic defect.

C, CT scan at the level of the herniated disc demonstrates the slightly asymmetric midline nature of the herniated disc. The nerve root sleeves continue to fill with contrast material and therefore illustrate why there is no abnormality on the PA view of the myelogram.

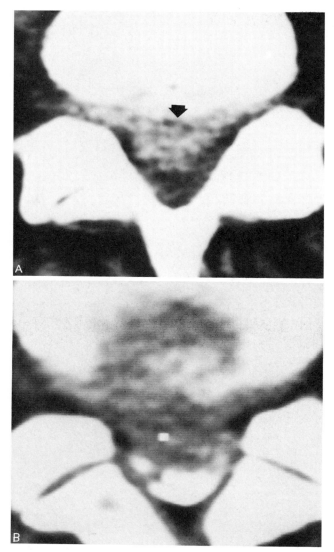

FIGURE 15–48. *Herniated Disc with Sequestered Fragment:* *A* and *B*, CT slice below the level of the disc (*A*) reveals that there is material of disc density (*arrow*) that extends below the disc and behind the vertebral body—a sequestered fragment. At the disc space level there is also disc density material—usual measurement 40 to 80 Hounsfield Units. The contrast-filled subarachnoid space is displaced posteriorly and almost completely obliterated.

C and *D*, AP and lateral views of the myelogram reveal a complete block to the flow of contrast material at the disc space level. The lateral view demonstrates that the contrast column is displaced posteriorly at the disc space level between L_4 and L_5. The displacement of the contrast column extends up to the level of the midbody of the L_4. There is disc space narrowing at the L_4–L_5 level, and while the appearance is consistent with a herniated nucleus pulposus, the L_5–S_1 level is not evaluated because of the complete block.

E and *F*, After the patient is turned into the supine position, the contrast material accumulates in the lumbar cul-de-sac. The posterior displacement of the contrast column extends from the midbody of L_4 to the upper third of L_5. There is an "hour-glass" deformity of the contrast column on the PA view. The L_5–S_1 disc is well outlined and appears normal. Thus the simple manipulation of the patient into the supine position allows, in almost all cases, the contrast to progress beyond the level of the block, making evaluation of the abnormal disc more accurate and allowing for evaluation of the lower disc levels. This facilitates surgical planning. In those cases where contrast material cannot be manipulated below the level of the initiated block, delayed CT scanning usually demonstrates that contrast material has reached the lumbar cul-de-sac and can therefore be evaluated with CT myelography.

Illustration continued on the following page

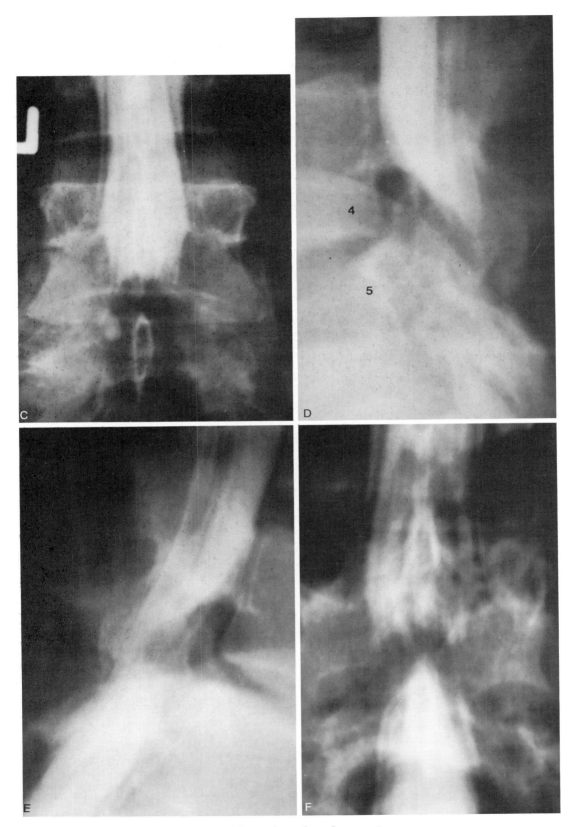

FIGURE 15–48. *See legend on the opposite page.*

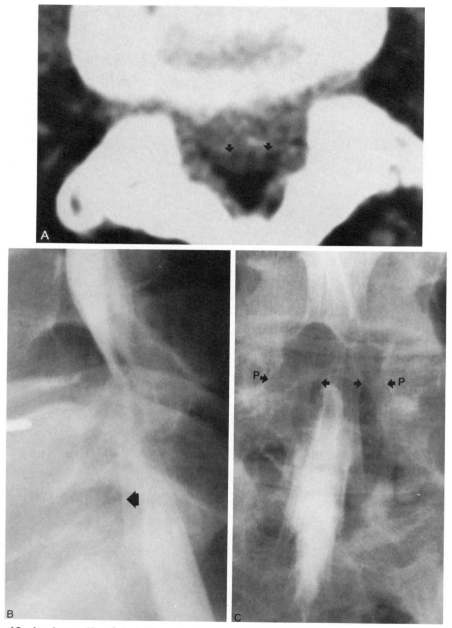

FIGURE 15–49. *Isodense Herniated Disc:* *A,* CT scan through the disc level appears normal. In actuality, there is a large herniated nucleus pulposus (HNP) in the midline that occupies the majority of the lumbar canal at this level. The herniated portion of the disc occupies the majority of the lumbar canal in such a way that it mimics the appearance of the thecal sac. Close inspection reveals a faint cleavage place (*arrows*) between the HNP and the subarachnoid space. If density measurements are not done on every case, then this type of abnormality can be overlooked.

B and *C,* Myelograms demonstrate a large ventral defect at the L_4–L_5 disc space level with associated disc space narrowing. The displacement of the contrast column extends to the level of the inferior end-plate of L_5 (*arrows*), because the disc fragment has been extruded inferiorly (*B*). On the PA view (*C*) the displacement of the contrast column away from the pedicle on the left side as compared to the pedicle (*P*) on the right side (*arrows*) allows one to say that the extruded portion of the disc rests in the left side of the vertebral canal, which facilitates the surgical approach.

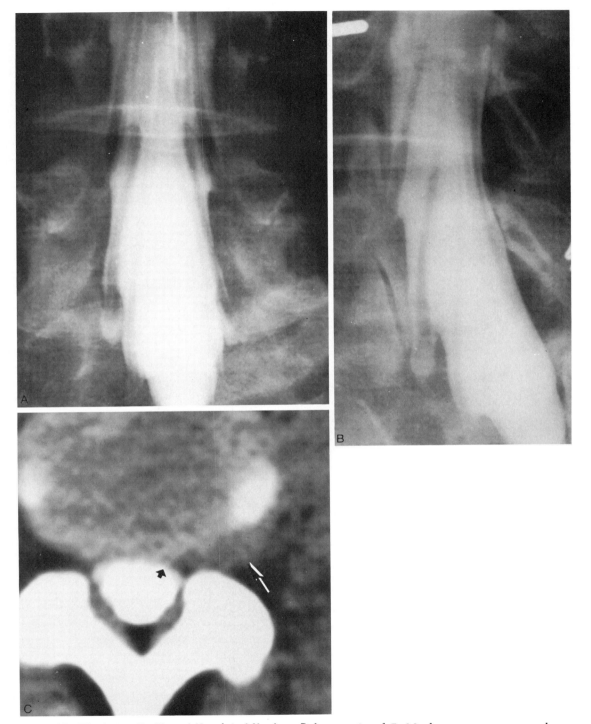

FIGURE 15–50. *Laterally Placed Herniated Nucleus Pulposus:* *A* and *B*, Myelograms appear normal.

C, Postmyelogram CT reveals only the very slightest effacement of the contrast column on the left side, and a large, laterally placed HNP. The HNP is disc density—40 to 80 Hounsfield Units—and obliterates the fat in the neural foramen and surrounding the nerve exiting at this level. The nerve itself is displaced posteriorly around the laterally herniated disc (*arrows*).

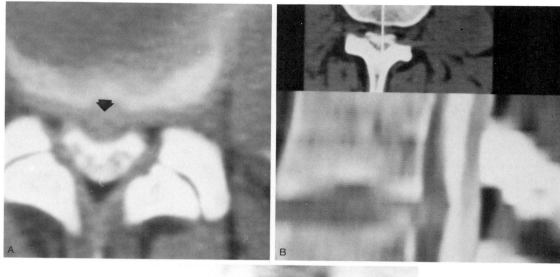

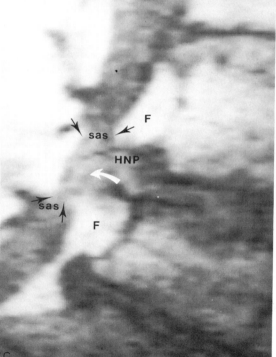

FIGURE 15–51. *Herniated Disc:* A, Axial CT demonstrates midline herniated disc (*arrow*).

B, Mid-sagittal reconstruction image of multiple parallel cuts through the lumbar region reveals the disc space narrowing, the ventral indentation upon the contrast column, and the HNP projecting just behind the disc space. Note that there is widening of the extradural space above and below the level of the HNP. This results in a widened appearance of the epidural fat, a change readily appreciated on MR scans.

C, MR scan in a different patient demonstrates the widening of the epidural fat (*F*) at the level of a herniated disc (*HNP*). This herniated disc is at the L_4–L_5 level and markedly compresses the subarachnoid space (*sas*) at this level. There is also a bulging disc at the L_5–S_1 level. These changes are best appreciated on this surface coil, TR530/TE30 SE sequence.

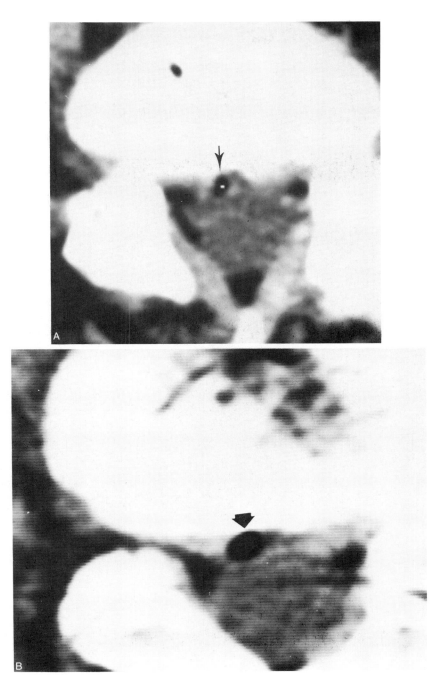

FIGURE 15–52. *Herniated Vacuum Disc:* *A,* Axial CT scan through a degenerated disc reveals that the gaseous portion of the disc is herniated posteriorly into the vertebral canal (*arrow*). The cursor measured in negative numbers. A small amount of gas can also be seen in the disc more anteriorly.

B, A magnified view at a slightly different level again demonstrated an HNP with a small amount of gas along the right side of the disc (*arrow*). A large amount of vacuum change is now visible anteriorly in the disc.

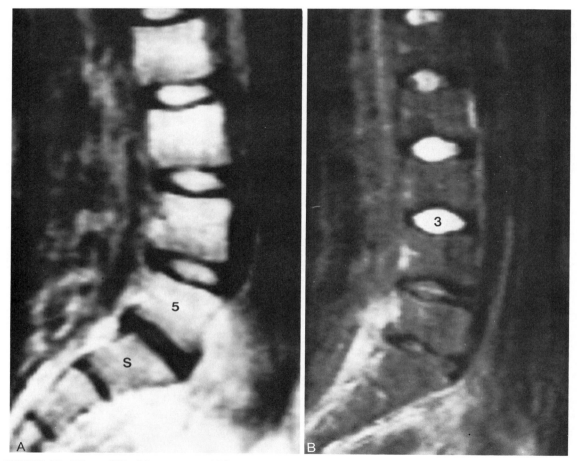

FIGURE 15–53. *A, **MR of Degenerated Disc:*** TR3120/TE120 SE reveals high signal intensity from the normal discs and low signal intensity from the L_5–S_1 disc that is degenerated following the injection of chymopapaine. The posterior margin of the disc bulges into the high signal intensity CSF at this level.

*B, **Degenerated Discs:*** TR3120/TE120 SE reveals degenerated discs at the L_4, L_5, and S_1 levels. The normal discs are of high signal intensity, and the degenerated discs are of low signal intensity, with associated disc space narrowing.

Illustration continued on the following page

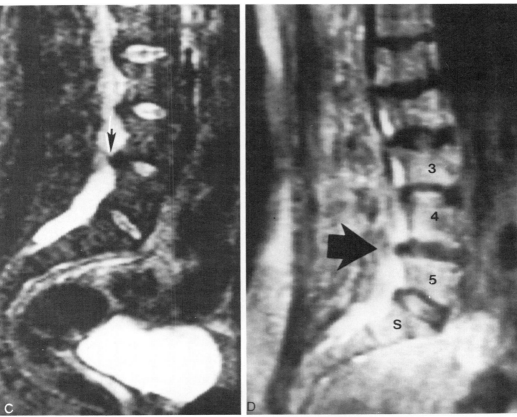

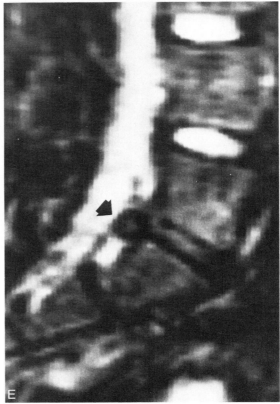

FIGURE 15–53 *Continued.*

*C, **Bulging Disc:*** TR3120/TE120 image demonstrates some decrease in signal intensity from the L_4–L_5 disc and posterior bulging of the disc into the high signal intensity of the CSF (*arrow*). If the disc were herniated, one would expect very low signal intensity; therefore, the findings are consistent with a bulging rather than a herniated disc.

*D, **Multiple Degenerated Discs:*** TR3120/TE120 SE image demonstrates that all the visualized discs are lower than normal signal intensity, with relative sparing of L_3–L_4 and L_5–S_1. There is bulging of several discs and a possible herniation at the L_4–L_5 level (*arrow*). The patient is a 64-year-old "normal" volunteer.

*E, **MR of Herniated HNP:*** There is a low signal intensity degenerated disc at the L_5–S_1 level. A large herniated portion of the disc is seen projecting posteriorly into the high signal intensity of the CSF (*arrow*).

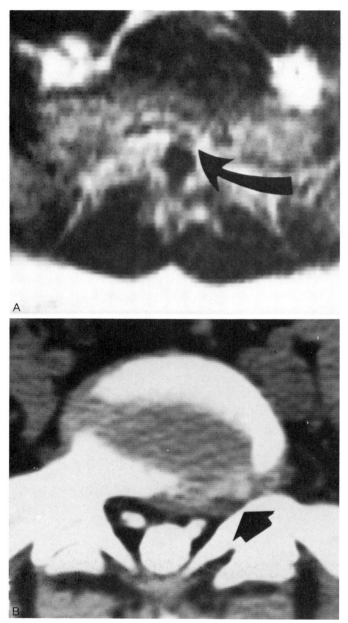

FIGURE 15–54. *Herniated Disc:* A, Axial MR TR530/TE30 SE image reveals the low signal intensity of the herniated portion of the disc (*arrow*) which has caused interruption of the epidural fat and slight effacement of the low signal intensity CSF in the thecal sac.

B, The axial CT scan at the same level also demonstrates the laterally herniated disc (*arrow*).

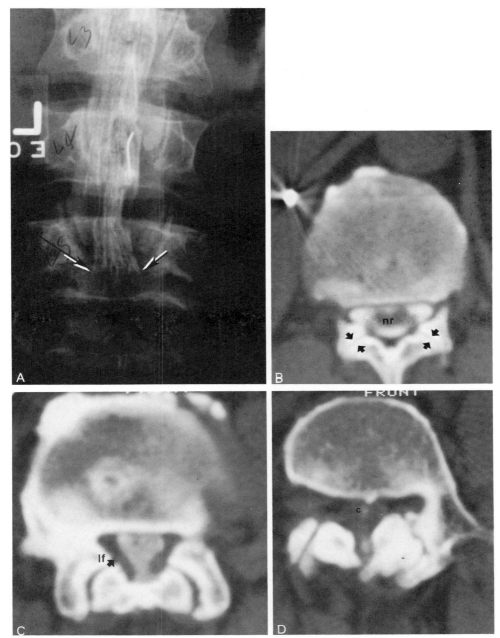

FIGURE 15–55. *Spinal Stenosis and Arachnoiditis:* A, Myelogram demonstrates a complete block to flow of contrast in the low lumbar region (*arrows*). There is circumferential narrowing of the contrast column secondary to interfacet degenerative change with facet overgrowth. In addition, there is a lacy, irregular appearance to the contrast material with adhesions between the nerve rootlets secondary to adhesive arachnoiditis.

B and C, Axial CT scans demonstrate clumping of the nerve rootlets (*nr*), hypertrophic changes involving the facets, and facet joint narrowing (*arrows*). There is also hypertrophy of the ligamentum flavum that encroaches upon the dorsal aspect of the contrast column bilaterally (*lf*).

D, At the level of the block to flow of contrast there is only a very faint amount of contrast visible in the subarachnoid space (*c*). There is marked encroachment upon the vertebral canal secondary to bony overgrowth of the facets. There is irregularity and narrowing of the facet joints as well. The appearance is that of acquired spinal stenosis secondary to degenerative arthritis.

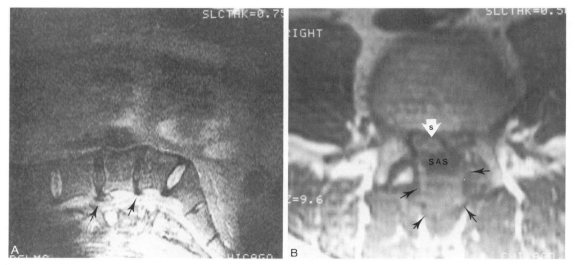

FIGURE 15–56. *Postoperative Scarring:* *A,* The T-2 weighted SE image with a TR2500/TE60 reveals degenerated discs at L$_3$–L$_4$ and L$_4$–L$_5$. There is also disc space narrowing, more marked at L$_4$–L$_5$, and focal areas of herniation of the disc at both these levels (*arrows*).

B, Axial T-1 weighted image reveals scarring posteriorly (*black arrows*), scar and/or herniated disc anterior to the subarachnoid space (*s*), and circumferential encroachment upon the lumbar subarachnoid space (*SAS*). The lamina has been surgically removed. The findings are consistent with postoperative changes and scar formation.

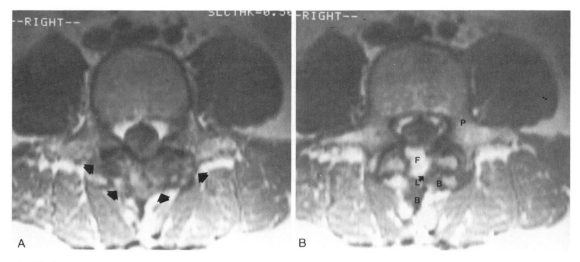

FIGURE 15–57. *Postoperative Spine:* *A,* There is an extensive bony fusion that obliterates the dorsal epidural fat normally present and extends from the facet joint on one side to the facet joint on the other side (*arrows*).

B, At the level of the pedicle (*P*), there is an increase in the amount of epidural fat (*F*) because this is put in place at the time of surgery. Fusion elements are present, as well as distortion of the laminae and facet joints because of the previous laminectomy (*L*) and fusion (*B*). These changes are normal findings that would be anticipated following a laminectomy and fusion.

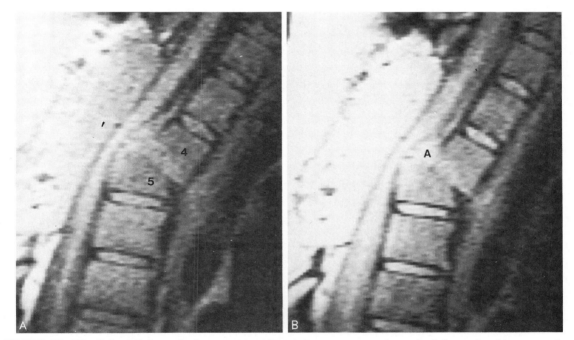

FIGURE 15–58. *Spinal Tuberculosis:* A, TR3120/TE60 SE image reveals marked forward subluxation of T_4 on T_5. There is complete loss of the intervertebral disc and destruction of the adjacent vertebral body endplates.

B, TR3120/TE120 SE image reveals that the abscess becomes increased in signal intensity (A). There is focal accentuation of the dorsal kyphosis and marked compression of the spinal cord at this level.

The involvement of the disc space and the adjacent vertebral bodies is typical of spinal tuberculosis. Note that on both echo sequences there is increased signal intensity material that extends behind the vertebral body of T_4 and T_3. This represents epidural extension of the inflammatory process.

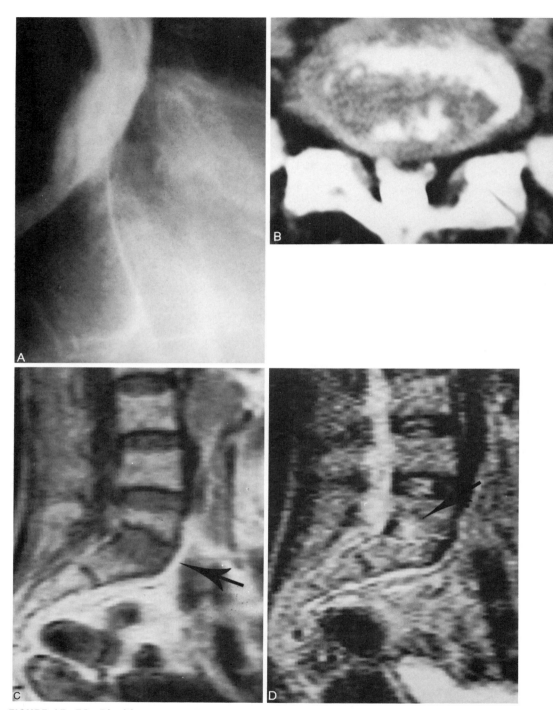

FIGURE 15–59. *Discitis:* A, Lateral view of the myelogram reveals widening of the extradural space behind the disc level of L_5–S_1. There is also widening of the disc space at this level and indistinctness of the inferior end-plate of L_5 and superior end-plate of S_1.

B, Postmyelogram CT reveals what appears to be a diffuse bulging of the disc.

C, MR TR530/TE30 reveals a widened disc space at L_5–S_1 and erosion of the adjacent end-plates (*arrow*).

D, TR3120/TE120 SE reveals increased signal intensity at the level of disc space (*arrow*). This finding is consistent with a discitis, which in this case is secondary to chymopapaine injection.

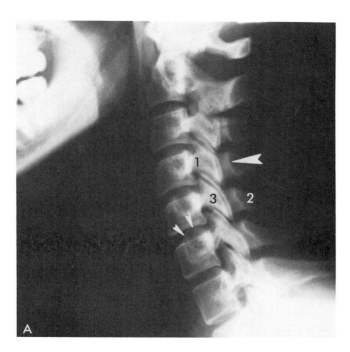

FIGURE 15–60. *Normal Lateral View of the Cervical Spine:* *A, 1,* Pedicle. *2,* Spinous process. *3,* Lateral mass. The small arrowheads indicate the uncinate process. The large arrowhead points to the posterior limitation of the subarachnoid space, the point where the laminae join to form the spinous process. A white line (the spinolaminar line) is visible radiographically.

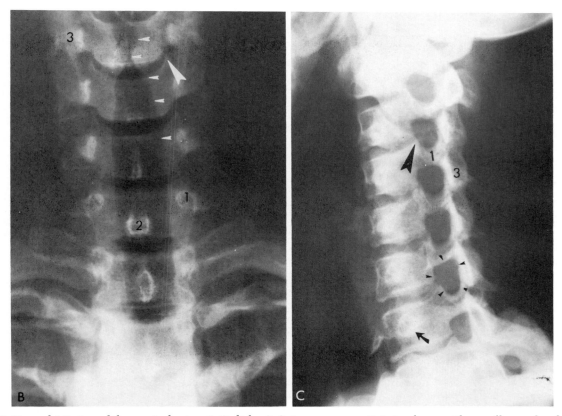

B, Normal AP view of the cervical spine: *1,* Pedicle. *2,* Spinous process. *3,* Lateral mass. The small arrowheads outline the tracheal air shadow. The large arrowhead demonstrates the uncinate process at the level of the joint of Luschka.

C, Normal oblique view of the cervical spine, LAO position: *1,* Pedicle. *3,* Lateral mass, viewed obliquely. The large arrowhead demonstrates the joint of Luschka, where osteophytes develop and may be noted to encroach upon the neural foramina. The black arrow indicates the right pedicle viewed on end; the small arrowheads outline the neural foramina at the C_6–C_7 level.

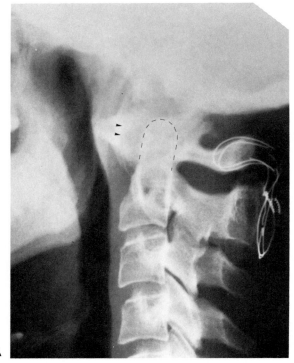

A

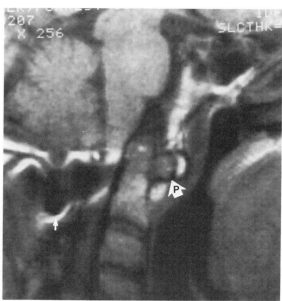

B

FIGURE 15–61. Rheumatoid Arthritis: *A,* There is atlantoaxial dislocation secondary to laxity of the ligaments that stabilize the odontoid process. The arrowheads mark the posterior margin of the anterior arch of C_1. Stabilization had been attempted by the use of wires surrounding the posterior elements of C_1 and C_2, but the wires subsequently broke.

B, MR TR530/TE30 SE sequence reveals that there has been further progression of the disease with upward mobility of the odontoid process through the foramen magnum—basilar invagination. There is narrowing of the medulla and upper spinal cord at the level of the foramen magnum. Pannus formation appears as an area of decreased signal intensity (*P*) and projects behind the high signal intensity of the marrow containing anterior arch of C_1. The fixating wires degrade the image by "warping" the field in a localized area (*small arrow*).

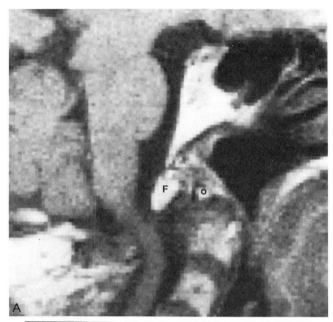

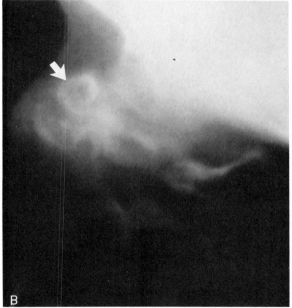

FIGURE 15–62. *Os Odontoideum:* *A,* TR530/TE30 SE demonstrates that the odontoid process is not seen, but there is only a small rounded area of high signal intensity surrounded by a low signal intensity cortical margin (*o*) that represents the os odontoideum, or separate ossification center of the odontoid process. The irregular area of increased signal represents the fat at the anterior margin of the foramen magnum (*F*). C_2 and the remainder of the cervical spine are displaced forward relative to the C_1 vertebral body and the skull base; this has resulted in curvilinear distortion of the medulla and upper cervical spinal cord, with slight compression just at the level of the foramen magnum. These changes are nicely demonstrated without the use of contrast material or the need for manipulation of the patient.

B, Lateral radiographic tomography reveals the os odontoideum (*arrow*) with its well-defined cortical margin.

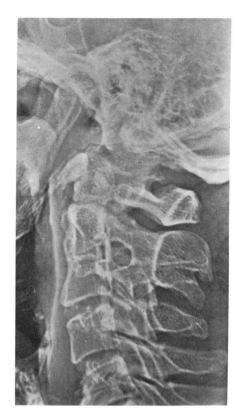

FIGURE 15–63. *Klippel-Feil Syndrome:* This congenital anomaly may occur alone or with other anomalies. The Klippel-Feil anomaly is fusion (failure of segmentation) of two or more cervical vertebral bodies. This fusion results in a decrease in the normal motility of the spine. There may be an associated Chiari malformation.

"Block vertebrae": A lateral xeroradiogram of the neck reveals fusion of the vertebral bodies and the spinous processes of the C_2 and C_3 vertebral bodies. The problem is really one of failure to segment, not one of fusion.

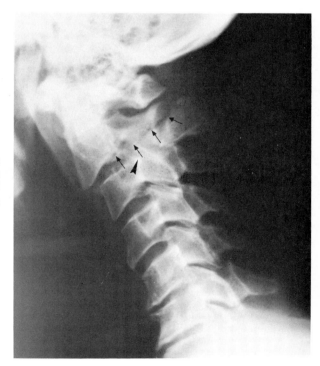

FIGURE 15–64. *Hangman's Fracture:* A fracture extends through the lateral masses and laminae as well as the spinous process of the C_2 vertebral body (*arrows*). There is forward subluxation of C_2 on C_3. (*Arrowhead* illustrates back of C_3.)

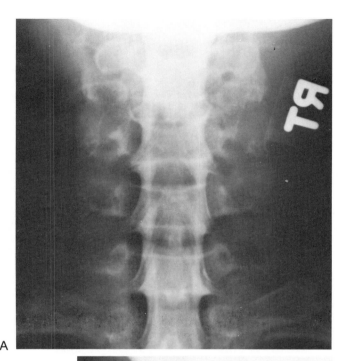

A

FIGURE 15–65. *Normal Cervical Myelogram:* *A*, PA view reveals the normal cervical cord widening extending from C3 to T3. There is good nerve root sleeve filling at all levels, revealing multiple thread-like nerve roots existing at each level.

B, PA oblique view better demonstrates the nerve root sleeves as they exit anteroventrally from the spinal cord. This view is best obtained by rotating the tube rather than the patient. One of the attachments of the dentate ligament is identified by the arrow.

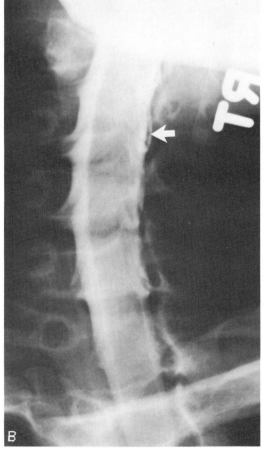

B

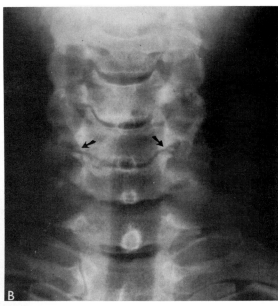

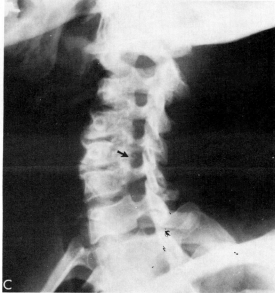

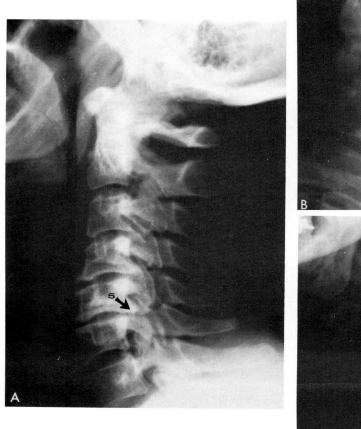

FIGURE 15–66. *Cervical Arthritis:* *A*, The lateral view reveals degenerative changes, with narrowing of the C_4–C_5 and C_5–C_6 disc spaces. There is anterior spur formation and large posterior osteophytes at these levels. The posterior osteophytes are marked at the C_5 level on all views but are readily visible at the C_4–C_5 level also.

B, The AP view demonstrates the bony overgrowth about the uncinate processes bilaterally. This extends posteriorly into the spurs, which impinge upon the neural foramina.

C, The oblique view allows visualization of the neural foramina and demonstrates the encroachment by the bony osteophytes (*arrow*). Note that the level above also demonstrates the osteophytes, while the remainder of the neural foramina are oval and without evidence of impingement by spur formation.

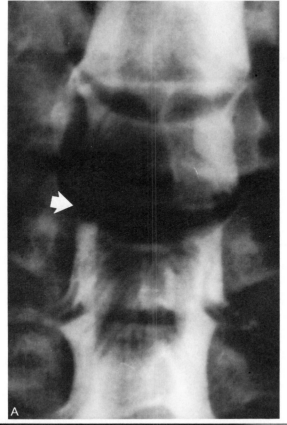

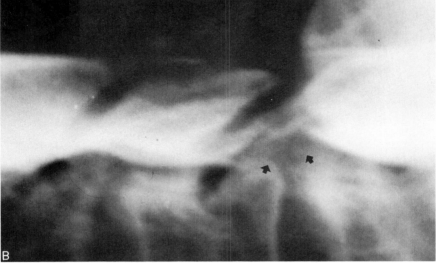

FIGURE 15–67. *Herniated Cervical Disc:* A, PA view of the myelogram with water-soluble contrast material reveals focal widening of the cord at the C₅–C₆ level, with interruption of nerve root sleeve filling on the left side at this level (*arrow*), and a wedge-shaped defect in the contrast column. There is also slight interruption of nerve root sleeve filling on the contralateral side.

B, The lateral view reveals bony osteophytes (*arrows*) with a ventral indentation upon the contrast column, but the defect in the contrast column extends beyond the bony spur, implying that there is also a component of herniated disc present.

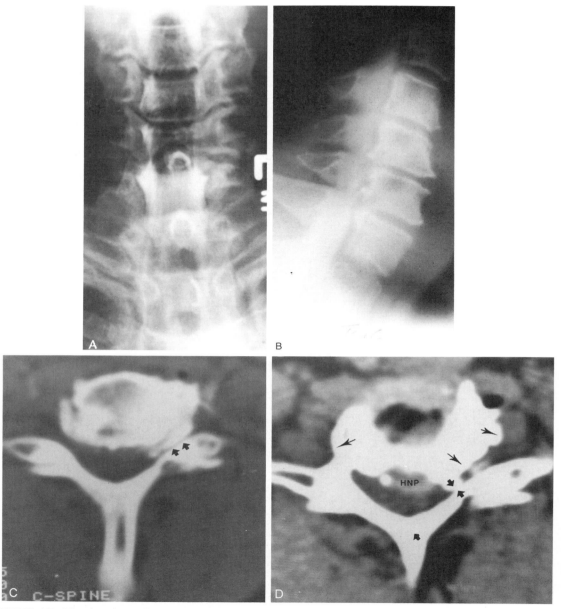

FIGURE 15–68. *Cervical Discs and Osteophytes:* A, PA view of the myelogram reveals poor nerve root sleeve filling at the C_4 to C_7 levels. There is also extradural encroachment upon the contrast column, most marked on the left side. There is slight widening of the cord at all these levels.

B, Lateral tomographic section reveals large osteophytes at all levels, with indentations upon the contrast column from C_4 to C_7. The canal measures 11 mm at the C_6–C_7 level.

C, CT scan at wide window widths reveals marked osteophyte formation, most marked on the left side with encroachment upon the neural foramen to a slit-like size (*arrows*).

D, CT at the C_6–C_7 disc level reveals a vacuum change because of a degenerated disc and multiple osteophytes (*long arrows*) with bilateral encroachment upon the neural foramina, more on the left than the right (*small arrows*). There is also a large herniated disc in the midline at the C_6–C_7 level (*HNP*).

The findings are consistent with cervical "spondylosis"—degenerative changes—and a herniated disc at C_6–C_7. The combination of these changes results in an acquired spinal stenosis in the cervical region.

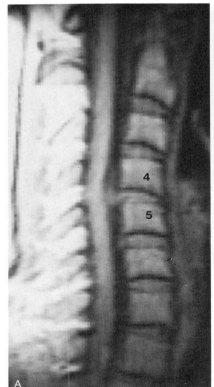

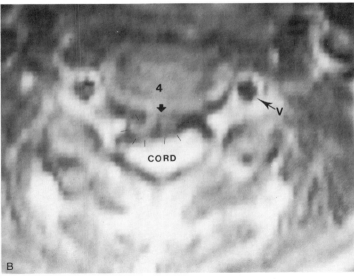

FIGURE 15–69. *Herniated Cervical Disc:* A, Mid-sagittal T-1 weighted TR530/TE30 SE image reveals a large herniated disc at the C_4–C_5 level. The intervertebral disc material can be seen to be contiguous with the disc and to extend posteriorly into the vertebral canal. There is obliteration of the CSF at this level and curvilinear compression of the cervical spinal cord. There is reversal of the curve of the cervical spine at this level. The posterior margin of the disc at the C_5–C_6 level is also prominent.

B, The axial T-1 weighted image through this same level reveals the disc density material as it extends posteriorly into the vertebral canal (*arrow*) and is contiguous with the intervertebral disc. The spinal cord (*CORD*) is compressed and displaced toward the left side. The vertebral artery (*V*) appears as a negative flow defect within the foramina transversaria.

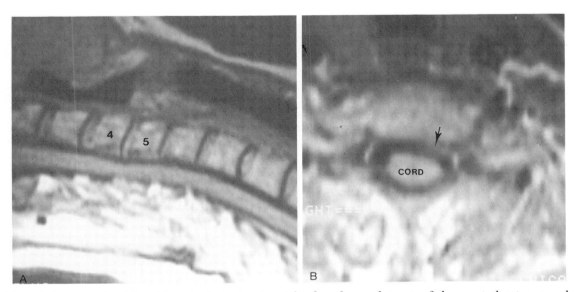

FIGURE 15–70. *Herniated Disc:* A, Sagittal T-1 weighted surface coil image of the cervical spine reveals reversal of the curve of the spine at the C_4–C_5 level. There is posterior displacement of the posterior margin of the C_4 and C_5 vertebral bodies with compromise of the CSF, displacement of the cervical spinal cord posteriorly, and compression of the spinal cord.

B, Axial T-1 weighted image at the C_4–C_5 level reveals a herniated cervical disc on the left side (*arrow*). The cord is effaced at the level of the herniated disc, and there is compromise of the CSF at this level.

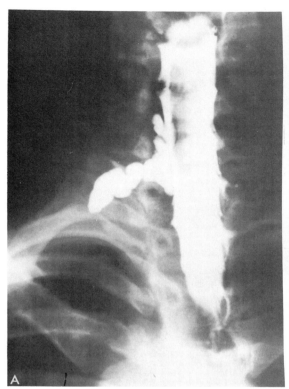

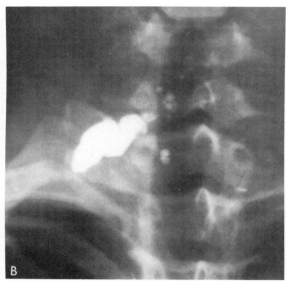

FIGURE 15–71. *Nerve Root Avulsion:* A, The Pantopaque collects in a sac made up of the arachnoid protruding through a dural tear. The end of the avulsed nerve, which is pulled from the cord, retracts distally in the arachnoid sac. In addition to the marked change at the C_7–T_1 level, there has also been a less marked avulsion at the C_6–C_7 level.

B, When the contrast material is drained from the cervical subarachnoid space, the rest of the contrast is still present in the sac. (Courtesy of the Carle Clinic Radiologists, Urbana, Illinois.)

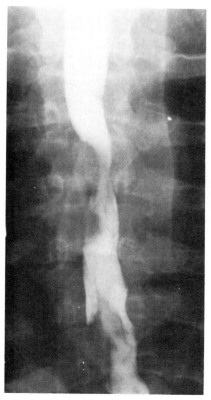

FIGURE 15–72. *Metastases:* There are multiple indentations on the contrast column secondary to multiple metastatic deposits in the extradural space. This patient had a lymphoma.

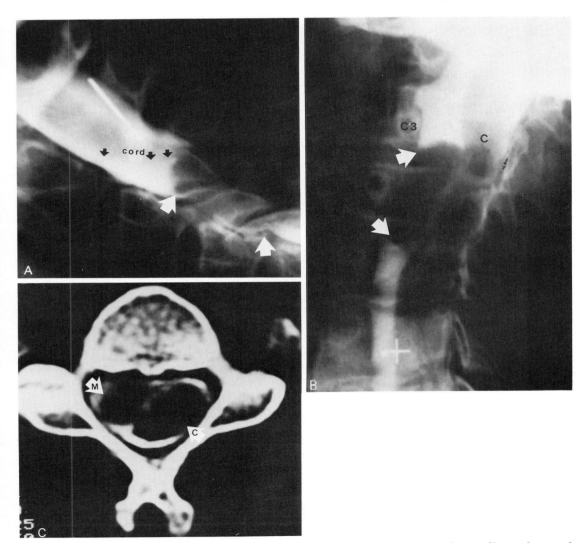

FIGURE 15–73. _Cervical Meningioma:_ _A_, Lateral view of the myelogram reveals the needle in place at the C₁–C₂ level. Contrast has been instilled and demonstrates a meniscus outlining the upper margin of the intradural meningioma at the C₃–C₄ level (_arrows_). The cervical spinal cord is displaced dorsally and compressed by the tumor.

_B_, Oblique view of the myelogram reveals the typical intradural tumor at the C₃–C₄ level. The cervical spinal cord (_C_) is displaced dorsally and to the contralateral side.

_C_, Postmyelogram CT scan reveals the meningioma (_M_) and the cervical cord displaced dorsally and to the contralateral side (_C_). An intradural schwannoma may have a similar appearance. Surgically proved.

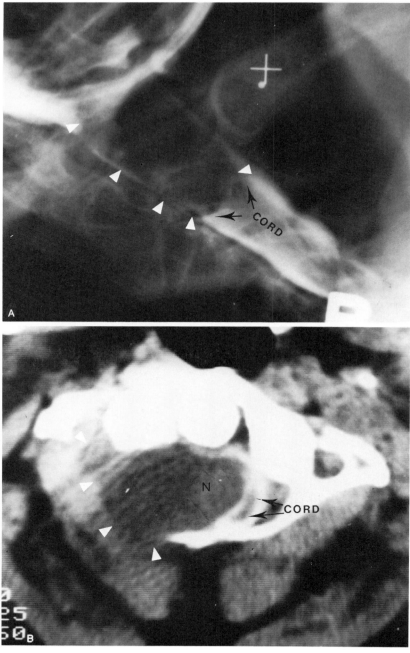

FIGURE 15–74. *Foramen Magnum Neurofibroma: A,* Lateral view of the myelogram reveals a large intradural mass at the level of the foramen magnum and extending down to the level of the superior end-plate of C_3 (*arrows*). The cervical spinal cord is visualized and is widened at the level of the tumor (*arrowheads*).

B, CT scan at the level of the odontoid process reveals the large mass (*N*) that has eroded the lamina and lateral mass of the C_1 vertebral body and extends into the soft tissues of the dorsal aspect of the right side of the neck (*arrowheads*). The cervical spinal cord is compressed and displaced markedly to the left, where it is flattened into a ribbon-like structure.

Surgically proved neurofibroma that extended through the foramen magnum.

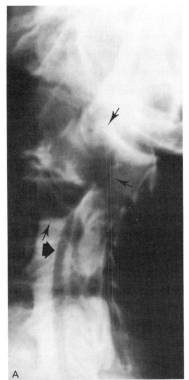

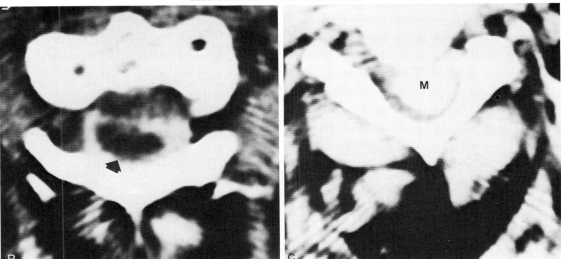

FIGURE 15–75. *Meningioma:* *A*, Myelogram reveals an intradural mass that arises along the left side of the cervical subarachnoid space (*small arrows*) and displaces the cervical cord (*large arrow*) to the contralateral side.

B, CT slice through the base of the odontoid process reveals that the cervical cord is flattened and displaced posteriorly (*arrow*). The mass is identified just behind the base of the odontoid process.

C, At the level of the meningioma (*M*) a densely calcified portion of the mass is seen. The spinal cord is compressed in a ribbon-like fashion and displaced posteriorly. Surgically proved meningioma.

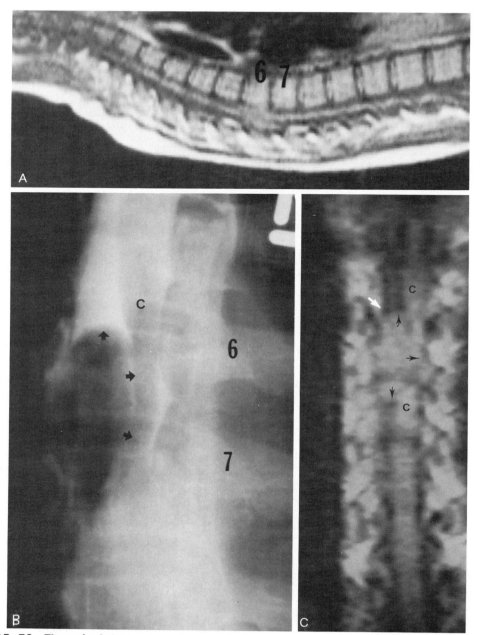

FIGURE 15–76. *Thoracic Schwannoma:* *A*, Sagittal T-1 weighted SE image obtained with the body coil reveals a mass at the C₆–C₇ level. There is interruption of the CSF surrounding the spinal cord and a mass that is isointense with the cord at this level.

B, The myelogram performed via C₁–C₂ tap reveals the typical appearance of an intradural mass (*black arrows*) beginning at the T₆ level, displacing the cord (*C*) to the contralateral side, and compressing it at the level of T₆–T₇.

C, T-1 weighted SE image obtained with the surface coil also demonstrated the intradural mass (*black arrows*) with displacement of the cord to the contralateral side. The CSF in the subarachnoid space above the mass is widened because the cord is displaced to the contralateral side (*white arrow*).

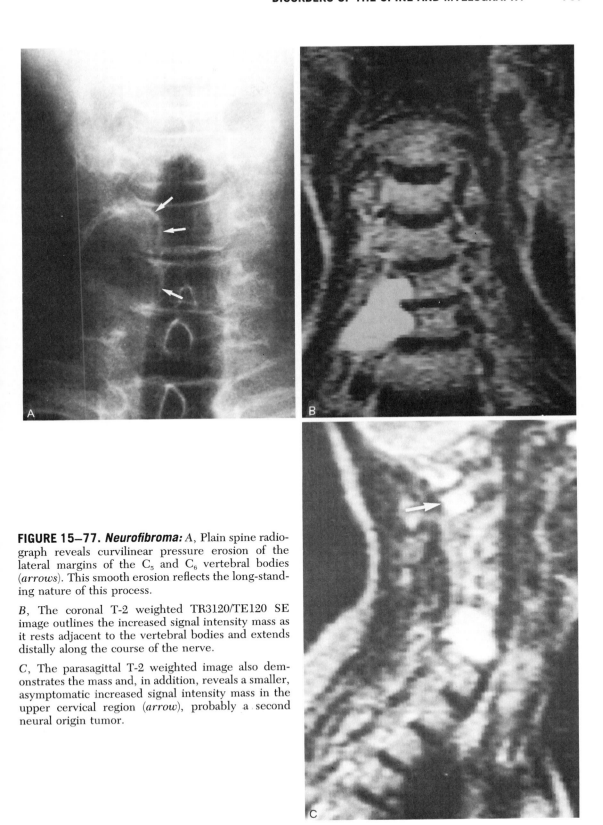

FIGURE 15–77. *Neurofibroma: A,* Plain spine radiograph reveals curvilinear pressure erosion of the lateral margins of the C_5 and C_6 vertebral bodies (*arrows*). This smooth erosion reflects the long-standing nature of this process.

B, The coronal T-2 weighted TR3120/TE120 SE image outlines the increased signal intensity mass as it rests adjacent to the vertebral bodies and extends distally along the course of the nerve.

C, The parasagittal T-2 weighted image also demonstrates the mass and, in addition, reveals a smaller, asymptomatic increased signal intensity mass in the upper cervical region (*arrow*), probably a second neural origin tumor.

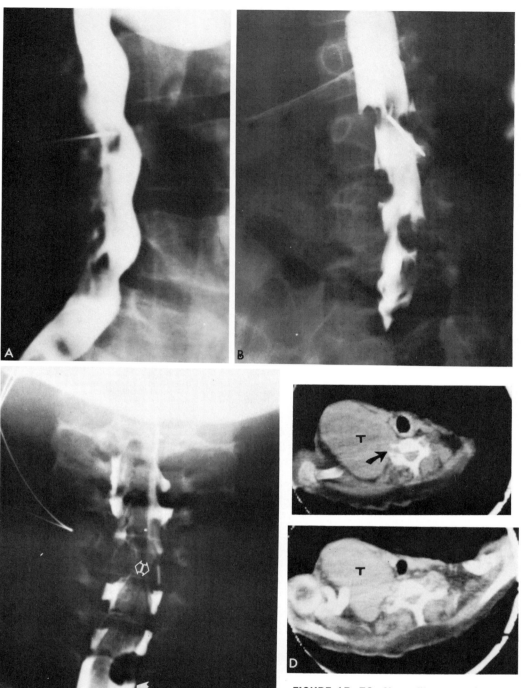

FIGURE 15–78. *Neurofibromatosis:* *A* to *C*, Views in both the lumbar and cervical regions reveal multiple rounded filling defects of the nerve rootlets. In the cervical region the cervical cord is displaced to the left by the large tumor (*white arrow*), while higher in the cervical region the cervical cord is compressed (*open white arrows*). These neurofibromas are the so-called "dumbbell tumors," which also have a soft tissue neurofibroma outside the neural foramina. At times the portion of the tumor outside the central canal is palpable in the neck.

D, The CT scan in another patient with neurofibromatosis demonstrates a dumbbell tumor (*T*) present in the soft tissues of the neck. The neurofibroma also extends into the spinal canal and widens the bony neural foramina (*arrow*).

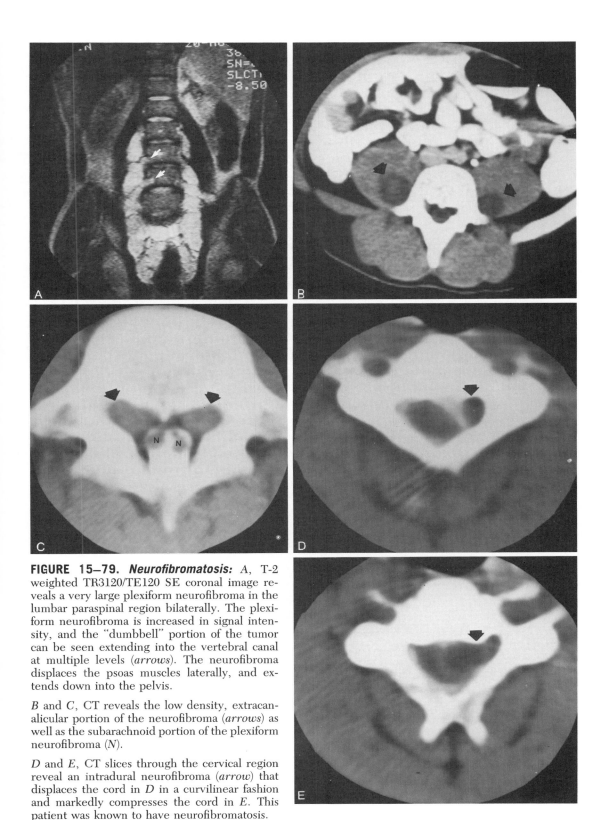

FIGURE 15–79. *Neurofibromatosis:* *A*, T-2 weighted TR3120/TE120 SE coronal image reveals a very large plexiform neurofibroma in the lumbar paraspinal region bilaterally. The plexiform neurofibroma is increased in signal intensity, and the "dumbbell" portion of the tumor can be seen extending into the vertebral canal at multiple levels (*arrows*). The neurofibroma displaces the psoas muscles laterally, and extends down into the pelvis.

B and *C*, CT reveals the low density, extracanalicular portion of the neurofibroma (*arrows*) as well as the subarachnoid portion of the plexiform neurofibroma (*N*).

D and *E*, CT slices through the cervical region reveal an intradural neurofibroma (*arrow*) that displaces the cord in *D* in a curvilinear fashion and markedly compresses the cord in *E*. This patient was known to have neurofibromatosis.

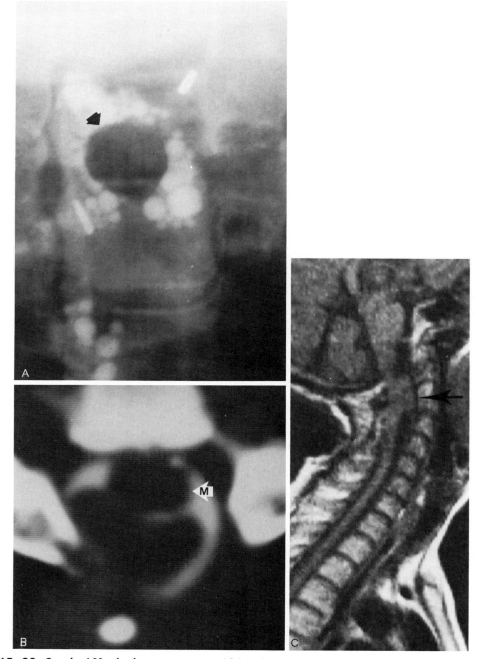

FIGURE 15–80. *Cervical Meningioma:* A 69-year-old female, previously operated on for cervical meningioma. A, Cervical myelogram in the prone position demonstrates a rounded 1.5-cm filling defect in the ventral aspect of the cervical subarachnoid space (*arrow*). There are surgical clips present and a small amount of Pantopaque from a previous myelogram.

B, CT scan following the myelogram at the level of C_2 reveals the mass (*M*) in the ventral aspect of the subarachnoid space. The cervical spinal cord is displaced posteriorly and distorted in a curvilinear fashion around the mass.

C, Mid-sagittal TR530/TE30 SE reveals the mass (*arrow*) projecting behind the body of C_2. The medulla and the spinal cord are displaced posteriorly, and the cervical subarachnoid space is widened above and below the mass. The appearance is typical of an intradural type of tumor. Major considerations in the differential diagnosis are neurofibroma and meningioma. The final diagnosis in this case was a meningioma; the tumor was successfully removed via an anterior approach with removal of the C_2 vertebral body.

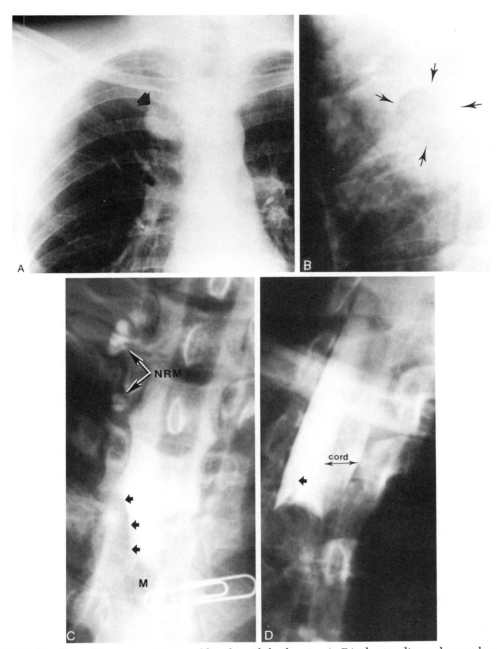

FIGURE 15–81. *Neurofibroma:* A 16-year-old male with back pain. *A,* PA chest radiograph reveals a mass in the right superior mediastinum (*arrow*).

B, Close examination of the lateral view of the chest x-ray reveals widening of the neural foramen (*arrows*) at the level of the mass.

C and *D,* Myelogram was performed via a C_1–C_2 tap. There is a complete block at the level of the widened neural foramen. In the oblique view (*D*), the cord can be seen displaced from right to left. The tumor is "capped" by the contrast material, and there is widening of the contrast-filled subarachnoid space on the side of the mass. Close inspection also reveals a small curvilinear filling defect in the subarachnoid space (*arrow*) just above the mass; this represents a dilated vein. *C,* AP supine view demonstrates the intradural component of the mass (*M*) with displacement of the spinal cord from right to left. In addition, there is also an extradural component with displacement of the contrast column from right to left (*arrows*) above the level of the mass. Incidentally noted are small nerve root meningoceles (*NRM*) in the upper thoracic region—they are of no pathologic significance. The paper clip is taped to the patient's back at the level of the abnormality to facilitate the surgical approach. Surgically proved "dumbbell" neurofibroma.

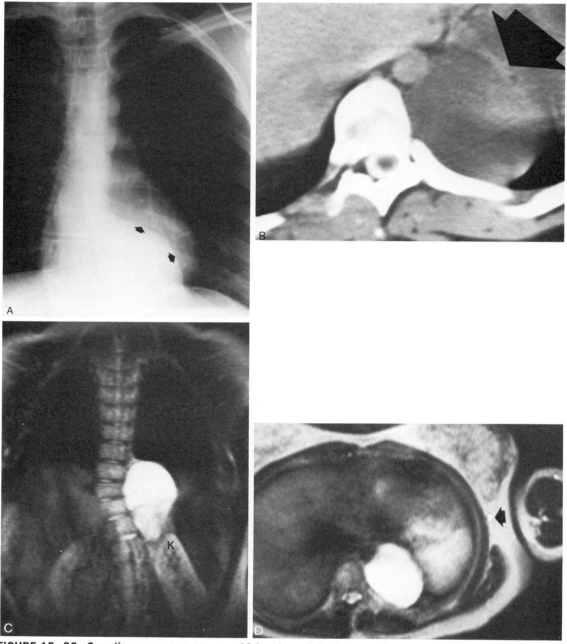

FIGURE 15–82. *Ganglioneuroma:* A 26-year-old female with back pain and progressive scoliosis. *A*, PA chest radiograph demonstrates a large, smoothly marginated retrocardiac mass (*arrows*). The mass is at the level of the thoracic scoliosis.

B, Axial CT scan following metrizamide myelography reveals the paraspinal mass (*arrow*). The left hemidiaphragm is displaced laterally around the mass. The abdominal aorta projects anteromedial to the mass. There was no communication with the subarachnoid space.

C, Coronal TR3120/TE120 SE demonstrates that the mass is well defined, and because of its increased signal intensity, its exact location is readily appreciated. The superior pole of the left kidney (*K*) is displaced laterally and rests just at the inferior end of the paraspinal mass.

D, Axial TR3120/TE120 SE again confirms the paraspinal location of the mass and the absence of any communication with the vertebral canal. The *arrow* points to the long thoracic nerve, which also became very high in signal intensity on this T-2 weighted image, as did other neural structures. Surgically proved ganglioneuroma.

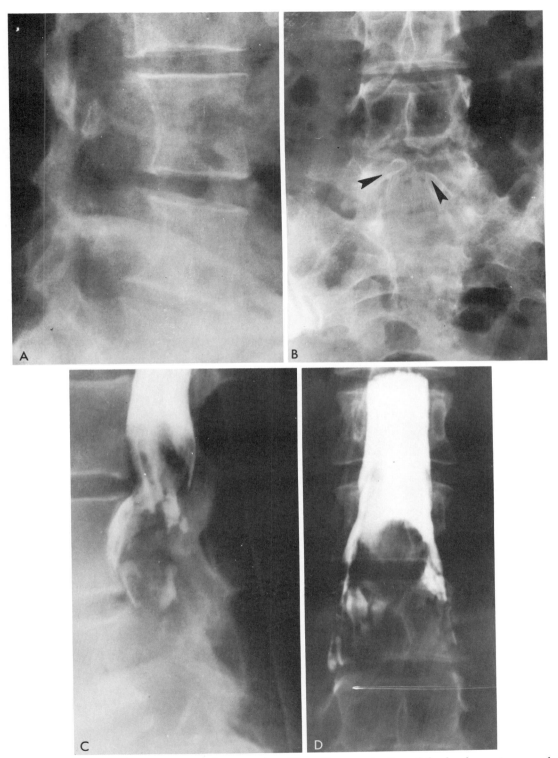

FIGURE 15–83. *Dermoid of Cauda Equina:* *A* and *B*, Plain film examination of the lumbar spine reveals a marked increase in the lateral and AP diameter of the subarachnoid space, with scalloping of the posterior aspects of all the lower vertebral bodies. In addition, there is a spina bifida of the L₅ vertebral bodies (*arrows*).

C and *D*, The myelogram reveals a large lobulated mass lesion that has expanded the lumbar subarachnoid space. The Pantopaque column outlines the upper border of the tumor.

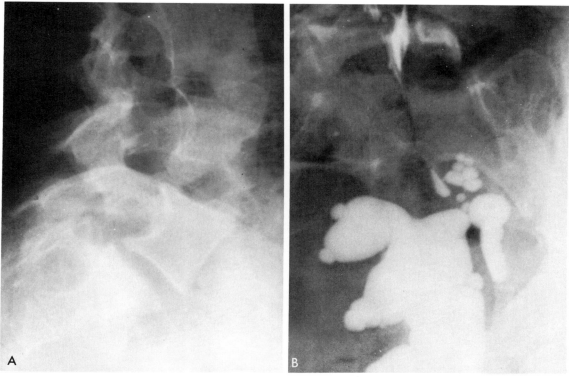

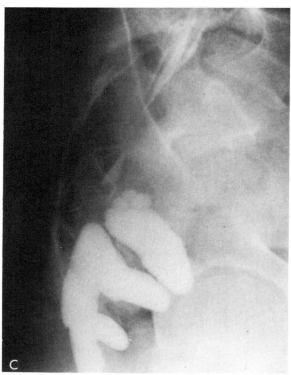

FIGURE 15–84. *Anterior Sacral Meningocele:* A, Plain film examination reveals marked scalloping of the posterior aspects of all of the lumbar and sacral vertebral bodies. There is an increase in the AP and lateral diameters of the subarachnoid space.

B and C, Following the instillation of Pantopaque, a large anterior sacral meningocele is filled with contrast material. On the lateral view, the meningocele projects into the pelvic canal. This may present as a pelvic mass on physical examination.

FIGURE 15–85. *Intramedullary Tumor:*
A, The cervical cord is widened and there is bilateral thinning of the contrast material in the subarachnoid space. There was a similar appearance on the lateral view. Surgery revealed an astrocytoma. (Courtesy of Drs. Oscar Sugar and Glen Dobben, University of Illinois.)

B, There is widening of the lower cervical and upper thoracic cord (*arrowheads*). Surgery revealed an astrocytoma.

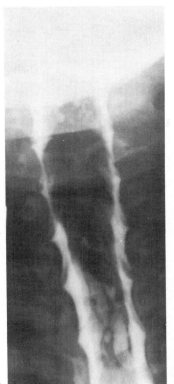
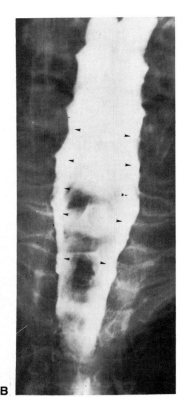

A B

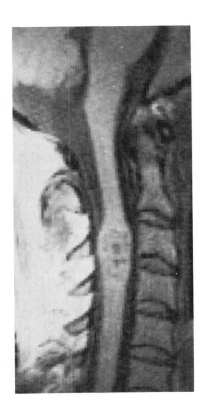

FIGURE 15–86. *Intramedullary Tumor:* This 36-year-old male presented with progressive arm and leg weakness. The TR530/TE30 (T-1 weighted) SE image reveals an area of focal expansion of the cord at the C_3–C_4 level that is very readily appreciated. The mass contains areas of decreased signal intensity that could represent either calcification or flowing blood (calcification was identified by CT). There is circumferential compromise of the subarachnoid space. Although not surgically proved, this is believed to be a calcified astrocytoma.

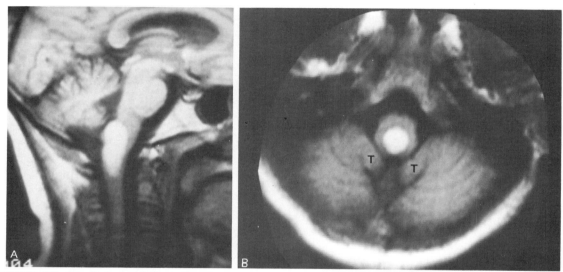

FIGURE 15–87. *Spinomedullary Hematoma:* A 23-year-old female with sudden onset of quadraparesis 10 days prior to examination. *A,* Mid-sagittal TR530/TE30 SE demonstrates a slightly lobulated, smoothly marginated, increased signal intensity mass involving the medulla and the upper cervical cord. There is slight expansion of the cord and medulla at this level.

B, Axial TR530/TE30 SE image at the level of the medulla reveals the acentric position of the increased signal intensity area in the posterior portion of the medulla. The cerebellar tonsils are clearly outlined (*T*). The increased signal on T-1 weighted image implies that this abnormality represents either fat or subacute hemorrhage. Because of the sudden onset it was believed that it represented an area of hemorrhage secondary to an arteriovenous malformation—a vascular malformation that had bled and obliterated itself (angiogram was normal). The hematoma was evacuated via a midline incision, and the patient recovered sufficiently to be able to walk out of the hospital.

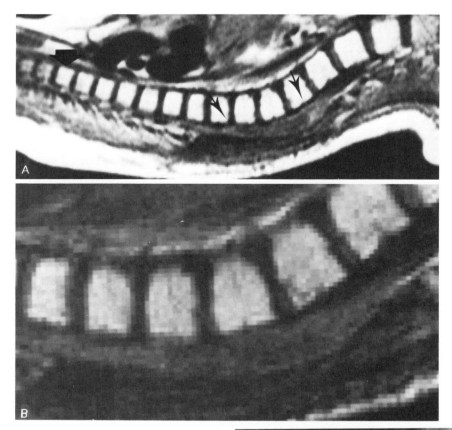

FIGURE 15–88. *Conus Medullaris Astrocytoma:* A 14-year-old female with previous surgery for partial removal of astrocytoma. *A,* Mid-sagittal TR530/TE30 SE demonstrates the tumor in the lower thoracic spinal cord (*arrows*), where it appears as an area of expansion of the cord and contains areas of decreased signal intensity. There is an extensive laminectomy at the T_8 and L_2 levels. The spinous processes are surgically absent, and there is disruption of the soft tissue planes. The increased signal intensity of the vertebral bodies of T_2 through the lowest lumbar segment is secondary to previous radiation therapy and to a relative increase in the amount of adipose tissue in the marrow of the vertebrae.

B, Magnified view better demonstrates the expanded cord with decreased signal intensity center.

C, TR3120/TE120 SE reveals that the CSF is increased in signal intensity, but there is an even greater increase in the signal intensity of the tumor (*arrow*). Note also the acute kyphosis of the spine and deformity of the vertebral bodies secondary to the radiation treatment. Known astrocytoma of the conus medullaris.

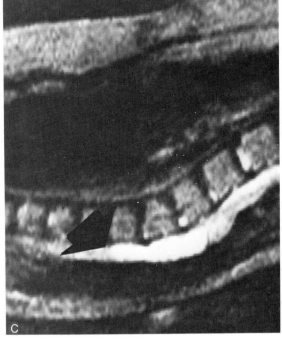

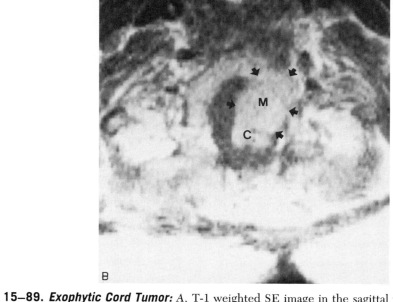

FIGURE 15–89. *Exophytic Cord Tumor: A*, T-1 weighted SE image in the sagittal plane reveals a large mass (*M*) at the C_6–C_7 level (where there has been a previous fusion), which arises from the cervical spinal cord (*C*). The cord is expanded above and below the tumor mass.

B, The T-1 weighted SE image in the axial plane reveals the relationship between the cervical spinal cord and the mass, although a true cleavage plane cannot be identified. The cervical canal is enlarged. The margins of the mass are outlined by the arrows. Biopsy reveals a teratomatous type of primitive tumor.

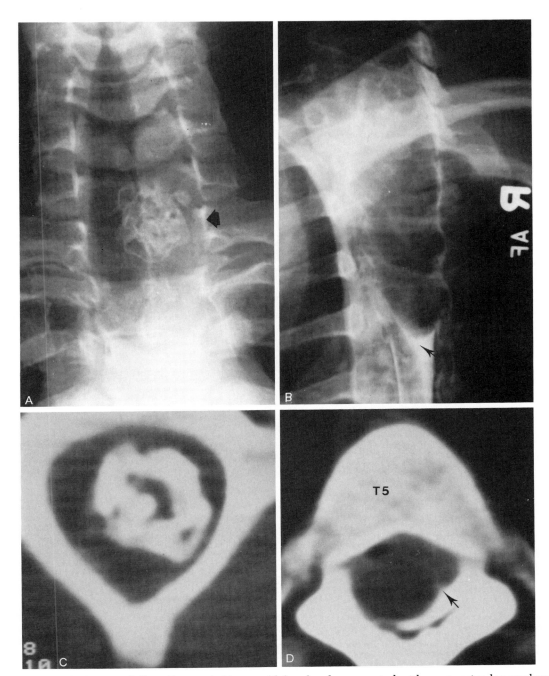

FIGURE 15–90. *Intramedullary Tumor:* A 14-year-old female who presented with progressive leg weakness.
A, Plain spine radiograph reveals marked expansion of the cervical spinal canal secondary to pressure from a
long-standing process. There is also a 2-cm densely but amorphously calcified mass at the C_7–T_1 level (*arrow*).

B, Myelogram reveals that while the mass is an intramedullary tumor, there is also a large exophytic
component along the dorsal aspect of the spinal cord that compresses the cord and displaces it anteriorly
(*arrow*). Note that the lower extent of the mass is at the T_5–T_6 level, well below the calcified portion.

C, CT through the calcified portion of the mass reveals the greatly expanded cord occupying the entire
cervical canal.

D, At the T5 level the cleavage plane between the cord anteriorly and the exophytic component of the tumor
posteriorly (*arrow*) can be faintly identified. Surgery revealed an astrocytoma.

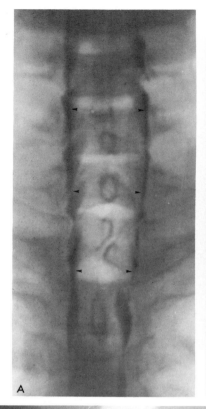

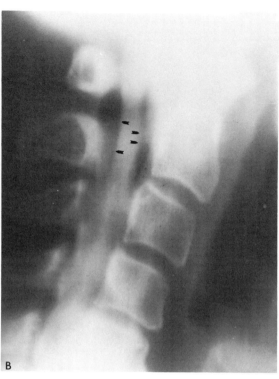

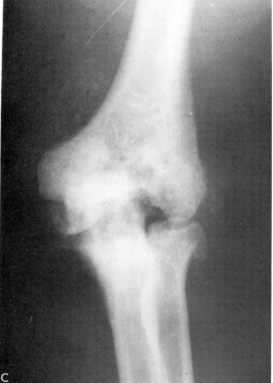

FIGURE 15–91. *Syringohydromyelia: A,* There is diffuse widening of the cord that extends throughout the entire cervical region and well down into the thorax. The cervical cord has almost obliterated the subarachnoid space bilaterally *(arrowheads).* Incidentally, there is a spina bifida of the T₁ spinous process.

B, Air myelography reveals that the cervical cord collapses and becomes very narrow *(arrowheads).* The cord is surrounded by the radiolucent shadow of the surrounding air. The collapse of the cervical cord occurs when the patient's head is elevated and the fluid in the hydromyelic sac flows by gravity to a more distal position in the cord.

C, Charcot joint: The elbow demonstrates a marked amount of soft tissue calcification and degenerative changes surrounding the elbow. The bony structures continue to be well ossified. The appearance is typical of a Charcot joint.

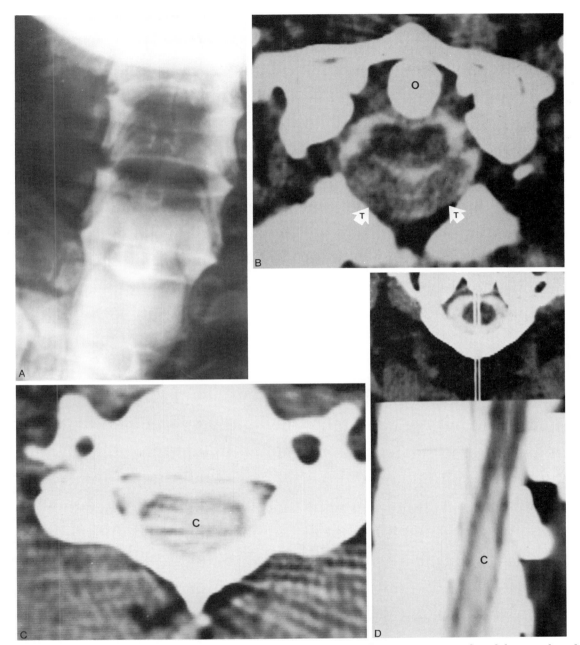

FIGURE 15–92. *Chiari Type I Malformation:* A 43-year-old male with progressive atrophy of the muscles of the hands. *A*, Myelogram demonstrates widening of the spinal cord throughout its entire visualized portion.

B, Postmyelogram CT at the level of the vertebral body of C$_1$ and the odontoid (*O*). The cerebellar tonsils are identified (*T*) dorsal to the cord and compressing the cord anteriorly. This represents herniated tonsils of the Chiari Type I malformation.

C, CT scan at the C$_4$ level obtained six hours following the myelogram demonstrates the large cystic cavity (*C*) that now contains contrast material, the surrounding ribbon-like spinal cord, and the contrast material in the cervical subarachnoid space.

D, Mid-sagittal reconstruction view reveals the contrast material in the cavity (*C*) and the thin surrounding cord. In most cases, MR can provide the same, or more accurate, information without the necessity of injecting contrast material. This is particularly helpful in pediatric cases.

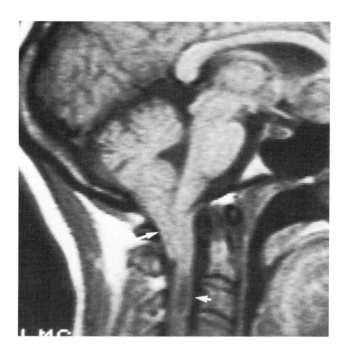

FIGURE 15–93. *Chiari Malformation and Small Cervical Syrinx:* The cerebellar tonsils are displaced inferiorly below the level of the foramen magnum and elongated (*large white arrow*). There is a small localized cavity within the upper cervical cord at the level of the C3 vertebral body (*small white arrow*).

FIGURE 15–94. *Syringohydromyelia:* A 38-year-old male with progressive arm and leg weakness. TR530/TE30 SE image demonstrates the syrinx cavity in the upper cervical cord (*arrows*), extending up to the level of the posterior arch of C_1. This study was performed using the head coil.

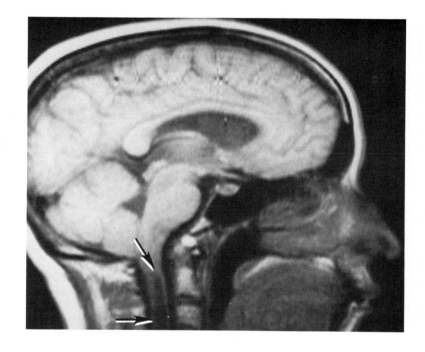

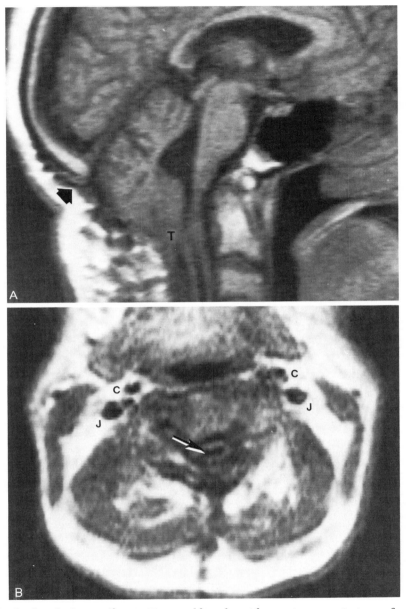

FIGURE 15–95. *Syringohydromyelia:* A 27-year-old male with previous craniectomy for Chiari Type I malformation. *A*, TR530/TE30 SE reveals the postoperative changes with surgical removal of the lower portion of the occipital bone. The bone of the calvarium ends at the midcerebellar level (*arrow*). The cerebellar hemispheres extend through the craniectomy level, and a portion of the cerebellum and the cerebellar tonsils extend below the anticipated position of the foramen magnum (*T*). The fourth ventricle is enlarged and the medulla is atrophic. The syrinx cavity is visible within the upper cervical cord.

B, The cavity is also demonstrated in the axial TR530/TE30 SE slice (*arrow*). The negative flow defect of blood is seen in the carotid arteries (*C*) and jugular veins (*J*) bilaterally.

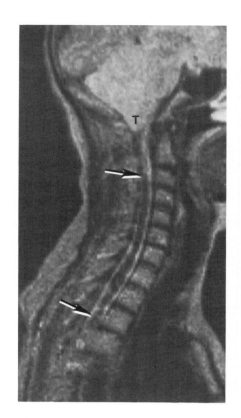

FIGURE 15–96. *Chiari Type I Malformation:* Mid-sagittal TR530/TE30 SE image demonstrates the typical appearance of the Chiari malformation, with the cerebellar tonsils extending below the level of the foramen magnum (*arrows*). There is a large and long loculated cavity extending throughout the entire cervical cord. The cord is enlarged. The cord is visualized in the thoracic region because the scoliosis often seen with these cases has resulted in the cord's moving out of the plane of section of this 1-cm thick slice. Other contiguous slices demonstrated the syrinx in the thoracic region. Axial sections may sometimes demonstrate the cavity to best advantage, particularly if there is a scoliosis.

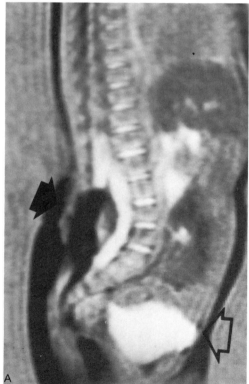

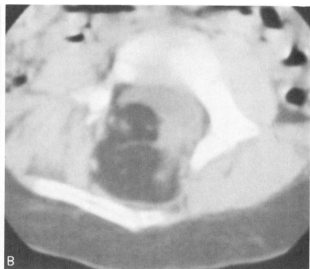

FIGURE 15–97. *Chiari Type II Malformation:* *A,* Inversion recovery image of the entire body obtained in the head coil reveals that the fat in the subcutaneous tissue and in the lipoma (normally high signal intensity) is of very low signal intensity with this sequence. A somewhat unusual bone island is seen in the subcutaneous tissue just anterior to the arrow, the lipoma just anterior to that, and the neural plaque between the lipoma and the high signal intensity of the CSF in the expanded lumbar vertebral canal. The dilated neurogenic bladder is also seen (*open arrow*), as well as a tethered cord.

B, Axial CT through the lipoma also demonstrates the dysraphic spine, the enlarged lumbar vertebral canal, and the bone island in the soft tissue of the back.

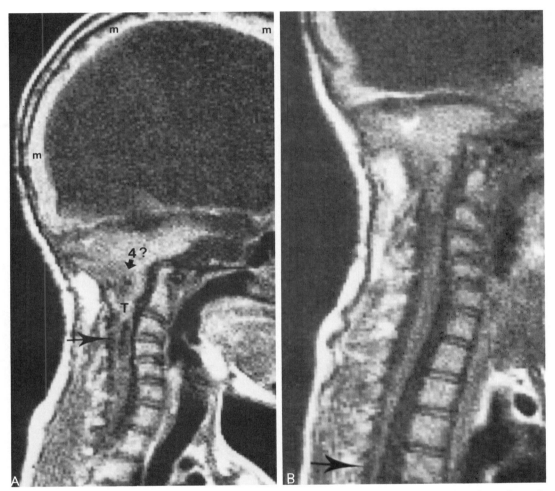

FIGURE 15–98. *Chiari Type II Malformation and Syrinx:* The patient is a 20-year-old male with a Chiari Type II malformation and previous repair of a meningomyelocele. *A,* Mid-sagittal TR530/TE30 SE image reveals the small posterior fossa with the fourth ventricle displaced into the upper cervical vertebral canal *(4?).* There is massive hydrocephalus secondary to aqueduct stenosis and only a very thin cortical mantel *(m)* of the brain. The cerebellar tonsils *(I)* are herniated into the cervical vertebral canal, and a small syrinx cavity is demonstrated in the cervical cord *(arrow).*

B, The patient had progressive lower extremity weakness, and the lower cervical/upper thoracic cord demonstrates marked atrophy *(arrow).* MR provides accurate, noninvasive evaluation of all of these changes.

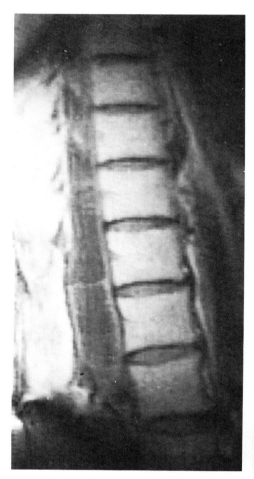

FIGURE 15–99. *Syrinx of the Conus Medullaris:* T-1 weighted SE image of the low thoracic cord reveals a multiseptated syrinx cavity involving the lower thoracic spinal cord. There is essentially complete obliteration of the subarachnoid space surrounding the cord at this level. (The entire spinal cord was abnormal.)

FIGURE 15–100. *Posterior Fossa Arachnoid Cyst and Cervical Syrinx:* There is a large, space-occupying posterior fossa arachnoid cyst that is of CSF signal intensity. The fourth ventricle is displaced forward (*black arrow*), and the cerebellar tonsils are displaced inferiorly (*T*) below the level of the foramen magnum (tonsilar herniation). The cervical spinal cord is involved with a cavity that begins just below the cerebellar tonsils and extends through the cervical cord. The syrinx is largest at the C_5–C_6 level (*white arrow*).

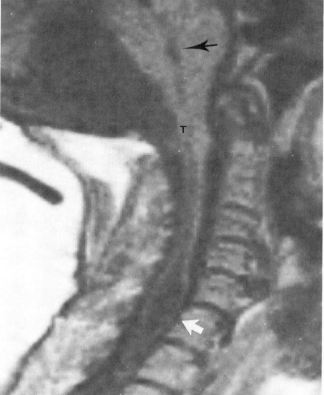

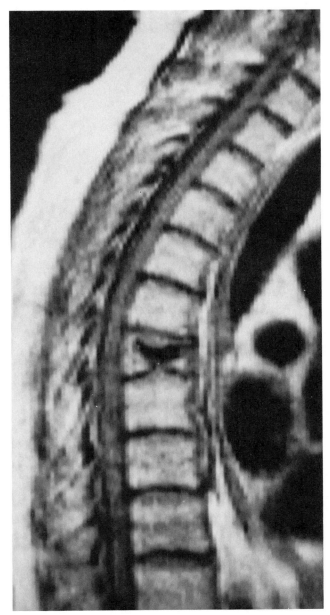

FIGURE 15–101. *Compression Fracture of the Thoracic Spine:* A 58-year-old female with back pain following a fall. MR TR530/TE30 SE demonstates the compression fracture of the thoracic vertebral body. Both the superior and inferior end-plates are compressed more centrally than elsewhere. There is slight accentuation of the thoracic kyphosis, but no compromise of the spinal cord or surrounding subarachnoid space. Note that there is no alteration of the signal intensity from the vertebral body marrow because this is a post-traumatic fracture rather than a pathologic fracture.

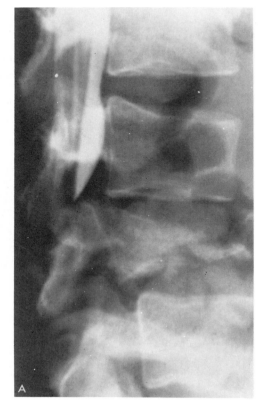

FIGURE 15–102. *Lumbar Spine Fracture with Amipaque Myelogram and CT Scan:* *A*, After the instillation of contrast material at the C_1–C_2 level, a complete block to the flow is encountered at the level of the fracture. The L_3 vertebral body is noted to be compressed and deformed. There is posterior displacement of the posterior aspect of L_3. The contrast column is displaced posteriorly, and the nerves of the cauda equina are compressed.

B, The true extent of the fracture is better appreciated on the CT scan:

#16: The thoracic cord is normal (*arrow*). Note the anterior and posterior roots as they enter and exit from the spinal cord. The subarachnoid space is filled with Amipaque.

#15: The transverse process demonstrates a comminuted fracture (*arrow*).

#12: The nerves of the cauda equina are distributed in the lumbar subarachnoid space and bathed by Amipaque.

#07: The comminuted fracture of L_3 can now be seen. Note that the Amipaque is no longer seen because there is a complete block to flow.

#06: A fracture is seen through the spinous process and articulating facet (*arrow*). Note the comminuted pieces of the L_3 vertebral body. A portion of the vertebral body has been displaced posteriorly into the spinal canal.

#05: There is diastasis of the interfacet articulation (*arrow*).

#04: There is a fracture through the lamina of the vertebral body and bilateral distraction of the interfacet joints.

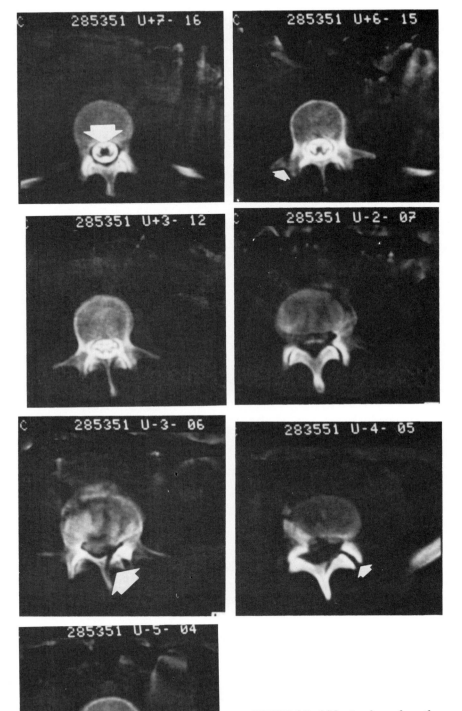

FIGURE 15–102. *See legend on the opposite page.*

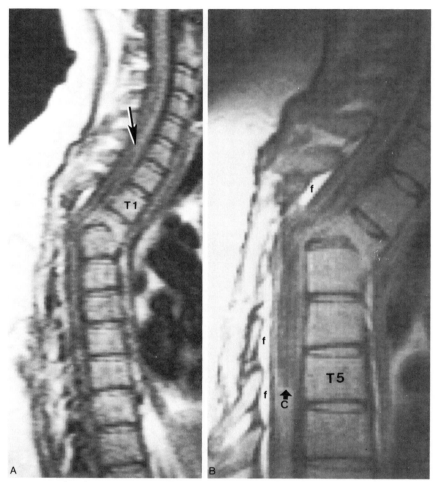

FIGURE 15–103. *Post-traumatic Fracture and Syringohydromyelia:* This 26-year-old female initially sustained a T_2 fracture following a motor vehicle accident approximately two years prior to this study. *A,* Body coil image in the mid-sagittal plane with T-1 weighted SE image reveals the fracture of the T_2 vertebral body with acute kyphosis at the level of the fracture. There is accentuation of the dorsal kyphosis at the fracture site. A syrinx cavity is faintly demonstrated (*arrow*).

B, Surface coil image better demonstrates the fracture. Note the preservation of the intervertebral disc and the kyphosis. A large, well-defined syrinx cavity (*C*) can be easily seen extending down to the T_5 level. The cavity extended superiorly up to the level of C_1 (not shown). Fat (*f*) is identified in the dorsal epidural space—a normal finding. This represents a post-traumatic syrinx cavity that develops following resorption of an intramedullary hematoma or an area of myelomalacia that progresses to cavitation. While a severe scoliosis may compromise the MR study, axial views will usually demonstate the syrinx cavity.

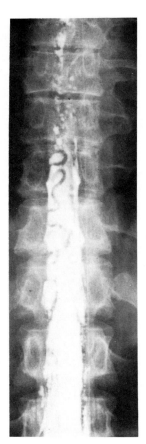

FIGURE 15–104. *Arteriovenous Malformation of the Thoracic Spinal Cord:* With the patient in the supine position, multiple, enlarged tortuous vessels can be readily demonstrated over the thoracic spinal cord. This appearance is very typical for the enlarged arteries and draining vessels asosciated with an arteriovenous malformation of the cord (see Chapter 6).

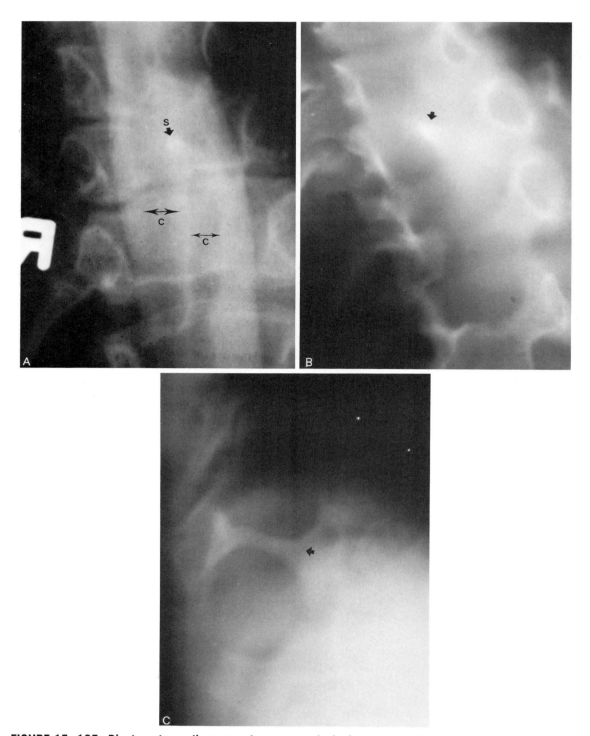

FIGURE 15–105. *Diastematomyelia: A,* Myelogram reveals the bony spur in the midportion of the vertebral canal (*S*); the spinal cord (*C*) is divided into two hemicords, and the subarachnoid space is widened and the vertebral bodies are abnormal at all the visualized levels. The vertebral bodies are deformed, and the interpedicular distance is widened.

B, AP radiographic tomography demonstrates the deformed vertebral bodies, and the bony spur (*arrow*) is viewed end on.

C, Lateral radiographic tomogram demonstrates the bony spur extending from front to back at the level of the midcanal (*arrow*).

Illustration continued on the following page

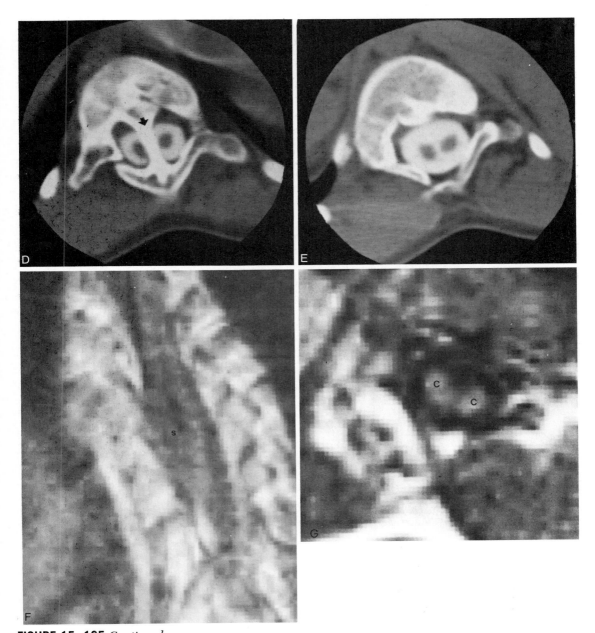

FIGURE 15–105 *Continued.*

D, Axial CT scan at the level of the bony spur also confirms the two hemicords, both surrounded by contrast-filled subarachnoid space.

E, CT at a slightly lower level reveals that there are still two hemicords, but there is now only one subarachnoid space. The deformed vertebral bodies that always accompany diastematomyelia are readily appreciated.

F, Coronal MR TR530/TE30 SE faintly visualizes the bony spur (*s*); the spinal hemicords are on either side, and there is focal widening of the vertebral canal. The bony abnormalities are better demonstrated on the radiographic tomograms and CT scan.

G, Axial TR530/TE30 SE demonstrates the two spinal cord segments (*C*).

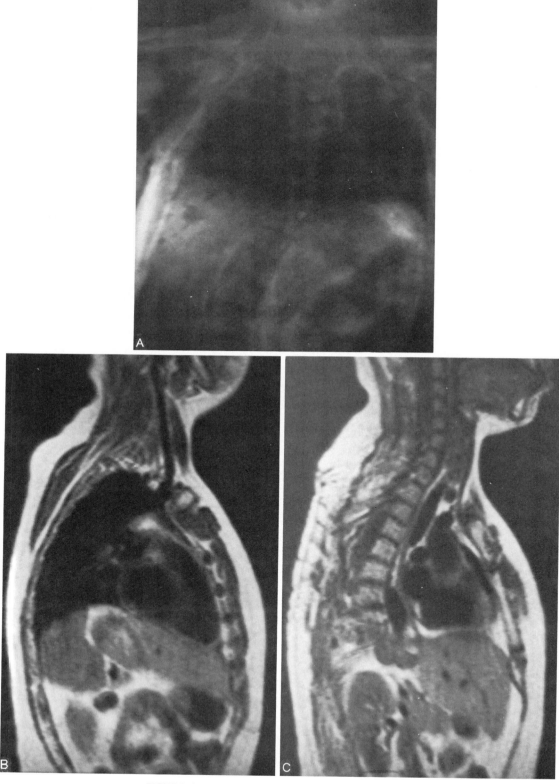

FIGURE 15–106. *See legend on the opposite page.*

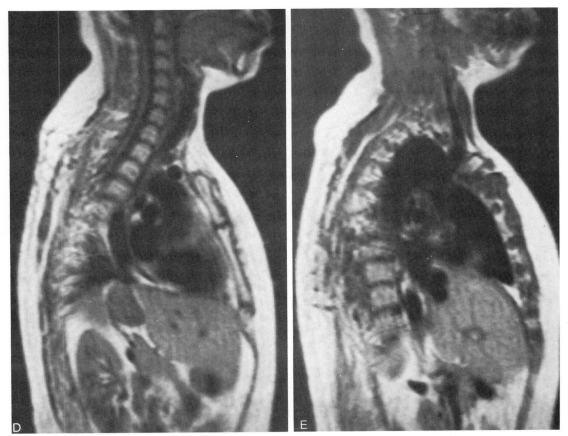

FIGURE 15–106. *Scoliosis:* *A*, Shadowgram in the AP projection reveals the marked scoliosis. This markedly compromises the MR study because it is a planar type of examination.

B to *E*, The vertebral column and the spinal cord can be demonstrated on the sequential images, but evaluation is markedly compromised. CT alone or CT following myelography is a better method of evaluation in this patient.

16

FUTURE ADVANCES IN NEURORADIOLOGY

Magnetic resonance is in its infancy, and future hardware and software developments will certainly expand the clinical usefulness of MR. Larger field strengths will allow spectroscopy to be performed. There is also extensive work being done in the development of MR contrast agents, both for the CNS and for other organ systems. Angled cuts, thin and/or overlapping cuts, accurate localization and repositioning, faster scanning, and new surface coils are or soon will be available. New low-osmolality and non-ionic contrast agents have recently become available for use as radiographic contrast agents. There will continue to be advances in CT scanning with automated processing and three-dimensional reconstruction of images.

New Intravascular Iodinated Radiographic Contrast Agents

A number of new contrast agents were released in 1985 and 1986 for clinical use. These include the low-osmolality contrast agent Hexabrix, as well as two non-ionic contrast agents, Omnipaque and Isovue.

Ioxaglate (Hexabrix, Mallinckrodt, Inc.). Hexabrix is a low-osmolality contrast agent that can be used for angiography, intravenous pyelography, digital subtraction angiography, and contrast-enhanced cranial computed tomography. Hexabrix has been shown to cause less pain and heat in clinical use and less alteration of the cardiovascular system than standard ionic contrast agents.

Iopamidol (Isovue, Mallinckrodt, Inc.). Iso-

vue is a new non-ionic contrast agent that is used for angiography and intravenous studies and can also be used as a myelographic contrast agent (see Chapter 15). Isovue can be used to evaluate the entire spinal column.

Iohexol (Omnipaque, Winthrop, Breon). Omnipaque is a new non-ionic contrast agent that is used for angiography and intravenous studies. Omnipaque can also be used as a contrast agent for study of the lumbar and thoracic subarachnoid space. As of this writing, Omnipaque is not approved for use in the cervical region.

ADVANCES IN MAGNETIC RESONANCE

Magnetic Resonance Flow Imaging

One of the unique properties of MR is the phenomenon of the absence of signal in those areas, such as blood vessels, where there is flowing fluid. Because of the multislice nature of the technique, the fluid does not remain in the slice being imaged long enough to return a signal. This results in a "negative flow defect," or area of signal void. As a general rule, the faster the flow, the darker the image or the more "negative" the defect. However, a paradoxic effect may occur because of slow or turbulent flow; a bright image occurs within the slice when the fluid happens to return a signal that can be detected. This paradoxic signal is variable in intensity and is commonly seen in the region of the jugular bulb with brain imaging and in the descending and thoracic aorta with imaging of these parts of the body.

The flow of CSF can also be evaluated and is useful in determining the patency of the cerebral aqueduct. Even in normal patients one can see the decrease in signal intensity when CSF flows rapidly through the aqueduct or occasionally the foramen of Monro. In Figure 16–1 this flow defect is identified in the foramen of Monro.

Subtraction Imaging

A technique has been developed by Drs. Van Vedeen and Brady at the Massachusetts General Hospital which uses a subtraction technique to image blood flowing in various blood vessels. This is demonstrated in Figure 16–2. This image was generated by first imaging the blood vessels in systole and then imaging these same blood vessels in diastole. The two images that are generated are then subtracted. The potential for clinical usefulness is readily apparent.

Gadolinium-DTPA

Gadolinium-DTPA (GD-DTPA) is an intravenous contrast agent that can be used with magnetic resonance imaging. GD-DTPA is used in a dose of approximately 0.1 mmol/kg of body weight and is not toxic at that dose. GD-DTPA crosses the blood-brain barrier in areas where there has been breakdown of the barrier and therefore reflects changes similar to those seen on CT where there is enhancement after intravenous infusion of iodinated contrast material. GD-DTPA causes a decrease in the T-1 of the abnormal area and therefore causes the tumor to appear bright on the T-1 weighted image. This allows differentiation of the tumor from surrounding edema. GD-DTPA should be very helpful for the evaluation of tumors such as meningioma and acoustic neuroma, although the exact role of this contrast agent has not yet been defined. GD-DTPA is currently an experimental contrast agent but should be available for clinical use in 1987 or 1988.

Other contrast materials are currently being studied.

Spectroscopy

It is in fields other than neuroradiology that spectroscopy will probably have its greatest impact. Because of the properties of magnetic resonance imaging, adenosine triphosphate (ATP) and adenosine diphosphate (ADP) each have different resonant frequencies. Myocardial infarction may be reflected in the varying levels of the compounds ATP and ADP as found in the Krebs cycle of metabolism. Therefore, if the level of ADT and ATP could be determined in an accurate and noninvasive way, it might be possible to easily identify the presence of a myocardial infarct with magnetic resonance imaging. The clinical benefits of this are readily apparent.

Surface Coils

The use and development of additional surface coils such as those used for the orbit (Fig. 16–3) will greatly aid magnetic resonance imaging. It is in the improvement and development of surface coils that magnetic resonance will see its greatest advances in the near future.

Higher Field Strengths

The ideal field strength has not yet been determined for either CNS or body imaging. Figure 16–4 illustrates a Kiwi fruit image at 4.7 Tesla.

Chemical Shift Imaging/Registration

Chemical shift misregistration occurs because water and lipid protons have different resonant frequencies. Because of this resonant frequency difference, bands of increased and decreased density occur at the edges of soft-tissue structures. This is particularly seen in the images of the lumbar spine, where the shift occurs in the direction of the frequency-encoding gradient. The "chemical shift" or false black line on one side of the tissue and a white line on the other occur because the computer interprets the different resonant frequencies as coming from different sources. With this technique one can image only fat or only water to some advantage, and this method of imaging should prove to be advantageous in some cases. One specific area of advantage is the study of an anatomic part such as the globe of the eye, in which selective suppression of the orbital fat allows better visualization of the water-containing extra-ocular muscles of the eye and optic nerve and will greatly aid evaluation of the orbit by magnetic resonance (Fig. 16–5).

The clinical availability and usefulness of MR could not have been anticipated 8 or even 5 years ago. It is impossible to predict what additional new instruments or procedures may become available for diagnosis.

I would like to express sincere appreciation to Mr. Barclay N. Dorman and the Technicare Corporation for their help and cooperation.

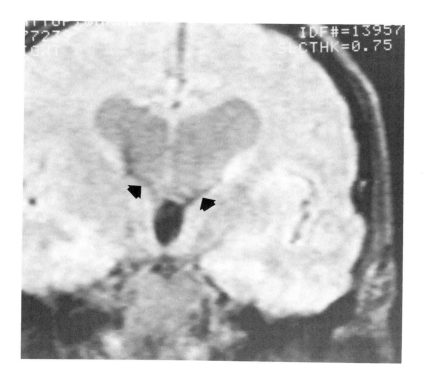

FIGURE 16–1. *CSF Flow Through Foramen of Monro:* This coronal view reveals that the CSF in the lateral ventricles is slightly lower in signal intensity than normal brain. The CSF in the third ventricle is much lower in signal intensity, and the laminar flow of the CSF from the lateral ventricles into the third ventricle (*arrows*) can be easily identified.

FIGURE 16–2. *MR Subtraction Imaging:* The image obtained in systole is subtracted from the image obtained in diastole. This results in an image of the blood vessels, in this example, of the distal superficial femoral artery, the trifurcation, and the blood vessels in the lower extremity. (Courtesy of Drs. Van Vedeen and Brady at the Massachusetts General Hospital.)

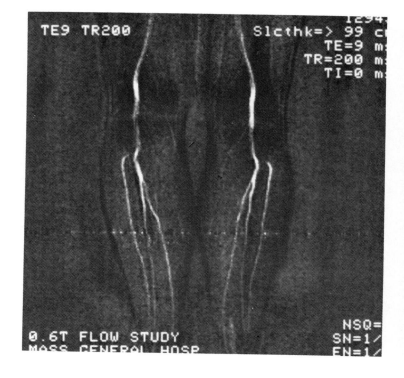

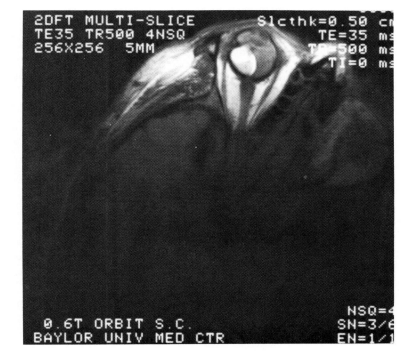

FIGURE 16–3. *Surface Coil, Orbit:* This surface coil image allows excellent visualization of the globe, the extraocular muscles, and a mass within the globe. (Courtesy of Baylor University Medical Center.)

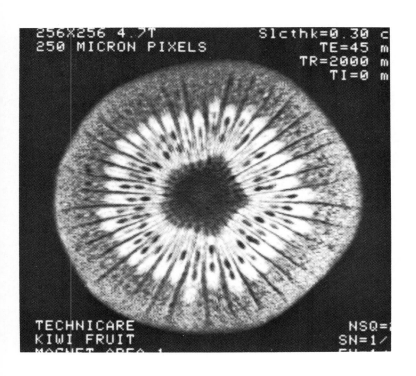

FIGURE 16–4. *4.7 Tesla Image:* This is an example of a 0.30-cm thick slice of a kiwi fruit at Harvard at 4.7 Tesla. (Courtesy of Mr. Barclay Dorman, Technicare Corporation.)

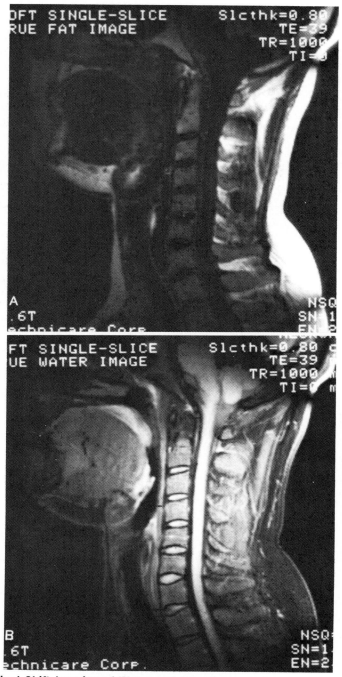

FIGURE 16–5. *Chemical Shift Imaging of Water and Fat:* There is selective suppression of water (*A*) and fat (*B*) to allow excellent visualization of the spinal cord. (Courtesy of Alan Stein, Ph.D., Technicare Corporation.)

BIBLIOGRAPHY

THE ORDER OF NEURORADIOLOGIC PROCEDURES

Abraham A: The Principles of Nuclear Magnetism. London, Oxford University Press, 1961, p 2.

Beall PT, Hazlewood CF, Rao PN: Nuclear magnetic resonance patterns of intracellular water as a function of hela cell cycle. Science 192:904–907, 1976.

Bobman SA, Riederer SJ, Lee JN, Suddarth SA, Wang HZ, MacFall JR: Synthesized MR images: Comparison with acquired images. Radiology 155:731–738, 1985.

Bottomley PA, Hart HR, Edelstein WA, et al: Anatomy and metabolism of the normal human brain studied by magnetic resonance at 1.5 tesla. Radiology 150:441–446, 1984.

Bracewell RN: The Fourier Transform and Its Applications. New York, McGraw-Hill, 1965.

Bradley WF, Open W, Kassabian JP: Magnetic resonance installation: Siting and economic considerations. Radiology 151:719–721, 1984.

Bradley WG, Crooks LE, Newton TH: Physical principles of NMR. In Newton TH, Potts DG (eds): Advanced Imaging Techniques. Vol 2. San Francisco, Clavadel Press, 1983.

Bradley WG, Newton TH, Crooks LE: Physical principles of nuclear magnetic resonance. In Newton T, Potts DG (eds): Modern Neuroradiology. Vol. 2. San Francisco, Clavadel Press, 1983, pp 15–61.

Brant-Zawadzki M, Bartowski HM, Ortendahl DA, et al: NMR in experimental cerebral edema: Value of T_1 and T_2 calculations. AJNR 5:125–129, 1983.

Brant-Zawadzki M, Davis PL, Crooks LE, Mills CM, Norman D, Newton TH, Sheldon P, Kaufman L: NMR demonstration of cerebral abnormalities: Comparison with CT. AJR 140:847–854, 1983.

Bydder GM, Steiner RE, Young IR, et al: Clinical NMR imaging of the brain: 140 cases. AJNR 3:459–480, 1982.

Cooke R, Wien R: Biophys J. 11:1002, 1971.

Crooks LE, Arakawa M, Hoenninger J, et al: Nuclear magnetic resonance whole-body imager operating at 3.5 K gauss. Radiology 143:169–174, 1982.

Davis PL, Crooks L, Arakawa M, et al.: Potential hazards in NMR imaging: Heating effects of changing magnetic fields and RF fields on small metallic implants. AJR 137:857–860, 1981.

Dixon WT: Simple proton spectroscopic imaging. Radiology 153:189–194, 1984.

Droege RT, Weiner SN, Rzeszotarski MS, et al: Nuclear magnetic resonance: A gray scale model for head images. Radiology 148:763–771, 1983.

Evans RG: Economic costs of nuclear magnetic resonance imaging. J. Comput. Assist Tomogr 8:200–203, 1984.

Flannigan BD, Bradley WG, Mazziotta JC, Rauschning W, Bentson JR: Magnetic resonance imaging of the brainstem: Normal structure and basic functional anatomy. Radiology 154:375–383, 1985.

Fullerton GD, Cameron IL, Ord VA: Frequency dependence of magnetic resonance spin-lattice relaxation of protons in biological materials. Radiology 151:135–138, 1984.

Hollis DP, Saryan LA, Economou JS, et al: Nuclear magnetic resonance study of cancer. V. Appearance and development of a tumor systemic effect in serum and tissues. J Natl Cancer Inst 53:807–815, 1974.

Hoult DI: Rotating frame zeugmatography. J Magnetic Res 3:183–198, 1979.

House WV: Introduction to the principles of NMR. IEEE Trans Nucl Sci NS-27:1220, 1980.

Kjos BO, Ehman RL, Brant-Zawadzki M, Kelly WM, Norman D, Newton TH: Reproducibility of relaxation times and spin density calculated from routine MR imaging sequences: Clinical study of the CNS. AJNR 6:271–276, 1985.

Koenig SH, Brown RD III, Adams D, et al: Magnetic field dependence of $1/T_1$ of protons in tissue. Invest Radiol 19:76–81, 1984.

Kramer DM: Imaging of elements other than hydrogen. In Crooks L, et al (eds): Nuclear Magnetic Resonance Imaging in Medicine. New York, Igaku-Shoin, 1981.

Kumar A, Welti D, Ernst RR: NMR Fourier zeugmatography. J Magnetic Res 18:69–83, 1975.

Lauterbur PC: Image formation by induced local interactions: Examples employing nuclear magnetic resonance. Nature 242:190–191, 1973.

Lauterbur PC, Lai CM: Zeugmatography by reconstruction from projections. IEEE Trans Nucl Sci NS-27:1227–1231, 1980.

Mills CM, Brant-Zawadzki M, Crooks LE, et al: Nuclear magnetic resonance: Principles of blood flow imaging. AJNR 4:1161–1166, 1983.

Mills CM, Crooks LE, Kaufman L, Brant-Zawadzki M: Cerebral abnormalities: Use of calculated T1 and T2 magnetic resonance images for diagnosis. Radiology 150:87–94, 1984.

New PFJ, Rosen BR, Brady TJ, et al: Potential hazards and artifacts of ferromagnetic and nonferromagnetic surgical and dental materials and devices in nuclear magnetic resonance imaging. Radiology 147:139–148, 1983.

NMR-Nuclear Magnetic Resonance Guideline Report AHA Hospital Technology Series. Vol. 2, No. 8, March 1983.

Pavlicek W, Geisinger M, Castle L, Borkowski GP, Meaney TF, Bream BL, Gallagher JH: The effects of nuclear magnetic resonance on patients with cardiac pacemakers. Radiology 147:149–153, 1983.

Posin JP, Arakawa M, Crooks LE, Feinberg DA, Hoenninger JC, Watts JC, Mills CM, Kaufman L: Hydrogen MR imaging of the head at 0.35 T and 0.7 T: Effects of magnetic field strength. Radiology 157:679–686, 1985.

Pykett IL, Buonanno FS, Brady TJ, et al: Techniques and approaches to proton imaging of the head. Comput Radiol 7:1–17, 1983.

Pykett IL, Newhouse JH, Buonanno FS, et al: Principles of nuclear magnetic resonance imaging. Radiology 143:157–168, 1982.

Shaw D: In vivo chemistry with NMR. In Crooks L, et al (eds): Nuclear Magnetic Resonance Imaging in Medicine. New York, Igaku-Shoin, 1981.

Wehrli FW, McFall JR, Glover GH, et al: The dependence of nuclear magnetic resonance (NMR) image contrast on intrinsic and pulse sequence timing parameters. Magnet Reson Imaging 2:3–16, 1984.

Wehrli FW, McFall JR, Newton T: Parameters determining the appearance of NMR images. In Newton T, Potts, DG (eds): Modern Neuroradiology, Vol. 2. San Francisco, Clavadel Press, 1983, pp. 81–117.

THE SKULL

Baker SR, Gaylord GM, Lantos G, Tabaddor K, Gallagher EJ: Emergency skull radiography: The effect of restrictive criteria on skull radiography and CT use. Radiology 156:409–414, 1985.

Banna M: Arachnoid cysts on computed tomography. AJR 127:979, 1976.

Bentson JR, Wilson GH, Newton TH: Cerebral venous drainage pattern of Sturge-Weber syndrome. Radiology 101:111–118, 1971.

Bradley WG, Waluch V, Yadley RA, et al: Comparison of CT and NMR in 400 cases of the brain and cervical cord. Radiology 152:695, 1984.

Bull JWD, Nixon WLB, Pratt RTC: The radiological criteria and familial occurrence of primary basilar impression. Brain 78:229, 1955.

Chamberlain WE: Basilar impression (platybasia). Yale J Biol Med 11:487, 1939.

Chirathivat S, Post MJD: CT demonstration of dural metastases in neuroblastoma. J Comput Assist Tomogr 4(3):316–319, 1980.

Dallair L, Fraser FC, Wiglesworth FW: Familial holoprosencephaly. Birth Defects 7(7):136, 1971.

Davidson HD, Abraham R, Steiner RE: Magnetic resonance imaging of agenesis of the corpus callosum. Radiology 155:371–373, 1985.

Felson B (ed): The normal skull and its variations. Sem Roentgenol 9:91, 1974.

Harwood-Nash DC, Fitz CR: Neuroradiology in Infants and Children. Vol 1. St. Louis, CV Mosby Company, 1976, pp 1–169.

Hawkes RC, Holland GN, Moore WS, Corston R, Kean DM, Worthington BS: Craniovertebral junction pathology: Assessment by NMR. AJNR 4:232–233, 1983.

Huckman MS, Russell EJ: Selecting the optimal plane for CT examination of the base of the skull, AJNR 5:333–334, 1984.

Kido DK, Gould R, Taasti F, Duncan A, Schnur J: Comparative sensitivity of CT scans, radiographs and radionuclide scans in detecting metastatic calvarial lesions. Radiology 128:371–375, 1978.

Kruff E, Jeffs R: Skull abnormalities associated with the Arnold-Chiari malformation. Acta Radiol [Diagn] (Stockh) 5:9, 1966.

Kushnet MW, Goldman RL: Lipoma of the corpus callosum associated with a frontal bone defect. AJR 131:517, 1978.

Larsen JL, Bassoe HH: Transsphenoidal meningocele with hypothalamic insufficiency. Neuroradiology 18:205, 1979.

Lee BCP, Deck MDF, Kneeland JB, Cahill PT: MR imaging of the craniocervical junction. AJNR 6:209–213, 1985.

Lee SH, Zimmerman RA, Bilaniuk LT, Woo V: Computed tomographic findings in basilar invagination. J Comput Assist Tomogr 2:255–266, 1978.

Lister J: Nasal glioma. J Laryngol Otol 77:34, 1963.

Ludwin SK, Malamud N: Pathology of congenital anomalies of the brain. In Newton TH, Potts DC (eds): Radiology of the Skull and Brain. Chapter 92. St. Louis, CV Mosby Company, 1977.

Manelfe C, Rochiccioli P: CT of septo-optic dysplasia. AJR 133:1157, 1979.

Manelfe C, Starling-Jardim D, Touibi S, et al: Case report: Transsphenoidal encephalocele associated with agenesis of corpus callosum: Value of metrizamide computed cisternography. J Comput Assist Tomogr 2:356, 1978.

McGregor M: The significance of certain measurements of the skull in the diagnosis of basilar impression. Br J Radiol 21:171, 1948.

McLaurin RL: Parietal cephaloceles. Neurology 14:764, 1964.

Mitnick JS, Pinto RS: Computed tomography in the diagnosis of eosinophilic granuloma. J Comput Assist Tomogr 4:791–793, 1980.

Naidich TP, Pudlowski RM, Naidich JB, et al: Computed tomography signs of the Chiari II malformation. I: Skull and dural partitions. Radiology 134:65, 1980.

Naidich TP, Pudlowski RM, Naidich JB: Computed tomographic signs of Chiari II malformation. II: Midbrain and cerebellum. Radiology 134:391, 1980.

Naidich TP, Pudlowski RM, Naidich JB: Computed tomographic signs of Chiari II malformation. III: Ventricles and cisterns. Radiology 134:657, 1980.

Newton TH, Potts DG: The skull. In Newton TH, Potts DG (eds): Radiology of the Skull and Brain. St. Louis, CV Mosby Company, 1971.

Nobler MP, Shapiro JH, Fine DI: The cerebral angiogram in agenesis of the corpus callosum. AJR 90(3):522, 1963.

Norman MG, Roberts M, Sirois J, et al: Lissencephaly. Can J Neurol Sci 3:39, 1976.

Tait MV, Gilday DL, Ash JM, et al: Craniosynostosis: Correlation of bone scans, radiographs, and surgical findings. Radiology 133:615, 1979.

Tjon-A-Tham RTO, Bloem JL, Falke THM, Bijroet OLM, Gohel VK, Harinck BIJ, Ziedses des Plates GB Jr: Magnetic resonance imaging in Paget disease of the skull. AJNR 6:879–882, 1985.

Warkany J: Congenital Malformations: Notes and Comments. Chicago, Year Book Medical Publishers, 1971.

Terrier F, Weber W, Ruefenacht D, Porcellini B: Pictorial essay anatomy of the ethmoid: CT, endoscopic, and macroscopic. AJNR 6:77–84, 1985.

Welch K, Naheedy MH, Abroms IF, Strand RD: Computed tomography of Sturge-Weber syndrome in infants. J Comput Assist Tomogr 4:33–36, 1980.

Wilson GH, Hanafee WN: Angiographic findings in 16 patients with juvenile nasopharyngeal angiofibroma. Radiology 92:279, 1969.

COMPUTED TOMOGRAPHY AND MAGNETIC RESONANCE

AAPM: Phantoms for Performance Evaluation and Quality Assurance of CT Scanners, Report Number 1. New York, AAPM, 1978.

Agarwal SK, Friesen EJ, Bhaduri D, Courlas G: Dose distribution from a delta 25 head scanner. Med Phys 6:302–304, 1979.

Alfidi RJ, Haaga JR, El Yousef SJ, et al: Preliminary experimental results in humans and animals with a superconducting, whole-body nuclear magnetic scanner. Radiology, 143:175–181, 1982.

Bailes DR, Young IR, Thomas DJ, et al: NMR imaging of the brain using spin-echo sequences. Clin Radiol 33:395–414, 1982.

Bottomley PA, Hardy CJ, Argersinger RE, Allen GR: A review of pathological Tissue ^{1}H NMR relaxation times from 1-100 MHz. Paper presented at the Society for Magnetic Resonance Imaging, San Diego, March 22–26, 1985.

Bottomley PA, Hart HR Jr, Edelstein WA, Schenck JF, Smith LS, Leue WM, Mueller OM, Redington RW: Anatomy and metabolism of the normal human brain studied by magnetic resonance at 1.5 Tesla. Radiology 150:441–446, 1984.

Brant-Zawadzki M, Davis PL, Crooks LE, et al: NMR demonstration of cerebral abnormalities: Comparison with CT. AJNR 4:117–124, 1983.

Brant-Zawadzki M, Norman D, Newton TH, Kelly WM, Kjos B, Mills CM, Dillon W, Sobel D, Crooks LE: Magnetic resonance of the brain: The optimal screening technique. Radiology 152:71–78, 1984.

Brooks RA, Dichiro G: Theory of image reconstruction in computed tomography. Radiology 117:561–572, 1975.

Budinger TF: Nuclear magnetic resonance (NMR) in vivo studies: Known thresholds for health effects. J Comput Assist Tomogr 5:800–811, 1981.

Bydder GM: Magnetic resonance imaging of the brain. Radiol Clin North Am 22:779–793, 1984.

Bydder GM, Steiner RE, Spencer DH, Soleimanpour C: NMR imaging of the brain: Current status and perspectives. Ann Radiol 26:39–47, 1983.

Crooks LE, Arakawa M, Hoenninger J, et al: Nuclear magnetic resonance whole-body imager operating at 3.5 K gauss. Radiology 143:169–174, 1982.

Davis PL, Crooks LE, Arakawa M, et al: Potential hazards in NMR imaging: Heating effects of changing magnetic fields and RF fields on small metallic implants. AJR 137:857, 1981.

Drayer B, Burger P, Darwin R, Riederer S, Herfkens R, Johnson GA: Magnetic resonance imaging of brain iron. AJNR 7:373, 1986.

Flannigan B, Bradley W, Mazziotta J, Rauschning W, Bentson J, Lufkin R, Hieshima G: Magnetic resonance imaging of the brainstem: Normal structure and basic functional anatomy. Radiology 154:375–383, 1985.

Gado M, Phelps M: Peripheral zone of increased density in computed tomography. Radiology 117:71–74, 1975.

Gado MH, Phelps ME, Coleman RE: Extravascular component of contrast enhancement in cranial computed tomography. Part I: Tissue-blood ratio of contrast enhancement. Radiology 117:589–594, 1975.

Gado MH, Phelps ME, Coleman RE: Extravascular component of contrast enhancement in cranial computed tomography. Part II: Contrast enhancement and the blood brain barrier. Radiology 117:595–597, 1975.

Gilderdale DJ, Young, IR, Pennock JM, et al: Color display in NMR imaging (Abstract.) In Scientific Program. Second Annual Meeting of the Society of Magnetic Resonance in Medicine. August 16–19, 1983, pp 136–137.

Glover GN, Pelc NJ: Nonlinear partial volume artefacts in x-ray computed tomography. Med Phys 7:238–248, 1980.

Gyldensted C: Gonadal thermoluminescence dosimetry in cranial computed tomography with the EMI scanner. Neuroradiology 14:111–112, 1977.

Isherwood I, Pullon BR, Ritchings RT: Radiation dose in neuroradiological procedures. Neuroradiology 16:477–481, 1978.

Joseph PM: Artefacts in computed tomography. In Radiology of the Skull and Brain: Technical Aspects of Computed Tomography. Vol 5. St. Louis, CV Mosby Company, 1981.

Joseph PM: Image noise and smoothing in computed tomography (CT) scanners. Opt Eng 17:396–399, 1978.

Joseph PM, Spital RD: A method for correcting bone induced artefacts in computed tomography scanners. J. Comput Assist Tomogr 2:100–108, 1978.

Kelly WM, Paglen PG, Pearson JA, San Diego AG, Solomon MA: Ferromagnetism of intraocular foreign body causes unilateral blindness after MR study. AJNR 7:243, 1986.

Kijewski PK, Biarngard B: Correction for beam hardening in computed tomography. Med Phys 5:209–214, 1978.

LeMay M: Radiologic changes of the aging brain and skull. AJNR 5:269–276, 1984.

Mamourian AC, Briggs RW: Appearance of Pantopaque on MR images. Radiology 158:457, 1986.

Maue-Dickson W, Trefler M, Dickson DR: Comparison of dosimetry and image quality in computed and conventional tomography: Radiology 131:509–514, 1979.

Naidich TP, Leeds NE, Kricheff II, et al: The tentorium in axial section. II. Lesion localization. Radiology 123:639, 1977.

New PFJ, Rosena BR, Brady RJ, et al: Potential hazards and artifacts of ferromagnetic and nonferromagnetic surgical and dental materials and devices in nuclear magnetic resonance imaging. Radiology 147:139–148, 1983.

Partain CL, James AE, Watson JT, Price RR, Coulam CM, Rollo FD: Nuclear magnetic resonance and computed tomography. Radiology 136:767–770, 1980.

Penn RD, Trinko B, Baldwin L: Brain maturation followed by computed tomography. J Comput Assist Tomogr 4(5):614, 1980.

Phelps ME, Gado MH, Hoffman EJ: Correlation of effective atomic number and electron density with attenuation coefficients. Radiology 117:585–588, 1975.

Quencer RM: Maturation of normal primate white matter: Computed tomographic correlation. AJNR 3:365–372, 1982.

Reed D, Robertson WD, Graeb DA, Lapointe JS, Nugent RA, Woodhurst WB: Acute subdural hematomas: Atypical CT findings. AJNR 7:417, 1986.

Shrivastava PN, Lynn SL, Ting JY: Exposures to patient and personnel in computed axial tomography. Radiology 125:411–415, 1977.

Simmonds D, Banks LM, Steiner RE, Young IR: NMR anatomy of the brain using inversion-recovery sequences. Neuroradiology 25:113–118, 1983.

Sze G, De Armond SJ, Brant-Zawadzki M, Davis RL, Norman D, Newton TH: Foci of MRI signal (pseudo lesions) anterior to the frontal horns: Histologic correlations of a normal finding. AJNR 7:381, 1986.

Thompson JR, Triolo PJ, Moore RJ, Hinshaw DB Jr, Hasso AN: CT scanning phantom for normalization of infant brain attenuation. AJNR 5:167–170, 1984.

Wall BF, Green DAC: Radiation dose to patients from EMI brain and body scanners. Br J Radiol 52:189–196, 1979.

Weisman ID, Bennett LH, Maxwell LR, et al: Recognition of cancer in vivo by NMR. Science 178:1288, 1972.

Zimmerman RD, Yurberg E, Leeds NE: The falx and interhemispheric fissure on axial computed tomography: I. Normal anatomy. AJNR 3:175–180, 1982.

Premedication and Sedation

Anderson RE, Osborn AG: Efficacy of simple sedation for pediatric computed tomography. Radiology 125:739, 1977.

Bachman DS, Hodges FJ III, Freeman JM: Computerized axial tomography in neurologic disorders of children. Pediatrics 59:352, 1977.

Boltshauser E, Hamalatha H, Grant DN, et al: Impact of computerized axial tomography on the management of posterior fossa tumors in childhood. J Neurol Neurosurg Psychiatry 40:209, 1977.

Byck R: Drugs and the treatment of psychiatric disorders. In Goodman LS, Gilman A (eds): The Pharmacological Basis of Therapeutics, 5th ed. New York, Macmillan, 1975, pp 160–161.

Byrd SE, Harwood-Nash DC, Barry JF, et al: Coronal computed tomography of the skull and brain in infants and children. I: Technique and results. Radiology 124:705, 1977.

Groover RV, Chutorian AM, Nellhaus G: Neuroradiologic procedures in children, comparison of heavy sedation and general anesthesia. Acta Radiol [Diagn] (Stockh) 5:179, 1966.

Harwood-Nash DC, Breckbill D: Computed tomography in children: A new diagnostic technique. J Pediatr 89:343, 1976.

Harwood-Nash DC, Fitz CR: Neuroradiology in Infants and Children. Vol 1. St. Louis, CV Mosby Company, 1976.

Hauser OW, Smith B, Gomez MR, Baker H Jr: Evaluation of intracranial disorders in children by computerized transaxial tomography: A preliminary report. Neurology 25:25, 1975.

Thompson JR, Schneider S, Ashwall S, et al: A choice of sedation for computed tomography in children: A prospective evaluation. Radiology 143:475, 1982.

ANGIOGRAPHIC TECHNIQUE

Andersen PE: The lenticulo-striate arteries and their diagnostic value; a preliminary report. Acta Radiol (Stockh) 50:84, 1958.

Bub B, Ferris EJ, Levy PS, et al: The cerebral venogram: A statistical analysis of the sequence of venous filling in cerebral arteriograms. Radiology 91:1112, 1968.

Chase NE, Kricheff II: The comparison of the complication rates of meglumine iothalamate and sodium diatrizoate in cerebral angiography. AJR 95:852, 1965.

Dilenge D, MeonM: The internal carotid artery. In Newton TH, Potts DG (eds): Radiology of the Skull and Brain. St. Louis, CV Mosby Company, 1974.

Earnest F IV, Forbes G, Sandok BA, et al: Complications of cerebral angiography: Prospective assessment of risk. AJNR 4:1191–1198, 1983.

Galloway JR, Greitz T: The medial and lateral choroid arteries; an anatomic and roentgenographic study. Acta Radiol (Stockh) 53:353, 1960.

Hacker H: Superficial supratentorial veins and dural sinuses: I. Normal superficial veins and dural sinuses. In Newton TH, Potts DG (eds): Radiology of the Skull and Brain. St. Louis, CV Mosby Company, 1974.

Hahreh SS: The ophthalmic artery. In Newton TH, Potts DG (eds): Radiology of the Skull and Brain. St. Louis, CV Mosby Company, 1974.

Hanafee W: Orbital venography. Radiol Clin North Am 10:63, 1972.

Hanafee W, Rosen LM, Weidner W, et al: Venography of the cavernous sinus, orbital veins and basal venous plexus. Radiology 84:751, 1965.

Mani RL, Eisenberg RL: Complications of catheter cerebral arteriography: Analysis of 5,000 procedures. III. Assessment of arteries injected, contrast medium used, duration of procedure, and age of patient. AJR 131:871, 1978.

Michotey P, Moscow N, Salamon G: Anatomy of the cortical branches of the middle cerebral artery. In Newton TH, Potts DG (eds): Radiology of the Skull and Brain. St. Louis, CV Mosby Company, 1974.

Miller JDR, Grace MG, Russel DB, et al: Complications of cerebral angiography and pneumoencephalography. Radiology 124:741, 1977.

Newton TH: The axillary artery approach to arteriography of the aorta and its branches. AJR 89:275, 1963.

Newton TH, Kramer RA: Clinical uses of selective external carotid arteriography. AJR 97:458, 1966.

Obenchain TG, Clark R, Hanafee W, et al: Complication rate of selective cerebral angiography in infants and children. Radiology 95:669, 1970.

Parkinson D: A surgical approach to the cavernous portion of the carotid artery; anatomical studies and case report. J Neurosurg 23:474, 1965.

Seldinger SI: Catheter replacement of the needle in percutaneous arteriography. A new technique. Acta Radiol (Stockh) 39:368, 1953.

Digital Subtraction Angiography

Ackerman RH: A perspective on noninvasive diagnosis of carotid disease. Neurology 29:615, 1979.

Anderson RE, Kruger RA, Sherry RG, Nelson JA, Liu P: Tomographic DSA using temporal filtration: Initial Neurovascular application. AJNR 5:277–280, 1984.

Brant-Zawadzki M, Gould R, Norman D, Newton TH, Lane B: Digital subtraction cerebral angiography in intraarterial injection: Comparison with conventional angiography. AJNR 3:593–600, 1982.

Brody WR, Enzmann DR, Deutsch L-S, et al: Intravenous carotid arteriography using line-scanned digital radiology. Radiology 139:297, 1981.

Chilcote WA, Modic MT, Pavlicek WA, et al: Digital subtraction angiography of the carotid arteries: A comparative study in 100 patients. Radiology 139:287, 1981.

Christenson PC, Ovitt TW, Fisher HD, et al: Intravenous angiography using digital video subtraction: Intravenous cervicocerebrovascular angiography. AJNR 1:379, 1980.

DeFilipp GJ, Pinto RS, Lin JP, Kricheff II: Intravenous digital subtraction angiography in the investigation of intracranial disease. Radiology 148:129–136, 1983.

Edwards JH, Kricheff II, Rilies T, et al: Angiographically detected ulceration of the carotid bifurcation as a cause of embolic stroke. Radiology 132:369, 1979.

Enzmann DR, Brody WR, Djang WT, Riederer S, Keyes G, Collins W, Pelc N: Intraarterial digital subtraction spinal angiography. AJNR 4:25–26, 1983.

Ergun DL, Mistretta CA, Kruger RA, et al: A hybrid computerized fluoroscopy technique for noninvasive cardiovascular imaging. Radiology 132:739, 1979.

Ford KK, Heinz ER, Johnson GA, et al: Low cost digital subtraction. AJNR 3:448, 1982.

Gomes AS, Hallinan JM: Intravenous digital subtraction angiography in the diagnosis of brain death. AJNR 4:21–24, 1983.

Kruger RA, Mistretta CA, Houk TL, et al: Computerized fluoroscopy in real time for noninvasive visualization of the cardiovascular system. Radiology 130:49, 1979.

MacIntyre WJ, Pavlicek W, Gallagher JH, et al: Imaging capability of an experimental digital subtraction angiography. Radiology 139:307, 1981.

McCreary JA, Schellhas KP, Brant-Zawadzki M, Norman D, Newton TH: Outpatient DSA in cerebrovascular disease using transbrachial arch injections. AJNR 6:795–801, 1985.

Meaney TF, Weinstein MA, Buonocore E, et al: Digital subtraction angiography of the human cardiovascular system. SPIE 233:272, 1980.

Meaney TF, Weinstein MA, Buonocore E, et al: Digital subtraction angiography of the human cardiovascular system. AJR 135:1153, 1980.

Mistretta CA, Crummy AB, Strother CM: Digital angiography: A perspective. Radiology 139:273, 1981.

Ovitt TW, Christenson PC, Fisher HD, et al: Intravenous angiography using digital video subtraction: X-ray imaging system. AJNR 1:387, 1980.

Pinto RS, Manuell M, Kricheff II: Complications of digital intravenous angiography: Experience in 2488 cervico-cranial examinations. AJNR 5:553–558, 1984.

Seeger JF, Carmody RF, Goldstone J: Intravenous digital subtraction angiography of the nearly occluded internal carotid artery. AJNR 5:35–40, 1984.

Sheldon JJ, Janowitz W, Leborgne JM, Sivina M, Rolo N: Intravenous DSA of extracranial carotid lesions: Comparison with other techniques and specimens. AJNR 5:547–552, 1984.

Sternglass EJ, Sashin D, Heinz ER: Electronic imaging in diagnostic radiology. In Potchen EJ (ed.): Current Concepts in Radiology. Vol 2. St. Louis, CV Mosby Company, 1975, pp 74–116.

Strother CM, Sackett JF, Crummy AB, et al: Clinical applications of computerized fluoroscopy. Radiology 136:781, 1980.

Weinstein MA, Chilcote WA, Modic MT, et al: Digital subtraction of the carotid arteries: A comparison study with conventional angiography in 100 patients. Radiology 139:287, 1981.

Wolverson MK, Heiberg E, Tantana S, Pilla TJ: Intravenous DSA and duplex sonography as screening examinations for carotid disease: Comparison in 102 vessels. AJNR 6:569–574, 1985.

Wood GW, Lukin RR, Tomsick TA, Chambers AA: Digital subtraction angiography with intravenous injection: Assessment of 1,000 carotid bifurcations. AJNR 4:125–130, 1983.

Worthington C, Peters TM, Ethier R, et al: Stereoscopic digital subtraction angiography in neuroradiologic assessment. AJNR 6:802–808, 1985.

THE ABNORMAL ANGIOGRAM

Afra D, Norman D, Levin CA: Cysts in malignant glioma identification by CT. J Neurosurg 53:821–825, 1980.

Altemus LR, Radvany J: Multifocal glioma visualized by contrast enhanced computed tomography: Report of a case with pathologic correlation. J Maine Med Assoc 68:324–327, 1977.

Amundsen P, Dugstad G, Syvertsen AH: The reliability of computer tomography for the diagnosis and differential diagnosis of meningiomas, gliomas, and brain metastasis. Acta Neurochirurgica 41:177–190, 1978.

Araki T, Inouye T, Suzuki H, Machida T, Iio M: Magnetic resonance imaging of brain tumors: Measurement of T1. Radiology 150:95–98, 1984.

Armington WG, Osborn AG, Cubberley DA, Harnsberger HR, Boyer R, Naidich TP, Sherry RG: Supratentorial ependymoma: CT appearance. Radiology 157:367–372, 1985.

Bradley WG, Waluch V, Yadley RA, Wycoff RR: Comparison of CT and MR in 400 patients with suspected disease of the brain and cervical spinal cord. Radiology 152:695–702, 1984.

Brant-Zawadzki M, Badami JP, Mills CM, Norman D, Newton TH: Primary intracranial tumor imaging: A comparison of magnetic resonance and CT. Radiology 150:435–440, 1984.

Brant-Zawadzki M, Bartowski HM, Ortendahl DA, et al: NMR in experimental cerebral edema: Value of T_1 and T_2 calculations. AJNR 5:125–129, 1983.

Butler AR, Horri SC, Kricheff II, Shannon MB, Budzilovich GN: Computed tomography in astrocytomas: A statistical analysis of the parameters of malignancy and the positive contrast-enhanced CT scan. Radiology 129:433–439, 1978.

Bydder GM, Steiner RE, Young IR, et al: Clinical NMR imaging of the brain: 140 cases. AJNR 3:459–480, 1982.

Davis DO: CT in the diagnosis of supratentorial tumor. Semin Roentgenol 12:97, 1977.

Dorsch JA, Wadsenheim A: Density of intracranial masses in computed tomography. J Belge Radiol 61:292–296, 1978.

Enzmann DR, et al: CT in primary reticulum cell sarcoma of the brain. Radiology 130:165–170, 1979.

Futrell NN, Osborne AQ, Cheson BD: Pineal region tumors: CT-pathologic spectrum. AJNR 2:415–420, 1981.

Gado MH, Phelps ME, Coleman RE: An extravascular component of contrast enhancement in cranial computed tomography. Radiology 177:589–593, 595–597, 1975.

Ganti SR, Antunes JL, Louis KM, Hilal SK: Computed tomography in the diagnosis of colloid cysts of the third ventricle. Radiology 138:385, 1981.

Gilbertson EL, Gooding CA: Roentgenographic signs of tumors of the brain. Am J Roentgenol 76:226, 1956.

Gore RM, Weinberg PE, Kim KS, Ramsey RG: Sphenoid sinus mucoceles presenting as intracranial masses on computed tomography. Surg Neurol 13:375, 1980.

Graif M, Bydder GM, Steiner RE, Niendorf P, Thomas DGT, Young IR: Contrast-enhanced MR imaging of malignant brain tumors. AJNR 6:855–862, 1985.

Guner M, Shaw M: Computed tomography in the diagnosis of colloid cyst. J Neurosurg 2:72–75, 1976.

Hanafee W, Shinnos JM: Second-order subtraction with simultaneous bilateral carotid, internal carotid injections. Radiology 86:334, 1966.

Hayman LA, Evans RA, Hinck VC: Delayed high iodine dose contrast computed tomography: Cranial neoplasms. Radiology 136:677–684, 1980.

Hayman LA, Evans RA, Hinck V: Rapid high dose cranial CT: A concise review of normal anatomy. J Comput Assist Tomogr 3:147–154, 1979.

Hilal SK, Chang CH: Sensitivity and specificity of CT in supratentorial tumors. J Comput Assist Tomogr 2:511, 1978.

Hilal SK, Chang CH: Specificity of computed tomography in the diagnosis of supratentorial neoplasms: Consideration of metastasis and meningiomas. Neuroradiology 16:537–539, 1978.

Holland BA, Kucharcyzk W, Brant-Zawadzki M, Norman D, Haas DK, Harper PS: MR imaging of calcified intracranial lesions. Radiology 157:353–356, 1985.

Huang PY, Wolf BS: Angiographic features of the pericallosal cistern. Radiology, 82:14, 1964.

Jacoby CG, Go RT, Beran RA: Cranial CT of neurofibromatosis. AJNR 1:311–315, 1980.

Kalan C, Burrows EH: Calcification in intracranial gliomata. Br J Radiol 35:589–602, 1962.

Kernohan JW, Mabon RS, Svein HJ, et al: A simplified classification of the gliomas. Proc Staff Meet Mayo Clin 24:71, 1949.

Kjos BO, Brant-Zawadzki M, Kucharczyk W, Kelly WM, Norman D, Newton TH: Cystic intracranial lesions: Magnetic resonance imaging. Radiology 155:363–369, 1985.

Kramer RA, Janetos GP, Perlstein G: An approach to contrast enhancement in computed tomography of the brain. Radiology 16:641–647, 1975.

Lee BCP, Kneeland JB, Cahill PT, Deck MDF: MR recognition of supratentorial tumors. AJNR 6:871–878, 1985.

Lee Y-Y, Castillo M, Nauert C, Moser RP: Computed tomography of gliosarcoma. AJNR 6:527–532, 1985.

Leeds NE: Image enhancement with magnification and subtraction. Radiol Clin North Am 12:241, 1974.

Leeds NE, Isard HJ, Goldberg H, et al: Serial magnification cerebral angiography. Radiology 90:1171, 1968.

Lin JP, Kricheff II: Abnormal anterior cerebral artery. In Newton TH, Potts DG (eds): Radiology of the Skull and Brain. St. Louis, CV Mosby Company, 1974.

Lin JP, Kricheff II: Effects of masses on cerebral vessels. In Newton TH, Potts DG (eds): Radiology of the Skull and Brain. St. Louis, CV Mosby Company, 1974.

Little JR, et al: Brain hemorrhage from intracranial tumor. Stroke 10:283–288, 1979.

Little JR, MacCarty CS: Colloid cysts of the third ventricle. J Neurosurg 40:230–235, 1974.

Mastri AR: Brain herniations. In Newton TH, Potts DG (eds): Radiology of the Skull and Brain. St. Louis, CV Mosby Company, 1974.

McCormack TJ, Plassche WM, Lin SR: Ruptured teratoid tumors in the pineal region. J Comput Assist Tomogr 2:499–501, 1978.

Neuwelt EA, et al: Malignant pineal region tumors. J Neurosurg 51:597–607, 1979.

Norman D, et al: Quantitative aspects of contrast enhancement in cranial computed tomography. Radiology 129:683–688, 1978.

North C, Segall HD, Stanley P, Zee C-S, Ahmadi J, McComb JG: Early CT detection of intracranial seeding from medulloblastoma. AJNR 6:11–14, 1985.

Osborn AG: Diagnosis of descending transtentorial herniation by cranial computed tomography. Radiology 123:93–96, 1977.

Osborn AG: The medical tentorium and incisura: Normal and pathological anatomy. Neuroradiology 13:109, 1977.

Osborn AG, Heaston DK, Wing SD: Diagnosis of ascending transtentorial herniation by cranial computed tomography. AJR 130:755–760, 1978.

Peterman SB, Steiner RE, Bydder GM: Magnetic resonance imaging of intracranial tumors in children and adolescents. AJNR 5:703–709, 1984.

Raimondi AJ, Guiterrez FA: Diagnosis and surgical treatment of choroid plexus papilloma. Child's Brain 1:81, 1975.

Reeves GI, Marks JE: Prognostic significance of lesion size for glioblastoma multiforme. Radiology 132:469–471, 1979.

Richards P, McKissock W: Intracranial metastases. Br Med J 1:15, 1963.

Russell DS, Rubenstein LJ: Pathology of Tumors of the Nervous System. Baltimore, Williams & Wilkins, 1977.

Smith AS, Weinstein MA, Modic MT, et al: Magnetic resonance with marked T2-weighted images: Improved demonstration of brain lesions, tumor, and edema. AJNR 6:691–698, 1985.

Steinhoff H, et al: CT in the diagnosis and differential diagnosis of glioblastomas. Neuroradiology 14:193–200, 1977.

Steinhoff H, Kazner E, Lanksch W, Grumme T, Meese W, Lange S, Aulich A, Wende S: The limitations of computerized axial tomography in the detection and differential diagnosis of intracranial tumours: A study based on 1304 neoplasms. In Bories J (ed): The Diagnostic Limitations of Computerized Axial Tompgraphy. New York, Springer-Verlag, 1978, pp 4–49.

Swartz JD, Zimmerman RA, Bilaniuk LT: Computed tomography of intracranial ependymomas. Radiology 143:97–101, 1982.

Tadmor R, Harwood-Nash DC, Savoiardo M, Scotti G,

Musgrave M, Fitz CR, Chuang S: Brain tumors in the first two years of life: CT diagnosis. AJNR 1:411–418, 1980.

Tans J, De Jongh IE: Computed tomography of supratentorial astrocytoma. Clin Neurol Neurosurg 80:156–168, 1978.

Taveras JM: The roentgen diagnosis of intracranial incisural space occupying lesions. AJR 84:52, 1960.

Thomson JLG: Computerized axial tomography and the diagnosis of glioma: A study of 100 consecutive histologically proven cases. Clin Radiol 27:431–441, 1976.

Vonosakos D, Marcu H, Hacker H: Oligodendrogliomas: CT patterns with emphasis on features indicating malignancy. J Comput Assist Tomogr 3:783, 1979.

Wende S, et al: A German multicentric study of intracranial tumors. In duBoulay GH, Moseley IF (eds): Computerized Axial Tomography in Clinical Practice. Heidelberg, Springer-Verlag, 1977.

Yang PJ, Knake JE, Gabrielsen TO, Latack JT, Gebarski SS, Mehta BA, Metes JJ: Primary and secondary histiocytic lymphoma of the brain: CT features. Radiology 154:683–686, 1985.

Ziedses des plantes BG: Application of the roentgenographic subtraction method in neuroradiology. Acta Radiol [Diagn] (Stockh) 1:961, 1963.

Zimmerman RA, et al: CT of pineal, paraspinal and histologically related tumors. Radiology 137:669–677, 1980.

Zimmerman RA, Bilaniuk LT: Computed tomography of acute intratumoral hemorrhage. Radiology 135:355–359, 1980.

Zimmerman RA, Bilaniuk LT: Computed tomography of choroid plexus lesions. CT: J Comput Tomogr 3:93–103, 1979.

ANEURYSMS AND VASCULAR MALFORMATIONS

Aalmaani WS, Richardson AE: Multiple intracranial aneurysms: Identifying the ruptured lesion. Surg Neurol 9:303–305, 1978.

Ahmadi J, Teal JS, Segall HD, Zee CS, Han JS, Becker TS: Computed tomography of carotid-cavernous fistula. AJNR 4:131–136, 1983.

Augustyn GT, Scott JA, Olson E, Gilmor RL, Edwards MK: Cerebral venous angiomas: MR imaging. Radiology 156:391–396, 1985.

Axel L: Blood flow effects in magnetic resonance imaging. AJR 143:1157–1166, 1984.

Bartlett JE, Kishore PRS: Intracranial cavernous angioma. AJR 128:653–656, 1977.

Bell BA, Kendall BE, Symon L: Angiographically occult A-V malformations of the brain. J Neurol Neurosurg Psychiatr 41:1057–1064, 1978.

Bjorkesten G, Halonen V: Incidence of intracranial vascular lesions in patients with subarachnoid hemorrhage investigated by four-vessel angiography. J Neurosurg 23:29–32, 1965.

Bradley WG Jr, Schmidt PG: Effect of methemoglobin formation on the MR appearance of subarachnoid hemorrhage. Radiology 156:99–103, 1985.

Bradley WG, Waluch V: Blood flow: Magnetic resonance imaging. Radiology 154:443–450, 1985.

Bradley WG, Waluch V, Lai K, Fernandez E, Spalter C: Magnetic resonance appearance of rapidly flowing blood. AJR 143:1167–1174, 1984.

Braun IF, Chambers E, Leeds NE, Zimmerman RD: The value of unenhanced scans in differentiating lesions producing ring enhancement. AJNR 3:643–647, 1982.

Bull JWD: Massive aneurysms at the base of the brain. Brain 92:535–570, 1969.

Byrd SE, Bentson JR, Winter J, Wilson GH, Joyce PW, O'Connor L: Giant intracranial aneurysms simulating brain neoplasms on computed tomography. J Comput Assist Tomogr 2:303–307, 1978.

Cammarata C, Han JS, Haaga JR, Alfidi RJ, Kaufman B: Cerebral venous angiomas imaged by MR. Radiology 155:639–644, 1985.

Chakeres DW, Bryan RN: Acute subarachnoid hemorrhage: In vitro comparison of magnetic resonance and computed tomography. AJNR 7:223, 1986.

Crooks L, Sheldon P, Kaufman L, Rowan W, Milter T: Quantification of obstructions in vessels by nuclear magnetic resonance. IEEE Trans Nucl Sci 29:1181, 1982.

Crooks LE, Mills CM, Davis PL, Brant-Zawadzki M, Hoenninger J, et al: Visualization of cerebral and vascular abnormalities by NMR imaging. The effects of imaging parameters on contrast. Radiology 144:843–852, 1982.

Davis JM, Davis KR, Crowell RM: Subarachnoid hemorrhage secondary to ruptured intracranial aneurysm: Prognostic significance of cranial CT. AJNR 1:17–21, 1980.

Deeb ZL, Janetta PJ, Rosenbaum AE, Kerber CW, Drayer BP: Tortuous vertebro-basilar arteries causing cranial nerve syndromes: Screening by computed tomography. J Comput Assist Tomogr 3:774–778, 1979.

Diebler C, et al: Aneurysms of the vein of Galen in infants aged 2 to 15 months. Diagnosis and natural evolution. Neuroradiology 21:185–197, 1981.

Duboulay GH: Some observations on the natural history of intracranial aneurysms. Br J Radiol 38:721–757, 1965.

Enzmann DR, Britt RH, Lyons BE, Buxton JL, Wilson DA: Natural history of experimental intracerebral hemorrhage: Sonography, computed tomography and neuropathology. AJNR 2:517–526, 1981.

Fernandez RE, Kishore PRS, Wilson M, Barker TE: Unusual manifestation of vein of Galen aneurysm. AJNR 3:440–441, 1982.

Fierstein SB, Pribram HW, Hieshima G: Angiography and computed tomography in the evaluation of cerebral venous malformations. Neuroradiology 52:246–250, 1979.

Grumme T, Lanksch W, Wende S: Diagnosis of spontaneous intracranial hemorrhage by computerized tomography. In Lanksch W, Kazner E (eds): Cranial computerized tomography. Berlin, Springer, 1976, pp 284–290.

Ishikawa M, et al: Computed tomography of cerebral cavernous hemangiomas. J Comput Assist Tomogr 4(5):587–591, 1980.

Ito J, Sato I, Tanimura K: Angiographic and computed tomography findings of a convexity cavernous hemangioma. Jpn J Clin Radiol 23:204–205, 1978.

Kase CS, Williams JP, Wyatt DA, Mohr JP: Lobar intracerebral hematomas: Clinical and CT analysis of 22 cases. Neurology 32:1146–1150, 1982.

Kendall BE, Claveria LE: The use of computed axial tomography for the diagnosis and management of intracranial angiomas. Neuroradiology 12:141–160, 1976.

Kendall BE, Lee BCP, Claveria E: Computerized tomography and angiography in subarachnoid hemorrhage. Br J Radiol 49:483–501, 1976.

Knaus WA, Wagner DP, Davis DO: CT for headache: Cost/benefit for subarachnoid hemorrhage. AJNR 1:567–572, 1980.

Kramer RA, Wing SD: Computed tomography of angiographically occult cerebral vascular malformations. Radiology 123:649–652, 1977.

Kucharczyk W, Lemme-Pleghos L, Uske A, Brant-Zawadzki M, Dooms G, Norman D: Intracranial vascular malformations: MR and CT imaging. Radiology 156:383–390, 1985.

Kumar AJ, Viñuela F, Fox AJ, Rosenbaum AE: Unruptured intracranial arteriovenous malformations do cause mass effect. AJNR 6:29–32, 1985.

Laster DW, Moody DM, Ball MR: Resolving intracerebral hematoma: Alteration of the "ring-sign" with steroids. AJR 130:935–939, 1978.

Lee BCP, Herzberg L, Zimmerman RD, Deck MDF: MR imaging of cerebral vascular malformations. AJNR 6:863–870, 1985.

Lee YY, Moser R, Bruner JM, Van Tassel P: Organized intracerebral hematoma with acute hemorrhage: CT patterns and pathologic correlations. AJNR 7:409, 1986.

Lemme-Plaghos L, Kucharczyk W, Brant-Zawadzki M, et al: MR imaging of angiographically occult vascular malformations. AJNR 7:217, 1986.

Locksley HB: Report on the cooperative study of intracranial aneurysms and subarachnoid hemorrhage. J Neurosurg 25:219–239, 1966.

Lotz PR, Quisling RG: CT of venous angiomas of the brain. AJNR 4:1124–1126, 1983.

Lukin RR, Chabers AA, McLaurin R, Tew J: Thrombosed giant middle cerebral aneurysms. Neuroradiology, 10:125–129, 1975.

McKissock W, Richardson A, Walsh L, Owe E: Multiple intracranial aneurysms. Lancet 1:623–626, 1964.

MacPherson P, Teasdale GM, Lindsay KW: Computed tomography in diagnosis and management of aneurysm of the vein of Galen. J Neurol Neurosurg Psychiatry 42:786–789, 1979.

Michels LG, Beavson JR, Winter J: Computed tomography of cerebral venous angiomas. J Comput Assist Tomogr 1:149–154, 1977.

Modesti LM, Binet EF: Value of computed tomography in the diagnosis and management of subarachnoid hemorrhage. Neurosurgery 3:151–156, 1978.

Moran PR, Moran RA, Karsaedt N: Verification and evaluation of internal flow and motion. Radiology 154:433–441, 1985.

Morley TP, Barr HWK: Giant intracranial aneurysms: Diagnosis, course and management. Clin Neurosurg 16:73–94, 1969.

Nadjmi M, Ratzka M, Wodarz M: Giant aneurysms in C.T. and angiography. Neuroradiology 16:284–286, 1978.

Osborn AG, Anderson RE, Wing SD: The false falx sign. Radiology 134:421–425, 1980.

Perret G, Nishioka H: Report on the cooperative study of intracranial aneurysms and subarachnoid hemorrhage. J Neurosurg 25:98–114, 1966.

Pinto RS, Cohen WA, Kricheff II, Redington RW, Berninger WH: Giant intracranial aneurysms: Rapid sequential computed tomography. AJNR 3:495–500, 1982.

Pressman BD, Gilbert GE, Davis DO: Computerized transverse tomography of vascular lesions of the brain: II. Aneurysms. AJR 124:215–219, 1976.

Pressman BD, Kirkwood JR, Davis DO: Computerized transverse tomography of vascular lesions of the brain: I. Arteriovenous malformations. AJR 124:208–215, 1975.

Ramina R, Ingunza W, Vonofakos D: Cystic cerebral cavernous angioma with dense calcification. J Neurosurg 52:259–262, 1980.

Rengachary SS, Szymanski DC: Subdural hematomas of arterial origin. Neurosurgery 8(2):166–172, 1981.

Richardson JC, Hyland HH: Intracranial aneurysms: Clinical and pathological study of subarachnoid and intracerebral hemorrhage caused by berry aneurysms. Medicine 20:1–83, 1941.

Richmond T, et al: Intraparenchymal blood fluid levels: New CT sign of arteriovenous malformation: Rupture. AJNR 2:577–579, 1981.

Roberson GH, Kase CS, Wolpow ER: Telangiectases and

cavernous angiomas of the brain stem: "Cryptic" vascular malformations. Neuroradiology 8:83–89, 1974.

Rothfus WE, Albright AL, Casey KF, Latchaw RE, Roppolo HMN: Cerebellar venous angioma: "Benign" entity? AJNR 5:61–66, 1984.

Russell DS, Rubinstein LJ: Pathology of Tumors of the Nervous System, 4th ed. Edinburgh, E. Arnold, 1977, pp 126–145.

Saito l, Shigenu T, Aritake K, Tanishima T, Sano K: Vasospasm assessed by angiography and computerized tomography. J Neurosurg 51:466–475, 1979.

Sartor K: Spontaneous closure of cerebral arteriovenous: Malformation demonstrated by angiography and computed tomography. Neuroradiology 15:95–98, 1978.

Savoiardo M, Strada L, Passerini A: Intracranial cavernous hemangiomas: Neuroradiologic review of 36 operated cases. AJNR 4:945–950, 1983.

Scott JA, Augustyn GT, Gilmor RL, Mealey J Jr, Olson EW: Magnetic resonance imaging of a venous angioma. AJNR 6:284–286, 1985.

Singer JR: Blood flow rates by nuclear magnetic resonance measurements. Science 130:1652–1653, 1959.

Singer JR, Crooks LE: Nuclear magnetic resonance blood flow measurements in the human brain. Science 221:654–656, 1983.

Sipponen JT, Sepponen RE, Sivula A: Nuclear magnetic resonance (NMR) imaging of intracerebral hemorrhage in the acute and resolving phases. J Comput Assist-Tomogr 7:954–959, 1983.

Solis OJ, Davis KR, Ellis GT: Dural arteriovenous malformation associated with subdural and intracerebral hematoma: A C.T. scan and angiographic correlation. Comput Tomogr 1:145–150, 1977.

Spalline A: Computed tomography in aneurysms of the vein of Galen. J Comput Assist Tomogr 3:779–782, 1979.

Takasugi S: Cause of ring enhancement in computed tomographic image of intracerebral hemorrhage—an experimental histological study. Neurol Med Chir (Tokyo) 20:689–700, 1980.

Terbrugge K, Scotti G, Ethier R, Melancon D, Tchang S, Milner C: Computed tomography in intracranial arteriovenous malformations, Radiology 122:703–705, 1977.

Waluch V, Bradley WG: NMR even echo rephasing in slow laminar flow. J Comput Assist Tomogr 8:594–598, 1984.

Weisberg LA: Peripheral rim enhancement in supratentorial intracerebral hematoma. Comput Radiol 4:145–154, 1980.

Worthington BS, Kean DM, Hawkes RC, et al: Nuclear magnetic resonance imaging in recognition of giant intracranial aneurysms. AJNR 4:835–836, 1983.

Wyburn-Mason R: The Vascular Abnormalities and Tumors of the Spinal Cord and Its Membranes. London, Kingston, 1943.

Yeakley JR, Patchall LL, Lee KF: Interpeduncular fossa sign: CT criterion of subarachnoid hemorrhage. Radiology 158:699, 1986.

Yock DH, Larson DA: Computed tomography of hemorrhage from anterior communicating artery aneurysms, with angiographic correlation. Radiology 134:399–407, 1980.

Young IR, Bydder GM, Hall AS, et al: Nuclear magnetic resonance imaging in the diagnosis and management of intracranial angiomas. AJNR 4:837–838, 1983.

Zimmerman RD, Norman EL, Naidich TP: Ring blush associated with intracranial hematoma. Radiology 122:707–711, 1977.

Zimmerman RD, Russell EJ, Yurberg E, Leeds NE: Falx and interhemispheric fissure on axial CT: II. Recognition and differentiation of interhemispheric subarachnoid and subdural hemorrhage. AJNR 3:635–642, 1982.

DEGENERATIVE, METABOLIC, AND INFLAMMATORY DISEASES

Degenerative Diseases

Aisen AM, Martel W, Gabrielsen TO, Glazer GM, Brewer G, Young AB, Hill G: Wilson disease of the brain: MR imaging. Radiology 157:137–142, 1985.

Aisen AM, Gabrielsen TO, McCune WJ: MR imaging of systemic lupus erythematosus involving the brain. AJNR 6:197–202, 1985.

Aita JF, Bennett DR, Anderson RE, et al: Cranial CT appearance of acute multiple sclerosis. Neurology (NY) 28:251–255, 1978.

Allen JH, Martin JT, McLain LW: Computed tomography in cerebellar atrophic processes. Radiology 130:379–382, 1979.

Allen JC, Thaler HT, Deck F, Rottenberg DA: Leukoencephalopathy following high dose intravenous methotrexate chemotherapy: Quantitative assessment of white matter attenuation using computed tomography. Neuroradiology 16:44–47, 1978.

Arrington JA, Murtagh FR, Martinez CR, Schnitzlein HN: CT of multiple intracranial cryptococcoma. AJNR 5:472–473, 1984.

Barnes DM, Enzmann DR: The evolution of white matter disease as seen on computed tomography. Radiology 138:379–383, 1981.

Barr AN, Heinze WJ, Dobben GD, Valvassori GE, Sugar O: Bicaudate index in computerized tomography of Huntington disease and cerebral atrophy. Neurology 28:1196–1200, 1978.

Bentson J, Reza M, Winter J, Wilson G: Steroids and apparent cerebral atrophy on computed tomography scans. J Comput Assist Tomogr 2:16–23, 1978.

Besson JAO, Corrigan FM, Foreman EI, et al: Differentiating senile dementia of Alzheimer type and multiinfarct dementia by proton NMR imaging. Lancet 2:789, 1983.

Bjorgen JE, Gold LHA: Computed tomographic appearance of methotrexate-induced necrotizing leukoencephalopathy. Radiology 122:377–378, 1977.

Bockman JM, Kingsbury DT, McKinley MP, Bendheim PE, Prusiner SB: Creutzfeldt-Jakob disease prion proteins in human brains. N Engl J Med 312:73–78, 1985.

Bosch EP, Cancilla PA, Cornell SH: Computerized tomography in progressive multifocal leukoencephalopathy. Arch Neurol 33:216, 1976.

Bosch EP, Hart MN: Late adult-onset metachromatic leukodystrophy. Arch Neurol 35:475–477, 1978.

Bradley WG, Waluch V, Brant-Zawadzki M, et al: Patchy periventricular white matter lesions in the elderly: A common observation during NMR imaging. Noninvasive Med Imaging 1:35–41, 1984.

Brant-Zawadzki M, Fein G, Van Dyke C, Kiernan R, Davenport L, de Groot J: MR imaging of the aging brain: Patchy white-matter lesions and dementia. AJNR 6:675–682, 1985.

Brant-Zawadzki M, Norman D, Newton TH, et al: Magnetic resonance of the brain: The optimal screening technique. Radiology 152:71–77, 1984.

Buonanno FS, Ball MR, Laster DW, Moody DM, McLean WT: Computed tomography in late-infantile metachromatic leukodystrophy. Ann Neurol 4:43–46, 1978.

Burszytn EM, Lee BCP, Bauman J: CT of acquired immunodeficiency syndrome. AJNR 5:711–714, 1984.

Campbell AMG, Evans M, Thomson JLG, et al: Cerebral atrophy in young cannabis smokers. Lancet 2:1219–1225, 1971.

Caplan LR, Schoene WC: Clinical features of subcortical

arteriosclerotic encephalopathy: (Binswanger disease). Neurology 28:1206–1215, 1978.

Carroll BA, Lane B, Norman D, Enzmann D: Diagnosis of progressive multifocal leukoencephalopathy by computed tomography. Radiology 122:137–141, 1977.

Co BT, Goodwin DW, Gado M, Mikhael M, Hill SY: Absence of cerebral atrophy in chronic cannabis users: Evaluation by computerized transaxial tomography. JAMA 237:1229–1230, 1977.

Courville CB, Myers RO: The process of demyelination in the central nervous system. II. Mechanism of demyelination and necrosis of the cerebral centum incident to x-radiation. J Neuropathol Exp Neurol 17:158–181, 1958.

Craelius W, Migdal MW, Luessenhop CP, Sugar A, Mihalakis I: Iron deposits surrounding multiple sclerosis plaque. Arch Pathol Lab Med 106:397–399, 1982.

Cumings JN: The copper iron content of brain and liver in the normal and hepatolenticular degeneration. Brain 71:410–415, 1948.

Cummings JL, Benson DF: Subcortical dementia: Review of an emerging concept. Arch Neurol 41:874–879, 1984.

Curnes JT, Laster DW, Ball MR, Moody DM, Witcofski RL: Magnetic resonance imaging of radiation injury to the brain. AJNR 7:389, 1986.

Di Chiro G: Differential diagnosis of hypodense white matter lesions. J Comput Assist Tomogr 3:562, 1979.

Dooms GC, Hecht S, Brant-Zawadski M, Berthiaume Y, Norman D, Newton TH: Brain radiation lesions: MR imaging. Radiology 158:149–156, 1986.

Drayer BP, Olanow W, Burger P, Johnson AG, Herfkens R, Riederer S: Parkinson plus syndrome: Diagnosis using high field MR imaging of brain iron. Radiology 159:493, 1986.

Duda EE, Huttenlocher PR: Computed tomography in adrenoleukodystrophy. Correlation of radiological and histological findings. Radiology 120:349–350, 1976.

Eiben RM, DiChiro G: Computer assisted tomography in adrenoleukodystrophy. J Comput Assist Tomogr 1:308–314, 1977.

Enzmann DR, Lane B: Cranial computed tomography findings in anorexia nervosa. J Comput Assist Tomogr 1:410–414, 1977.

Escourolle R, Poirier J: Manual of Basic Neuropathology, 2nd ed. Philadelphia, WB Saunders Company, 1978.

Fog T: The topography of plaques in multiple sclerosis. Acta Neurol Scand 41(Suppl 15):1–161, 1965.

Fox JF, Ramsey RG, Huckman MS, Proske AE: Cerebral ventricular enlargement: Chronic alcoholics examined by computed tomography. JAMA 236:365–368, 1976.

Friedland RP, Budinger TF, Brant-Zawadzki M, Jagust WJ: The diagnosis of Alzheimer-type dementia. JAMA 252:2750–2752, 1984.

Friedland RP, Budinger TF, Ganz E, et al: Regional cerebral metabolic alterations in dementia of the Alzheimer type: Positron emission tomography with [18F] fluorodeoxyglucose. J Comput Assist Tomogr 7:590–598, 1983.

Furuse M, Obayashi T, Tsuji S, Miyatake T: Adrenoleukodystrophy. Radiology 126:707–710, 1978.

Gebarski SS, Gabrielsen TO, Gilman S, et al: The initial diagnosis of multiple sclerosis: Clinical impact of magnetic resonance imaging. Ann Neurol 17:469–474, 1985.

Gebarski SS, Gabrielsen TO, Knake JE, Latack JT: Cerebral CT findings in methylmalonic and propionic acidemias. AJNR 4:955–957, 1983.

Gilroy J, Lynn GE: Computerized tomography and auditory-evoked potentials: Use in the diagnosis of olivopontocerebellar degeneration. Arch Neurol 35:143–147, 1978.

Glydensted C: Computed tomography of the cerebrum in multiple sclerosis. Neuroradiology 12:33–42, 1976.

Greenberg HS, Halverson D, Lane B: CT scanning and diagnosis of adrenoleukodystrophy. Neurology 27:884–886, 1977.

Hahn FJY, Rim K: Frontal ventricular dimensions on normal computed tomography. Am J Roentgenol 126:593, 1976.

Harik SI, Post MJD: Computed tomography in Wilson's disease. Neurology 31:107–110, 1981.

Haug G: Age and sex dependence of the size of normal ventricles on computed tomography. Neuroradiology 14:201–204, 1977.

Haughton VM, Ho KC, Williams AL, Eldevik OP: CT detection of demyelinated plaques in multiple sclerosis. AJR 132:213–215, 1979.

Hayman LA, Evans RA, Hinck VC: Delayed high iodine dose contrast computed tomography. Radiology 136:677, 1980.

Hayman LA, Evans RA, Hinck VC: Rapid high dose (RHD) contrast cranial computed tomography: A concise review of normal anatomy. J Comput Assist Tomogr 3:147, 1979.

Heinz ER, Drayer BP, Haenggeli CA, Painter HJ, Crumrine P: Computed tomography in white-matter disease. Radiology 130:371–378, 1979.

Heinz ER, Martinez J, Haenggeli A: Reversibility of cerebral atrophy in anorexia nervosa and Cushing's syndrome. J Comput Assist Tomogr 1:415–418, 1977.

Hershey LA, Gado MH, Trotter JL: Computerized tomography in the diagnostic evaluation of multiple sclerosis. Ann Neurol 5:32–39, 1979.

Holland IM, Kendall BE: Computed tomography in Alexander's disease. Neuroradiology 20:103–106, 1980.

Hopkins LN, Bakay L, Kinkel WR, Grand W: Demonstration of transventricular CSF absorption by computerized tomography. Acta Neurochir (Wien) 39:151–157, 1977.

Huckman MS, Fox JH, Ramsey RG: Computed tomography in the diagnosis of degenerative disease of the brain. Semin Roentgenol 12:63–75, 1977.

Hughes CP, Gado M: Computed tomography and aging of the brain. Radiology 139:391–396, 1981.

Inoue Y, Fukuda T, Takashima S, Ochi H, Onoyama Y, Kusuda S, Matsuoka O, Murata R: Adrenoleukodystrophy: New CT findings. AJNR 4:951–955, 1983.

Jackson JA, Leake DR, Schneiders NJ, et al: Magnetic resonance imaging in multiple sclerosis: Results in 32 cases. AJNR 6:171–176, 1985.

Jacobs L, Kinkel WR: Computerized axial transverse tomography in multiple sclerosis. Neurology (Minneap) 26:390–391, 1976.

Jacobs L, Kinkel WR, Polachini I, et al: Clinical-nuclear magnetic resonance (NMR) correlations in multiple sclerosis (MS). Neurology (Cleve) 34 (Suppl 1):141, 1984.

Jacobson PL, Farmer TW: The "hypernormal" CT scan in dementia: Bilateral isodense subdural hematoma. Neurology 29:1522–1524, 1979.

Johnson MA, Desai S, Hugh-Jones K, Starer F: Magnetic resonance imaging of the brain in Hurler syndrome. AJNR 5:816–819, 1984.

Johnson MA, Pennock JM, Bydder GM, et al: Clinical NMR imaging of the brain in children: Normal and neurologic disease. AJNR 4:1013–1026, 1983.

Kendall B: Cranial CT scans in metabolic diseases involving the CNS of children. Resident Staff Physician 28:33–42, 1982.

Kendall BE, Pollock SS, Bass NM, Valentine AR: Wilson's disease—Clinical correlation with cranial computed tomography. Neuroradiology 22:1–5, 1981.

Kim KS, Weinberg PE, Suh JH, Ho SU: Acute carbon

monoxide poisoning: Computed tomography of the brain. AJNR 1:399–402, 1980.

Kingsley DPE, Kendall BE: Cranial computed tomography in leukemia. Neuroradiology 16:543–546, 1978.

Kingsley DPE, Kendall BE: Review: CT of the adverse effects of therapeutic radiation of the central nervous system. AJNR 2:453–460, 1981.

Kinkel WR, Jacobs L, Polachini I, et al: Computerized tomography (CT) and nuclear magnetic resonance (NMR) in multiple sclerosis (MS): A comparative study. Neurology (Cleve) 34 (Suppl 1):136, 1984.

Kinkel WR, Jacobs L, Polachini I, et al: Subcortical arteriosclerotic encephalopathy (Binswanger's disease): Computerized tomographic, nuclear magnetic resonance and clinical correlations. Arch Neurol 42:951–959, 1985.

Klintworth GK: Huntington's chorea—morphologic contributions of a century. In Advances in Neurology. New York, Raven Press, 1973, pp 353–368.

Koller WC, Glatt SL, Perlik S, et al: Cerebellar atrophy demonstrated by computed tomography. Neurology 31:405, 1981.

Kuehnle J, Mendelson J, Davis K, New P: Computed tomographic examination of heavy marijuana smokers. JAMA 237:1231–1232, 1977.

Kwan E, Drace J, Enzmann D: Specific CT findings in Krabbe disease. AJNR 5:453–458, 1984.

Lagenstein I, Willig RP, Kuhne D: Cranial computed tomography (CCT) findings in children treated with ACTH and dexamethasone: First results. Neuropadiatrie 10:370, 1979.

Lane B, Carroll BA, Pedley TA: Computerized cranial tomography in cerebral diseases of white matter. Neurology 28:534–544, 1978.

Lawler GA, Pennock JM, Steiner RE, Jenkins WJ, Sherlock S, Young IR: NMR imaging in Wilson disease. J Comput Assist Tomogr 7:1–8, 1983.

Lebow S, Anderson DC, Mastri A, Larson D: Acute multiple sclerosis with contrast-enhancing plaques. Arch Neurol 35:435–439, 1978.

LeMay M, Abramowicz A: The pneumoencephalographic findings in various forms of cerebellar degeneration. Radiology 85:284, 1965.

Loizou LA, Kendall BE, Marshall J: Subcortical arteriosclerotic encephalopathy: A clinical and radiological investigation. J Neurol Neurosurg Psychiatry 44:294–304, 1981.

Lukes SA, Aminoff MJ, Mills C, et al: Nuclear magnetic resonance imaging of multiple sclerosis. J Comput Assist Tomogr 7:180, 1983.

Lynch MJC: Brain lesions in chronic alcoholism. Arch Pathol 69:342–353, 1960.

Malone MJ, Szoke MC, Looney GL: Globoid leukodystrophy: Clinical and enzymatic studies. Arch Neurol 32:606–612, 1975.

Maravilla KR, Weinreb JC, Suss R, Nunnally RL: Magnetic resonance demonstration of multiple sclerosis plaques in the cervical cord. AJNR 5:685–689, 1984.

Masucci EF, Borts FT, Smirniotopoulos JG, Kurtzke JF, Schellinger D: Thin-section CT of midbrain abnormalities in progressive supranuclear palsy. AJNR 6:767–772, 1985.

Maxwell RE, Long DM, French LA: The effects of glucosteroids on experimental cold-induced brain edema. J Neurosurg 34:477, 1971.

McCrea ES, Rao KCUG, Diaconis JN: Roentgenographic changes during long-term diphenylhydantoin therapy. South Med J 73:310–311, 1980.

McDonald WI: What is multiple sclerosis: Clinical criteria for diagnosis. In Davison AN, Humphrey JH, Liversedge LA, et al (eds): Multiple Sclerosis Research. New York, Elsevier, North Holland, 1975, p 5.

McGeachie RE, Fleming JO, Sharer LR, et al: Case report: Diagnosis of Pick's disease by computed tomography. J Comput Assist Tomogr 3:113, 1979.

McLain LW Jr, Martin JT, Allen JH: Cerebral degeneration due to chronic phenytoin therapy. Ann Neurol 7:18–23, 1980.

Mikhael MA: Radiation necrosis of the brain: Correlation between computed tomography, pathology, and dose distribution. J Comput Assist Tomogr 2:71–80, 1978.

Miura T, Mitomo M, Kawai R, Harada K: CT of the brain in acute carbon monoxide intoxication: Characteristic features and prognosis. AJNR 6:739–742, 1985.

Morariu MA, Wilkins DE, Patel S: Multiple sclerosis and serial computerized tomography, delayed contrast enhancement of acute and early lesions. Arch Neurol 37:189–190, 1980.

Nardizzi LR: Computerized tomographic correlate to carbon monoxide poisoning. Arch Neurol 36:38–39, 1979.

Novetsky GJ, Berlin L: Aqueductal stenosis: Demonstration by MR imaging. J Comput Assisted Tomogr 8:1170–1171, 1984.

Okuno T, Ito M, Yoshioka M, Nakano Y: Cerebral atrophy following ACTH therapy. J Comput Assist Tomogr 4:20–23, 1980.

Peylan-Ramu N: Abnormal CT scans of the brain in asymptomatic children with acute lymphocytic leukemia after prophylactic treatment of the central nervous system with radiation and intrathecal chemotherapy. N Engl J Med 293:815–818, 1978.

Peylan-Ramu N, Poplack DG, Blei CL, et al: Computer assisted tomography in methotrexate encephalopathy. J Comput Assist Tomogr 1:216–221, 1977.

Post MJD, Kursunoglu SJ, Hensley GT, Chan JC, Moskowitz LB, Hoffman TA: Cranial CT in acquired immunodeficiency syndrome: Spectrum of diseases and optimal contrast enhancement technique. AJNR 6:743, 1985.

Radue EW, Kendall BE: Iodide and xenon enhancement of computed tomography (CT) in multiple sclerosis (MS). Neuroradiology 15:153–158, 1978.

Rambaugh CL, et al: Cerebral CT findings in drug abuse: Clinical and experimental observations. J Comput Assist Tomogr 4:330–334, 1980.

Ramsey RG: Neuroradiology with Computed Tomography. Philadelphia, WB Saunders Company, 1981.

Ramsey RG, Huckman MS: Computed tomography of proencephaly and other cerebrospinal fluid–containing lesions. Radiology 123:73–77, 1977.

Rosenbloom S, Buchholz D, Kumar AJ, Kaplan RA, Moses H III, Rosenbaum AE: Evolution of central pontine myelinolysis on CT. AJNR 5:110–113, 1984.

Rottenberg DA, Chernik NL, Deck MDF, et al: Cerebral necrosis following radiotherapy of extracranial neoplasms. Ann Neurol 1:339–357, 1977.

Rowland LP: Merritt's Textbook of Neurology, 7th ed. Philadelphia. Lea & Febiger, 1984.

Rubinstein LJ: Pathology of white matter disease of the brain. Keynote Lecture, 16th Annual Meeting, American Society of Neuroradiology, New Orleans, LA, 1978.

Runge VM, Price AC, Kirshner HS, et al: Magnetic resonance imaging of multiple sclerosis: A study of pulse-technique efficacy. AJR 143:1015–1026, 1984; AJNR 5:691–702, 1984.

Schellinger D, Grant EG, Richardson JD: Cystic periventricular leukomalacia: Sonographic and CT findings. AJNR 5:439–446, 1984.

Sears ES, McCammon A, Bibelow R, Hayman LA: Maximizing the harvest of contrast enhancing lesions in multiple sclerosis. Neurology 32:815–820, 1982.

Sears ES, Tindall RSA, Zarnow H: Active multiple sclerosis. Enhanced computerized tomographic imaging of lesions and the effect of corticosteroids. Arch Neurol 35:426–434, 1978.

Seay AR, Bray PF, Wing SD, et al: CT scans in Menkes disease. Neurology 29:304, 1979.

Sheldon JJ, Siddharthan R, Tobias J, Sheremata WA, Soila K, Viamonte M Jr: MR imaging of multiple sclerosis: Comparison with clinical and CT examinations in 74 patients. AJNR 6:683, 1985.

Shenkin HA, Greenberg J, Bouzarth WF, Gutterman P, Morales JO: Ventricular shunting for relief of senile symptoms. JAMA 225:1486–1489, 1973.

Skomer C, Stears J, Austin J: Adult metachromatic leukodystrophy with focal lesions by computed tomography. Arch Neurol 40:354–355, 1983.

Spiegel SM, Viñuela F, Fox AJ, Pelz DM: CT of multiple sclerosis: Reassessment of delayed scanning with high doses of contrast material. AJNR 6:533–536, 1985.

Stober T, Wussow W, Schimrigk K: Bicaudate diameter—the most specific and simple CT parameter in the diagnosis of Huntington's disease. Neuroradiology 26:25–28, 1984.

Suzuki K, Suzuki Y: Globoid leukodystrophy (Krabbe disease) deficiency of galactocerebroside-beta-galactosidase. Proc Natl Acad Sci (USA) 66:302–308, 1970.

Telfer RB, Miller EM: Central pontine myelinolysis following hyponatremia, demonstrated by computerized tomography. Ann Neurol 6:455–456, 1979.

Terrence CF, Delaney JF, Alberts MC: Computed tomography for Huntington's disease. Neuroradiology 13:173–175, 1977.

Tomlinson BE: Brainstem lesions after head injury. J Clin Pathol 23(Suppl 4):154, 1970.

Valenstein E, Rosman NP, Carter AP: Schilder's disease. Positive brain scan. JAMA 217:1699–1700, 1971.

Van Dongen KJ, Braakman R: Late computed tomography in survivors of severe head injury. Neurosurgery 7:14–21, 1980.

Wagle WA, Smith TW, Weiner M: Intracerebral hemorrhage caused by cerebral amyloid angiopathy: Radiographic-pathologic correlation. AJNR 5:171–176, 1984.

Wang AM, Morris JH, Hickey WF, Hammerschlag SB, O'Reilly GV, Rumbaugh CL: Unusual CT patterns of multiple sclerosis. AJNR 4:47–50, 1983.

Weingarten KL, Zimmerman RD, Pinto RS, Whelan MA: Computed tomographic changes of hypertensive encephalopathy. AJNR 6:395–398, 1985.

Wendling LR, Bleyer WA, DiChiro G, McIlyanic SK: Transient, severe periventricular hypodensity after leukemic prophylaxis with cranial irradiation and intrathecal methotrexate. J Comput Assist Tomogr 2:502–505, 1978.

Young IR, Hall AS, Pallis CA, et al: Nuclear magnetic resonance imaging of the brain in multiple sclerosis. Lancet 2:1963–1966, 1981.

Young IR, Randell CP, Kaplan PW, et al: Nuclear magnetic imaging in white matter disease of the brain using spin-echo sequences. J Comput Assist Tomogr 7:290–294, 1983.

Zatz LM, Jernigan TL, Ahumada AJ Jr: Changes on computed cranial tomography with aging: Intracranial fluid volume. AJNR 3(1):1–12, 1982.

Zimmerman HM, Netsky MG: The pathology of multiple sclerosis. Res Publ Assoc Res Nerv Ment Dis 28:271–312, 1950.

Inflammatory Diseases

Bentson JR, Wilson GH, Helmer E, et al: Computed tomography in intracranial cysticercosis. J Comput Assist Tomogr 1:464, 1977.

Bhardari T, Sarkan N: Subdural empyema: A review of 37 cases. J Neurosurg 32:35–39, 1970.

Bilaniuk LT, Zimmerman RA, Brown L, et al: Computed tomography in meningitis. Neuroradiology 16:13, 1978.

Carbajal JR, Palacios E, Azar-Kia B, et al: Radiology of cysticercosis of the central nervous system including computed tomography. Radiology 125:127, 1977.

Danziger A, Price H, Schechter MM: An analysis of 113 intracranial infections. Neuroradiology 19:31, 1980.

Davis JM, Davis KR, Kleinman GM, et al: Computed tomography of herpes simplex encephalitis, with clinicopathological correlation. Radiology 129:409–417, 1978.

Domingue JN, Wilson CB: Pituitary abscesses: Report of seven cases and review of the literature. J Neurosurg 46:601, 1977.

Dublin AB, Merten DF: Computed tomography in the evaluation of herpes simplex encephalitis. Radiology 125:133, 1977.

Dublin AB, Phillips HE: CT of disseminated cerebral coccidioidomycosis. Radiology 135:361–368, 1980.

Enzmann DR, Brant-Zawadzki M, Britt RH: CT of central nervous system infections in immunocompromised patients. AJR 135:263, 1980.

Enzmann DR, Ranson B, Norman D, et al: Computed tomography of herpes simplex encephalitis. Radiology 129:419, 1978.

Frazee JG, Cahan LD, Winter J: Bacterial intracranial aneurysms. J. Neurosurg 53:633, 1980.

Harwood-Nash DC, et al: Massive calcification of the brain in a newborn infant. AJR 108:528–532, 1970.

Karlin CA, Robinson RG, Hinthorn DR, et al: Radionuclide imaging in herpes simplex encephalitis. Radiology 126:181, 1978.

Kaufman D, Leeds NE: Computed tomography (CT) in the diagnosis of intracranial abscesses. Neurology 27:1069, 1977.

Kerr FWL, King RB, Meagher JN: Brain abscess: A study of 47 consecutive cases. JAMA 168:868–872, 1958.

Kobrine A, Davis DO, Rizzoli HV: Multiple abscesses of the brain: Case report. J Neurosurg 54:93–97, 1981.

Labeau J, et al: Surgical treatment of brain abscess and subdural empyema. J Neurosurg 38:198, 1973.

Moskowitz MA, Rosenbaum AE, Tyler HR: Angiographically monitored resolution of cerebral mycotic aneurysms. Neurology 24:1103, 1974.

New PFJ, Davis KR, Ballantine HT Jr: Computed tomography in cerebral abscess. Radiology 121:641, 1976.

Nielsen H, Gyldenstadt C: CT in the diagnosis of cerebral abscess. Neuroradiology 12:207–217, 1977.

Ozgen T, et al: The use of CT in the diagnosis of cerebral hydatid cysts. J Neurosurg 50:339–342, 1979.

Post MJD, Hensley GT, Moskowitz LB, Fischl M: Cytomegalic inclusion virus encephalitis in patients with AIDS: CT, clinical, and pathologic correlation. AJNR 7:275, 1986.

Post MJD, Sheldon JJ, Hensley GT, Soila K, Tobias JA, Chan JC, Quencer RM, Moskowitz LB: Central nervous system disease in acquired immunodeficiency syndrome: Prospective correlation using CT, MR imaging, and pathologic studies. Radiology 158:141, 1986.

Rosenbaum ML, et al: Decreased mortality from brain abscesses since advent of CT. J Neurosurg 49:659–668, 1978.

Rosenblum ML, Hoff JT, Norman D, et al: Nonoperative treatment of brain abscesses in selected high-risk patients. J Neurosurg 52:217, 1980.

Stephanov S: Experience with multiloculated brain abscesses. J Neurosurg 49:199, 1978.

Stevens DL, Everett ED: Sequential computerized axial tomography in tuberculous meningitis. JAMA 239:642, 1978.

Stevens EA, Norman D, Kramer RA, et al: Computed

tomographic brain scanning in intraparenchymal pyogenic abscesses. AJR 130:111, 1978.

Swartz MN, Dodge PR: Bacterial meningitis—A review of selected aspects. N Engl J Med 272:725–731, 779–787, 842–848, 898–902, 954–960, 1003–1010, 1965.

Zee C-S, Segall HD, Miller C, et al: Unusual neuroradiological features of intracranial cysticeriosis. Radiology 130:397, 1980.

Zilkha A, Diaz AS: Computed tomography in the diagnosis of superior sagittal sinus thrombosis. J Comput Assist Tomogr 4(1):124, 1980.

Zimmerman RA, Patel S, Bilaniuk LT: Demonstration of purulent bacterial intracranial infections by computed tomography. AJR 127:155–165, 1976.

Infections

Benator RM, Magill HL, Gerald B, Igarashi M, Fitch SJ: Herpes simplex encephalitis: CT findings in the neonate and young infant. AJNR 6:539–544, 1985.

Brant-Zawadzki M, Enzmann DR, Placone RC Jr, et al: NMR imaging of experimental brain abscess: Comparison with CT. AJNR 4:250–253, 1983.

Britt RH, Enzmann DR: Clinical stages of human brain abscesses on serial CT scans after contrast infusion: Computerized tomography, neuropathological and clinical correlations. J Neurosurg 59:972–989, 1983.

Bursztyn, EM, Lee BCP, Bauman J: CT of acquired immunodeficiency syndrome. AJNR 5:711–714, 1984.

Byrd SE, Locke GE, Biggers S, Percy AK: The computed tomographic appearance of cerebral cysticercosis in adults and children. Radiology 144:819–823, 1982.

Davidson HD, Steiner RE: Magnetic resonance imaging of central nervous system infections. AJNR 6:499–504, 1985.

Edwards MG, Pordell GR: Ocular toxocariasis studied by CT scanning. Radiology 157:685–686, 1985.

Enzmann DR, Britt RH, Placone RC, Obana W, Lyons B, Yeager AS: The effect of short-term corticosteroids on the CT appearance of experimental brain abscess. Radiology 145:79–84, 1982.

Enzmann DR, Britt RH, Placone R: Staging of human brain abscess by computed tomography. Radiology 146:703–708, 1983.

Enzmann DR, Britt RH, Yeager AS: Experimental brain abscess evolution, computed tomographic and neuropathologic correlation. Radiology 133:113–122, 1979.

Grossman RI, Joseph PM, Wolf G, Biery D, McGrath J, Kundel HL, Fishman JE, Zimmerman RA, Goldberg HI, Bilaniuk LT: Experimental intracranial septic infarction: MR enhancement. Radiology 155:649–654, 1985.

Lukes SA, Norman D, Mills C: Acute disseminated encephalomyelitis: CT and NMR findings. J Comput Assist Tomogr 7:182, 1983.

Post MJD, Chan JC, Hensley GT, Hoffman TA, Moskowitz LB, Lippmann S: Toxoplasma encephalitis in Haitian adults with acquired immunodeficiency syndrome: A clinical-pathologic-CT correlation. AJNR 4:155–162, 1983.

Post MJD, Kursunoglu SJ, Hensley GT, Chan JC, Moskowitz LB, Hoffman TA: Cranial CT in acquired immunodeficiency syndrome: Spectrum of diseases and optimal contrast enhancement technique. AJNR 6:743–754, 1985.

Post MJD, Sheldon JJ, Hensley GT, Soila K, Tobias JA, Chan JC, Quencer RM, Moskowitz LB: Central nervous system disease in acquired immunodeficiency syndrome: Prospective correlation using CT, MR imaging, and pathologic studies. Radiology 158:141–148, 1986.

Rodriquez-Carbajal J, Salgado P, Gutierrez-Alvarado R, Escobar-Izquierdo A, Aruffo C, Palacios E: The acute encephalitic phase of neurocysticercosis: Computed tomographic manifestations. AJNR 4:51–56, 1983.

Runge VM, Clanton JA, Price AC, et al: Dyke award. Evaluation of contrast-enhanced MR imaging in a brain-abscess model. AJNR 6:139–148, 1985.

Ruskin JA, Haughton VM: CT findings in adult Reye syndrome. AJNR 6:446–447, 1985.

Sadhu VK, Handel SF, Pinto RS, Glass TF: Neuroradiologic diagnosis of subdural empyema and CT limitations. AJNR 1:39–44, 1980.

MENINGIOMAS

Cushing H, Eisenhardt L: The Meningiomas. Springfield, IL, Charles C Thomas, 1938.

Frugoni P, Nori A, Galligioni F, et al: A particular angiographic sign in meningiomas of the tentorium; the artery of Bernasconi and Cassinari. Neurochirurgia 2:142, 1960.

New PFJ, Hesselink JR, O'Carroll CP, Kleinman GM: Malignant meningiomas: CT and histologic criteria, including a new sign. AJNR 3:267–276, 1982.

Russell DS: Meningeal tumors: A review. J Clin Pathol 3:191, 1950.

Russell DS, Rubinstein LJ: Pathology of Tumors of the Nervous System. 4th ed. Baltimore, Williams & Wilkins, 1977.

Shapir J, Coblentz C, Malanson D, Ethier R, Robitaille Y: New CT finding in aggressive meningioma. AJNR 6:101–102, 1985.

Soffer D, Pittaluga S, Feiner M, Beller AJ: Intracranial meningiomas following low-dose irradiation to the head. J Neurosurg 59:1048–1053, 1983.

Wilson G, Weidner W, Hanafee W: The demonstration and diagnosis of meningiomas by selective carotid angiography. Am J Roentgenol 95:858, 1965.

Zimmerman RD, Fleming CA, Saint-Louis LA, Lee BCP, Manning JJ, Deck MDF: Magnetic resonance imaging of meningiomas. AJNR 6:149–157, 1985.

DEEP MIDLINE TUMORS

Bonneville JF, Cattin F, Moussa-Bacha K, et al: Dynamic computed tomography of the pituitary gland: The "tuft sign." Radiology 149:145–148, 1983.

Bundinger TF: Nuclear magnetic resonance (NMR) in vivo studies: Known thresholds for health effects. J Comput Assist Tomogr 5:800–811, 1981.

Burrow G, Wortzman G, Rewcastle N, et al: Microadenomas of the pituitary and abnormal sellar tomograms in an unselected autopsy series. N Engl J Med 301:156–158, 1981.

Cohen WA, Pinto RS, Kricheff II: Dynamic CT scanning for visualization of the parasellar carotid arteries. AJNR 3:185, 1982.

Drayer BD, Kattah J, Rosenbaum A, et al: Diagnostic approaches to pituitary adenoma. Neurology 29:161, 1979.

Drayer BD, Rosenbaum AE, Kennerdell JS, et al: Computed tomographic diagnosis of suprasellar masses by intrathecal enhancement. Radiology 123:339, 1977.

Earnest F IV, McCullough EC, Frank DA: Fact or artifact: An analysis of artifact in high-resolution computed tomographic scanning of the sella. Radiology 140:109, 1981.

Futrell NN, Osborn AG, Cheson BD: Pineal region tumors: Computed tomographic-pathologic spectrum, AJNR 2:415–420, 1981.

Hawkes RC, Holland GN, Moore WS, et al: The application

of NMR imaging to the evaluation of pituitary and juxtasellar tumours. AJNR 4:221–222, 1983.

Hemminshytt S, Kalkoff RK, Daniels DL, et al: Computed tomographic study of hormone-secreting microadenomas. Radiology 146:65–79, 1983.

Kaufman B: Diagnostic radiology. In Ezrin C, Horvath E, Kaufman B, et al (eds): Pituitary Diseases. Boca Raton, CRC Press, Inc, 1980, pp 129–133.

Kaufman B, Arafan BM, Brodkey JS, et al: NMR in evaluation of pituitary tumors: Radiology 149:177, 1983.

Mark L, Peck P, Daniels D, et al: The pituitary fossa: A correlative anatomic and MR study. Radiology 153:453–457, 1984.

Martins AN, Hayes GJ, Kempe LG: Invasive pituitary adenomas. J Neurosurg 22:268, 1971.

Miller JH, Pena AM, Segall HD: Radiological investigation of sellar region masses in children. Radiology 134:81, 1980.

Naidich TP, Pinto RS, Kushner MJ, Lin JP, Kricheff II, Leeds NE, Chase NE: Evaluation of sellar and parasellar masses by computed tomography. Radiology 120:91, 1976.

Rao KCVG, Harwood-Nash DC, Fitz CR: Neurodiagnostic studies in craniopharyngiomas in children. Rev Interam Radiol 2:149–159, 1977.

Reich NE, Zelch JV, Alfidi RJ: Computed tomography in the detection of juxtasellar lesions. Radiology 118:333–335, 1976.

Rovit RI, Fein JM: Pituitary apoplexy: A review and reappraisal. J Neurosurg 37:280, 1972.

Pituitary Lesions

Ahmadi J, North CM, Segall HD, Zee C-S, Weiss MH: Cavernous sinus invasion by pituitary adenomas. AJNR 6:893–898, 1985.

Armstrong EA, Harwood-Nash DCF, Hoffman H, Fitz CR, Chuang S, Pettersson H: Benign suprasellar cysts: The CT approach. AJNR 4:163–166, 1983.

Banna M, Schatz SW: Intraoperative delineation of lesions in the sellar region with metrizamide. AJNR 2:461–464, 1981.

Bonneville J-F, Cattin F, Portha C, Cuenin E, Clere P, Bartholomot B: Computed tomographic demonstration of the posterior pituitary. AJNR 6:889–892, 1985.

Bursztyn EM, Lavyne MH, Aisen M: Empty sella syndrome with intrasellar herniation of the optic chiasm. AJNR 4:167–168, 1983.

Chernow B, Buck DR, Early CB, Ray J, O'Brian JT: Rapid shrinkage of a prolactin-secreting pituitary tumor with bromocriptine: CT documentation. AJNR 3:442–443, 1982.

Davis PC, Hoffman JC Jr, Tindall GT, Braun IF: CT-surgical correlation in pituitary adenomas: Evaluation of 113 patients. AJNR 6:711–716, 1985.

Davis PC, Hoffman JC Jr, Tindall GT, Braun IF: Prolactin-secreting pituitary microadenomas: Inaccuracy of high-resolution CT imaging. AJNR 5:721–726, 1984.

Drayer BP, Rosenbaum AE, Kennerdell JS, et al: Computed tomographic diagnosis of suprasellar masses by intrathecal enhancement. Radiology 123:339, 1976.

Eisenberg HM, Sarwar M, Schochet S: Symptomatic Rathke's cleft cysts. J Neurosurg 45:585–588, 1976.

Enzmann DR, Sieling RJ: CT of pituitary abscess. AJNR 4:79–80, 1983.

Fitz CR, Wortzman G, Hardwood-Nash DC, Holgate RC, Barry JF, Boldt DW: Computed tomography in craniopharyngioma. Radiology 127:687–691, 1978.

Futrell NN, Osborne AG, Cheson BD: Pineal region of tumors: CT—pathological spectrum. AJNR 2:415–420, 1981.

Haughton VM, Prost R: Pituitary fossa: Chemical shift effect in MR imaging. Radiology 158:461, 1986.

Haughton VM, Rosenbaum AE, Williams AL, et al: Recognizing the empty sella by CT: The infundibulum sign. AJNR 1:527, 1980.

Hawkes RC, Holland GN, Moore WS, Corston R, Kean DM, Worthington BS: The application of NMR imaging to the evaluation of pituitary and juxtasellar tumors. AJNR 4:221–222, 1983.

Kaplan HC, Baker HL Jr, Houser OW, Laws ER Jr, Abboud CF, Scheithauer BW: CT of the sella turcica after transsphenoidal resection of pituitary adenomas. AJNR 6:723–732, 1985.

Kilgore DP, Strother CM, Starshak RJ, Haughton VM: Pineal germinoma: MR imaging. Radiology 158:435, 1986.

Kokoris N, Rothman LM, Wolintz AH: CT and angiography in the diagnosis of suprasellar mass lesions. Am J Ophthalmol 89:278–283, 1980.

Lee BCP, Deck MDF: Sellar and juxtasellar lesion detection with MR. Radiology 157:143–148, 1985.

Lipper MH, Rad FF, Kishore PRS, Ward JD: Craniopharyngioma: Unusual computed tomographic presentation. Neurosurgery 9:76–78, 1981.

Messina AV, Potts DG, Sigel RM: Computed tomography evaluation of the posterior third ventricle. Radiology 119:581–592, 1978.

Miller JH, Pena AM, Segall HD: Radiological investigation of sellar region masses in children. Radiology 134:81, 1980.

Naidich TP, Pinto RS, Kushner MJ, et al: Evaluation of sellar and parasellar masses by computed tomography. Radiology 120:91, 1976.

Neuwelt EA, Glasberg M, Frenkel E, et al: Malignant pineal region tumors. J Neurosurg 51:597, 1979.

Newton DR, Witz S, Norman D, Newton TH: Economic impact of CT scanning on the evaluation of pituitary adenomas. AJNR 4:57–60, 1983.

Numaguchi Y, Kishikawa T, Ikeda J, et al: Neuroradiological manifestations of suprasellar pituitary adenomas, meningiomas, and craniopharyngiomas. Neuroradiology 21:67, 1981.

Peyster RG, Hoover ED: CT of the abnormal pituitary stalk. AJNR 5:49–52, 1984.

Peyster RG, Hoover ED, Adler LP: CT of the normal pituitary stalk. AJNR 5:45–48, 1984.

Pojunas KW, Daniels DL, Williams AL, Haughton VM: MR imaging of protacin-secreting microadenomas. AJNR 7:2093, 1986.

Post MJD, David NJ, Glazer JS, Safran A: Pituitary apoplexy: Diagnosis by computed tomography. Radiology 134:665–670, 1980.

Richmond IL, Newton TH, Wilson CB: Prolactin secreting pituitary adenomas: Correlation of radiographic and surgical findings. AJNR 1:13, 1980.

Robertson WB, Newton TH: Radiologic assessment of pituitary microadenomas. AJR 131:489–492, 1978.

Roppolo HMN, Latchaw RE, Meyer JD, Curtin HD: Normal pituitary gland: 1. Macroscopic anatomy-CT correlation. AJNR 4:927–936, 1983.

Roppolo HMN, Latchaw RE: Normal pituitary gland: 2. Microscopic anatomy-CT correlation. AJNR 4:937–944, 1983.

Rozario R, et al: Diagnosis of empty sella with CT scan. Neuroradiology 13:85–88, 1977.

Seidel FG, Towbin R, Kaufman RA: Normal pituitary stalk size in children: CT study. AJNR 6:733–738, 1985.

Sondheimer FK: Basal foramina and canals. In Newton TH, Potts DG (eds): Radiology of the Skull and Brain. Vol 2. St. Louis, CV Mosby Company, 1971, pp 333–341.

Syvertsen A, Haughton VM, Williams AL, Cusick JF: The computed tomographic appearance of the normal pituitary gland and pituitary microadenomas. Radiology 133:385–391, 1979.

Wiener SN, Rzeszotarski MS, Droege RT, Pearlstein AE, Shafron M: Measurement of pituitary gland height with MR imaging. AJNR 6:717–722, 1985.

Wolpert SM, et al: The value of computed tomography in evaluating patients with prolactinomas. Radiology 131:117–119, 1979.

Wolpert SM, Molitch ME, Goldman JA, Wood JB: Size, shape, and appearance of the normal female pituitary gland. AJNR 5:263–268, 1984.

Wortzman G, Rewcastle NB: Tomographic abnormalities simulating pituitary microadenomas. AJNR 3:505–512, 1982.

Zimmerman RA, Bilaniuk LT, Wood JH, et al: Computed tomography of pineal, papapineal, and histologically related tumors. Radiology 137:669, 1980.

HYDROCEPHALUS, PORENCEPHALY, AND METASTASES

Hydrocephalus

Adams RD, Fisher CM, Hakim S, et al: Symptomatic occult hydrocephalus with "normal" cerebrospinal fluid pressure. N Engl J Med 273:117, 1965.

Adams RD, Greenburg JO: The mega cisterna magna. J Neurosurg 48:190–192, 1978.

Adapon BD, Braunstein P, Lin JP, et al: Radiologic investigations of normal pressure hydrocephalus. Radiol Clin North Am 12:353, 1974.

Altman NR, Altman DH, Sheldon JJ, Leborgne J: Holoprosencephaly classified by computed tomography. AJNR 5:433–438, 1984.

Archer C, Darwish H, Smith K Jr: Enlarged cisternae magnae and posterior cysts simulating Dandy-Walker syndrome on computed tomography. Radiology 127:681–686, 1978.

Belloni G, DiRocco C, Focacci C, et al: Surgical indications in normotensive hydrocephalus. A retrospective analysis of the relations of some diagnostic findings to the results of surgical treatment. Acta Neurochir (Wein) 33:1, 1976.

Benson DF, LeMay M, Patten DH, et al: Diagnosis of normal pressure hydrocephalus. N Engl J Med 283:609, 1970.

Black PM: Idiopathic normal-pressure hydrocephalus. J Neurosurg 52:371, 1977.

Bradley WG Jr, Kortman KE, Burgoyne B: Flowing cerebrospinal fluid in normal and hydrocephalic states: Appearance on MR images. Radiology 159:611, 1986.

Bush JA, Bajanda FJ: Septo-optic dysplasia (deMorsier's). Am J Ophthalmol 86:202–205, 1978.

Byrd SE, Harwood-Nash DC, Fitz CR: Absence of corpus callosum: Computed tomographic evaluation in infants and children. J Can Assoc Radiol 20:108–112, 1978.

Byrd SE, Harwood-Nash DC, Fitz CR, Rogovitz DM: Computed tomography in the evaluation of encephaloceles in infants and children. J Comput Assist Tomogr 2:81–87, 1978.

Byrd SE, Harwood-Nash DC, Fitz CR, Rogovitz DM: Computed tomography evaluation of holoprosencephaly in infants and children. J Comput Assist Tomogr 1:456–463, 1977.

Dandy WE: Congenital cerebral cysts of the cavum septi pellucidi (fifth ventricle) and the cavum vergae (sixth ventricle). Arch Neurol Psychiatry 25:44–66, 1931.

Di Rocco C, Caldarelli M, Di Trapani G: Infratentorial arachnoid cysts in children. Child's Brain 8:119–133, 1981.

Drayer BP, Rosenbaum AE, Higman HB: Cerebrospinal fluid imaging using serial metrizamide CT cisternography. Neuroradiology 13:7, 1977.

Drayer BP, Rosebaum AE, Maroon JC, Bank WO, Woodford JE: Posterior fossa extra-axial cyst: Diagnosis by metrizamide CT cisternography. AJR 128:431–436, 1977.

Dublin AB, French BN: Diagnostic image evaluation of hydranencephaly and pictorially similar entities with emphasis on computed tomography. Radiology 137:81, 1980.

Enzmann DR, Norman D, Price DC, et al: Metrizamide and radionuclide cisternography in communicating hydrocephalus. Radiology 130:681, 1979.

Fishman RA: Occult hydrocephalus. N Engl J Med 274:466, 1966.

Flodmark O, et al: Correlation between computed tomography and autopsy in premature and full-term neonates that have suffered perinatal asphyxia. Radiology 137:93–103, 1980.

Hahn FJY, Rim K: Frontal ventricular dimensions on normal computed tomography. Am J Roentgenol 126:593, 1976.

Hahn FJY, Schapiro RL: The excessively small ventricle on computed axial tomography of thhe brain. Neuroradiology 12:137, 1976.

Hakim S, Adams RD: The special clinical problem of symptomatic hydrocephalus with normal cerebrospinal fluid pressure. J Neurol Sci 2:307, 1965.

Hakim S, Venegas JG, Burton JD: The physics of the cranial cavity, hydrocephalus and normal pressure hydrocephalus: Mechanical interpretation and mathematical model. Surg Neurol 5:187, 1976.

Halsey JA, Allen N, Chamberlin HR: The morphogenesis of hydraencephaly. J Neurol Sci 12:187–217, 1971.

Hart MN, Malamud N, Ellis WG: The Dandy-Walker syndrome: A clinicopathological study based on 28 cases. Neurology 22:771–780, 1972.

Hartmann A, Alberti E: Differentiation of communicating hydrocephalus and presenile dementia by continuous recording of cerebrospinal fluid pressure. J Neurol Neurosurg Psychiatry 40:630, 1977.

Harwood-Nash DC: Congenital cranio-cerebral abnormalities and computed tomography. Semin Roentgenol 12:39–51, 1977.

Harwood-Nash DC, Fitz CR: Neuroradiology in Infants and Children. St. Louis, CV Mosby Company, 1976.

Haug G: Age and sex dependence of the size of normal ventricles on computed tomography. Neuroradiology 14:201, 1977.

Hayashi T, Yoshida M, Kuramoto S, Takya S, Hashimoto T: Radiological features of holoprosencephaly. Surg Neurol 12:261–265, 1979.

Heinz ER, Davis DO: Clinical, radiological, isotopic and pathologic correlation in normotensive hydrocephalus. In Harbert JC, McCullough DC, Luessenhop AJ, et al (eds): Cisternography and Hydrocephalus: A Symposium. Springfield, IL, Charles C Thomas, 1972, p. 217.

Heinz ER, Davis DO, Karp HR: Abnormal isotope cisternography in symptomatic occult hydrocephalus. Radiology 95:109, 1970.

Heinz ER, Ward A, Drayer BP, Dubois PJ: Distinction between obstructive and atrophic dilatation of ventricles in children. J Comput Assist Tomog 4:320–325, 1980.

Hindmarsh T, Greitz T: Hydrocephalus, atrophy and their differential diagnosis—CSF dynamics investigated by computer cisternography. In DuBoulay GH, Moseley IF (eds): Computerized Axial Tomography in Clinical Practice. Berlin, Springer, 1977, pp 205–217.

Hiratsuka H, et al: Modification of periventricular hypodensity in hydrocephalus with ventricular reflux in metrizamide CT cisternography. J Comput Assist Tomog 2:204–208, 1979.

Huckman MS: Normal pressure hydrocephalus: Evaluation of diagnostic and prognostic tests. AJNR 2:385, 1981.

Huckman MS, Fox JS, Ramsey RG, et al: Computed tomography in the diagnosis of pseudotumor cerebri. Radiology 119:593, 1976.

Hughes CP, Siegel BA, Coxe WS, et al: Adult idiopathic communicating hydrocephalus with and without shunting. J Neurol Neurosurg Psychiatry 41:961, 1978.

Hungerford GH, Ross P, Robertson HJK: CT in lead encephalopathy. Radiology 123:91, 1977.

Jacobs L, Conti D. Kinkel WR, et al: "Normal-pressure" hydrocephalus. Relationship of clinical and radiographic findings to improvement following shunt surgery. JAMA 235:510, 1976.

Jacobs L, Kinkel W: Computerized axial transverse tomography in normal pressure hydrocephalus. Neurology 26:501, 1976.

Lightfoote WE, Pressman BD: Increased intracranial pressure: Evaluation by CT. Am J Roentgenol 124:195, 1975.

Lipton HL, Preziosi TJ, Moses H: Adult onset of the Dandy-Walker syndrome. Arch Neurol 35:672–674, 1978.

Lynn RB, Buchanan DC, Fenichel GM, Freemon FR: Agenesis of the corpus callosum. Arch Neurol 37:478, 1980.

Messert B, Wannamaker BB: Reappraisal of the adult occult hydrocephalus syndrome. Neurology 24:224, 1974.

Mori K, Handa H, Itoh M, Okuno T: Benign subdural effusions in infants. J Comput Assist Tomgr 4:466–471, 1980.

Naidich TP, Pudlowski MR, Naidich JB, Gornish M, Rodriguez FJ: Computed tomographic signs of the Chiari II malformation: I. Skull and dural portions. Radiology 134:65–71, 1980.

Naidich TP, Pudlowski RM, Naidich JB: Computed tomography signs of Chiari II malformation: II. Midbrain and cerebellum. Radiology 134:391–398, 1980.

Naidich TP, Pudlowski RM, Naidich JB: Computed tomography signs of Chiari II malformation: III. Ventricles and cisterns. Radiology 134:657–663, 1980.

Naidich TP, Leeds NE, Krichett II, Pudlowski RM, Naidich JB, Zimmerman RD: The tentorium in axial section: I. Normal CT appearance and non-neoplastic pathology. Radiology 123:631–638, 1977.

New PFJ, Scott WR, Schnur JA: Computerized axial tomography with EMI scanner. Radiology 110:109, 1974.

Ojemann RG, Fisher CM, Adams RD, et al: Further experience with the syndrome of "normal" pressure hydrocephalus. J Neurosurg 31:279, 1969.

Pretorius DH, Davis K, Manco-Johnson ML, Manchester D, Meier PR, Clewell WH: Clinical course of fetal hydrocephalus: 40 cases. AJNR 6:23–28, 1985.

Ramsey RG, Huckman MS: Computed tomography of porencephaly and other cerebrospinal fluid-containing lesions. Radiology 123:73–77, 1977.

Shenkin HA, Greenberg J, Bouzarth WF, et al: Ventricular shunting for relief of senile symptoms. JAMA 225:1486, 1973.

Strother CM, Harwood-Nash DC: Congenital malformations in radiology of the skull and brain. In Newton TH, Potts DG (eds): Radiology of the Skull and Brain: Ventricles and cisterns. Vol 4. St. Louis, CV Mosby Company, 1978, pp 3712–3748.

Taggart JK, Walker AE: Congenital atresia of the foramens of Luschka and Magendie. Arch Neurol Psychiatr 48:583–594, 1942.

Tans JTJ: Differentiation of normal pressure hydrocephalus and cerebral atrophy by computed tomography and spinal infusion test. J Neurol 222:109, 1979.

Udvarhelyi GB, Wood JH, James AE, et al: Results and complications in 55 shunted patients with normal pressure hydrocephalus. Surg Neurol 3:271, 1975.

Weisberg L, Nice CN: Computed tomographic evaluation of increased intracranial pressure without localizing signs. Radiology 122:133, 1977.

Weisberg LA, Pierce JF, Jabbari B: Intracranial hypertension resulting from a cerebrovascular malformation. South Med J 70:624, 1977.

Wing SD, Osborn AG: Normal and pathological anatomy of the corpus callosum by computed tomography. Comput Tomogr 1:183–192, 1977.

Yamada F, Fukuda S, Samejima H, et al: Significance of pathognomonic features of normal pressure hydrocephalus on computerized tomography. Neuroradiology 16:212, 1978.

Zettner A, Netsky MG: Lipoma of the corpus callosum. J Neuropathol Exp Neurol 19:305–319, 1960.

Zimmerman RD, et al: Cranial CT findings in patients with meningomyelocele. AJR 132:623–629, 1979.

Metastases

Aronson SM, Garcia JH, Aaronson BE: Metastatic neoplasms of the brain: Their frequency in relation to age. Cancer 17:558–563, 1964.

Baker HI, Houser OW, Campbell JK: National Cancer Institute study: Evaluation of computed tomography in diagnosis of intracranial neoplasms. Radiology 136:91–96, 1980.

Becker H, Norman D, Boyd DP, Hattner RS, Newton TH: Computed tomography in detecting calvarial metatases: A comparison with skull radiography and radionuclide scanning. Neuroradiology 16:504–505, 1978.

Bradfield PA, Passalaque AM, Braunstein P, Raghauendra BN, Leeds NE, Kricheff II: A comparison of radionuclide scanning and computed tomography in metastatic lesions of the brain. J Comput Asst Tomogr 1:315–318, 1977.

Butler AR, Kricheff II: Noncontrast CT scanning: Limited value in suspected brain tumors. Radiology 126:689–693, 1978.

Butler AR, Leo JS, Lin JP, Boyd AD, Kricheff II: The value of routine cranial computed tomography in neurologically intact patients with primary carcinoma of the lung. Radiology 131:399–401, 1979.

Claussen C, Laniado M, Schorner W, et al: Gadolinium-DTPA in MR imaging of glioblastomas and intracranial metastases. AJNR 6:669–674, 1985.

Crocker EF, Zimmerman RA, Phelps ME, Kuhl DE: The effect of steroids on the extra-vascular distribution of radiographic contrast material and technetium pertechnetate in brain tumors as determined by computed tomography. Radiology 119:471–476, 1976.

Deck MDF: Computed tomography of metastatic disease of the brain. In Weiss L, Gilbert H, Posner J (eds): Workshop on Brain Metastasis. Memorial Sloan-Kettering Cancer Center, 1978. Boston, GK Hall, 1980.

Deck MDF, Messina AV, Sackett JF: Computed tomography in metastatic disease of the brain. Radiology 119:115–120, 1976.

Dubois PJ, Martine AJ, Myerowitz RL, Rosenbaum AE: Subependymal and leptomeningeal spread of systemic malignant lymphoma demonstrated by cranial computed tomography. J Comput Assist Tomogr 2:218–221, 1978.

Enzmann DR, Kramer R, Norman D, Pollock J: Malignant melanoma metastatic to the central nervous system. Radiology 127:177–180, 1978.

Enzmann DR, Kricorian J, Yorke C, Haywood R: Computed tomography in leptomeningeal spread of tumor. J Comput Assist Tomogr 2:448–455, 1978.

Gildersleeve N, Koo AH, McDonald CJ: Metastatic tumor presenting as intracerebral hemorrhage. Radiology 124:109, 1977.

Ginaldi S, Wallace S, Shalen P, Luna M, Handel S: Cranial computed tomography of malignant melanoma. AJNR 1:531–536, 1980.

Healy JF, Rosenkontz H: Intraventricular metastases demonstrated by cranial computed tomography. Radiology 136:124, 1980.

Kazner E, Wilske J, Steinoff H, Stockdorph O: Computer assisted tomography in primary malignant lymphoma of the brain. J Comput Assist Tomgr 2:125–134, 1978.

Lee Y-Y, Glass JP, Geoffray A, Wallace S: Cranial computed tomographic abnormalities in leptomeningeal metastasis. AJNR 5:559–564, 1984.

Mandybur TI: Intracranial hemorrhage caused by metastatic tumors. Neurology 27:650–655, 1977.

Naheedy MH, Kido DK, O'Reilly GV: Computed tomography evaluation of subdural and epidural metastases. J Comput Assist Tomgr 4:311–315, 1980.

Olderberg E: The hemorrhage into glioma: A review of eight hundred and thirty-two consecutive verified cases of glioma. Arch Neurol Psychiatry 30:1061–1073, 1933.

Pagani JJ, Hayman LA, Bigelow RH, Libshitz HI, Lepke RA, Wallace S: Diazepam prophylaxis of contrast media–induced seizures during computed tomography of patients with brain metastases. AJNR 4:67–72, 1983.

Posner JB: Brain metastases: A clinician's view. In Weiss L, Gilbert H, Posner JB (eds): Brain metastases. Boston, GK Hall, 1980.

Ranshoff J: Surgical management of metastatic tumors. Semin Oncol 2:21–27, 1975.

Rao KCVG, Levine H, Sajore E, Itani A, Walker R: CT in multicentric glioma: Radiological-pathological correlation. CT: J Comput Tomogr 4:187–192, 1980.

Russcalleda J: Clinical symptomatology and computerized tomography in brain metastases. Comput Tomogr 2:69–77, 1978.

Sears ES, Tindall RSA, Zarnow H: Active multiple sclerosis: Enhanced computerized tomographic imaging of lesions and effects of corticosteroids. Arch Neurol 35:426–436, 1978.

Simionescue MD: Metastatic tumors of the brain: A follow-up study of 195 patients with neurosurgical considerations. J Neurosurg 17:361–373, 1960.

Solis OJ, Davis KR, Adair LB, Robertson AR, Kleinman G: Intracerebral metastatic melanoma—CT evaluation. Comput Tomogr 1:135–143, 1977.

Steinhoff H, Kazner E, Lauksch W, Grumme T, Meese W, Lange S, Aulich A, Wende S: The limitation of computerized axial tomography in the detection and differential diagnosis of intracranial tumors: A study based on 1304 neoplasms. In Bories J (ed): Diagnostic Limitations of Computerized Axial Tomography. New York, Springer-Verlag, 1978.

Vaneck JHM, Go KG, Ebels EJ: Metastatic tumors of the brain. Neurol Neurochir 68:443–462, 1965.

Vannucci RC, Baten M: Cerebral metastatic disease in childhood. Neurology 24:981–985, 1974.

Vieth RG, Odom GL: Intracranial metastases and their neurosurgical treatment. J Neurosurg 23:375–383, 1965.

Weisberg LA, Nice CN: Intercranial tumors simulating the presentation of cerebrovascular syndromes. JAMA 63:517, 1977.

Zimmerman RA, Bilaniuk LT: Computed tomography of acute intratumoral hemorrhage. Radiology 135:355–359, 1980.

TRAUMA

Ahmadi J, Weiss MH, Segall HD, Schultz DH, Zee C, Giannotta SL: Evaluation of cerebrospinal fluid rhinorrhea by metrizamide computed tomographic cisternography. Neurosurgery 16:54–60, 1985.

Amendola MA, Ostrum BJ: Diagnosis of isodense subdural hematomas by computed tomography. AJR 129:693–697, 1977.

Auer L, et al: Relevance of CAT-scan for the level of ICP in patients with severe head injury. In Shulman K, et al (eds): Intracranial Pressure IV. Berlin, Springer-Verlag, 1980, pp 45–47.

Auh YH, Lee SH, Toglia JU: The excessively small ventricle on cranial computed tomography: Clinical correlation in 75 patients. J Comput Assist Tomogr 4:325–329, 1980.

Bakay L. Glasauer FE: Head Injury. Boston, Little, Brown and Company, 1980.

Baratham G, Dennyson WG: Delayed traumatic intracerebral hemorrhage. J Neurol Neurosurg Psychiatry 35:698–706, 1972.

Bergstrom M, et al: Computed tomography of cranial subdural and epidural hematomas: Variation of attenuation related to time and clinical events such as rebleeding. J Comput Assist Tomogr 1:449–455, 1977.

Bhimani S, Virapongse C, Sabshin JK, Sarwar·M, Paterson RH: Intracerebral pneumatocele: CT findings. Radiology 154:111–114, 1985.

Brown FD, Mullan S, Duda EE: Delayed traumatic intracerebral hematomas: Report of 3 cases. J Neurosurg 48:1019–1022, 1978.

Bruce DS, Alavi A, Bilaniuk LT, et al: Diffuse cerebral swelling following head injuries in children: The syndrome of "malignant brain edema." J Neurosurg 54:170, 1981.

Buonanno FS, Moody DM, Ball MR, Laster DW: Computed cranial tomographic findings in cerebral sinovenous occlusion. J Comput Assist Tomogr 2:281–290, 1978.

Caffey J: The whiplash-shaken-infant syndrome: Manual shaking by the extremities with whiplash-induced intracranial and intraocular bleeding, linked with residual permanent brain damage and mental retardation. Pediatrics 54:396, 1974.

Clifton GL, Grossman RG, Makela ME, Miner ME, Handel S, Sadhu V: Neurological course and correlated computerized tomography findings after severe closed head injury. J Neurosurg 52:611–624, 1980.

Cohen RA, Kaufman RA, Myers PA, Towbin RB: Cranial computed tomography in the abused child with head injury. AJNR 6:883–888, 1985.

Cooper PR, Maravilla K, Kirkpatrick J, Moody SF, Sklar FH, Diehl J, Clark WK: Traumatically induced brainstem hemorrhage and the computerized tomographic scan: Clinical pathological and experimental observations. Neurosurgery 4:115–124, 1979.

Cooper PR, Maravilla K, Moody S, Clark WK: Serial computerized tomographic scanning and the prognosis of severe head injury. Neurosurgery 5:566–569, 1979.

Cordobés F, Lobato RD, Rivas JJ, et al: Observations on 82 patients with extradural hematoma. J Neurosurg 54:179, 1981.

Cowan RJ, Maynard CD: Trauma to brain and extracranial structures. Semin Nucl Med 4:319, 1974.

Cromwell LD, Mack LA, Loop JW: CT scout view for skull fracture: Substitute for skull films? AJNR 3:421–425, 1982.

Cummins RO: Clinicians' reasons for overuse of skull radiographs. Am J Neuroradiology 1:339–342, 1980.

Davis JM, Zimmerman RA: Vascular injury: Head and neck. In Rosenkrantz H, Oleaga J (eds): Angiography of Trauma. Mt. Kisco, NY, Futura, 1982.

Desmet AA, Fryback DG, Thornbury JR: A second look at the utility of radiographic skull examination for trauma. AJR 132:95–99, 1979.

Diaz FG, Yock DH Jr, Larson D, Roskwold GL: Early diagnosis of delayed posttraumatic intracerebral hematomas. J Neurosurg 50:217–223, 1979.

Dolinskas CA, Bilaniuk LT, Zimmerman RA, et al: Computed tomography of intracerebral hematomas. I. Transmission CT observations on hematoma resolution. AJR 129:681, 1977.

Dolinskas CA, Zimmerman RA, Bilaniuk LT: A sign of subarachnoid bleeding on cranial computed tomograms of pediatric head trauma patients. Radiology 126:409–411, 1978.

Drayer BP, Wilkins RH, Boehnke M, Horton JA, Rosenbaum AE: Cerebrospinal fluid rhinorrhea demonstrated by metrizamide CT cisternography. AJR 129:149–151, 1977.

Forbes GS, et al: Computed tomography in the evaluation of subdural hematomas. Radiology 126:143–148, 1978.

Fox JL, Schiebel FG: Intracranial air bubbles localizing cerebrospinal fluid fistula. J Comput Assist Tomogr 3:832–833, 1979.

French BN: Limitations and pitfalls of computed tomography in the evaluation of craniocerebral injury. Surg Neurol 10:395–401, 1978.

French BN, Dublin AB: The value of computerized tomography in the management of 1000 consecutive head injuries. Surg Neurol 7:171–183, 1977.

George AE, Russell EJ, Kricheff II: White matter buckling: CT sign of extra-axial intracranial mass. AJNR 1:425, 1980.

Ghoshohajra K: Metrizamide CT cisternography in the diagnosis and localization of cerebrospinal fluid rhinorrhea. J Comput Assist Tomogr 4:306–310, 1980.

Gudeman SK, Kishore PRS, Becker DP, Lipper MH, Girevendulis AK, Jeffries BF, Butterworth J: Computerized tomography in the evaluation of incidence and significance of post-traumatic hydrocephalus. Radiology 141:397–402, 1981.

Han JS, Kaufman B, Alfidi RJ, et al: Head trauma evaluated by magnetic resonance and computed tomography: A comparison. Radiology 150:71–77, 1984.

Harwood-Nash DC, Hendrick EB, Hudson AR: The significance of skull fractures in children; A study of 1,187 patients. Radiology 101:151, 1971.

Heinz RE, Ward A, Drayer BP, Dubois PJ: Distinction between obstructive and atrophic dilatation of ventricles in children. J Comput Assist Tomogr 4:320–325, 1980.

Horikawa Y, Naruse S, Tanaka C, et al: 1H-nuclear magnetic resonance studies on brain edema: Effects of Mn-EDTA on proton relaxation time and consideration of the location of water molecules and edematous brain. Neurotraumatology (Tokyo) 4:97–102, 1981 (in Japanese, with English abstract).

Kim KS, Hemmati M, Weinberg PE: Computed tomography in isodense subdural hematoma. Radiology 128:71, 1978.

Levander B, Stattin S, Svendsen P: Computer tomography of traumatic intra and extracerebral lesions. Acta Radiol [Suppl. 346] (Stockh) pp 107–118, 1975.

Levin HS, Meyers CA, Grossman RG, Sarwar M: Ventricular enlargement after closed head injury. Arch Neurol 38:623–629, 1981.

Lipper MH, Kishore PRS, Girevendulis AK, Miller JD, Becker DP: Delayed intracranial hematoma in patients with severe head injury. Radiology 133:645–649, 1979.

Manelfe C, Cellerier P, Sobel D, Prevost C, Bonafe A: Cerebrospinal fluid rhinorrhea: Evaluation with metrizamide cisternography. AJNR 3:25–30, 1982.

Masters SJ: Evaluation of head trauma: Efficacy of skull films. AJNR 1:329–338, 1980.

Mendelsohn DB, Hertzanu Y: Intracerebral pneumatoceles following facial trauma: CT findings. Radiology 154:115–118, 1985.

Messina AV: Computed tomography: Contrast media within subdural hematomas. A preliminary report. Radiology 119:725, 1976.

Messina AV, Chernick NL: Computed tomography: The "resolving" intracerebral hemorrhage. Radiology 118:609–613, 1975.

Moon KL Jr, Brant-Zawadzki M, Pitts LH, Mills CM: Nuclear magnetic resonance imaging of CT-isodense subdural hematomas. AJNR 5:319–322, 1984.

Naidich T, Moran CJ: Precise anatomic localization of atraumatic sphenoethmoidal cerebrospinal fluid rhinorrhea by metrizamide CT cisternography. J Neurosurg 53:222–228, 1980.

Naidich TP, Moran CJ, Pudlowski RM, et al: CT diagnosis of the isodense subdural hematoma. In Thompson RA, Green JR (eds): Advances in Neurology. Vol 22. New York, Raven Press, 1979, pp 73–105.

Osborn AG, Anderson RE, Wing SD: The false falx sign. Radiology 134:421, 1980.

Osborn AG, Daines JH, Wing SD, et al: Intracranial air on computerized tomography. J Neurosurg 48:355, 1978.

Patronas NJ, Duda EE, Mirfakhraee M, Wollman RL: Superior sagittal sinus thrombosis diagnosed by computed tomography. Surg Neurol 15:11–14, 1981.

Sipponen JT, Sepponnen RE, Suvula A: Chronic subdural hematoma demonstration by magnetic resonance. Radiology 150:79–85, 1984.

Smith WP Jr, Bainitzky S, Rengachary SS: Acute isodense subdural hematomas: A problem in anemic patients. AJNR 2:37–40, 1981.

Strich SJ: Shearing of nerve fibers as a cause of brain damage due to head injury. A pathological study of twenty cases. Lancet 2:433, 1961.

Taveras JM, Ransohoff J: Leptomeningeal cysts of the brain following trauma, with erosion of the skull. J Neurosurg 10:233, 1953.

Wendling LR: Intracranial venous sinus thrombosis: Diagnosis suggested by computed tomography. AJR 130:978–980, 1978.

Zimmerman RA, Bilaniuk LT, Bruce D, et al: Computed tomography of craniocerebral injury in the abused child. Radiology 130:687, 1979.

Zimmerman RA, Bilaniuk LT, Bruce D, et al: Computed tomography of pediatric head trauma: Acute general cerebral swelling. Radiology 126:403, 1978.

Zimmerman RA, Bilaniuk LT, Dolinskas C, et al: Computed tomography of acute intracerebral hemorrhagic contusion. CT 1:271, 1977.

Zimmerman RA, Bilaniuk LT, Gennarelli T: Computed tomography of shearing injuries of the cerebral white matter. Radiology 127:393, 1978.

Zimmerman RA, Bilaniuk LT, Gennarelli T, et al: Cranial computed tomography in diagnosis and management of acute head trauma. AJR 131:27, 1978.

THE ORBIT

Bacon KT, Duchesneau PM, Weinstein MA: Demonstration of the superior ophthalmic vein by high resolution computed tomography. Radiology 124:129, 1977.

Bernardino ME, Danziger J, Young SE, Wallace S: Computed tomography in ocular neoplastic disease. AJR 131:111–113, 1978.

Bernardino ME, Zimmerman RD, Citrin CM, Davis DO:

Scleral thickening: A sign of orbital pseudotumor. AJR 129:703–706, 1977.

Brant-Zawadzki M, Badami JM, Mills CM, Norman D, Newton, TH: Primary intracranial tumor imaging: Comparison of magnetic resonance and CT. Radiology 150:435–440, 1984.

Byrd SE, Harwood-Nash DC, Fitz CR, et al: Computed tomography of intra-orbital optic nerve gliomas in children. Radiology 129:73, 1978.

Cabanis EA, Salvolini U, Radallec A, et al: Computed tomography of the optic nerve: II. Size and shape modifications in papilledema. J Comput Assist Tomogr 2:150, 1978.

Char DM, Norman D: The use of computer tomography and ultrasonography in the evaluation of orbital masses. Surv Ophthalmol 17:49–63, 1982.

Daniels DL, Herfkins R, Gager WE, Meyer GA, Koehler PR, Williams AL, Haughton VM: Magnetic resonance imaging of the optic nerves and chiasm. Radiology 152:79–83, 1984.

Daniels DL, Kneeland JB, Shimakawa A, et al: MR imaging of the optic nerve and sheath: Correcting the chemical shift misregistration effect. AJNR 7:249, 1986.

Danziger A, Price HI: CT findings in retinoblastoma. AJR 133:783, 1979.

deRaad R: The ophthalmic artery: Radiology. In Newton TH, Potts DG (eds): Radiology of the Skull and Brain. St. Louis, CV Mosby Company, 1974.

Dubois PJ, Kennerdell JS, Rosenbaum AE: Advantages of a fourth generation CT scanner in the management of patients with orbital mass lesions. Comput Tomogr 3:279, 1979.

Edwards JH, Hyman RA, Vacirca SJ, Boxer MA, Packer S, Kaufman IH, Stein HL: 0.6T magnetic resonance imaging of the orbit. AJNR 6:253–258, 1985.

Enzmann D, et al: Computed tomography in Graves' ophthalmopathy. Radiology 118:615–620, 1976.

Enzmann DR, Donaldson SS, Kriss JP: Appearance of Graves' disease on orbital computed tomography. J Comput Assist Tomogr 3:815–819, 1979.

Enzmann D, Donaldson SS, Marshall WH, Kriss JP: Computed tomography in orbital pseudotumor (idiopathic orbital inflammation). Radiology 120:597–601, 1976.

Forbes GS, Sheedy PF II, Waller RR: Orbital tumors evaluated by computed tomography. Radiology 136:101, 1980.

Gomori JM, Grossman RI, Shields JA, Augsburger JJ, Joseph PM, DeSimeone D: Choroidal melanomas: Correlation of NMR spectroscopy and MR imaging. Radiology 158:443, 1986.

Grove AS Jr, Tadmor R, New PFJ, Momose KJ: Orbital fracture evaluation by coronal computed tomography. Am J Ophthalmol 85:679–685, 1978.

Gyldensted C, Lester J, Fledelius H: Computed tomography of orbital lesions. Neuroradiology 13:141–150, 1977.

Hall K, McAllister VL: Metrizamide cisternography in pituitary and juxtapituitary lesions. Radiology 134:101, 1980.

Han JS, Benson JE, Bonstelle CT, Alfidi RJ, Kaufman B, Levine B: Magnetic resonance imaging of the orbit: A preliminary experience. Radiology 150:755–759, 1984.

Hawkes RC, Holland GN, Moore WS, Rizk S, Worthington BS, Kean DM: NMR imaging in the evaluation of orbital tumors. AJNR 4:254–256, 1983.

Hesselink JR, et al: Computed tomography of the paranasal sinus and face: I. Normal anatomy. Comput Assist Tomogr 2:559–567, 1978.

Hesselink JR, Davis KR, Weber AL, et al: Radiological evaluation of orbital metastases, with emphasis on computed tomography. Radiology 137:363, 1980.

Hesselink JR, Weber AL, New PFJ, et al: Evaluation of mucoceles of the paranasal sinuses with computed tomography. Radiology 133:397, 1979.

Hilal SK, Trokel SL: Computerized tomography of the orbit using thin sections. Semin Roentgenol 12:137, 1977.

Hilal SK, Trokel SL, Kreps SM: Diseases of the orbit; computerized tomography. In Duane TD (ed): Clinical Ophthalmology. Vol 2. Hagerstown, Maryland, Harper and Row, 1976.

Hurwitz BS, Citrin CM: Use of computerized axial tomography (CAT scan) in evaluating therapy of orbital pseudotumor. Ann Ophthalmol 11:217, 1979.

Li KC, Poon PY, Hinton P, Willinsky R, Pavlin CJ, Hurwitz JJ, Buncic JR, Henkelman RM: MR imaging of orbital tumors with CT and ultrasound correlations. J Comput Assist Tomogr 8:1039–1047, 1984.

Mafee M, Peyman GA, McKusick MA: Malignant uveal melanoma and similar lesions studied by computed tomography. Radiology 156:403–408, 1985.

Moseley I, Brant-Zawadzki M, Mills C: Nuclear magnetic resonance imaging of the orbit. Br J Ophthalmol 67:333–342, 1983.

Mottow LS, Jakobiec FA: Idiopathic inflammatory orbital pseudotumor in childhood. I. Clinical characteristics. Arch Ophthalmol 96:1410, 1978.

Peyster RG, Hoover ED, Hershey BL, Haskin ME: Special article: High-resolution CT of lesions of the optic nerve. AJNR 4:169–174, 1983.

Post MJD, David NJ, Glaser JS, et al: Pituitary apoplexy: Diagnosis by computed tomography. Radiology 134:665, 1980.

Ramirez H, Blatt ES, Hibri NS: Computed tomographic identification of calcified optic nerve drusen. Radiology 148:137–140, 1983.

Rothfus WE, Curtin HD, Slamovits TL, Kennerdell JS: Optic nerve sheath enlargement: A differential approach based on high-resolution CT morphology. Radiology 150:409–415, 1984.

Rucker CW: The causes of paralysis of the third, fourth and sixth cranial nerves. Am J Ophthalmol 61:1293, 1966.

Sassani JW, Osbakken MD: Anatomic features of the eye disclosed with nuclear magnetic resonance imaging. Arch Ophthalmol 102:541–546, 1984.

Schenck JF, Hart HR Jr, Foster TH, Edelstein WA, Bottomley PA, Redington RW, Hardy CJ, Zimmerman RA, Bilaniuk LT: Improved MR imaging of the orbit at 1.5T with surface coils. AJNR 6:193–196, 1985.

Sobel DF, Kelly W, Kjos B, Char D, Brant-Zawadzki M, Norman D: MR imaging of orbital and ocular disease. AJNR 6:259–264, 1985.

Sobel DF, Mills C, Char D, Norman D, Brant-Zawadzki M, Kaufman L, Crooks L: NMR of the normal and pathologic eye and orbit. AJNR 5:345–350, 1984.

Som PM, Lawson W, Biller HF, Lanzieri CF: Ethmoid sinus disease: CT evaluation in 400 cases: Part 1. Nonsurgical patients. Radiology 159:591, 1986.

Som PM, Shugar MA: The CT classification of ethmoid mucoceles. J Comput Assist Tomogr 4:199, 1980.

Spoor TC, Kennerdell JS, Martinez AJ: Malignant gliomas of the optic nerve pathways. Am J Ophthalmol 89:284, 1980.

Stern J, Jakobiec FA, Housepian EM: The architecture of optic nerve gliomas with and without neurofibromatosis. Arch Ophthalmol 98:505, 1980.

Stewart WB, Krohel GB, Wright JE: Lacrimal gland and fossa lesions: An approach to diagnosis and management. Ophthalmology 86:886, 1979.

Tadmor R, New PFJ: Computed tomography of the orbit with special emphasis on coronal sections. I. Normal anatomy. J Comput Assist Tomogr 2:24, 1978.

Tewfik HH, Platz CE, Corder MP, et al: A clinicopathologic study of orbital and adnexal non-Hodgkin's lymphoma. Cancer 44:1022, 1979.

Towbin R, Han BK, Kaufman RA, Burke M: Postseptal cellulitis: CT in diagnosis and management. Radiology 158:735, 1986.

Trokel SL, Hilal SK: Recognition and differential diagnosis of enlarged extraocular muscles in computed tomography. Am J Ophthalmol 87:503, 1979.

Trokel SL, Hilal SK: Submillimeter resolution CT scanning of orbital diseases. Ophthalmology 87:412, 1980.

Turner RM, Gutman I, Hilal SK, Behrens M, Odel J: CT of drusen bodies and other calcific lesions of the optic nerve: Case report and differential diagnosis. AJNR 4:175–178, 1983.

Unsold R, Newton TH, Hoyt WF: CT examination technique of the optic nerve. J Comput Assist Tomogr 4:560, 1980.

Unsold R, Safran E, Hoyt WF: Metastatic infiltration of nerves in the cavernous sinus. Arch Neurol 37:59, 1980.

Wende S, Aulich A, Nover A, Lanksch W, Kazner E, Steinhoff H, Meese W, Lange S, Grummet T: Computed tomography of orbital lesions. Neuroradiology 13:123–134, 1977.

Zimmerman RA, Bilaniuk LT: Computed tomography in the evaluation of patients with bilateral retinoblastomas. CT: J Comput Tomogr 3:251–257, 1979.

Zimmerman RA, Bilaniuk LT: Ct of orbital infection and its cerebral complications. AJR 134:45–50, 1980.

THE POSTERIOR FOSSA

Adair LB, Ropper AH, Davis KR: Cerebellar hemangioblastoma: CT, angiographic and clinical condition in seven cases. CT: J Comput Tomogr 2:281–294, 1978.

Archer C, Darwish H, Smith K Jr: Enlarged cisternae magnae and posterior cysts simulating Dandy-Walker syndrome on computed tomography. Radiology 127:681, 1978.

Bosley TM, Cohen DA, Schatz NJ, Zimmerman RA, et al: Comparison of metrizamide computed tomography and magnetic resonance imaging in evaluation of lesions at the cervicomedullary junction. Neurology 35:485–492, 1985.

Bradac GB, Schramm J, Grumme T, Simon RS: CT of the base of the skull. Neuroradiology 17:1–5, 1978.

Britton BH: Glomus tympanicum and glomus jugulare. Radiol Clin North Am 12:543–551, 1974.

Curati WL, Graif M, Kingsley DPE, Niendorf HP, Young IR: Acoustic neuromas: Gd-DTPA enhancement in MR imaging. Radiology 158:447, 1986.

Daniels DL, Herfkens R, Koehler PR, et al: Magnetic resonance imaging of the internal auditory canal. Radiology 151:105–108, 1984.

Davis DO, Roberson GH: Angiographic diagnosis of posterior fossa mass lesions. Semin Roentgenol 6:89, 1971.

De La Paz RL, Brady TJ, Buonanno FS, et al: Nuclear magnetic resonance (NMR) imaging of Arnold-Chiari type I malformation with hydromyelia. J Comput Assist Tomogr 7:126–129, 1983.

Enzmann DR, Krikorian J, Norman D, et al: Computed tomography in primary reticulum cell sarcoma of the brain. Radiology 130:165, 1979.

Enzmann DR, Norman D, Levin V, et al: Computed tomography in the followup of medulloblastomas and ependymomas. Radiology 128:57, 1978.

Flannigan BD, Bradley WG Jr, Mazziotta JC, Rauschnig W, Bentson JR, Lufkin RB, Hieshima GB: Magnetic resonance imaging of the brainstem: Normal structure and basic functional anatomy. Radiology 154:375, 1985.

George AE: A systematic approach to the interpretation of posterior fossa angiography. Radiol Clin North Am 12:371, 1974.

Glanz S, Geehr RB, Duncan CC, Piepmeier JM: Metrizamide-enhanced CT for evaluation of brainstem tumors. AJNR 1:31–34, 1980.

Greitz T, Sjorgen S: The posterior inferior cerebellar artery. Acta Radiol (Stockh) 1:284, 1963.

Guild SR: The glomus jugulare, a nonchromaffin paraganglion in man. Ann Otolaryngol 62:1045–1071, 1953.

Haller JS, Wolpert SM, Rabe EF, et al: Cystic lesions of the posterior fossa in infants: A comparison of the clinical, radiological, and pathological findings in Dandy-Walker syndrome and extra-axial cysts. Neurology 21:494, 1971.

Han JS, Bonstelle CT, Kaufman B, et al: Magnetic resonance imaging in the evaluation of the brainstem. Radiology 150:705–712, 1984.

Han JS, Huss RG, Benson JE, et al: MR imaging of the skull base. J Comput Assist Tomogr 8:944–952, 1984.

Hart MN, Malamud N, Ellis WG: The Dandy Walker syndrome: A clinicopathological study based on 28 cases. Neurology 22:771, 1972.

Hatam A, Bergstrom M, Moller A, Olivecrona H: Early contrast enhancement of acoustic neuroma. Neuroradiology 17:31–33, 1978.

Hatam A, Moller A, Olivecrona H: Evaluation of the internal auditory meatus with acoustic neuromas using computed tomography. Neuroradiology 17:197–200, 1978.

Hawkes RC, Holland GN, Moore WS, et al: Craniovertebral junction pathology: Assessment by NMR. AJNR 4:232–233, 1983.

Hoffman HB, Margolis MJ, Newton TH: The superior cerebellar artery. I. Normal, gross, and radiographic anatomy. In Newton TH, Potts DG (eds): Radiology of the Skull and Brain. St. Louis, CV Mosby Company, 1974.

Howieson J, Megison LC Jr: Complications of vertebral artery catheterization. Radiology 91:1109, 1968.

Howland WJ, Curry JL: Transient cerebral blindness—A hazard of vertebral artery catheterization. Radiology 83:828, 1964.

Huang PY, Wolf BS: Precentral cerebellar vein in angiography. Acta Radiol [Diagn] (Stockh) 5:250, 1966.

Huang PY, Wolf BS: The veins of the posterior fossa—Superior or galenic draining group. AJR 95:808, 1965.

Huang PY, Wolf BS, Antin SP, et al: The veins of the posterior fossa—Anterior or petrosal draining group. AJR 103:36, 1968.

Kingsley DPE, Brooks GB, Leung AW-L, Johnson MA: Acoustic neuromas: Evaluation by magnetic resonance imaging. AJNR 6:1–5, 1985.

Koenig H. Lenz M, Sauter R: Temporal bone region: High-resolution MR imaging using surface coils. Radiology 159:191, 1986.

Kricheff II, et al: Air CT cisternography and canalography for small acoustic neuromas. AJNR 1:57–63, 1980.

LaMasters DL, Watanabe TJ, Chambers EF, Norman D, Newton TH: Multiplanar metrizamide-enhanced CT imaging of the foramen magnum. AJNR 3:485–494, 1982.

Latack JT, Kartush JM, Kemink JL, Graham MD, Knake JE: Epidermoidomas of the cerebellopontine angle and temporal bone: CT and MR aspects. Radiology 157:361–366, 1985.

Lee BCP, Deck MDF, Kneeland JB, Cahill PT: MR imaging of the craniocervical junction. AJNR 6:209–214, 1985.

Lee BCP, Kneeland JB, Deck MDF, Cahill PT: Posterior fossa lesions: Magnetic resonance imaging. Radiology 153:137–143, 1984.

Lee BCP, Kneeland JB, Walker RW, Posner JB, Cahill

PT, Deck MDF: MR imaging of brainstem tumors. AJNR 6:159–164, 1985.

Lee YY, Glass JP, van Eys J, Wallace S: Medulloblastoma in infants and children: Computed tomographic follow-up after treatment. Radiology 154:677–682, 1985.

Littman P, Jarrett P, Bilaniuk LT, et al: Pediatric brainstem gliomas. Cancer 45:2787, 1980.

Mawad ME, Silver AJ, Hilal SK, Ganti SR: Computed tomography of the brain stem with intrathecal metrizamide. Part I: The normal brain stem. AJNR 4:1–12, 1983.

Mawad ME, Silver AJ, Hilal SK, Ganti SR: Computed tomography of the brain stem with intrathecal metrizamide. Part II: Lesions in and around the brain stem. AJNR 4:13–20, 1983.

Mikhael MA, Ciric IS, Wolf AP: Differentiation of cerebellopontine angle neuromas and meningiomas with MR imaging. JCAT 9:852, 1985.

Naidich TP: Infratentorial masses. In Norman D, Korobkin M, Newton TH (eds): Computed Tomography. St. Louis, CV Mosby Company, 1977.

Naidich TP, et al: The anterior inferior cerebellar artery in mass lesions. Preliminary findings with emphasis on the lateral projection. Radiology 119:375, 1976.

Naidich TP, et al: The normal contrast-enhanced computed tomogram of the brain. J Comput Assist Tomogr 1:16, 1977.

Naidich TP, Lin JP, Leeds NE, et al: Computed tomography in the diagnosis of extra-axial posterior fossa masses. Radiology 120:333, 1976.

Naidich TP, Lin JP, Leeds NP, Pudlowski RM, Naidich JB: Primary tumors and other masses of the cerebellum and fourth ventricle: Differential diagnosis by computed tomography. Neuroradiology 14:153–174, 1977.

New PFJ, Bachow TB, Wismer GL, Rosen BR, Brady TJ: MR imaging of the acoustic nerves and small acoustic neuromas at 0.6 T: Prospective study. AJNR 6:164–170, 1985.

Newton TH: The vertebral artery. In Newton TH, Potts DG (eds): Radiology of the Skull and Brain. St. Louis, CV Mosby Company, 1974.

Newton TH, Margolis MT: The superior cerebellar artery: Pathology involving the superior cerebellar artery. In Newton TH, Potts DG (eds): Radiology of the Skull and Brain. St. Louis, CV Mosby Company, 1974.

Pelz DM, Vinuela F, Fox AJ: Unusual radiologic and clinical presentations of posterior fossa venous angiomas. AJNR 4:81–84, 1983.

Randell CP, Collins AG, Hayward R, et al: Nuclear magnetic resonance imaging of posterior fossa tumours. AJR 141:489–496, 1983.

Randell CP, Collins AG, Young IR, et al: Nuclear magnetic resonance imaging of posterior fossa tumors. AJNR 4:1027–1034, 1983.

Roukkula M: Roentgenological findings in chrondromas of the pontine angle. Acta Radiol (Diagn) 2:120–128, 1964.

Saltzman GF: Angiographic demonstration of the posterior communicating and posterior cerebral arteries. I. Normal angiography. Acta Radiol (Stockh) 51:1, 1959; II. Pathologic angiography. Acta Radiol (Stockh) 52:114, 1959.

Sarwar M, Swischuk LE, Schechter MM: Intracranial chrondromas. AJR 127:973–977, 1976.

Solti-Bohman LG, Magram DL, Lo WM, et al: Gas-CT cisternography for detection of small acoustic tumor. Radiology 150:403–407, 1984.

Spinos E, Laster DW, Moody DM, Ball MR, Witcolski RL, Kelly DL Jr: MR evaluation of Chiari I malformations at 0.15 T. AJNR 6:203–208, 1985.

Steele JR, Hoffman JC: Brainstem evaluation with CT cisternography. AJNR 1:521, 1980.

Takahashi M: The anterior inferior cerebellar artery. In Newton TH, Potts DG (eds): Radiology of the Skull and Brain. St. Louis, CV Mosby Company, 1974.

Takahashi M, Wilson G, Hanafee W: The anterior inferior cerebellar artery: Its radiographic anatomy and significance in the diagnosis of extra-axial tumors of the posterior fossa. Radiology 90:281, 1968.

Takahashi M, Wilson G, Hanafee W: Catheter vertebral angiography: A review of 300 examinations. J Neurosurg 30:722, 1969.

Tsai FY, Teal JS, Quinn MF, Itabashi HH, Huprich JE, Ahmadi J, Segall HD: CT of brainstem injury. AJNR 1:23–30, 1980.

Wolf BS, Newman CM, Khilnani MT: The posterior inferior cerebellar artery on vertebral angiography. AJR 87:322, 1962.

Young IR, Burl M, Clarke GJ, et al: Posterior fossa: Magnetic resonance properties. AJR 137:895–901, 1981.

Young IR, Bydder GM, Hall AS, et al: The role of nuclear magnetic resonance imaging in the diagnosis and management of acoustic neuroma. AJNR 4:223–224, 1983.

Zimmerman RA, Bilaniuk LT: Spectrum of medulloblastomas demonstrated by computed tomography. Radiology 126:137, 1978.

Zimmerman RA, Bilaniuk LT, Bruno L, Rosenstock J: Computed tomography of cerebellar astrocytoma. AJR 130:929–933, 1978.

ATHEROSCLEROSIS

Alcala H, Gado M, Torack RM: The effect of size, histologic elements, and water content on the visualization of cerebral infarcts. Arch Neurol 35:1, 1978.

Anderson DC, Coss DT, Jacobson RL, Meyer MW: Tissue pertechnetate and iodinated contrast material in ischemic stroke. Stroke 11:617–622, 1980.

Bauer RB, Boulos RS, Meyer JS: Natural history and surgical treatment of occlusive cerebrovascular disease evaluated by serial arteriography. AJR 104:1, 1968.

Berman SA, Hayman LA, Hinck VC: Correlation of CT cerebral vascular territories with function: 3. Middle cerebral artery. AJNR 5:161–166, 1984.

Bradac GM, Oberson R: CT and angiography in cases with occlusive disease of supratentorial cerebral vessels. Neuroradiology 19:193–200, 1980.

Brant-Zawadzki M, Gould R, Norman D, et al: Digital subtraction cerebral angiography by intraarterial injection: Comparison with conventional angiography. AJNR 3:593, 1982.

Buonanno FS, Pykett IL, Brady TJ, et al: Proton NMR imaging in experimental ischemic infarction. Stroke 14:178–184, 1983.

Buonnano FS, Pykett IL, Kistler JP, et al: Cranial anatomy and detection of ischemic stroke in the cat by nuclear magnetic resonance imaging. Radiology 143:187–193, 1982.

Campbell JK, Houser OW, Stevens JC, Wahner HW, Baker HL, Folger WN: Computed tomography and radionuclide imaging in the evaluation of ischemic stroke. Radiology 126:695–702, 1978.

Chilcote WA, Modic MT, Pavlicek WA, et al: Digital subtraction angiography of the carotid arteries: A comparative study in 100 patients. Radiology 139:287, 1981.

Christenson PC, Ovitt TW, Fisher HD, et al: Intravenous angiography using digital video subtraction: Intravenous cervicocerebrovascular angiography. AJNR 1:379, 1980.

Clark WM, Hatten HP Jr: Noninvasive screening of extracranial carotid disease: Duplex sonography with angiographic correlation. AJNR 2:443–448, 1981.

Crooks LE, Mills CM, Davis PL, et al: Visualization of cerebral and vascular abnormalities of NMR imaging.

The effects of imaging parameters on contrast. Radiology 144:843, 1982.

Davis KR, Ackerman RH, Kistler JP, Mohr JP: Computed tomography of cerebral infarction: Hemorrhagic, contrast enhancement, and time of appearance. Comput Tomogr 1:71–86, 1977.

Davis KR, Taveras JM, New PFJ, Schnur JA, Roberson GH: Cerebral infarction diagnosis by computerized tomography: Analysis and evaluation of findings. AJR 124:643–660, 1975.

Dyken ML, Klatte E, Kolar OJ, et al: Complete occlusion of common or internal carotid arteries. Arch Neurol 30:343, 1974.

Edwards JH, Kricheff II, Gorstein F, et al: Atherosclerotic subintimal hematoma of the carotid artery. Radiology 133:123, 1979.

Gado MH, Phelps ME, Coleman RE: An extravascular component of contrast enhancement in cranial computed tomography. I. The tissue-blood ratio of contrast enhancement. Radiology 117:589, 1975.

Gado MH, Phelps ME, Coleman RE: An extravascular component of contrast enhancement in cranial computed tomography. II. Contrast enhancement and the blood-tissue barrier. Radiology 117:595, 1975.

Hayman LA, Evans RA, Bastion FO, Hinck VC: Delayed high dose contrast CT; Identifying patients at risk of massive hemorrhagic infarction. AJNR 2:139–147, 1981.

Herfkens RJ, Higgins CB, Hricak H, Lipton MJ, Crooks LE, Sheldon PE, Kaufman L: Nuclear magnetic resonance imaging of atherosclerotic disease. Radiology 148:161–166, 1983.

Hilal SK, Maudsley AA, Simon HE, et al: In vivo NMR imaging of tissue sodium in the intact cat before and after acute cerebral stroke. AJNR 4:245–249, 1983.

Houser OW, Sundt TM Jr, Holman CB, et al: Atheromatous disease of the carotid artery: Correlation of angiographic, clinical, and surgical findings. J Neurosurg 41:321, 1974.

Jorgensen L, Torbik A: Ischaemic cerebrovascular diseases in an autopsy series: II. Prevalency, location, pathogenesis and clinical course of cerebral infarcts. J Neurol Sci 9:285–320, 1969.

Kendall BE, Pullicino P: Intravascular contrast injection in ischemic lesions. II. Effect on prognosis. Neuroradiology 19:241, 1980.

Kendt GW, Youmans JR, Albrand O: Factors influencing the autoregulation of cerebral blood flow during hypotension and hypertension. J Neurosurg 26:299–305, 1967.

Kishore PRS, Chase NE, Kricheff II: Carotid stenosis and intracranial emboli. Radiology 100:351, 1971.

Lassen NA: The luxury-perfusion syndrome and its possible relation to acute metabolic acidosis localized within the brain. Lancet 2:1113–1115, 1966.

Lassen NA, Agnoli A: The upper limit of autoregulation of cerebral blood flow in the pathogenesis of hypertensive encephalopathy. Scand J Clin Lab Invest 30:113–115, 1972.

Laster DW, Moody DM, Ball MR: Resolving intracerebral hematoma: Alteration of the "ring sign" with steroids. AJR 130:935–939, 1978.

Levy RM, Mano I, Brito A, et al: NMR imaging of acute experimental cerebral ischemia: Time course and pharmacologic manipulations. AJNR 4:238–241, 1983.

Lhermitte F, Gautier JC, Derousne C: Nature of occlusion of the middle cerebral artery. Neurology 20:82, 1970.

Mani RL, Eisenberg RL: Complications of catheter cerebral arteriography: Analysis of 5,000 procedures. II. Relation of complication rates to clinical and arteriographic diagnoses. AJR 131:867, 1978.

Mani RL, Eisenberg RL: Complications of catheter cerebral arteriography: Analysis of 5,000 procedures. III. Assessment of arteries injected, contrast medium used, duration of procedure, and age of patient. AJR 131:871, 1978.

Mani RL, Eisenberg RL, McDonald EJ Jr, et al: Complications of catheter cerebral arteriography: Analysis of 5,000 procedures. I. Criteria and incidence. AJR 131:861, 1978.

Modic MT, Weinstein MA, Chilcote WA, et al: Digital subtraction angiography of the intracranial vascular system: Comparative study in 55 patients. AJR 138:299, 1982.

Moore WS, Hall AD: Importance of emboli from carotid bifurcation in pathogenesis of cerebral ischemic attacks. Arch Surg 101:708, 1970.

Norman D, Axel L, Berninger WH, Edward MS, Cann C, Redington RW, Cox L: Dynamic computed tomography of the brain: Techniques, data analysis, and applications. AJNR 2:1–12, 1981.

Norton GA, Kishore PRS, Lin J: CT contrast enhancement in cerebral infarction. AJR 131:881–885, 1978.

O'Leary DH, Persson AV, Clouse ME: Noninvasive testing for carotid artery stenosis: I. Prospective analysis of three methods. AJNR 2:437–442, 1981.

Prineas J, Marshall J: Hypertension and cerebral infarction. Br Med J 1:14–17, 1966.

Pullicino P, Kendall BE: Contrast enhancement in ischaemic lesions: I. Relationship to prognosis. Neuroradiology 19:235–239, 1980.

Rosenberg GA, Kornfeld M, Stovring J, Bicknell JM: Subcortical arteriosclerotic encephalopathy (Binswanger): Computerized tomography. Neurology 29:1102–1106, 1979.

Rueck JD, Crevits L, Coster WD, Sieben G, Ecken H: Pathogenesis of Binswanger chronic progressive subcortical encephalopathy. Neurology 30:920–928, 1980.

Ruff RL, Talman WT, Petito F: Transient ischemic attacks associated with hypotension in hypertensive patients with carotid artery stenosis. Stroke 12:353–355, 1981.

Rumbaugh CL, Bergeron RT, Fang HCH, et al: Cerebral angiographic change in the drug abuse patient. Radiology 101:335, 1971.

Runge VM, Foster MA, Clanton JA, Jones MM, Lukehart CM, Hutchison JMS, Mallard JR, Smith FW, Partain CL, James AE Jr: Contrast enhancement of magnetic resonance images by chromium EDTA: An experimental study. Radiology 152:123–126, 1984.

Sipponen JT, Kasle M, Ketonen L, et al: Serial nuclear magnetic resonance (NMR) in patients with cerebral infarction. J Comput Assist Tomogr 7:585–589, 1983.

Spetzler RF, Zabramski JM, Kaufman B, et al: Acute NMR changes during MCA occlusion: Preliminary study in primate. Stroke 14:185–191, 1983.

Stockman JA, Nigro MA, Mishkin MM, et al: Occlusion of large cerebral vessels in sickle-cell anemia. N Engl J Med 287:846, 1972.

Strother CM, Sackett JF, Crummy AB, et al: Clinical applications of computerized fluoroscopy. The extracranial carotid arteries. Radiology 136:781, 1980.

Takahashi M, Miyauchi T, Kowada M: Computed tomography of moyamoya disease: Demonstration of occluded arteries and collateral vessels as important diagnostic signs. Radiology 134:671, 1980.

Taveras JM: Angiographic observations in occlusive cerebrovascular disease. Neurology 11:86, 1961.

Wing SD, Norman D, Pollock JA, Newton TH: Contrast enhancement of cerebral infarcts in computed tomography. Radiology 121:89–92, 1976.

Wood EH, Correll JW: Atheromatous ulceration in major neck vessels as a cause of cerebral embolism. Acta Radiol [Diagn] (Stockh) 9:520, 1969.

Yock D, Marshall WH: Recent ischemic brain infarcts at

cranial computed tomography: Appearance pre and post contrast infusion. Radiology 117:599, 1975.

Zeumer H, Schonsky B, Strum KW: Predominant white matter involvement in subcortical arteriosclerotic encephalopathy (Binswanger disease). J Comput Assist Tomogr 4:14–19, 1980.

THE SPINE

Aguila LA, Piraino DW, Modic MT, Dudley AW, Duchesneau PM, Weinstein MA: The intranuclear cleft of the intervertebral disk: Magnetic resonance imaging. Radiology 155:155, 1985.

Anand AK, Lee BCP: Plain and metrizamide CT of lumbar disk disease: Comparison with myelography. AJNR 3:567–571, 1982.

Aubin ML, Vignaud J, Jardin C, et al: Computed tomography in 75 clinical cases of syringomyelia. AJNR 2:199–204, 1981.

Badami JP, Baker RA, Scholz FJ, McLaughlin M: Outpatient metrizamide myelography: Prospective evaluation of safety and cost effectiveness. Radiology 158:175, 1986.

Barnes PD: Progress in cost-effective radiologic evaluation of pediatric and adolescent neurologic spine disease. Presented at the annual meeting of the Society for Pediatric Radiology, Atlanta, April 1983. AJR (abstract) 141:851–852, 1983.

Barnes PD, Reynolds AF, Galloway DC, Pollay M, Leonard JC, Prince JR: Digital myelography of spinal dysraphism in infancy: Preliminary results. AJNR 5:208–211, 1984; 142:1249–1252, 1984.

Barnett HJM, Jousse AT: Syringomyelia as a late sequel to traumatic paraplegia and quadriplegia—clinical features. In Barnett HJM, Foster JB, Hudgson P (eds): Major problems in neurology, Syringomyelia. Vol 1. London, WB Saunders Company, 1973, pp 129–153.

Batnitsky S, Price HI, Gaughan MJ, et al: The radiology of syringomyelia. Radiographics 3:585–611, 1983.

Bonafe A, Manelfe C, Espagno J, et al: Evaluation of syringomyelia with metrizamide computed tomographic myelography. J Comput Assist Tomogr 4:797–802, 1980.

Bradley WG, Waluch V, Yadley RA, et al: Comparison of CT and MR in 400 patients with suspected disease of the brain and cervical spinal cord. Radiology 152:695–702, 1984.

Brant-Zawadzki M, Davis PL, Crooks LE, et al: NMR demonstration of cerebral abnormalities: Comparison with CT. AJNR 4:117–124, 1983.

Brant-Zawadzki M, Jeffrey RB, Minagi H, et al: High resolution CT of thoracolumbar fractures. AJR 138:699–704, 1982.

Brant-Zawadzki M, Miller ER, Federle MP: CT in the evaluation of spinal trauma. AJR 136:369, 1981.

Braun IF, Lin JP, Benjamin MV, Kricheff II: Computed tomography of the asymptomatic postsurgical lumbar spine: Analysis of the physiologic scar. AJNR 4:1213–1216, 1983.

Braun IF, Hoffman JC Jr, Davis PC, Landman JA, Tindall GT: Contrast enhancement in CT differentiation between recurrent disk herniation and postoperative scar: Prospective study. AJNR 6:607–612, 1985.

Brown BM, Brant-Zawadzki M, Cann CE: Dynamic CT scanning of spinal column trauma. AJNR 3:461–466, 1982.

Brown HA: Enlargement of the ligamentum a cause of low back pain with sciatic radiation. J Bone Joint Surg 20:325, 1938.

Burrows EH: Myelography with iohexol (Omnipaque): Review of 300 cases. AJNR 6:349–352, 1985.

Cacayorin ED, Kieffer SA: Applications and limitations of computed tomography of the spine. Radiol Clin North Am 20:185–206, 1982.

Carrera GF, Williams AL, Haughton VM: Computed tomography in sciatica. Radiology 137:433, 1980.

Chafetz N: Computed tomography of lumbar disc disease. In Genant HK, Chafetz N, Helms CA (eds): Computed Tomography of the Lumbar Spine. Berkeley, University of California Press, 1982.

Chafetz NI, Genant HK, Moon KL, et al: Recognition of lumbar disc herniation with NMR. AJR 141:1153–1156, 1983.

Chafetz NI, Genant HK, Moon KL, Helms CA, Morris JM: Recognition of lumbar disk herniation with NMR. AJNR 5:23–26, 1984.

Crolla D, Hens L, Wilms G, et al: Metrizamide enhanced CT in hydrosyringomyelia. Neuroradiology 19:39, 1980.

Crooks LE, Arakawa M, Hoenninger J, et al: Nuclear magnetic resonance whole-body imager operating at 3.5 gauss. Radiology 143:169–174, 1982.

Crooks LE, Hoenninger J, Arakawa M, et al: High resolution magnetic resonance imaging. Radiology 150:163–171, 1984.

Daneman A, Mancer K, Sonley M: CT appearance of thickened nerves in neurofibromatosis. AJR 141:899–900, 1983.

Deeb ZL, Schimel S, Daffner RH, Lupetin AR, Hryshko FG, Blakley JB: Intervertebral disk-space infection after chymopapain injection. AJNR 6:55–58, 1985.

Di Chiro G, Doppman J, Ommaya AK: Selective arteriography of arteriovenous aneurysms of spinal cord. Radiology 88:1065, 1967.

Djindjian R: Angiography of spinal cord. Surg Neurol 2:179, 1974.

Dublin AB, McGahan JP, Reid MH: Value of computed tomographic metrizamide myelography in the neuroradiological evaluation of the spine. Radiology 146:79–86, 1983.

Edelman R, Shoukimas G, Stark D, et al: High-resolution surface-coil imaging of lumbar disk disease. AJNR 6:479–485, 1985.

Ellertsson AB: Syringomyelia and other cystic spinal cord lesions. Acta Neurol Scand 45:403, 1969.

Elsberg CA, Dyke CG: The diagnosis and localization of tumors of the spinal cord by means of measurements made on the x-ray films of the vertebrae, and the correlation of clinical and x-ray findings. Bull Neurol Inst 3:359, 1934.

Epstein BS: Spinal canal mass lesions. Radiol Clin North Am 4:185, 1961.

Feinberg SB: The place of discography in radiology as based on 20 cases. AJR 92:1275, 1964.

Fox A, Vinuela F, Debrun G: Complete myelography with metrizamide. AJNR 2:79, 1981.

Gabrielsen TO, Gebarski SS, Knake JE, Latack JT, Yang PJ, Hoff JT: Iohexol versus metrizamide for lumbar myelography: Double-blind trial. AJNR 5:181–184, 1984.

Gebarski SS, Gabrielsen TO, Knake JE, Latack JT, Yang PJ, Hoff JT: Iohexol versus metrizamide for cervical myelography: Double-trial. AJNR 6:923–926, 1985.

Gebarski SS, Maynard FW, Gabrielsen TO, Knake JE, Latack JT, Hoff JT: Posttraumatic progressive myelopathy: Clinical and radiologic correlation employing MR imaging, delayed CT metrizamide myelography, and intraoperative sonography. Radiology 157:379–386, 1985.

Gehweiler JA, Osborne R, Becker R: The Radiology of Vertebral Trauma. Philadelphia, WB Saunders Company, 1980.

Golimbu C, Firooznia H, Rafii M: CT of osteomyelitis of the spine. AJNR 4:1207–1212, 1983.

Griffiths HED, Jones DM: Pyogenic infection of the spine.

A review of twenty-eight cases. J Bone Joint Surg (Br) 53:383, 1971.

Grogan JP, Hemminghytt S, Williams AL, Carrera GF, Haughton VM: Spondylolysis studied by CT. Radiology 145:737–742, 1982.

Han JS, Benson JE, Kaufman B, et al: Demonstration of diastematomyelia and associated abnormalities with MR imaging. AJNR 6:215–220, 1985.

Han JS, Benson JE, Yoon YS: Magnetic resonance imaging in the spinal column and craniovertebral junction. Radiol Clin North Am 22:805–827, 1984.

Han JS, Bonstelle CT, Kaufman B, et al: Magnetic resonance imaging in the evaluation of the brain stem. Radiology 150:705–712, 1984.

Han JS, Kaufman B, Yousef SJE, et al: NMR imaging of the spine. AJNR 4:1151–1160, 1983; AJR 141:1137–1145, 1983.

Helms CA, Dorwart RH, Gray M: The CT appearance of conjoined nerve roots and differentiation from a herniated nucleus pulposus. Radiology 144:808, 1982.

Hemminghytt S, Daniels DL, Williams AL, Haughton VM: Intraspinal synovial cysts: Natural history and diagnosis by CT. Radiology 145:375–376, 1982.

Hilal SK, Marton D, Pollack E: Diastematomyelia in children. Radiology 112:609, 1974.

Hoddick WK, Helms CA: Bony spinal canal changes that differentiate conjoined nerve roots from herniated nucleus pulposus. Radiology 154:119–120, 1985.

Hyman RA, Edwards JH, Vacirca SJ, Stein HL: MR imaging of the cervical spine: Multislice and multiecho techniques. AJNR 6:229–236, 1985.

Kan S, Fox AJ, Viñuela F, Barnett HJM, Peerless SJ: Delayed CT metrizamide enhancement of syringomyelia secondary to tumor. AJNR 1:73–78, 1983.

Kangarloo H, Gold RH, Diament MJ, Boechat MI, Barrett C: High resolution spinal sonography in infants. AJNR 5:191–195, 1984; AJR 142:1243–1247, 1984.

Kendall B, Russell J: Haemangioblastomas of the spinal cord. Clin Radiol 39:817, 1966.

Klatte EC, Franken EA, Smith JA: The radiographic spectrum in neurofibromatosis. Semin Roentgenol 11:17–33, 1976.

Kostiner AI, Krook PM: Outpatient lumbar myelography with metrizamide. Radiology 155:383–386, 1985.

Landman JA, Hoffman JC Jr, Braun IF, Barrow DL: Value of computed tomographic myelography in the recognition of cervical herniated disk. AJNR 5:391–394, 1984.

Lardé D, Mathieu D, Frija J, Gaston A, Vasile N: Vertebral osteomyelitis: Disk hypodensity on CT. AJNR 3:657–662, 1982.

Latchaw RE, Hirsch WL Jr, Horton JA, Bissonette D, Shaw DD: Iohexol vs. metrizamide: Study of efficacy and morbidity in cervical myelography. AJNR 6:931–934, 1985.

Lee BCP, Deck MDF, Kneeland JB, Cahill PT: MR imaging of the craniocervical junction. AJNR 6:209–213, 1985.

Lee BCP, Zimmerman RD, Manning JJ, Deck MDF: MR imaging of syringomyelia and hydromyelia. AJNR 6:221–228, 1985.

Lefkowitz DM, Quencer RM: Vacuum facet phenomenon: A CT sign of degenerative spondylolisthesis (case report). Radiology 44:562, 1982.

Lester PD, Barnes PD, Yamanashi WS, Maulsby GO: Magnetic resonance imaging in infants and children with spinal dysraphism. Presented at the annual meeting of the Society for Pediatric Radiology. Las Vegas, April 1984. AJR (abstract) 143:694, 1984.

Lipson SJ, Muir H: Experimental intervertebral disc degeneration. Morphologic and proteoglycan changes over time. Arthritis Rheum 24:12–21, 1981.

Maravilla KR, Lesh P, Weinreb JC, Selby DK, Mooney V: Magnetic resonance imaging of the lumbar spine with CT correlation. AJNR 6:237–246, 1985.

Maravilla KR, Weinreb JC, Suss R, Nunnally RL: Magnetic resonance demonstration of multiple sclerosis plaques in the cervical cord. AJNR 5:685–690, 1984.

Masdeu JC, Glista GG, Rubina FA, Martinez-Lage JM, Maravi E: Transient motor aphasia following metrizamide myelography. AJNR 4:200–202, 1983.

Modic MT, Feiglin DH, Piraino DW, Boumphrey F, Weinstein MA, Duchesneau PM, Rehm S: Vertebral osteomyelitis: Assessment using MR. Radiology 157:157–166, 1985.

Modic MT, Hardy RW, Weinstein MA, et al: Nuclear magnetic resonance of the spine: Clinical potential and limitation. Neurosurgery 15:288–292, 1984.

Modic MT, Pavlicek W, Weinstein MA, et al: Nuclear magnetic resonance of intervertebral disc disease: Clinical and pulse sequence considerations. Radiology 152:103–111, 1984.

Modic MT, Weinstein MA, Pavlicek W, et al: Magnetic resonance imaging of the cervical spine: Technical and clinical observations. AJR 141:1129–1136, 1983.

Modic MT, Weinstein MA, Pavlicek W, et al: Nuclear magnetic resonance imaging of the spine. Radiology 148:757–762, 1983.

Modic MT, Weinstein MA, Pavlicek W, Boumphrey F, Starnes D, Duchesneau PM: Magnetic resonance imaging of the cervical spine: Technical and clinical observations. AJNR 5:15–22, 1984.

Naidich TP, Fernbach SK, McLone DG, Shkolnik A: Sonography of the caudal spine and back: Congenital anomalies in children. AJNR 5:221–234, 1985; AJR 142:1229–1242, 1984.

Nakagawa H, Huang YP, Malis LI, et al: Computed tomography of intraspinal and paraspinal neoplasms. J Comput Assist Tomogr 1:377, 1977.

Norman D, Mills CM, Brant-Zawadzki M, Yeates A, Crooks LE, Kaufman L: Magnetic resonance imaging of the spinal cord and canal: Potentials and limitations. AJNR 5:9–14, 1984; AJR 141:1147–1152, 1983.

Numaguchi Y, Weems AM, Mizushima A, et al: Myelography with metrizamide: Effects of contrast removal on side effects. AJNR 7:498, 1986.

Nykamp PW, Levy JM, Christensen F, et al: Computed tomography for a bursting fracture of the lumbar spine: A case report. J Bone Joint Surg 60A:1108, 1978.

Panshter DM, Dengel FH, Modic MT, et al: Clinical applications of nuclear magnetic resonance: Central nervous system, brain stem and cord. Radiographics 4:97–112, 1984.

Pendleton B, Barton C, Pollay M: Spinal extradural benign synovial or ganglion cyst: Case report and review of the literature. Neurosurg 13:322–325, 1983.

Petterson H, Harwood-Nash DC: CT and Myelography of the Spine and Cord. New York, Springer-Verlag, 1982, pp 9–21, 32–33.

Pojunas K, Williams AL, Daniels DL, Haughton VM: Syringomyelia and hydromyelia: Magnetic resonance evaluation. Radiology 153:679–683, 1984.

Quencer RM, Green BA, Eismont FJ: Posttraumatic spinal cord cysts: Clinical features and characterization with metrizamide computed tomography. Radiology 146:415–423, 1983.

Quencer RM, Morse BMM, Green BA, Eismont FJ, Brost P: Intraoperative spinal sonography: An adjunct to metrizamide CT in the assessment and surgical decompression of posttraumatic spinal cord cysts. AJNR 5:71–79, 1984; AJR 142:593–601, 1984.

Quencer RM, Sheldon JJ, Post MJD, Diaz RD, Montalvo BM, Green BA, Eismont FJ: Magnetic resonance imaging of the chronically injured cervical spinal cord. AJNR 7:457, 1986.

Ramsey RG, Zacharias CE: MR imaging of the spine after radiation therapy: Easily recognizable effects. AJNR 6:247–253, 1985.

Resjo IM, Harwood-Nash DC, Fitz CR, et al: Computed tomographic metrizamide myelography in spinal dysraphism in infants and children. J Comput Assist Tomogr 2:549, 1978.

Rogers LF, Thayer C, Weinberg PE, Kim KS: Acute injuries of the upper thoracic spine associated with paraplegia. AJNR 1:89–96, 1980.

Rossier AB, Foo D, Naheedy MH, Wang AM, Rumbaugh CL, Levine H: Radiography of posttraumatic syringomyelia. AJNR 4:637–640, 1983.

Sarno JB: Transient expressive (nonfluent) dysphasia after metrizamide myelography. AJNR 6:945, 1985.

Sarwar M, Virapongse C, Bhimani S: Primary tethered cord syndrome. AJNR 5:235–242, 1984.

Scatliff JH, Till K, Hoare RD: Incomplete, false, and true diastematomyelia. Radiology 116:349, 1975.

Scotti G, Musgrave MA, Harwood-Nash DC, et al: Diastematomyelia in children: Metrizamide and CT metrizamide myelography. AJNR 1:403, 1980.

Stauffer RN: Pyogenic vertebral osteomyelitis. Orthop Clin North Am 6:1015, 1975.

Stein BM, Leeds NE, Taveras J, et al: Meningiomas of the foramen magnum. J Neurosurg 20:740, 1963.

Stevens JM, Olney JS, Kendall BE: Posttraumatic cystic and noncystic myelopathy. Neuroradiology 27:48–56, 1985.

Stratemeier PH: Evaluation of the lumbar spine. A comparison between computed tomography and myelography. Radiol Clin North Am 21:221–257, 1983.

Swanson HS, Barnett JC: Intradural lipomas in children. Pediatrics 29:911, 1962.

Tabaddor K: Unusual complications of iophendylate injection myelography. Arch Neurol 29:435–436, 1973.

Teplick JG, Haskin ME: Intravenous contrast-enhanced CT of the postoperative lumbar spine: Improved identification of recurrent disk herniation, scar, arachnoiditis, and diskitis. AJNR 5:373–384, 1984.

Teplick JG, Laffey PA, Berman A, Haskin ME: Diagnosis and evaluation of spondylolisthesis and/or spondylolysis on axial CT. AJNR 7:479, 1986.

Traub SL: Mass lesions in the spinal canal. Semin Rad 7:240, 1972.

Williams AL, Haughton VM, Daniels DL, Grogan JP: Differential CT diagnosis of extruded nucleus pulposus. Radiology 148:141–148, 1983.

Williams AL, Haughton VM, Meyer GA, et al: Computed tomographic appearance of the bulging annulus. Radiology 142:403, 1982.

Williams AL, Haughton VM, Syvertsen A: CT in the diagnosis of herniated nucleus pulposus. Radiology 135:95, 1980.

Williams B: The distending force in the production of "communicating syringomyelia." Lancet 2:189–193, 1969.

Wilson DH, MacCarly WC: Discography: Its role in the diagnosis of lumbar disc protrusions. J Neurosurg 31:520, 1969.

Yeates A, Brant-Zawadzki M, Norman D, Kaufman I, Crooks LE, Newton TH: Nuclear magnetic resonance imaging of syringomyelia. AJNR 4:234–237, 1983.

Zinreich SJ, Wang H, Updike ML, Kumar AJ, Ahn HS, North RB, Rosenbaum AE: CT myelography for outpatients: An inpatient/outpatient pilot study to assess methodology. Radiology 157:387–390, 1985.

FUTURE ADVANCES IN NEURORADIOLOGY

Brasch RC, Weinmann H-J, Wesbey GE: Contrast-enhanced NMR imaging: Animal studies using gadolinium-DTPA complex. AJR 142:625–630, 1984.

Brooks BS, El Gammal T, Van Tassel P, Stevenson TC: C1-C2 myelography with iohexol and metrizamide: Comparative study. AJNR 6:935, 1985.

Burt CT, Glonek T, Barany M: Analysis of phosphate metabolites, the intracellular pH, and the state of adenosine triphosphate in intact muscle by phosphorus nuclear magnetic resonance. J Biol Chem 251:2584–2591, 1976.

Carr DH, Brown J, Bydder GM, et al: Clinical use of intravenous gadolinium-DTPA as a contrast agent in NMR imaging of cerebral tumours. Lancet 1:484–486, 1984.

Carr DH, Brown J, Bydder GM, et al: Gadolinium-DTPA as a contrast agent in MRI: Initial clinical experience in 20 patients. AJR 143:215–224, 1984.

Carr DH, Brown JB, Bydder GM, et al: Intravenous chelated gadolinium as a contrast agent in NMR imaging of cerebral tumours. Lancet 1:484–486, 1984.

Claussen C, Laniado M, Schörner W, et al: Gadolinium-DTPA in MR imaging of glioblastomas and intracranial metastases. AJNR 6:669, 1985.

Gebarski SS, Gabrielsen TO, Knake JE, Latack JT, Yang PJ, Hoff JT: Iohexol versus metrizamide for cervical myelography: Double-blind trial. AJNR 6:923, 1985.

Graif M, Bydder GM, Steiner RE, Niendorf P, Thomas DGT, Young IR: Contrast-enhanced MR imaging of malignant brain tumors. AJNR 6:855, 1985.

Kramer DM: Imaging elements other than hydrogen. In Kaufman L, Crooks LE, Margulis AR (eds): Nuclear Magnetic Resonance in Medicine. New York, Igaku-Shoin, 1981.

Kaufman, L, Crooks LE, Sheldon PE, et al: Evaluation of NMR imaging for detection and quantification of obstructions in vessels. Invest Radiol 17:554, 1982.

Latchaw RE, Hirsch WL Jr, Horton JA, Bissonette D, Shaw DD: Iohexol vs. metrizamide: Study of efficacy and morbidity in cervical myelography. AJNR 6:931, 1985.

Latchaw RE, Sackett JF, Turski PA, Shaw DD: Iohexol for cervical myelography via C1-C2 puncture: Study of efficacy and adverse reactions. AJNR 6:927, 1985.

Maudsley AA, Hilal DK, Simon HE, Wittekoek S: In-vivo MR spectroscopic imaging with P-31. Radiology 153:745–750, 1984.

McNamara MT, Brant-Zawadzki M, Berry I, Pereira B, Weinstein P, Derugin N, Moore S, Kucharczyk W, Brasch RC: Acute experimental cerebral ischemia: MR enhancement using Gd-DTPA. Radiology 158:701, 1986.

Nakstad PH, Bakke SJ, Kjartansson O, von Krogh J: Omnipaque Vs. Hexabrix in intravenous DSA of the carotid arteries: Randomized double-blind crossover study. AJNR 7:303, 1986.

Ortendahl DA, Posin JP, Hylton NM, Mills CM: Optimal visualization of the cerebrospinal fluid on MRI. AJNR 7:403, 1986.

INDEX